Prognosis of Surgical Disease

BEN EISEMAN, M.D.

Professor of Surgery,
University of Colorado Medical Center,
Denver, Colorado

1980

W. B. SAUNDERS COMPANY   PHILADELPHIA • LONDON • TORONTO

W. B. Saunders Company: West Washington Square
                           Philadelphia, Pa.   19105

                           1 St. Anne's Road
                           Eastbourne, East Sussex BN21 3UN, England

                           1 Goldthorne Avenue
                           Toronto, Ontario M8Z   5T9, Canada

Library of Congress Cataloging in Publication Data

Eiseman, Ben.

Prognosis of surgical disease.

1. Surgery. 2. Prognosis. I. Title.

RD31.5.E37   617'.075   79-92615

ISBN 0-7216-3342-0

Prognosis of Surgical Disease   ISBN 0-7216-3342-0

Last digit is the print number: 9   8   7   6   5   4   3   2   1

To

F.C.S.,

whose superb surgical judgment has
always been based on
"numbers"

Contributors

FREDRICK R. ABRAMS, M.D., Assistant Clinical Professor of Obstetrics and Gynecology, University of Colorado School of Medicine, Denver, Colorado. Attending Physician, Rose Medical Center and Colorado General Hospital, Denver, Colorado.

JAMES T. ANDERSON, M.D., Associate Professor of Surgery, University of Colorado Health Sciences Center, Denver, Colorado. Chief of Cardiothoracic Surgery, Veterans' Administration Hospital, Denver, Colorado.

DONALD W. APTEKAR, M.D., Clinical Instructor, Department of Obstetrics and Gynecology, University of Colorado Medical Center, Denver, Colorado. Attending Obstetrician/Gynecologist, Rose Medical Center, Denver, Colorado.

G. E. ARAGON, M.D., Clinical Associate Professor of Surgery, University of Colorado Health Sciences Center, Denver, Colorado. Attending Surgeon, Denver General Hospital and Mercy Hospital, Denver, Colorado.

RICHARD R. AUGSPURGER, M.D., Assistant Professor of Surgery, Division of Urology, University of Colorado Health Sciences Center, Denver, Colorado. Active Staff, Children's Hospital, Colorado General Hospital, and Denver Veterans' Administration Hospital, Denver, Colorado. Courtesy Staff, Denver General Hospital,

Rose Medical Center, St. Anthony Hospital, Denver, Colorado; Lutheran Medical Center, Wheat Ridge, Colorado.

SYLVAN B. BAER, M.D., Associate Clinical Professor of Surgery, University of Colorado School of Medicine, Denver, Colorado. Attending Physician, Rose Medical Center and Mercy Hospital, Denver, Colorado.

WILLIAM CARL BAILEY, M.D., M.M.Sci. (Surg.), Associate Clinical Professor of Surgery, University of Colorado School of Medicine, Denver, Colorado. Director, Burn Center, and Attending Pediatric Surgeon, Children's Hospital, Denver, Colorado.

THOMAS J. BALKANY, M.D., Assistant Professor, Department of Otolaryngology, University of Colorado Health Sciences Center, Denver, Colorado. Director of Pediatric Otolaryngology, Children's Hospital; Attending Surgeon, Porter Memorial Hospital–Swedish Medical Center, Denver, Colorado.

R. S. BAUM, M.D., Assistant Clinical Professor of Medicine, University of Colorado School of Medicine, Denver, Colorado. Associate Director, Division of Cardiology, Rose Medical Center, Denver, Colorado.

ROBERT BEART, M.D., Assistant Professor of Surgery, Mayo Medical School, Rochester, Minnesota. Staff, Mayo Clinic, Rochester, Minnesota.

CONTRIBUTORS

JOHN A. BOSWICK, JR., M.D., Professor of Surgery, University of Colorado Health Sciences Center, Denver, Colorado. Chief, Hand Surgery Service, Colorado General Hospital, Denver, Colorado.

HARRY R. BOYD, M.D., Active Staff, St. Joseph Hospital, Denver, Colorado.

ROBERT K. BROWN, M.D., Clinical Professor of Surgery, University of Colorado School of Medicine, Denver, Colorado. Active Staff, Presbyterian Hospital, St. Luke's Hospital, St. Joseph Hospital, and Children's Hospital, Denver, Colorado.

WILLIAM A. BRYANS, M.D., Clinical Instructor, Department of Neurosurgery, University of Colorado School of Medicine, Denver, Colorado. Attending Neurosurgeon, St. Joseph Hospital, Children's Hospital, Denver, Colorado; Lutheran Hospital, Wheat Ridge, Colorado.

CHARLES A. BUERK, M.D., Associate Professor of Surgery, University of Colorado School of Medicine, Denver, Colorado. Director, Burn Unit, Colorado General Hospital, Denver, Colorado.

JACK H. T. CHANG, M.D., Assistant Clinical Professor of Surgery, University of Colorado Health Sciences Center, Denver, Colorado. Chairman, Department of General Pediatric Surgery, Children's Hospital, Denver, Colorado.

DAVID M. CHARLES, M.D., Ch.B., F.C.S.(S.A.), Assistant Clinical Professor of Surgery, University of Colorado Health Sciences Center, Denver, Colorado. Consultant in Plastic Surgery, Veterans' Administration Hospital, Denver, Colorado; Active Staff, St. Joseph Hospital, Presbyterian Medical Center, Children's Hospital, and University Hospital, Denver, Colorado.

DAVID CLARKE, M.D., Assistant Professor of Surgery, University of Colorado Health Sciences Center, Denver, Colorado. Attending Cardiac Surgeon, University Hospital, Veterans' Administration Hospital, and Children's Hospital, Denver, Colorado.

MACK L. CLAYTON, M.D., Clinical Professor of Surgery; Associate Clinical Professor of Orthopedic Surgery, University of Colorado School of Medicine, Denver, Colorado. Attending Orthopedic Surgeon, St. Joseph Hospital and General Rose Memorial Hospital, Denver, Colorado.

HENRY C. CLEVELAND, M.D., Clinical Professor of Surgery, University of Colorado Medical Center, Denver, Colorado. Medical Director of Patient Care Services, St. Anthony Hospital, Denver, Colorado.

R. COHEN, M.D., Assistant Clinical Professor of Surgery, University of Colorado School of Medicine, Denver, Colorado. Staff, General Rose Memorial Hospital, St. Anthony Hospital, Denver, Colorado; Lutheran Hospital, Wheat Ridge, Colorado.

STEPHEN R. COLEN, M.D., D.D.S., Clinical Instructor (Plastic Surgery), New York University School of Medicine, New York, New York. Resident in Plastic Surgery, Institute of Reconstructive Plastic Surgery, New York University Hospital, Bellevue Hospital, and Veterans' Administration Hospital, New York, New York.

THEODORE COOPER, M.D., Attending Obstetrician/Gynecologist, General Rose Memorial Hospital, Denver, Colorado; Swedish Medical Center, Englewood, Colorado.

THOMAS K. CRAIGMILE, M.D., Associate Clinical Professor of Neurological Surgery, University of Colorado School of Medicine, Denver, Colorado, Attending Neurosurgeon, St. Joseph Hospital, Children's Hospital, Colorado General Hospital, and Veterans' Administration Hospital, Denver, Colorado.

ROSS S. DAVIES, M.D., Chief of General and Thoracic Surgery, Dwight David Eisenhower Medical Center, Augusta, Georgia.

ALFRED JOHN DEFALCO, M.D., Associate Clinical Professor of Surgery (Urology), University of Colorado School of Medicine, Denver, Colorado. Active Staff, St. Anthony Hospital, Children's Hospital, Denver,

Colorado; Lutheran Hospital, Wheat Ridge, Colorado. Consultant, Fitzsimons Army Medical Center, Denver, Colorado.

ROBERT E. DONOHUE, M.D., Associate Professor of Surgery, Division of Urology, University of Colorado School of Medicine, Denver, Colorado. Chief of Urology, Veterans' Administration Hospital, Denver, Colorado. Staff, University Hospital, Denver General Hospital, and Children's Hospital, Denver, Colorado.

STEVEN L. DUBOVSKY, M.D., Associate Professor of Psychiatry, University of Colorado School of Medicine, Denver, Colorado. Attending Psychiatrist, University of Colorado Hospital and Veterans' Administration Hospital, Denver, Colorado. Consulting Psychiatrist, Fitzsimons Army Medical Center, Denver, Colorado.

ERNEST L. DUNN, M.D., Assistant Professor of Surgery, University of Colorado School of Medicine, Denver, Colorado. Director, Critical Care Unit, Denver General Hospital, Denver, Colorado.

T. K. EARLEY, M.D., Associate Clinical Professor of Surgery, University of Colorado School of Medicine, Denver, Colorado. Attending Surgeon, Presbyterian Hospital and St. Joseph Hospital, Denver, Colorado.

EDWARD L. EHRICHS, M.D., Assistant Clinical Professor of Surgery, University of Colorado School of Medicine, Denver, Colorado. Chief of Surgery, Aurora Community Hospital, Aurora, Colorado.

EIBERT EINARSSON, M.D., Department of Surgery, University of Lund, Lund, Sweden.

BEN EISEMAN, M.D., Professor of Surgery, University of Colorado School of Medicine, Denver, Colorado. Chairman, Department of Surgery, Rose Medical Center, Denver, Colorado.

BO EKLÖF, M.D., Ph.D., Associate Professor of Surgery, University of Lund, Lund, Sweden. Chairman, Department of Surgery, Helsingborg Hospital, Helsingborg, Sweden.

DONALD P. ELLIOTT, M.D., Associate Clinical Professor of Surgery, University of Colorado Health Sciences Center, Denver, Colorado. Chief, Cardiac Surgery, Rose Medical Center; Chief, Cardiovascular Surgery, St. Anthony Hospital Systems, Denver, Colorado.

STEPHEN ENGLE, M.D., M.S. (Surg.), Associate Clinical Professor of Surgery, University of Colorado School of Medicine, Denver, Colorado. Attending Surgeon, Rose Medical Center and St. Luke's Hospital, Denver, Colorado.

TIBOR ENGEL, M.D., Associate Clinical Professor, Department of Obstetrics and Gynecology, University of Colorado School of Medicine, Denver, Colorado. Active Staff, Rose Medical Center, Denver, Colorado.

ROBERT P. FARACI, M.D., Assistant Clinical Professor of Surgery, University of Colorado School of Medicine, Denver, Colorado. Director of Oncology, St. Anthony Hospital Systems, Denver, Colorado.

TANOUS FARIS, M.D., Associate Clinical Professor of Surgery, University of Colorado School of Medicine, Denver, Colorado. Active Staff, St. Joseph Hospital and Presbyterian Medical Center, Denver, Colorado.

DONALD C. FERLIC, M.D., Assistant Clinical Professor, University of Colorado School of Medicine, Denver, Colorado.

BARRY W. FRANK, M.D., Associate Clinical Professor of Internal Medicine, University of Colorado School of Medicine, Denver, Colorado. Attending Gastroenterologist, St. Joseph Hospital and Rose Medical Center, Denver, Colorado.

VERNER FRIEDMAN, M.D., Assistant Professor of Surgery (Neurosurgery), University of Colorado Medical Center. Active Staff, Rose Medical Center; Courtesy Staff, St. Joseph Hospital, Presbyterian Hospital, Mercy Hospital, Children's Hospital, St. Luke's Hospital, St. Anthony Hospital, Porter Memorial Hospital, Denver,

CONTRIBUTORS

Colorado; Lutheran Hospital, Wheat Ridge, Colorado; Swedish Medical Center, Englewood, Colorado.

WILLIAM E. FULLER, M.D., Associate Professor of Obstetrics and Gynecology, University of Colorado School of Medicine, Denver, Colorado. Attending Obstetrician/Gynecologist, University Hospital, Rose Medical Center, and Veterans' Administration Hospital, Denver, Colorado.

JACK GALLAGHER, M.D., Associate Clinical Professor of Surgery, University of Colorado School of Medicine, Denver, Colorado. Attending Surgeon, St. Joseph Hospital and Presbyterian Medical Center, Denver, Colorado.

ROBERT GERNER, M.D., Associate Professor of Surgery, University of Colorado Health Sciences Center, Denver, Colorado.

ERNESTO GOLDMAN, M.D., Instructor in Anesthesiology, University of Colorado Health Sciences Center, Denver, Colorado.

STANLEY N. GOODMAN, M.S., M.D., Associate Clinical Professor, University of Colorado Medical Center, Denver, Colorado. Attending Staff, Rose Medical Center, Denver, Colorado.

JOHN B. GRAMLICH, M.D., Clinical Professor of Surgery, University of Colorado School of Medicine, Denver, Colorado. Attending Surgeon, Colorado General Hospital, Denver, Colorado; DePaul Hospital and Memorial Hospital, Cheyenne, Wyoming.

JOSEPH C. GREER, M.D., Clinical Instructor in Surgery, University of Colorado Medical Center, Denver, Colorado. Attending Staff, Colon and Rectal Surgery, Presbyterian Medical Center, Denver, Colorado.

JOHN A. GROSSMAN, M.D., Instructor in Surgery (Plastic), University of Colorado Medical Center, Denver, Colorado. Vice Chairman, Department of Surgery, Rose Medical Center, Denver, Colorado.

WILLIAM L. HALSETH, M.D., Assistant Clinical Professor of Surgery, University of Colorado Medical Center, Denver, Colorado. Attending Surgeon, Rose Medical Center and St. Anthony Hospital, Denver, Colorado.

WILLIAM R. HAMAKER, M.D., Staff, St. Luke's Hospital and Mid-America Heart Institute, Kansas City, Missouri. Formerly, Associate Clinical Professor, University of Colorado Medical Center; Chief, Cardiothoracic Surgery Service, Fitzsimons Army Medical Center, Denver, Colorado.

JOHN F. HANSBROUGH, M.D., Assistant Professor of Surgery, University of Colorado School of Medicine, Denver, Colorado. Director, Emergency Department, University of Colorado Health Sciences Center, Denver, Colorado.

BRACK HATTLER, M.D., Ph.D., Attending Physician, Porter-Swedish Medical Centers, Denver, Colorado.

JOHN C. HEISER, M.D., Resident in Surgery, University of Colorado Medical Center, Denver, Colorado.

EUGENE HELLER, M.D., Clinical Professor of Surgery (Urology), University of Colorado School of Medicine, Denver, Colorado. Attending Urologist, Rose Medical Center, Children's Hospital, Mercy Hospital, Veterans' Administration Hospital, and Porter-Swedish Medical Centers, Denver, Colorado.

GILBERT HERMANN, M.D., Clinical Professor of Surgery, University of Colorado School of Medicine, Denver, Colorado. Attending Surgeon, Rose Medical Center, Colorado General Hospital, and Veterans' Administration Hospital, Denver, Colorado.

TRACY E. HICKS, M.D., F.R.C.S.(Can.), Private Practitioner; Attending Staff, Langley Memorial Hospital, Langley, British Columbia, Canada. Formerly, Fellow, Department of Hand Surgery, University of Colorado Medical Center, Denver, Colorado.

ALAN D. HILGENBERG, M.D., Assistant Clinical Professor of Surgery, University of Colorado School of Medicine, Denver, Colorado. Attending Thoracic Surgeon, St. Joseph Hospital, Presbyterian Medical Center, and Children's Hospital, Denver, Colorado.

RICHARD M. HIRATA, M.D., Associate Professor of Surgery, Uniformed Services University of the Health Sciences, Bethesda, Maryland. Chief, General Surgery Service; Chief, Head and Neck Surgery Service, Walter Reed Army Medical Center, Washington, D.C.

DAVID C. HITCH, M.D., Assistant Professor of Surgery; Assistant Clinical Professor of Pediatrics, University of Oklahoma College of Medicine, Oklahoma City, Oklahoma. Attending Pediatric Surgeon, Oklahoma Children's Memorial Hospital, Oklahoma City, Oklahoma.

W. HOWARD HUDSON, M.D., Orthopedic and Hand Surgeon, University Hospital and Doctor's Hospital, Augusta, Georgia. Formerly, Fellow, Arthritis Surgery, Denver Orthopedic Clinic, Denver, Colorado.

DAVID E. HUTCHISON, M.D., Associate Clinical Professor, University of Colorado School of Medicine, Denver, Colorado. Chief of Surgery; Member of Executive Board, St. Anthony Hospital and Mercy Hospital, Denver, Colorado. Member of Credentials Committee, St. Anthony Hospital, Denver, Colorado.

BRUCE W. JAFEK, M.D., Professor and Chairman, Department of Otolaryngology, University of Colorado Health Sciences Center, Denver, Colorado. Chairman, Department of Otolaryngology, Colorado General Hospital; Attending Otolaryngologist, Denver General Hospital, Veterans' Administration Hospital, Rose Medical Center, and Children's Hospital, Denver, Colorado.

ARTHUR F. JONES, M.D., Assistant Clinical Professor of Surgery, University of Colorado Health Sciences Center, Denver, Colorado. Attending Staff, Lutheran Hospital, Wheat Ridge, Colorado.

GLENN KELLY, M.D., Associate Professor of Surgery, University of Colorado School of Medicine, Denver, Colorado. Staff, Porter-Swedish Hospitals, Denver, Colorado.

RICHARD F. KEMPCZINSKI, M.D., Associate Professor of Surgery, University of Cincinnati College of Medicine, Cincinnati, Ohio. Chief of Vascular Surgery and Director of the Vascular Diagnostic Laboratory, University Hospitals of Cincinnati, General Division and Holmes Division; Attending Surgeon, Veterans' Administration Hospital, Cincinnati, Ohio.

WOLFF M. KIRSCH, M.D., Professor and Program Director, Division of Neurosurgery, University of Colorado Health Sciences Center, Denver, Colorado.

LAWRENCE J. KOEP, M.D., Associate Professor of Surgery, University of Colorado Health Sciences Center, Denver, Colorado.

JOSEPH L. KOVARIK, M.D., Associate Clinical Professor of Surgery, University of Colorado School of Medicine, Denver, Colorado.

ROBERT LATTES, M.D., Assistant Professor of Radiology, University of Colorado Medical Center, Denver, Colorado.

RALPH A. W. LEHMAN, M.D., Professor of Surgery, The Milton S. Hershey Medical Center of The Pennsylvania State University, Hershey, Pennsylvania. Chief, Division of Neurosurgery, The Milton S. Hershey Medical Center, Hershey, Pennsylvania.

R. D. LEICHTY, M.D., Professor of Surgery, University of Colorado School of Medicine, Denver, Colorado, Staff, Colorado General Hospital; Consultant, Veterans' Administration Hospital, Fitzsimons Army Medical Center, and Denver General Hospital, Denver, Colorado.

CONTRIBUTORS

JOHN R. LILLY, M.D., Professor of Surgery, University of Colorado School of Medicine, Denver, Colorado. Chief of Pediatric Surgery, University Hospital, Denver, Colorado.

C. A. LUEKENS, JR., M.D., Assistant Clinical Professor of Orthopedics, University of Colorado School of Medicine, Denver, Colorado. Attending Staff, St. Anthony Hospital, St. Luke's Hospital, Denver, Colorado; Lutheran Medical Center, Wheat Ridge, Colorado.

JAMES McGREGOR, M.D., C.M., Assistant Professor, University of Colorado School of Medicine, Denver, Colorado. Attending Obstetrician/Gynecologist, University of Colorado Medical Center, Denver, Colorado.

WINONA R. MACKEY, M.D., Assistant Professor of Radiology, University of Colorado Medical Center, Denver, Colorado. Radiotherapist, St. Mary-Corwin Hospital, Pueblo, Colorado.

FRANCIS J. MAJOR, M.D., Associate Clinical Professor of Obstetrics and Gynecology, University of Colorado School of Medicine, Denver, Colorado. Chief, GYN Tumor Service, Denver General Hospital, Denver, Colorado.

JOYCE A. MAJURE, M.D., Resident in Surgery, University of Colorado Health Sciences Center, Denver, Colorado.

EDGAR L. MAKOWSKI, M.D., Professor and Chairman, Department of Obstetrics and Gynecology, University of Colorado School of Medicine, Denver, Colorado. Chairman, Department of Obstetrics and Gynecology, University Hospital, Denver, Colorado.

FRANK MANART, M.D., Resident in Cardiothoracic Surgery, University of Colorado Medical Center, Denver, Colorado.

ARLEN D. MEYERS, M.D., Assistant Professor of Otolaryngology, University of Colorado Health Sciences Center, Denver, Colorado. Chief, Division of Oto-laryngology, Veterans' Administration Hospital, Denver, Colorado.

GERALD M. MILLER, M.D., Clinical Professor of Surgery (Urology), University of Colorado School of Medicine, Denver, Colorado. Chief, Department of Urology, Rose Medical Center; Attending Urologist, Children's Hospital, Veterans' Administration Hospital, St. Joseph Hospital, Mercy Hospital, and Porter-Swedish Hospitals, Denver, Colorado.

DANIEL MIRELMAN, M.D., Attending Surgeon, Brookwood Medical Center and South Highlands Hospital, Birmingham, Alabama.

BARRY L. MOLK, M.D., Assistant Clinical Professor of Medicine, University of Colorado Health Sciences Center, Denver, Colorado. Staff Cardiologist, Rose Medical Center, Denver, Colorado. Chairman, Department of Internal Medicine, Aurora Community Hospital, Aurora, Colorado.

LEWIS A. MOLOGNE, M.D., Chief, Department of Surgery; Attending General and Peripheral Vascular Surgeon, Fitzsimons Army Medical Center, Aurora, Colorado.

ELLEN L. MONCY, M.D., Clinical Instructor, University of Colorado Medical Center, Denver, Colorado. Active Staff, Lutheran Medical Center, Wheat Ridge, Colorado; Courtesy Staff, St. Anthony Hospital System, Denver, Colorado.

ERNEST E. MOORE, M.D., Assistant Professor of Surgery, University of Colorado Health Sciences Center, Denver, Colorado. Chief, Trauma Surgery, Denver General Hospital, Denver, Colorado.

GEORGE E. MOORE, M.D., Professor of Surgery, University of Colorado Medical Center, Denver, Colorado. Staff, Denver General Hospital, Denver, Colorado.

JOHN B. MOORE, M.D., Chief Surgery Resident, Denver General Hospital; Senior Surgery Resident, University of Colorado Health Sciences Center, Denver, Colorado.

CONTRIBUTORS

PETER C. MURR, M.D., Resident in Surgery, University of Colorado School of Medicine, Denver, Colorado.

WILLIAM R. NELSON, M.D., Associate Clinical Professor of Surgery, University of Colorado School of Medicine, Denver, Colorado. Active Staff, Presbyterian Medical Center, St. Joseph Hospital, St. Luke's Hospital; Courtesy Staff, Children's Hospital, General Rose Memorial Hospital, and Mercy Hospital, Denver, Colorado.

MELVIN M. NEWMAN, M.D., Associate Professor of Surgery, University of Colorado Medical Center, Denver, Colorado. Attending Surgeon, University Hospital; Courtesy Staff, General Rose Memorial Hospital, Denver, Colorado.

LAWRENCE W. NORTON, M.D., Professor of Surgery, University of Arizona College of Medicine, Tucson, Arizona. Chief, General Surgery Section, University of Arizona Health Sciences Center, Tucson, Arizona.

GEORGE PAPPAS, M.D., Associate Clinical Professor of Surgery, University of Colorado Medical Center, Denver, Colorado. Chief, Thoracic and Cardiovascular Surgery, Children's Hospital, Denver, Colorado.

RICHARD K. PARKER, M.D., Vice Chairman, Department of Surgery, St. Luke's Hospital, Denver, Colorado.

ROBERT M. PASH, M.D., Assistant Clinical Instructor, University of Colorado Medical Center, Denver, Colorado. Staff, Rose Medical Center, Mercy Hospital, Denver, Colorado; Aurora Community Hospital, Aurora, Colorado.

WILLIAM PEARCE, M.D., Surgical Resident, University of Colorado Medical Center, Denver, Colorado.

NATHAN W. PEARLMAN, M.D., Assistant Professor of Surgery, University of Colorado School of Medicine, Denver, Colorado. Surgical Oncologist, University of Colorado Hospital and Veterans' Administration Hospital, Denver, Colorado.

MORDANT E. PECK, M.D., Associate Clinical Professor of Surgery, University of Colorado School of Medicine, Denver, Colorado, Attending Surgeon, University of Colorado Medical Center, Rose Medical Center, St. Joseph Hospital, and Presbyterian Medical Center, Denver, Colorado.

ISRAEL PENN, M.D., F.R.C.S. (Eng.), F.R.C.S. (Can.), Professor of Surgery, University of Colorado Health Sciences Center, Denver, Colorado. Chief of Surgery, Veterans' Administration Hospital; Surgical Staff, University of Colorado Hospital, General Rose Memorial Hospital, and Children's Hospital, Denver, Colorado.

GEORGE PETERS, M.D., Assistant Clinical Professor of Surgery, University of Colorado School of Medicine, Denver, Colorado. Staff, Children's Hospital and St. Joseph Hospital, Denver, Colorado.

NORMAN E. PETERSON, M.D., Associate Professor of Surgery, University of Colorado Medical Center, Denver, Colorado. Chief, Division of Urology and Assistant Director of Surgery, Denver General Hospital; Attending Urologist, Veterans' Administration Hospital; Consultant in Urology, Fitzsimons Army Medical Center, Denver, Colorado.

RONALD R. PFISTER, M.D., Associate Professor of Surgery (Urology), University of Colorado School of Medicine, Denver, Colorado. Chief, Division of Urology, University of Colorado Medical Center; Staff, University Hospital, Children's Hospital, St. Anthony Hospital, Denver, Colorado; Lutheran Hospital, Wheat Ridge, Colorado.

MARVIN POMERANTZ, M.D., Associate Clinical Professor of Surgery, University of Colorado Medical Center, Denver, Colorado.

CHARLES F. PRATT, M.D., Resident in Surgery, University of Colorado Medical Center, Denver, Colorado.

W. GERALD RAINER, M.D., M.S. (Surg.), Clinical Professor of Surgery, University of Colorado Health Sci-

CONTRIBUTORS

ences Center, Denver, Colorado. Chief, Section of Thoracic and Cardiovascular Surgery, St. Joseph Hospital, Denver, Colorado.

M. P. REICH, M.D., Associate Clinical Professor of Surgery, University of Colorado Medical Center, Denver, Colorado. Attending Physician, Rose Medical Center, Denver, Colorado; Aurora Community Hospital, Aurora, Colorado.

SCOTT L. REPLOGLE, M.D., Resident in General Surgery, University of California, San Francisco, Medical Center, San Francisco, California.

ROBERT S. RICHARDSON, M.D., Attending Surgeon, Grays Harbor Community Hospital and St. Joseph Hospital, Aberdeen, Washington.

BENSON B. ROE, M.D., Professor of Surgery, University of California, San Francisco, School of Medicine, San Francisco, California. Co-chief, Cardiothoracic Surgery, University of California Hospitals; Consultant, Veterans' Administration Hospital and San Francisco General Hospital, San Francisco, California.

ROBERT R. ROKICKI, M.D., Associate Staff, St. Joseph Hospital, Presbyterian Medical Center, and Children's Hospital, Denver, Colorado.

DAVID B. ROOS, M.D., Associate Clinical Professor of Surgery, University of Colorado School of Medicine, Denver, Colorado. Staff, Presbyterian Medical Center, St. Joseph Hospital, and University Hospital, Denver, Colorado.

ROBERT B. RUTHERFORD, M.D., Professor of Surgery, University of Colorado School of Medicine, Denver, Colorado. Attending Staff, University of Colorado Health Sciences Center, Denver, Colorado.

FRANK A. SCOTT, M.D., F.R.C.S. (Can.), Assistant Professor of Surgery, University of Colorado Medical Center, Denver, Colorado. Chief, Hand Surgery Service, Veterans' Administration Hospital; Attending Surgeon,

Colorado General Hospital and Rose Medical Center, Denver, Colorado.

ROBERT G. SCRIBNER, M.D., Assistant Clinical Professor of Surgery, Stanford University School of Medicine, Stanford, California. Consultant in Vascular Surgery, Veterans' Administration Hospital, Palo Alto, California.

D. SHANDER, M.D., Assistant Clinical Professor of Medicine, University of Colorado School of Medicine, Denver, Colorado. Associate Director of Cardiology, Rose Medical Center, Denver, Colorado.

JOEL B. SIGDESTAD M.D., Staff, St. Joseph Hospital, Denver, Colorado.

JOHN S. SIMON, M.D., Assistant Clinical Professor of Surgery, University of Colorado School of Medicine, Denver, Colorado. Staff Surgeon, Rose Medical Center, Denver, Colorado; Aurora Community Hospital, Aurora, Colorado.

DANIEL L. SMITH, M.D., Assistant Clinical Professor of Surgery, University of Colorado School of Medicine, Denver, Colorado. Cardiovascular and Thoracic Surgeon, St. Luke's Hospital, Denver, Colorado.

GEORGE W. B. STARKEY, M.D., Assistant Clinical Professor of Surgery, Harvard Medical School, Boston, Massachusetts. Active Senior Staff, New England Deaconess Hospital and Faulkner Hospital, Boston, Massachusetts.

THOMAS E. STARZL, M.D., Professor and Chairman, Department of Surgery, University of Colorado Health Sciences Center, Denver, Colorado. Staff, University of Colorado Health Sciences Center, Denver, Colorado.

KARL STECHER, JR., M.D., Assistant Professor of Neurosurgery, University of Colorado School of Medicine, Denver, Colorado. Active Teaching Staff, Denver General Hospital, Colorado General Hospital, Veterans' Administration Hospital; Active Staff, Porter-Swedish

CONTRIBUTORS

Medical Centers, Denver, Colorado; Consulting Staff, Craig Hospital (Rocky Mountain Spinal Injury Center), Englewood, Colorado.

GREGORY VAN STEIGMANN, M.D., Resident in Surgery, University of Colorado Medical Center, Denver, Colorado.

MORRIS H. SUSMAN, M.D., Clinical Instructor, Department of Orthopedic Surgery, University of Colorado School of Medicine, Denver, Colorado. Attending Physician, St. Joseph Hospital and Rose Medical Center, Denver, Colorado.

ROY L. TAWES, JR., M.D., Assistant Professor of Surgery (Clinical), University of California, San Francisco, School of Medicine, San Francisco, California. Staff, Peninsula Hospital, Burlingame, California; Mills Memorial Hospital, San Mateo, California; Mary's Help Hospital, Daly City, California; San Francisco General Hospital, San Francisco, California; and Sequoia Hospital, Redwood City, California.

JERRY TEMPLER, M.D., Associate Professor of Surgery (Otolaryngology), University of Missouri Medical Center, Columbia, Missouri, Staff, University of Missouri Medical Center and Harry S Truman Memorial Veterans' Hospital, Columbia, Missouri.

JOHN TERBLANCHE, Ch.M., F.R.C.S., F.C.S. (S.A.), Professor of Surgery, University of Cape Town Medical School, Cape Town, South Africa. Co-director, Medical Research Council, Liver Research Group, University of Cape Town, Cape Town, South Africa. Chief Surgeon, Groote Schuur Hospital, Cape Town, South Africa.

JON S. THOMPSON, M.D., Senior Resident in General Surgery, University of Colorado Health Sciences Center, Denver, Colorado.

NINH N. TRAN, M.D., Teaching Fellow in Pediatric Surgery, University of Pittsburgh School of Medicine and Children's Hospital, Pittsburgh. Formerly, Professor of Pediatric Surgery, University of Saigon Med-

ical School, and Chief of Surgery, Children's Hospital, Saigon, Vietnam.

LILIA E. USUBIAGA, M.D., Assistant Professor of Anesthesiology, University of Colorado School of Medicine, Denver, Colorado. Staff Anesthesiologist, Veterans' Administration Hospital, Denver, Colorado.

GARY D. VANDER ARK, M.D., Staff, St. Joseph Hospital and Porter Memorial Hospital, Denver, Colorado; Swedish Medical Center, Englewood, Colorado.

CHARLES W. VAN WAY, III, M.D., Associate Professor of Surgery, University of Colorado School of Medicine, Denver, Colorado. Director of Surgery, Denver General Hospital; Staff Surgeon, Colorado General Hospital and Rose Medical Center, Denver, Colorado.

HAROLD VOGEL, M.D., Associate Professor of Surgery, University of Colorado Medical Center, Denver, Colorado. Chief, Division of Neurosurgery, Denver General Hospital, Denver, Colorado.

E. LANCE WALKER, M.D., Associate Clinical Professor of Surgery, University of Colorado Medical Center, Denver, Colorado. Cardiovascular and Thoracic Surgeon, St. Anthony Hospital, Mercy Hospital, and Rose Medical Center, Denver, Colorado.

RICHARD WEIL, III, M.D., Professor of Surgery, University of Colorado Health Sciences Center, Denver, Colorado.

JOHN N. WETTLAUFER, M.D., Director and Associate Professor, Division of Urology, University of Colorado Medical Center, Denver, Colorado. Courtesy Staff, Rose Medical Center, Children's Hospital, St. Anthony Hospital, Denver General Hospital, Denver, Colorado; Lutheran Hospital, Wheat Ridge, Colorado.

PAUL WEXLER, M.D., Associate Clinical Professor, Department of Obstetrics and Gynecology, University of Colorado Health Sciences Center, Denver, Colorado. Chairman, Department of Obstetrics and Gynecology, Rose Medical Center, Denver, Colorado.

xiii

CONTRIBUTORS

JEROME D. WIEDEL, M.D., Associate Professor, University of Colorado Health Sciences Center; Associate Professor, Department of Orthopedics, University Hospital, Denver, Colorado. Associate Staff, Denver General Hospital; Courtesy Staff, Veterans' Administration Hospital and General Rose Memorial Hospital, Denver, Colorado.

WILLIAM B. WILSON, JR., M.D., Assistant Professor of Obstetrics and Gynecology, University of Colorado School of Medicine, Denver, Colorado. Assistant Director of Obstetrics and Gynecology; Director of Family Planning and OB/GYN Outpatient Services, Denver General Hospital, Denver, Colorado.

IAN WINSPUR, M.D., F.R.C.S. (Ed.), Assistant Clinical Professor of Surgery, Hand Surgery Service, University of Colorado School of Medicine, Denver, Colorado. Attending Plastic Surgeon, University of Colorado Medical Center, St. Anthony Hospital, and Beth Israel Hospital, Denver, Colorado.

WILLIAM G. WINTER, M.D., Associate Professor, Department of Orthopedic Surgery and Department of Physical Medicine and Rehabilitation, University of Colorado School of Medicine, Denver, Colorado. Chief, Orthopedic Section, Veterans' Administration Hospital; Active Staff, University of Colorado Medical Center; Courtesy Staff, Rose Medical Center, Denver General Hospital, and Children's Hospital, Denver, Colorado.

P. S. WOLF, M.D., Associate Clinical Professor of Medicine, University of Colorado Health Sciences Center, Denver, Colorado. Associate Director, Division of Cardiology, Rose Medical Center, Denver, Colorado.

ROGER S. WOTKYNS, M.S., M.D., Associate Clinical Professor of Surgery, University of Colorado School of Medicine, Denver, Colorado. Chief of Staff, Lutheran Hospital and Medical Center, Wheat Ridge, Colorado; Attending Staff, University of Colorado Hospitals, Denver, Colorado.

FRANCIS K. YAMAMOTO, M.D., Assistant Clinical Instructor, University of Colorado School of Medicine, Denver, Colorado. Active Staff, Rose Medical Center, Denver, Colorado.

Preface

Surgeons seldom deny that they are logical. But with equal vehemence they usually protest that they are not statisticians. In fact, logical clinical decisions necessarily involve weighing the probability for good or evil of available options. Good can be measured by the probability of such things as cure of pain, improved physical activity, length of life, and increased earning power. Harm, on the contrary, can be measured by the probability of death, pain, hospitalization, and physical or mental incapacitation. In a world in which expensive medical technology has outpaced our knowledge of how most efficiently to use it, the cost in dollars to the individual or to society also must be considered in the numerator of a cost/benefit analysis.

A surgeon who denies an interest in or reliance on statistics and probabilities merely takes refuge behind his or her own exquisite computer—the brain—which regardless of conscious effort in the scientifically trained person subconsciously compares probabilities of good and bad outcome for the reasonable options. Surgeons are therefore intuitive if not overt statisticians. The best ones, who ultimately become known as wise, consciously record probabilities.

A surgeon gains knowledge of probabilities in several ways. Most important is his or her own experience. Unfortunately, it takes a lifetime to gather a statistically significant number of cases in order to use this source—by which time it is often too late to use these data. In addition, one usually inappropriately overweighs one's own experience—particularly one's recent experience. Another source of data is what one hears or reads. This is clearly the best way to analyze carefully the experience of others.

In a previous book (*Surgical Decision Making*, Saunders, 1978) we defined in diagramatic form using decision trees how pertinent data could develop a series of logical clinical options. This book is designed to present the statistical data base upon which choice can be made with the greatest probability of doing the maximum good and the least probability of doing harm. For each quoted number the reference source is cited.

Given the need for precise data concerning the probability of a good or bad outcome following surgical decisions, it is astounding how difficult it is to find such statistics for many common surgical diseases. For example, we had to omit the chapter on general anesthesia for lack of data using modern techniques!

Throughout the preparation of this book, the authors who had so gallantly volunteered to prepare the chapters came to the editor white-faced and shaken with variations of the complaint, "But in this particular field you would be amazed how little hard data is available." What was first thought to be a simple job for quick literature review inevitably turned out to be much more difficult. For their long hours of library searching, I am sincerely grateful.

Having made obeisance to numbers, let a caveat be added: Numbers are not everything. Data from two papers concerning the same disease are seldom totally comparable. Case selection and subjectivity in recording beneficial results, for example, are notoriously dependent on the bias of the author. Even length of life

PREFACE

is not invariably a good way to judge the benefit of operation. Life has depth as well as length. When the book was started, we tried to quantitate depth of life following certain operative procedures but gave up largely because we could find no good way to quantitate benefit with hard data. However, the principle is important, even though it is not faced in this book except indirectly by recording when possible good/excellent results or the incidence and severity of complications. Four pain-free months with good physical activity terminating in sudden death seems superior to six months of misery—but how do you quantitate it?

Finally, I thank the contributors for their tolerance during the necessary débridement and plastic reconstructive operations performed on their chapters as originally submitted. Being surgeons, they are individualists and are unaccustomed to being forced into even an editorial conformity. I hope the value of the book will compensate for bruised egos. Fortunately, all are colleagues and friends.

B. Eiseman

Contents

CONTENTS

CONTENTS

CONTENTS

CONTENTS

CONTENTS

xxii

CONTENTS

CONTENTS

Section **A**

Neurosurgery

CLOSED HEAD INJURY BY GARY VANDER ARK, M.D.

Comments

A. Incidence of symptoms is not related to severity of injury.[2, 3]

INJURY	SYMPTOM	INCIDENCE
Head injury without amnesia	Headache	72%
Head injury with amnesia	Headache	80%
Head injury without amnesia	Vertigo	42%
Head injury with amnesia	Vertigo	54%

B. Incidence of seizures for all head injuries is 10 per cent. When compound injuries are subtracted, the incidence is 5 per cent. For adults who have amnesia for less than 24 hours and no intracranial hematoma, the incidence is zero. If an intracranial hematoma develops, the incidence of seizures increases to 28.5 per cent.

C. Incidence of intracranial hematoma is expressed in per cent of patients having a closed head injury that requires hospital care.[5, 9]

D. Although acute subdural hematoma should mean only those clots that require surgery within 24 hours of injury, many series in the literature include all hematomas that develop within 72 hours of injury.[5]

Subacute = 3 days to 3 weeks postinjury

Chronic = more than 3 weeks postinjury

E. As survival rates for traumatic intracranial hemorrhage improve, the percentage of patients recovering completely also increases. Patients are not being saved only to vegetate. In one large series on acute subdural hematoma, 24 per cent of the patients returned to work, 23 per cent had some neurologic dysfunction that restricted their activity, and only 6 per cent were vegetating in nursing homes.[1, 5, 8, 10]

F. The rare patient who reaccumulates a chronic subdural hematoma following burr hole evacuation may then be treated by craniotomy or by subdural-peritoneal shunting. Shunting procedures are reserved for patients with significant craniocerebral disproportion.

References

1. Britt, R. H., and Hamilton, R. D.: Large decompressive craniotomy in the treatment of acute subdural hematoma. Neurosurgery, 2:195–200, 1978.
2. Friedman, A. P.: The so-called post-traumatic headache. In Walker, A. E., Caveness, W. F., and Critchley, M. (eds.): The Late Effects of Head Injury. Springfield, Ill., Charles C Thomas, 1969, pp. 55–70.
3. Jacobsen, S. A.: Mechanisms of the sequalae of minor craniocervical trauma. In Walker, A. E., Caveness, W. F., and Critchley, M. (eds.): The late Effects of Head Injury. Springfield, Ill., Charles C Thomas, 1969, pp. 35–45.
4. Jamieson, K. G., and Yelland, J. D. N.: Extradural hematoma. Report of 167 cases. J. Neurosurg., 29:13–23, 1968.
5. Jamieson, K. G., and Yelland, J. D. N.: Surgically treated traumatic subdural hematoma. J. Neurosurg., 37:137–149, 1972.
6. Jamieson, K. G., and Yelland, J. D. N.: Traumatic intracerebral hematoma. Report of 63 surgically treated cases. J. Neurosurg., 37:528–532, 1972.
7. Jennett, W. B.: Traumatic epilepsy after closed head injuries. J. Neurol. Neurosurg. Psychiatry, 23:295–301, 1960.
8. Moiel, R. H., and Caram, P. C.: Acute subdural hematoma: a review of 84 cases, a six year evaluation. J. Trauma, 7:660–66, 1967.
9. Thomas, L. M., and Gurdjian, E. S.: Intracranial hematomas of traumatic origin. In Youmans, J. R. (ed.): Neurological Surgery, Vol. II. Philadelphia, W. B. Saunders Co., 1973, pp. 960–968.
10. Vander Ark, G. D.: Cardiovascular changes with acute subdural hematoma. Surg. Neurol., 3:305–308, 1975.

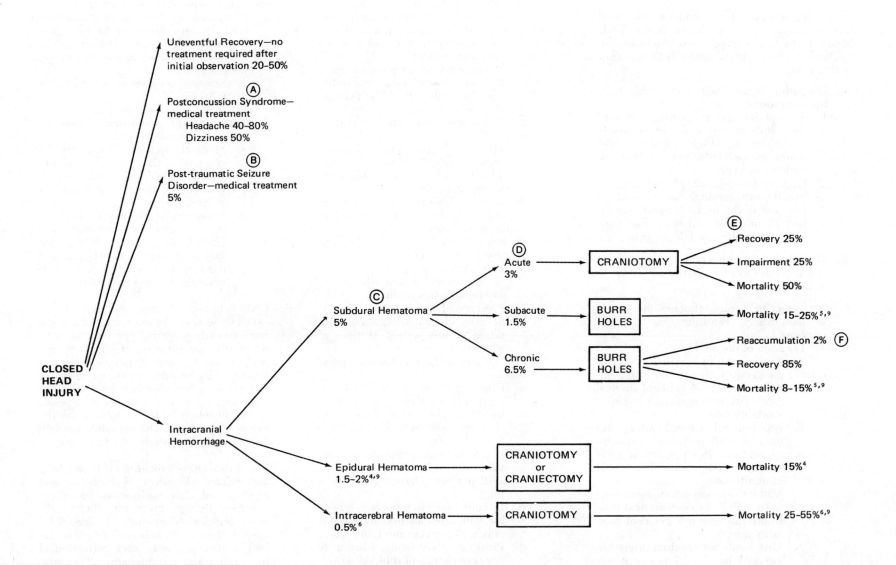

Uneventful Recovery—no treatment required after initial observation 20–50%

(A)
Postconcussion Syndrome—medical treatment
    Headache 40–80%
    Dizziness 50%

(B)
Post-traumatic Seizure Disorder—medical treatment 5%

CLOSED HEAD INJURY

Intracranial Hemorrhage

(C)
Subdural Hematoma 5%

(D)
Acute 3% → CRANIOTOMY (E)
→ Recovery 25%
→ Impairment 25%
→ Mortality 50%

Subacute 1.5% → BURR HOLES → Mortality 15–25%[5,9]

Chronic 6.5% → BURR HOLES
→ Reaccumulation 2% (F)
→ Recovery 85%
→ Mortality 8–15%[5,9]

Epidural Hematoma 1.5–2%[4,9] → CRANIOTOMY or CRANIECTOMY → Mortality 15%[4]

Intracerebral Hematoma 0.5%[6] → CRANIOTOMY → Mortality 25–55%[6,9]

SPONTANEOUS INTRACRANIAL HEMORRHAGE BY VERNER FRIEDMAN, M.D.

Comments

Vascular disease of the brain is the third most common cause of death in the USA. Spontaneous hemorrhage (versus ischemic infarctions, emboli, etc.) constitutes 28 per cent of this group.[8]

A. Idiopathic hemorrhage can result from two conditions:
  1. Arteriosclerosis: Hemorrhage is into the white matter of the brain and is of unknown source. Mortality and morbidity rate is 90 per cent with or without surgery.
  2. Cryptic hamartoma: Hemorrhage is usually intracerebral and is fatal 30 per cent of the time. Surgical evacuation is indicated and has a low morbidity-mortality rate (23 per cent).

B. Hypertensive intracranial hemorrhage has a 90 per cent mortality rate with or without surgery.

C. A number of factors influence the course of hemorrhage resulting from an aneurysm.[2, 8]
  1. Location of the aneurysm:
    a. In the anterior cerebral artery, an aneurysm with anterior communication has a 27.4 per cent surgical morbidity rate and a 15 per cent mortality rate.
    b. An internal carotid artery aneurysm with posterior communication has a 26.4 per cent surgical morbidity rate and a 3 per cent mortality rate.
    c. Middle cerebral artery aneurysms have a 19.7 per cent surgical morbidity rate and a 7 per cent mortality rate.
    d. Distal anterior cerebral artery aneurysms have a 2.7 per cent sur-

gical morbidity rate and a 5 per cent mortality rate.
    e. Vertebral and basilar artery aneurysms have a 3.6 per cent surgical morbidity rate and a 5 per cent mortality rate.
    f. Multiple-artery aneurysms have a 14 per cent surgical morbidity rate. Mortality rate is the average of those just described.
  2. Incidence of bleeding and rebleeding is as follows:[8]
    a. Fifty per cent of rebleeding occurs within the first two weeks.
    b. Twenty per cent of rebleeding occurs thereafter.
  3. Prognosis without surgery: 88 per cent of patients died of recurrent bleeding within three years.
  4. Factors influencing prognosis prior to surgical intervention are:
    a. Parenchyma damage.[2]
      1) Intracerebral hemorrhage.
      2) Remote infarction.
    b. Presence of spasm.
    c. Severity of hemorrhage and condition of the patient at time of surgery.
  5. The type of surgery influences prognosis.
    a. Clipping of the neck of the anerusym is possible 75 per cent of the time. There is a 95 per cent chance of prevention of rebleeding.
    b. Reinforcement of the dome with adhesives or by other means has a 10 per cent chance of rebleeding.
    c. Intraluminal thrombosis is possible with large aneurysms and has only a 10 per cent mortality rate.
    d. Proximal artery ligation has a 20 per cent chance of rebleeding.

D. Arteriovenous malformation can cause spontaneous intracranial hemorrhage.
  1. The incidence of rebleeding is 90 per cent. This usually is not fatal but produces neurologic deterioration.
  2. Factors influencing prognosis prior to treatment are:
    a. Size and number of major feeding vessels.
    b. Location within the brain.
  3. Treatment of hemorrhage from arteriovenous malformation:
    a. Medical treatment consists of supportive therapy plus anticonvulsants when indicated. It usually does not affect overall mortality rate.
    b. Surgical excision has a 7 to 8 per cent mortality and morbidity rate.
    c. Embolization has a 20 per cent morbidity and mortality rate, and the surgeon rarely is able to obliterate the lesion completely.

E. CNS neoplasms rarely (less than 1 per cent of the time) present with spontaneous hemorrhage. Fifty per cent of such neoplasms are primary, of which 80 per cent are benign and 20 per cent are malignant. The remaining 50 per cent are metastatic tumors. Surgical removal is the only treatment, and prognosis depends on the histology of the neoplasm and the extent of removal.[7] The operative mortality and morbidity rate is 2 to 3 per cent.

F. Blood dyscrasias[10] include (1) hemophilia and related disorders of bleeding and clotting and (2) complications of anticoagulation therapy given for other conditions. Surgical treatment is indicated for mass lesions, e.g., subdural or intracerebral hematomas, only after correction of the underlying coagulopathy. The mor-

SPONTANEOUS INTRACRANIAL HEMORRHAGE

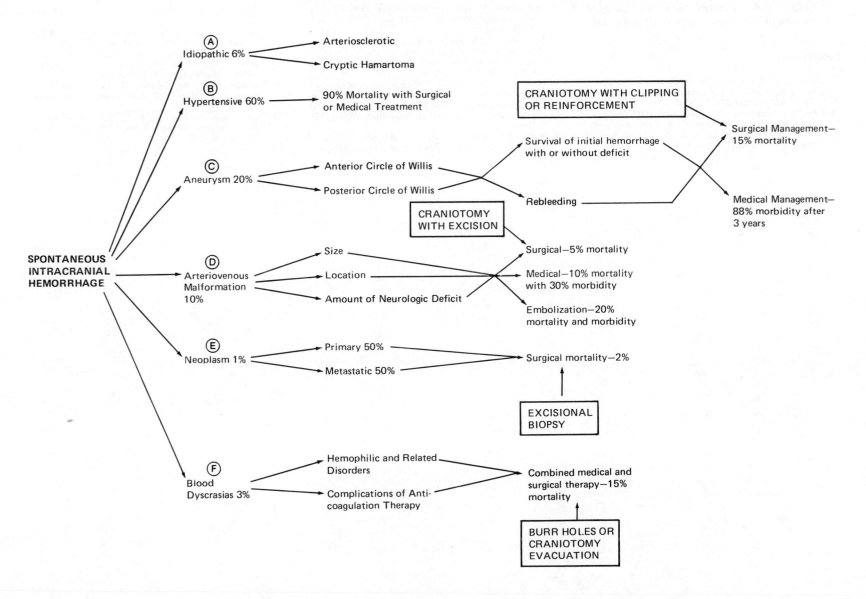

(A) Idiopathic 6%
→ Arteriosclerotic
→ Cryptic Hamartoma

(B) Hypertensive 60%
→ 90% Mortality with Surgical or Medical Treatment

(C) Aneurysm 20%
→ Anterior Circle of Willis
→ Posterior Circle of Willis

Survival of initial hemorrhage with or without deficit

Rebleeding

CRANIOTOMY WITH CLIPPING OR REINFORCEMENT

Surgical Management— 15% mortality

Medical Management— 88% morbidity after 3 years

SPONTANEOUS INTRACRANIAL HEMORRHAGE

(D) Arteriovenous Malformation 10%
→ Size
→ Location
→ Amount of Neurologic Deficit

CRANIOTOMY WITH EXCISION

Surgical—5% mortality

Medical—10% mortality with 30% morbidity

Embolization—20% mortality and morbidity

(E) Neoplasm 1%
→ Primary 50%
→ Metastatic 50%

Surgical mortality—2%

EXCISIONAL BIOPSY

(F) Blood Dyscrasias 3%
→ Hemophilic and Related Disorders
→ Complications of Anti-coagulation Therapy

Combined medical and surgical therapy—15% mortality

BURR HOLES OR CRANIOTOMY EVACUATION

SPONTANEOUS INTRACRANIAL HEMORRHAGE *Continued*

bidity and mortality rate for surgical treatment of these lesions is 10 per cent.

References

1. Drake, C. G.: Ligation of the vertebral or basilar artery in the treatment of large intracranial aneurysms. J. Neurosurg., *43*:255–274, 1975.
2. Graf, C. J.: Prognosis for patient with more surgically treated aneurysms. Analysis of the cooperative study of intracranial aneurysms and subarachnoid hemorrhage. J. Neurosurg., *35*:438–443, 1971.
3. Jamieson, K. D.: Aneurysms of the vertebrobasilar system: Surgical intervention in 19 cases. J. Neurosurg., *21*:781–797, 1964.
4. McKissock, W., Richardson, A., and Taylor, J.: Primary intradural hemorrhage: A controlled study of surgical and conservative treatment in 180 unselected cases. Lancet, 2:221–226, 1961.
5. Nishioka, H.: Evaluation of the conservative management of ruptured intracranial aneurysms. Report on the cooperative study of intracranial aneurysms and subarachnoid hemorrhage. J. Neurosurg., 25:574–592, 1966.
6. Paillas, J. E., and Alliez, B.: Surgical treatment of spontaneous intracerebral hemorrhage: Immediate and long-term results in 250 cases. J. Neurosurg., 39:145–151, 1973.
7. Posner, J. B., Management of central nervous system metastases. Semin. Oncol., 4:81–91, 1977.
8. Sahs, A. L., Perret, G., et al.: Intracranial Aneurysms and Subarachnoid Hemorrhage. A Cooperative Study. Philadelphia, J. B. Lippincott, 1969.
9. Sedzimin, C. B., and Robinson, J.: Intracranial hemorrhage in children and adolescents. J. Neurosurg., 38:296–281, 1973.
10. Seeler, R. A., and Imana, R. B.: Intracranial hemorrhage in patients with hemophilia. J. Neurosurg., 39:181–185, 1973.

SPINAL CORD INJURY

SPINAL CORD INJURY BY THOMAS CRAIGMILE, M.D.

Comments

SPINAL CORD INJURY I

A. General factors affecting prognosis include:
1. Accuracy of initial neurologic assessment.[13]
2. Initial management that avoids conversion of spinal injury to cord injury.
3. Pre-existence of lesions that encroach on cord space, such as spondylosis, rheumatoid spondylitis, congenital fusion (Klippel-Feil syndome), and other.
4. Avulsion of nerve root.
5. Decreased blood flow to cord (from hypotension, atherosclerosis, or vertebral artery injury).
6. Delayed cystic degeneration or traumatic syringomyelia months or years after injury.

B. Although their benefit is unproved, steroids[7, 12, 19] and osmotic diuretics[10, 14] are usually administered to decrease cord swelling. Local spine cooling is still experimental and of unproved benefit.[1, 13, 16, 17]

C. Physiologically complete lesions: In lower lesions no improvement will occur after 24 hours except for some return of nerve root function.[13, 15]

D. Physiologically incomplete lesions are determined by the presence of deep reflexes or of motor or sensory function. This implies physiologically reversible injuries. Improvement will continue for up to one month.

E. Stress bleeding (often minor) occurs in 10 per cent of cervical cord injuries.

SPINAL CORD INJURY II

F. High complete cervical lesions are immediately fatal.

G. Physiotherapy will achieve some functional improvement in ± 33 per cent of cases.

H. Motivation and intelligence are important determinants. In England, 80 per cent of all cord injury patients are employed. This includes 50 per cent of all quadriplegic patients.

I. Death was associated with inadequate ventilation.

J. Open injuries have a worse prognosis than do closed injuries. Débridement of gunshot wound minimizes infection (meningitis). Stab wounds may not require débridement.

K. This rate is associated with lethal vascular injuries.

L. Aortic rupture is occasionally associated with this injury.

M. Laminectomy is rarely indicated except for incomplete lesions that show radiologic signs of encroachment on the cord.

N. Débridement and early decompression laminectomy are indicated with these compound injuries: (1) injuries involving the abdomen, in order to avoid fecal contamination of the subarachnoid space; (2) injuries of cauda equina; (3) progressive defects; (4) pleural injury, in order to prevent pleural-subarachnoid fistula; (5) injury from intraspinal missiles or bone fragments; and (6) injuries whose entrance wound is near the spinal cord, in order to avert subarachnoid cutaneous fistula.

O. Injuries to heart, aorta, and vena cava are frequently associated with this condition.

P. Socially acceptable bladder and bowel control is achieved in about 50 per cent of all spinal cord injuries. This does not correlate with level of injury.

Q. Flaccid paraplegia means no motor function of lower extremities.

R. Some uncommon cord injuries are shown in the table.

LESION	CAUSE	TREATMENT	PROGNOSIS
Radiation myelopathy	Radiation therapy	None	Gradually progressive; no improvement
Occlusion of anterior spinal artery	Aortic aneurysmectomy	None	Occasionally slight improvement
Complications of aortic angiography	Overdose or injection of angiographic contrast material into anterior spinal artery	None	Occasionally slight improvement
Spinal concussion	Trivial cervical injury; more common in patient with congenital anomalies	Steroids	Full recovery in minutes to hours

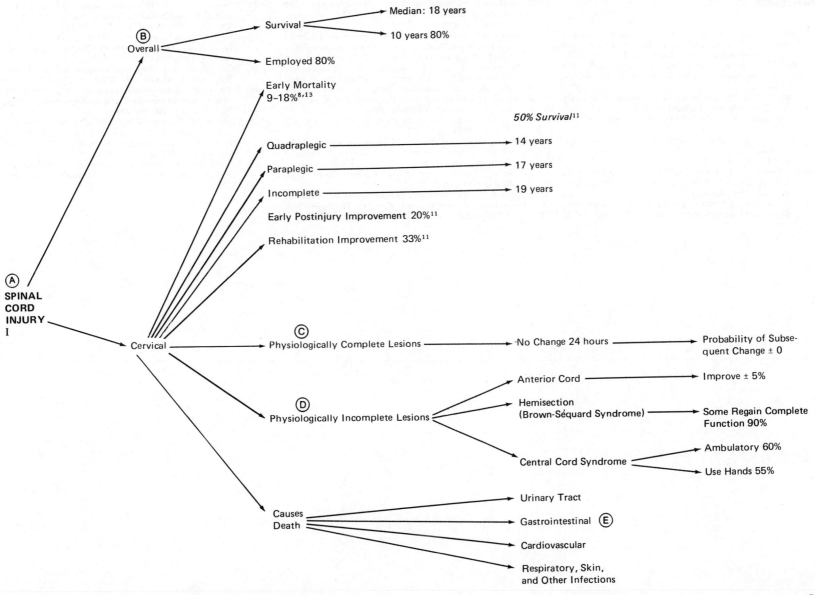

SPINAL CORD INJURY *Continued*

References

1. Albin, M. S., et al.: Study of functional recovery produced by delayed localized cooling after spinal cord injury in primates. J. Neurosurgy., *24*:113–130, 1968.
2. Barnett, H. J. M., et al.: Progressive myelopathy as a sequel to traumatic paraplegia. Brain, *89*:159–174, 1966.
3. Barnett, H. J. M.: Syringomyelia consequent on minor to moderate trauma. *In* Barnett, H. J. M., et al. (eds.): Syringomyelia. Philadelphia, W. B. Saunders Co., 1973.
4. Bosch, A., Stauffer, S., and Nickel, V. L.: Incomplete traumatic quadriplegia. A ten year review. JAMA, *216*:473–478, 1971.
5. Braithaupt, D. J., Jousse, A. T., and Wynn-Jones, M.: Late causes of death and life expectancy in paraplegia. Can. Med. Assoc. J., *85*:73–77, 1961.
6. Comarr, A. E.: Intermittent catheterization for the traumatic cord bladder patient. J. Urol., *108*:79–81, 1972.
7. Ducker, T. B., and Hamit, H. F. Experimental treatments of acute spinal cord injury. J. Neurosurg., *30*:693–697, 1969.
8. Harris, P.: Some neurosurgical aspects of traumatic paraplegia. *In* Harris, P. (ed.): Spinal Injuries. Edinburgh, Morris and Gibb, Ltd., 1965, pp. 101–112.
9. Herandeen, T. L., and King, H.: Transient anuria and paraplegia following traumatic rupture of the thoracic aorta. J. Thorac. Cardiovasc. Surg., *56*:599–602, 1968.
10. Joyner, J., and Freeman, L. W.: Urea and spinal cord trauma. Neurology, *13*:69–72, 1963.
11. Kurtzka, J. F.: Epidemiology of spinal cord injury. Exper. Neurol., *48*:163–236, 1975.
12. Lewin, M. G., Pappius, H. M., and Hansebout, R. R.: Effects of steroids on edema associated with injury of the spinal cord. *In* Reulen, H. J., and Schurmann, K. (eds.): Steroids and Brain Edema. New York, Springer-Verlag, 1972.
13. Norrell, H.: Fractures and dislocations of the spine. *In* Rothman, R., and Simeone, F. (eds.): The Spine, Vol. 2. Philadelphia, W. B. Saunders, 1975, pp. 529–566.
14. Parker, A. J., Park, R. D., and Stowater, J. L.: Reduction of trauma-induced edema of spinal cord in dogs given mannitol. Am. J. Vet. Res., *34*:1355–1357, 1973.
15. Ruge, D.: Spinal cord injuries. *In* Ruge, D. and Wiltse, L. L. (eds.): Spinal Disorders: Diagnosis and Treatment. Philadelphia, Lea and Febiger, 1977.
16. Selker, R. G.: Ice water irradiation of the spinal cord. Surg. Forum, *22*:411–413, 1971.
17. Tator, C. H.: Acute spinal cord injury: a review of recent studies of treatment and pathophysiology. Can. Med. Assoc. J., *107*:143–150, 1972.
18. Verbiest, H.: Surgery of the cervical vertebral body in cases of traumatic deformity or dislocation. *In* Harris, P. (ed.): Spinal Injuries. Edinburgh, Morris and Gibb, Ltd., 1965, pp. 112–120.
19. Yashon, D.: Pharmacologic treatment. *In* Yashon, D.: Spinal Injury. New York, Appleton-Century-Crofts, 1978.

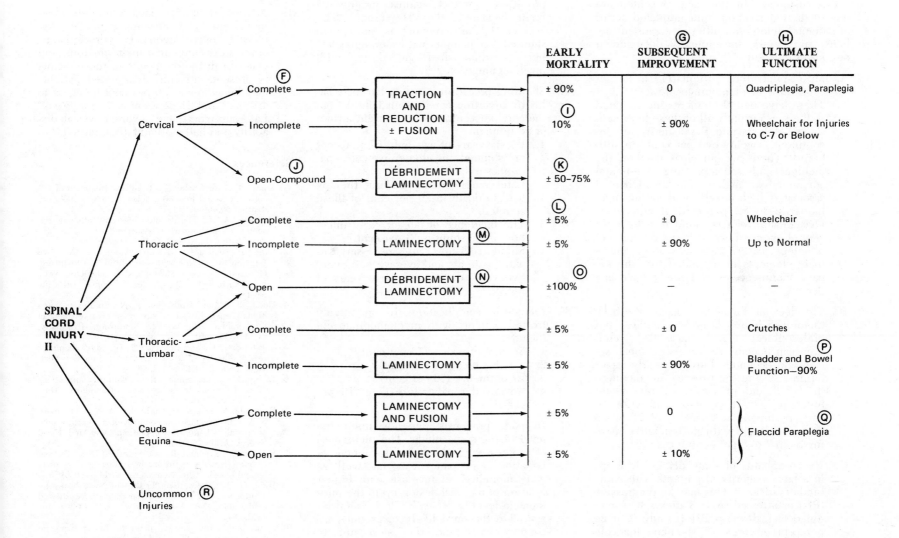

	EARLY MORTALITY	SUBSEQUENT IMPROVEMENT Ⓖ	ULTIMATE FUNCTION Ⓗ

Cervical
- Complete Ⓕ → TRACTION AND REDUCTION ± FUSION → ± 90% — 0 — Quadriplegia, Paraplegia
- Incomplete → 10% Ⓘ — ± 90% — Wheelchair for Injuries to C-7 or Below
- Open-Compound Ⓙ → DÉBRIDEMENT LAMINECTOMY → ± 50–75% Ⓚ

Thoracic
- Complete → ± 5% Ⓛ — ± 0 — Wheelchair
- Incomplete → LAMINECTOMY Ⓜ → ± 5% — ± 90% — Up to Normal
- Open → DÉBRIDEMENT LAMINECTOMY Ⓝ → ±100% Ⓞ — — — —

Thoracic-Lumbar
- Complete → ± 5% — ± 0 — Crutches
- Incomplete → LAMINECTOMY → ± 5% — ± 90% — Bladder and Bowel Function—90% Ⓟ

Cauda Equina
- Complete → LAMINECTOMY AND FUSION → ± 5% — 0
- Open → LAMINECTOMY → ± 5% — ± 10%
} Flaccid Paraplegia Ⓠ

Uncommon Injuries Ⓡ

SPINAL CORD INJURY II

SPINA BIFIDA CYSTICA BY RALPH A. W. LEHMAN, M.D.

Comments

Inconsistencies in the data presented are due to their derivation from unrelated series of patients undergoing differing treatment policies and having incompletely documented periods of followup.

A. Most spina bifida patients (73 to 95 per cent) have myelomeningoceles.[4, 12, 15, 19, 20] These have neural elements incorporated in the sac. Virtually all of these have neurologic deficits and the majority are incontinent. Twenty-five per cent are stillborn.[14] There are no clear data on the incidence of accompanying non-neural congenital anomalies. The incidence of associated hydromyelia and syringomyelia is 43 to 82 per cent at autopsy.[2, 6] Diastematomyelia is found in 4 to 5 per cent of operated cases[4, 19] and 50 per cent of autopsy cases.[2] Patients without neurologic elements incorporated into the sac have meningoceles and rarely have any deficits.

B. The decision for early repair of the back (before 48 hours) is both a medical and philosophical one, because these children can become enormous personal, social, and economic burdens. Early repair minimizes the occurrence of meningitis[4, 7, 20, 24] and preserves existing motor function.[4, 7, 24] It is associated with an early postoperative mortality of 2.3 to 4.5 per cent[7, 24] and with postoperative meningitis in 7 to 8 per cent of cases.[7, 24]

C. Hydrocephalus of some degree develops in a large majority of patients with spina bifida cystica.[5, 16] This may be progressive (PH) or arrested (AH). Patients with meningoceles develop PH in only 0 to 25 per cent of cases.[4, 19] Myelomeningocele patients develop PH in 71 to 77 per cent of cases.[1, 5, 18, 19, 23-25]

D. Without hydrocephalus, the average IQ of these patients is normal.[3] Shunting procedures protect against progressive brain damage in the PH patient.[17] The average IQ of survivors is normal in shunted PH patients with meningocele[19] but is diminished in those with myelomeningocele.[1, 17-19]

E. Shunting procedures correct hydrocephalus by diverting cerebrospinal fluid from the cerebral ventricles to the right atrium or peritoneum.
   1. By six years of age only 67 per cent of shunted myelomeningocele patients survive.[17]
   2. Late complications of shunt therapy lead to death in 20 per cent of those shunted.[19]
   3. The incidence of late or early infection of the shunt is 13 per cent.[5, 18]
   4. Shunt revisions are necessary in many patients and average one every two years during the early years of life.[17]

F. Long-term complications in operatively treated patients with myelomeningocele include:
   1. Seizure disorders (13 per cent)[19]
   2. Trophic ulcers (3 per cent)[19]
   3. Incontinence (63 per cent)[11]
   4. Advanced renal failure (7 to 16 per cent)[19, 24, 26]

G. In part, prognosis depends upon the level of the spina bifida. The incidences of progressive hydrocephalus, mental retardation, and paraparesis (as well as early mortality) all increase with higher location of the back lesion up to the mid-thoracic level.[1, 5, 7, 8, 11, 12, 16, 18, 19] Sacral lesions are the most likely to produce incontinence[12, 15] and the most apt to develop meningitis after repair of the back.[18] Patients with paralysis above the L2 level seldom lead an independent existence.[10, 11, 19, 21]

H. Adverse prognostic factors include meningitis and/or ventriculitis, marked kyphosis, severe neonatal hydrocephalus, other gross congenital malformations, and major birth trauma. If one of these factors is present, survival of operated patients may be as low as 39 per cent by age 2 to 4 years[18] and 21 per cent at 7 to 9 years.[19] Late survivors have severe physical disability and half are mentally retarded.[19]

References

1. Ames, M. D., and Schut, L.: Results of treatment of 171 consecutive myelomeningoceles — 1963 to 1968. Pediatrics, 50:466–470, 1972.
2. Cameron, A. H.: The Arnold-Chiari and other neuroanatomical malformations associated with spina bifida. J. Pathol. Bacteriol., 73:195–211, 1957.
3. Diller, L., Swinyard, C. A., and Epstein, F. J.: Cognitive function in children with spina bifida. In Swinyard, C. A. (ed.): Decision Making and the Defective Newborn. Springfield, Ill., Charles C Thomas, 1978, pp. 34–48.
4. Doran, P. A., and Guthkelch, A. N.: Studies in spina bifida cystica. I. General survey and reassessment of the problem. J. Neurol. Neurosurg. Psychiatry, 24:331–345, 1961.
5. Eckstein, H. B., and Macnab, G. H.: Myelomeningocele and hydrocephalus. The impact of modern treatment. Lancet, 1:842–845, 1966.
6. Emery, J. L., and Lendon, R. G.: Clinical implications of cord lesions in neurospinal dysraphism. Dev. Med. Child Neurol., 27:45–51, 1972.
7. Fernandez-Serrats, A. A., Guthkelch, A. N., and Parker, S. A.: The prognosis of open myelocele with a note on a trial of Laurence's operation. Dev. Med. Child Neurol., 13:65–74, 1967.
8. Foltz, E. L., Kronmal, R., and Shurtleff, D. B. To treat or not to treat: A neurosurgeon's perspective of myelomeningocele. Clin. Neurosurg., 20:147–160, 1973.
9. Hide, D. W.: The outlook for the child with a myelomeningocele for whom early surgery was considered inadvisable. Dev. Med. Child Neurol., 14:304–307, 1972.
10. Hunt, G. M.: Implications of the treatment of myelomeningocele for the child and his family. Lancet, 2:1308–1310, 1973.
11. Hunt, G. M., et al.: Predictive factors in open myelo-

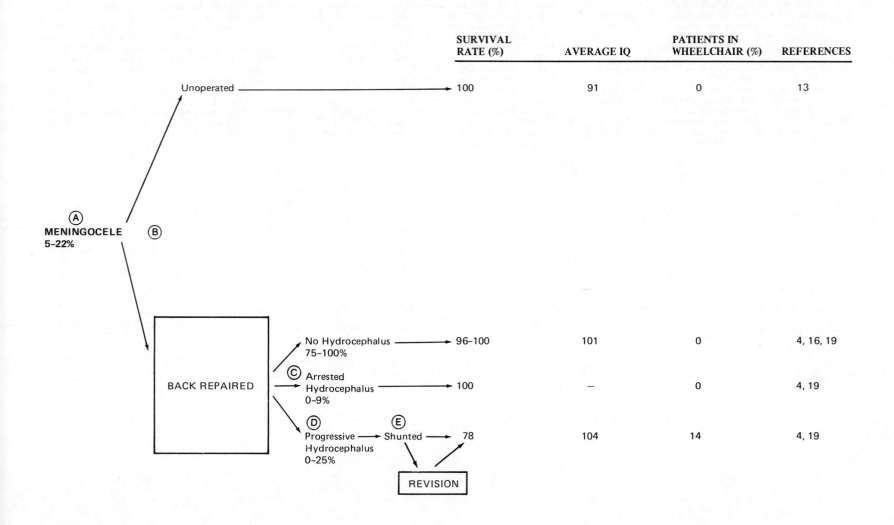

	SURVIVAL RATE (%)	AVERAGE IQ	PATIENTS IN WHEELCHAIR (%)	REFERENCES
Unoperated	100	91	0	13
No Hydrocephalus 75–100%	96–100	101	0	4, 16, 19
Arrested Hydrocephalus 0–9%	100	—	0	4, 19
Progressive Hydrocephalus 0–25% → Shunted	78	104	14	4, 19

Ⓐ
**MENINGOCELE
5–22%**   Ⓑ

BACK REPAIRED

Ⓒ
Ⓓ Ⓔ

REVISION

13

meningocele with special reference to sensory level. Br. Med. J., *4*:197–201, 1973.

12. Laurence, K. M.: The natural history of spina bifida cystica. Proc. R. Soc. Med., *53*:1055–1056, 1960.

13. Laurence, K. M.: Effect of early surgery for spina bifida cystica on survival and quality of life. Lancet, *1*:301–304, 1974.

14. Laurence, K. M., and Tew, B. J.: Follow-up of 65 survivors from the 425 cases of spina bifida born in South Wales between 1956 and 1962. Dev. Med. Child Neurol., *13*:1–3, 1967.

15. Laurence, K. M., and Tew, B. J.: Natural history of spina bifida cystica and cranium bifidum cysticum. Arch. Dis. Child., *46*:127–138, 1971.

16. Lorber, J.: Systematic ventriculographic studies in infants born with meningomyelocele and encephalocele. Arch. Dis. Child., *36*:381–389, 1961.

17. Lorber, J.: Medical and surgical aspects in the treatment of congenital hydrocephalus. Neuropaediatrie, *2*:239–246, 1971.

18. Lorber, J.: Results of treatment of myelomeningocele. An analysis of 524 unselected cases, with special reference to possible selection for treatment. Dev. Med. Child Neurol., *13*:279–303, 1971.

19. Lorber, J.: Spina bifida cystica. Results of treatment of 270 consecutive cases with criteria for selection for the future. Arch. Dis. Child., *47*:854–873, 1972.

20. Sharrard, W. J. W., Zachary, R. B., and Lorber, J.: Survival and paralysis in open myelomeningocele with special reference to the time of repairs of the spinal lesion. Dev. Med. Child Neurol., *13*:35–50, 1967.

21. Shurtleff, D. B., et al.: Myelodysplasia. Problems of long-term survival and social function. West. J. Med., *122*:199–205, 1975.

22. Shurtleff, D. B., et al.: Myelodysplasia: Decision for death or disability. N. Engl. J. Med., *291*:1005–1011, 1974.

23. Shurtleff, D. B., Kronmal, R., and Foltz, E. L. Follow-up comparison of hydrocephalus with and without myelomeningocele. J. Neurosurg., *42*:61–68, 1975.

24. Smith, G. K., and Smith, E. D.: Selection for treatment in spina bifida cystica. Br. Med. J., *4*:189–197, 1973.

25. Soare, P. L., and Raimondi, A. J.: Quality of survival in treated myelomeningocele children. A prospective study. *In* Swinyard, C. A. (ed.): Decision Making and the Defective Newborn. Springfield, Ill., Charles C Thomas, 1978, pp. 68–94.

26. Stark, G. D., and Drummond, M.: Results of selective early operation in myelomeningocele. Arch. Dis. Child., *48*:676–683, 1973.

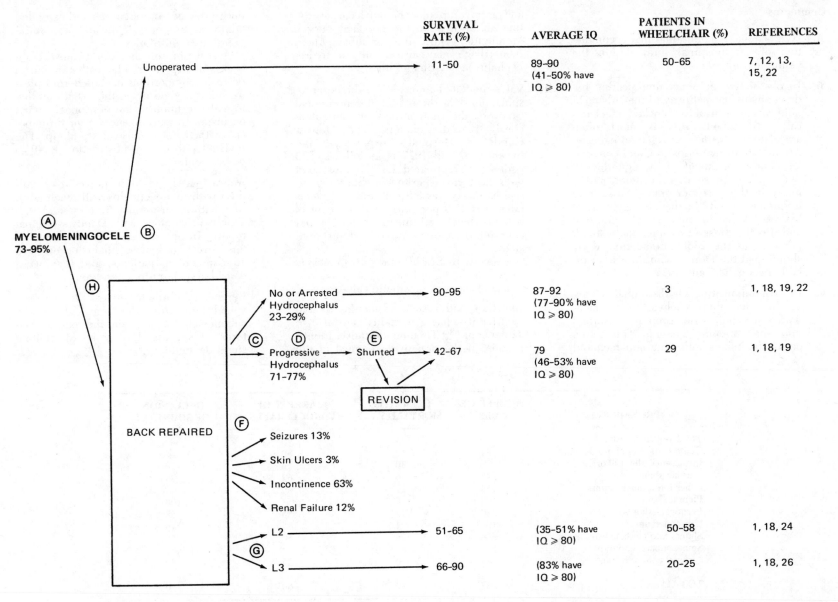

	SURVIVAL RATE (%)	AVERAGE IQ	PATIENTS IN WHEELCHAIR (%)	REFERENCES
Unoperated	11–50	89–90 (41–50% have IQ ⩾ 80)	50–65	7, 12, 13, 15, 22
No or Arrested Hydrocephalus 23–29%	90–95	87–92 (77–90% have IQ ⩾ 80)	3	1, 18, 19, 22
Progressive Hydrocephalus 71–77% → Shunted	42–67	79 (46–53% have IQ ⩾ 80)	29	1, 18, 19
L2	51–65	(35–51% have IQ ⩾ 80)	50–58	1, 18, 24
L3	66–90	(83% have IQ ⩾ 80)	20–25	1, 18, 26

Ⓐ Ⓑ MYELOMENINGOCELE 73–95%

Ⓗ

BACK REPAIRED

Ⓒ Ⓓ Ⓔ

REVISION

Ⓕ Seizures 13%

Skin Ulcers 3%

Incontinence 63%

Renal Failure 12%

Ⓖ

15

HYDROCEPHALUS BY WILLIAM A. BRYANS, M.D.

Comments

A. Hydrocephalus is an abnormal accumulation of cerebrospinal fluid within the ventricular system.

B. In obstructive or noncommunicating hydrocephalus the pathway to the subarachnoid space is usually blocked mechanically. In infants this is most often associated with myelomeningocele, Arnold-Chiari malformation, and congenital stenosis or atresia of the aqueduct of Sylvius. The presence of a tumor, particularly in the posterior cranial fossa, also frequently results in the development of hydrocephalus in infants and children and was the cause of hydrocephalus in 10 per cent of the 235 patients treated by shunting at the Denver Children's Hospital between 1967 and 1977.[4]

C. In communicating hydrocephalus the cerebrospinal fluid reaches the subarachnoid space but is not properly absorbed into the vascular system. This often occurs in infants following subarachnoid and intraventricular hemorrhage at the time of birth or in the neonatal period. Meningitis, ventriculitis, or subarachnoid hemorrhage may also result in hydrocephalus at any time of life.

D. Valve-regulated shunts allow the cerebrospinal fluid to drain into the peritoneal cavity or the right atrium via subcutaneously placed catheters. The Denver Children's Hospital's experience between 1967 and 1977 is as follows: 235 patients were treated for the most part with the Denver peritoneal shunt. Operative mortality was 3.8 per cent; case mortality was 11.9 per cent; 10.6 per cent of patients developed infections; and 50 per cent required one or more shunt revisions.[4]

A review by Scarff[19] of results to 1963 is shown in the table below. This was prior to use of modern prosthetic valves.

E. Infection, with associated meningitis and ventriculitis, has a mortality rate of 3 to 42 per cent.[2,4,5] Treatment requires identification of the organism, removal of the entire device, and vigorous and extended administration of systemic and often intraventricular antibiotics.

Obstruction of the shunt most often occurs at the ventricular catheter due to occlusion by portions of the choroid plexus, but it also occurs at the distal end due to malabsorption in the peritoneal cavity, occlusion by peritoneal cyst, or thrombosis in the ventriculocaval shunt tip. The revision rate due to obstruction is 40 to 50 per cent.[2,4,7]

F. Approximately 14 to 36 per cent of children with hydrocephalus will reach adult life with near-normal intelligence.[2,6,18] This is at variance with Dandy's original report.[1] In one reported series, spontaneous "arrest" of hydrocephalus occurred in 15 per cent of patients, and they were considered shunt-independent.[17]

G. Renewed efforts to divert the cerebrospinal fluid from the ventricles to the subarachnoid space via the basilar cisterns, if successful, may avoid lifelong shunt dependency.[9-12]

PROCEDURE	NUMBER OF CASES	OPERATIVE MORTALITY (%)	ARREST OF HYDROCEPHALUS (%)	OCCLUSION OF SHUNT (%)
Third ventriculostomy	529	15	70	—
Cauterization of choroid plexus	91	15	60	—
Intracranial shunt (TorKildson)	36	30	58	50
Cardiac shunts	345	6	62	28
Other intracranial shunts	118	21	60	—
Pleural shunts	108	8	53	100
Peritoneal shunts	230	13	55	58
Ureteral shunts	108	1	65	16
Shunts into epithelialized ducts	29	6	50	50
Spinal subarachnoid to spinal epidural shunts	13	0	75	50
TOTAL	1607	10	60	50

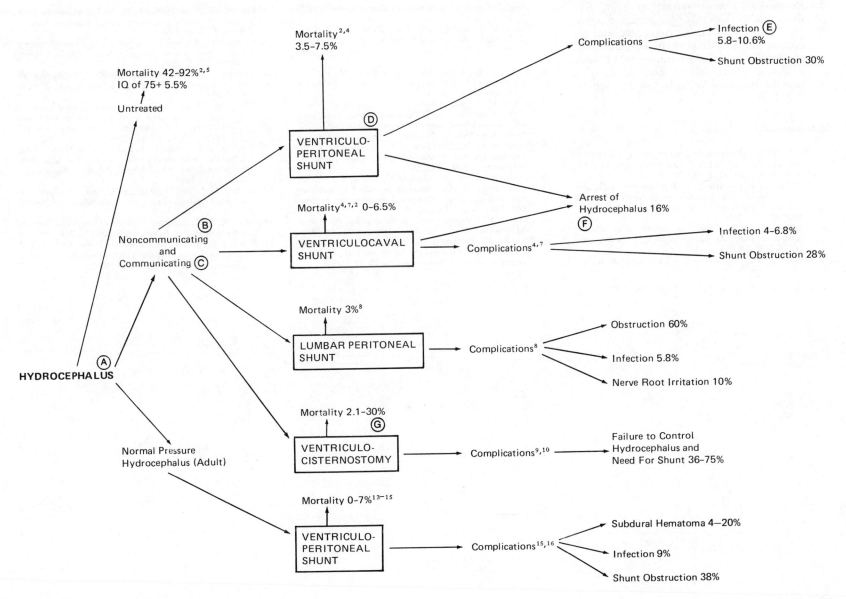

HYDROCEPHALUS (A)

Mortality 42-92%[2,5]
IQ of 75+ 5.5%

Untreated

Noncommunicating and Communicating (B) (C)

Normal Pressure Hydrocephalus (Adult)

Mortality[2,4] 3.5-7.5%

VENTRICULO-PERITONEAL SHUNT (D)

Complications → Infection (E) 5.8-10.6%
→ Shunt Obstruction 30%

Arrest of Hydrocephalus 16%

Mortality[4,7,2] 0-6.5%

VENTRICULOCAVAL SHUNT (B)

Complications[4,7] (F) → Infection 4-6.8%
→ Shunt Obstruction 28%

Mortality 3%[8]

LUMBAR PERITONEAL SHUNT

Complications[8] → Obstruction 60%
→ Infection 5.8%
→ Nerve Root Irritation 10%

Mortality 2.1-30%

VENTRICULO-CISTERNOSTOMY (G)

Complications[9,10] → Failure to Control Hydrocephalus and Need For Shunt 36-75%

Mortality 0-7%[13-15]

VENTRICULO-PERITONEAL SHUNT

Complications[15,16] → Subdural Hematoma 4-20%
→ Infection 9%
→ Shunt Obstruction 38%

17

HYDROCEPHALUS *Continued*

H. Prognosis in adult normal pressure hydrocephalus depends on accurate diagnosis. The triad of ataxia, dementia, and incontinence also is seen in organic brain syndromes with other causes. CAT scan evidence of significant cortical atrophy may be the most reliable test in predicting shunt success.[13]

References

1. Dandy, W. E.: Diagnosis and treatment of strictures of the aqueduct of Sylvius (causing hydrocephalus). Arch. Surg., 51:1–14, 1945.
2. Foltz, E. L., and Shurtleff, D. B.: Five year comparative study of hydrocephalus in children with and without operation (113 cases). J. Neurosurg., 20:1064–1079, 1963.
3. Hammon, W. M.: Evaluation and use of the ventriculoperitoneal shunt in hydrocephalus. J. Neurosurg., 34:792–795, 1971.
4. Bryans, W. A., et al.: Results of treatment of hydrocephalus at Denver Children's Hospital, 1967–1977. In preparation.
5. Nulsen, F. E., and Becker, D. P.: Shunt control of hydrocephalus. *In* Clinical Neurosurgery, vol. 14. Baltimore, The Williams & Wilkins Co., 1967, pp. 256–273.
6. Mealey, J., Jr., Gilmor, R. L., and Bubb, M. P.: The prognosis of hydrocephalus overt at birth. J. Neurosurg., 39:348–355, 1973.
7. Becker, D. P., and Nulsen, F. E.· Control of hydrocephalus by valve regulated venous shunt: Avoidance of complications in prolonged maintenance. J. Neurosurg., 28:215–226, 1968.
8. Eisenberg, H. M., Davidson, R. I., and Shillito, J., Jr.: Lumboperitoneal shunts, review of 34 cases. J. Neurosurg., 35:427–431, 1971.
9. Crosby, R. M. N., Henderson, C. M., and Parl, R.: Catheterization of the cerebral aqueduct for obstructive hydrocephalus in infants. J. Neurosurg., 38:596–601, 1973.
10. Vries, J. K.: An endoscopic technique for third ventriculostomy. Surg. Neurol. 9(3):165–168, March 1978.
11. Elvidge, A.: Treatment of obstructive lesions of the aqueduct of Sylvius and the fourth ventricle by interventriculostomy. J. Neurosurg., 24:11–23, 1966.
12. Sayers, M. P., and Kosnik, E. J.: Percutaneous third ventriculostomy: experience and technique. Child's Brain, 2:24–30, 1976.
13. Gunasekera, L., and Richardson, A. E.: Computerized axial tomography in idiopathic hydrocephalus. Brain, 100(IV):749, Dec. 1977.
14. Salmon, J. H.: Adult hydrocephalus: Evaluation of shunt therapy in 80 patients. J. Neurosurg., 37:423–428, 1978.
15. Illingworth, R. D., et al.: The ventriculocaval shunt in the treatment of adult hydrocephalus. Results and complications in 101 patients. J. Neurosurg., 35:681–685, 1971.
16. Samuelson, S., Long, D. M., and Chou, S. N.: Subdural hematoma as a complication of shunting procedure for normal pressure hydrocephalus. J. Neurosurg., 37:548–551, 1972.
17. Holtzer, G. J., and DeLange, S. A.: Shunt independent arrest of hydrocephalus. J. Neurosurg., 39:698–701, 1973.
18. Jones, K. F. C.: Long term results in various treatments of hydrocephalus. J. Neurosurg., 26:313–315, 1967.
19. Scarff, J. E.: Treatment of hydrocephalus: An historical and critical review of methods and results. J. Neurol. Neurosurg. Psychiatry, 26:1–26, 1963.

RUPTURED INTERVERTEBRAL DISC

RUPTURED INTERVERTEBRAL DISC BY HARRY R. BOYD, M.D.

Comments

A. Location:[1,2]

L4–5	47%
L5–S1	48%
Other	5%

B. The key to nonoperative care is bed rest. Exercise and back support may be helpful, but traction is of no advantage.[3]

C. The decision about discectomy depends upon the severity of disease. When neurologic deficit is present, 20 per cent of cases will clear with nonoperative therapy[4,5] and 20 per cent will ultimately require surgery.

D. Myelography is indicated in essentially all cases that will require operation.[1-6] The incidence of complication depends on the contrast medium. Pantopaque is prone to produce long-term complications, including arachnoiditis. Water-soluble compounds are more likely to produce acute symptoms, such as seizures, meningeal irritation, and radicular reactions (hyperalgesia, abdominal pain, urinary retention).[7,8]

E. Indications for performing spinal fusion in addition to discectomy are debatable.[10]

	FUSION	NO FUSION
Bed rest	7–10 days	2–3 days
Hospitalization	14 days	7 days
Limited activity	28 weeks	10 weeks
Fusion failure	10–15%	
Recurrence of symptoms	38%	38%

F. Morbidity of discectomy[1,2] includes increased neurologic deficit (less than .01 per cent) and vascular injury (also less than .01 per cent).

G. Recurrent pain (recurrence) may be caused by new disc herniation (22 per cent of cases), recurrent disc herniation (31 per cent), adhesions (12 per cent), bony compression (5 per cent), or spinal instability (30 per cent).[12,13] Lumbar adhesive arachnoiditis related to previous myelography using Pantopaque is increasingly recognized as a cause of recurrent pain.[13]

H. Prognosis is related to pending litigation and the contemplated size of settlement.[1,2]

I. Costs:[9]

	TOTAL AVERAGE COST
First operation	$12,061
Second operation	26,298
Third operation	51,652

These costs include compensation benefits.

J. Prognosis for a second disc operation is comparable to that of the first operation but is worse if fusion has been done previously.[10] For a third and subsequent discectomies, the prognosis for cure rapidly diminishes:
Third operation — 37 per cent of cases have good to excellent results.[11]
More than three operations — less than 10 per cent have good to excellent results.[9]

References

1. Mixter, W. J., and Barr, J. S.: Rupture of the intervertebral disc with involvement of the spinal canal. N. Engl. J. Med., 211:210–15, 1934.
2. Burton, C. V.: Lumbosacral arachnoiditis. Spine, 3:24–30, 1978.
3. Finneson, B. E.: Low Back Pain. Philadelphia, J. B. Lippincott Co., 1973.
4. Davis, C. H., Jr.: Extradural spinal cord and nerve root compression from benign lesions of the lumbar area. In Youmans, J. (ed.): Neurological Surgery, vol. II. Philadelphia. W. B. Saunders Co., 1973, pp. 1165–1183.
5. Semmes, R. E.: Ruptures of the Lumbar Intervertebral Disc. Springfield, Ill., Charles C Thomas, 1964.
6. Shapiro, R.: Myelography, 3rd ed. Chicago, Year Book Medical Publishers, 1975.
7. Burton, C., and Wiltsee, L.: Guest editor comment. Spine, 3:23, 1978.
8. Irstam, L.: Lumbar myelography with amipaque. Spine, 3:70–81, 1978.
9. McGrath, C., Asst. Manager, Colorado State Compensation Insurance Fund: Personal communication.
10. Frymoyer, J. W., et al.: Failed lumbar disc surgery requiring second operation. Spine, 3:7–11, 1978.
11. Kelley, J. H., et al.: Multiple operations for protruded lumbar intervertebral disc. Mayo Clin. Proc., 29:546–50, 1954.
12. Epstein, J. A., Lanine, L. S., and Epstein, B. S.: Recurrent herniation of the lumbar intervertebral disc. Clin. Orthop., 52:169–78, 1967.
13. Johnston, J. D. H., and Matheny, J. B.: Microscopic lysis of lumbar adhesive arachnoiditis. Spine, 3:36–40, 1978.
14. Barr, J. S., et al.: Evaluation of end results in treatment of ruptured lumbar intervertebral disc with protrusion of nucleus pulposus. Surg. Gynecol. Obstet., 125:250–56, 1967.
15. White, J. C.: Results of surgical treatment of herniated lumbar intervertebral discs. Clin. Neurosurg., 13:42–54, 1968.
16. Greenwood, J., Jr., McGuire, T. H., and Fariss, K.: A study of causes of failure in the herniated intervertebral disc operation. J. Neurosurg., 9:15–20, 1952.

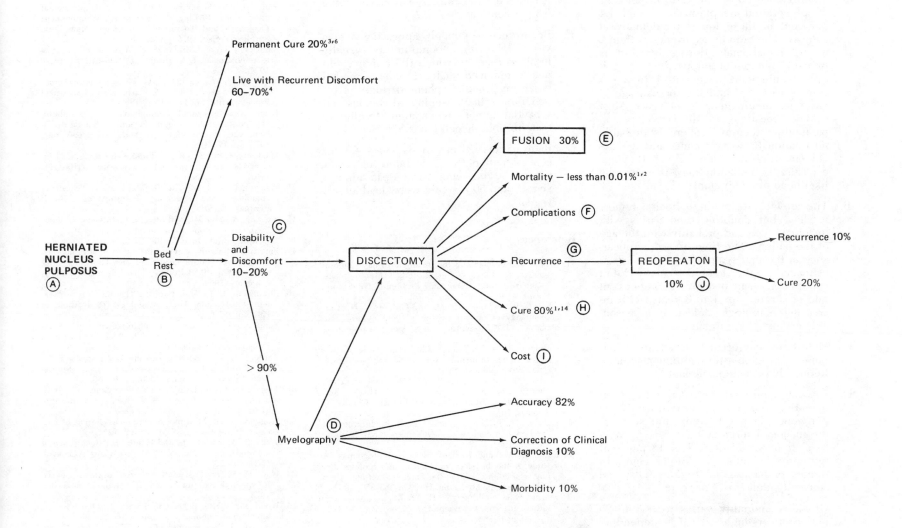

Permanent Cure 20%[3,6]

Live with Recurrent Discomfort
60–70%[4]

FUSION 30% Ⓔ

Mortality — less than 0.01%[1,2]

Complications Ⓕ

Recurrence Ⓖ

Cure 80%[1,14] Ⓗ

Cost Ⓘ

HERNIATED
NUCLEUS
PULPOSUS
Ⓐ

Bed
Rest
Ⓑ

Disability
and
Discomfort
10–20%
Ⓒ

DISCECTOMY

REOPERATON

Recurrence 10%

Cure 20%

10% Ⓙ

> 90%

Myelography
Ⓓ

Accuracy 82%

Correction of Clinical
Diagnosis 10%

Morbidity 10%

MENINGIOMA BY KARL STECHER, JR., M.D.

Comments

A. Meningiomas constitute 12 to 18 per cent of all cerebral neoplasms[4, 12, 26] and 1.4 per cent of those found incidentally at autopsy. The ratio of occurrence is from 2 to 4:1 female:male during life but is probably random at autopsy.[4, 6, 19, 29] Multiple meningioma occurs in 1 to 2 per cent of cases,[4, 22] and the median age of onset for meningioma is 44 years. Most common locations are the convexity and parasagittal regions.[17] There is probably no relation between trauma and the development of meningioma.[4, 21, 26] Previous exposure to radiation may increase the likelihood of meningioma.[2, 7]

B. The growth rate of these benign tumors is slow, but doubling time varies with histologic type and probably with the age of the patient. The time from the appearance of the first symptoms to diagnosis is estimated to be 1 to 3 years[5, 6, 10] but could be 40 years or more.[8] A 50 per cent rate of survival for 1 to 3 years, with increasing neurologic deficit, is a reasonable estimate for untreated cases.

C. Metastases may occur to lungs, liver, and bone.[4, 11] Angioblastic meningiomas more frequently become malignant.[15]

D. Ultimate neurologic deficit resulting from operative removal is approximately 22 per cent.[9] Tumor location and size are the major determinants.[1, 13, 14, 17, 20] With basal tumors, deficit is 7 to 18 per cent (formerly, as much as 53 per cent). In tumors of parasagittal regions, falx, and convexity, deficit is 3 per cent.

E. Operative mortality varies from 3 to 25 per cent or higher,[1, 13, 14, 20] depending primarily on the site and size of the tumor. Medial basal tumors involving the arteries of the circle of Willis have the highest mortality (as high as 53 per cent), yet lateral basal tumors may have only a 6.3 per cent rate.[1]

F. Recurrence, commonly appearing 5 to 6 years following operation, is usually local, in cases in which the tumor could not be removed totally (tumors of medial basal area, medial sphenoid ridge, or tuberculum sellae). Meningiotheliomas and syncytial tumors recur more frequently than fibroblastic cell types.[3, 23]

G. Rates of survival in various series: 26 per cent of patients died at home of recurrence,[4] 30 per cent were dead after 4 years,[17] and 50 per cent were dead after 5 years.[19]

References

1. Arnold, H.: Problems in the treatment of basal meningiomas. *In* Klug, W., et al. (eds.): Meningiomas: Diagnostic and Therapeutic Problems. New York, Springer-Verlag, 1975, pp. 75–78.
2. Choi, N. W., Schuman, L. M., and Gullen, W. H.: Epidemiology of primary central nervous system neoplasms. II. Case-control study. Am. J. Epidemiol., 91:467–485, 1970.
3. Crompton, R., and Gautier-Smith, P. C.: The prediction of recurrence in meningiomas. J. Neurol. Neurosurg. Psychiatry, 33:80–87, 1970.
4. Cushing, H., and Eisenhardt, L.: Meningiomas: Their Classification, Regional Behavior, Life History, and Surgical End Results. Springfield, Ill., Charles C Thomas, 1938.
5. Daly, D. D., Svien, H. J., and Yoss, R. E.: Intermittent cerebral symptoms with meningioma. Arch. Neurol., 5:69–75, 1961.
6. Earle, K. M., and Richany, S. F.: Meningiomas: A study of the histology, incidence, and biologic behavior of 243 cases from the Frazier-Grant collection of brain tumors. Med. Ann. D.C., 38:353–356, 1969.
7. Feiring, E. H., and Foer, W. H.: Meningioma following radium therapy. Case report. J. Neurosurg., 29:192–194, August 1968.
8. Fowler, G. W.: Meningioma and intermittent aphasia of 44 years' duration. Case report. J. Neurosurg., 33:100–102, July 1970.
9. Gregorius, F. K., Hepler, R. S., and Stern, W. E.: Loss and recovery of vision with suprasellar meningiomas. J. Neurosurg., 42:69–75, January 1975.
10. Kalm, H.: On the course of the disease of intracranial meningioma. *In* Klug, W., et al. (eds.): Meningiomas: Diagnostic and Therapeutic Problems. New York, Springer-Verlag, 1975, pp. 31–36.
11. Karasick, J. L., and Mullan, S. F.: A survey of metastatic meningiomas. J. Neurosurg., 39:206–212, February 1974.
12. Kernohan, J. W., and Sayre, G. P.: *In* Atlas of Tumor Pathology, Sec. 10, fas. 35. Washington, U.S. Armed Forces Institute of Pathology, 1952.
13. Logue, V.: Parasagittal meningiomas. *In* Krayenbuhl, H. (ed.): Advances and Technical Standards in Neurosurgery, vol. 2. New York, Springer-Verlag, 1975, pp. 171–198.
14. MacCarty, C. S.: Surgical techniques for removal of intracranial meningiomas. Clin. Neurosurg., 7:100–111, 1961.
15. Palacios, E., and Azar-Kia, B.: Malignant metastasizing angioblastic meningiomas. J. Neurosurg., 42:185–187, February 1975.
16. Rausing, A., Ybo, W., and Stenflo, J.: Intracranial meningioma — a population study of ten years. Acta Neurol. Scand., 46:102–110, 1970.
17. Ray, B. S.: Surgery of recurrent intracranial tumors. *In* Congress of Neurological Surgeons: Clinical Neurosurgery, Vol. 10. Baltimore, The Williams & Wilkins Company, 1964.
18. Rubinstein, L. J.: Tumors of the Central Nervous System. Washington, D.C., Armed Forces Institute of Pathology, 1970.
19. Simpson, D.: The recurrence of intracranial meningiomas after surgical treatment. J. Neurol. Neurosurg. Psychiatry, 20:22–39, 1957.
20. Taren, J. A.: Meningiomas. *In* Kahn, E. A., Crosby, E. C., and Taren, J. A.: Correlative Neurosurgery. Springfield, Charles C Thomas, 1969, pp. 68–86.
21. Turner, O. A., and Laird, A. T.: Meningioma with traumatic etiology. Report of a case. J. Neurosurg., 24:96–98, 1966.
22. Waga, S., et al.: Multiple meningiomas. Report of four cases. J. Neurosurg., 37:348–351, 1972.
23. Waga, S., Yamashita, J., and Handa, H.: Recurrence of meningiomas. Neurol. Med. Chir. (Tokyo), 17(II):203–208, 1977.
24. Wara, W. M., et al.: Radiation therapy of meningiomas. Roentgenol. Radium Ther. Nucl. Med., 123:453–458, 1975.
25. Wood, M., White, R., and Kernohan, J.: One hundred intracranial meningiomas found incidentally at necropsy. J. Neuropathol. Exp. Neurol., 16:337–340, 1957.
26. Zulch, K. J.: Brain Tumors. New York, Springer, 1957.

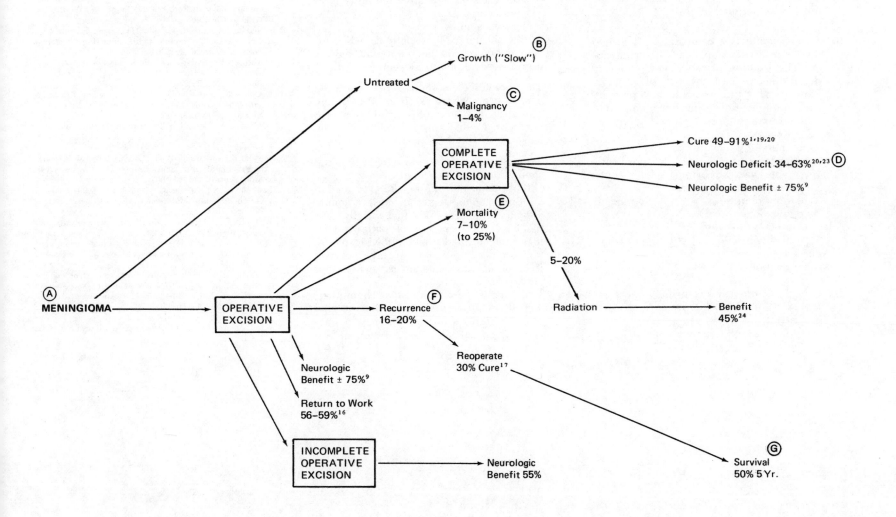

GLIOMAS BY WOLFF M. KIRSCH, M.D., AND HAROLD VOGEL, M.D.

Comments

A. This term refers to primary brain tumors of neuroectodermal origin.

B. *Slow-growing* is a comparative term and does not always imply lack of malignancy. The location of the tumor obviously determines in part the risk of excision. Slow-growing tumors, with their percentage frequency of occurrence compared with all brain tumors, include:[1-3, 8, 11]

Astrocytomas
Optic nerve glioma an-
terior to chiasm   <1 per cent
Subependymal astrocytoma <1 per cent
Cystic astrocytoma of cere-
bellum (children)   2 per cent
Ependymomas
Colloid cyst of anterior
third ventricle   <1 per cent
Neuronal tumors
Ganglioglioma   Rare

C. Other infrequently occurring tumors not included in the intermediate growth group are:[5, 9, 10]

Optic nerve glioma involving chiasm
Choroid plexus papilloma

Infratentorial ependymoma with a 45 per cent 5-year survival rate following excision (operative mortality is 14 per cent).
Neuroblastoma

D. Of the 90 per cent of patients who survive operation, 34 per cent will have a useful survival of 5 to 31 years.[5]

E. The operative mortality for attempted cure of a pinealoma is 35 to 50 per cent. Mortality for shunt plus irradiation is 8 per cent. Median survival of those who leave the hospital is 4 years.[12]

F. Average survival for a high-grade brain stem glioma is 3 to 4 months.[7]

G. Glioblastoma multiforme (23 per cent of all brain tumors) is the most common glioma of neuroectodermal origin. For the 85 to 90 per cent of patients who leave the hospital alive following operation for decompression, average survival is 8 months after diagnosis, and 10 per cent of patients live 2 years.[6, 7]

H. Evidence is inconclusive that chemotherapy alters the course of malignant glial tumors. Steroids are temporarily beneficial but do not alter the duration of survival.

References

1. Walsh, F. B., and Hoyt, W. F.: Clinical Neuro-opthalmology, 3rd ed. Vol. III Baltimore, Williams & Wilkens Co., 1969.
2. Hehman, K., Norrell, H., and Howieson, J.: Subependymomas of the septum pellucidum. Report of two cases. J. Neurosurg., 29:640, 1968.
3. Cushing, H.: Experiences with cerebellar astrocytomas; critical review of 76 cases. Surg. Gynecol. Obstet., 51:129, 1931.
4. Levy, L. F., and Elvidge, A. R.: Astrocytoma of brain and spinal cord; review of 176 cases, 1940–1949. J. Neurosurg., 13:413, 1956.
5. Bouchard, J.: Radiation Therapy of Tumors and Diseases of the Nervous System. Philadelphia, Lea & Febiger, 1966.
6. Jelsma, R., and Bucy, P. C.: Glioblastoma multiforme: its treatment and some factors effecting survival. Arch. Neurol., 26:161, 1969.
7. Panitch, H. S., and Berg, B. O.: Brain stem tumors of childhood and adolescence. Am. J. Dis. Child., 119:465, 1970.
8. Kelly, R.: Colloid cysts of third ventricle: analysis of 29 cases. Brain, 74:23, 1951.
9. Walker, J. C., and Horrax, G.: Papilloma of choroid plexus with report of unusual case. J. Neurosurg., 4:387, 1947.
10. Kricheff, I. I., et al.: Intracranial ependymomas: a study of survival in 65 cases treated by surgery and irradiation. Am. J. Roentgenol., 91:167, 1964.
11. Robertson, D. M., Hendry, W. S., and Vogel, F. S.: Central ganglioneuroma: a case study using electron microscopy. J. Neuropathol. Exp. Neurol., 23:692, 1964.

GLIOMAS

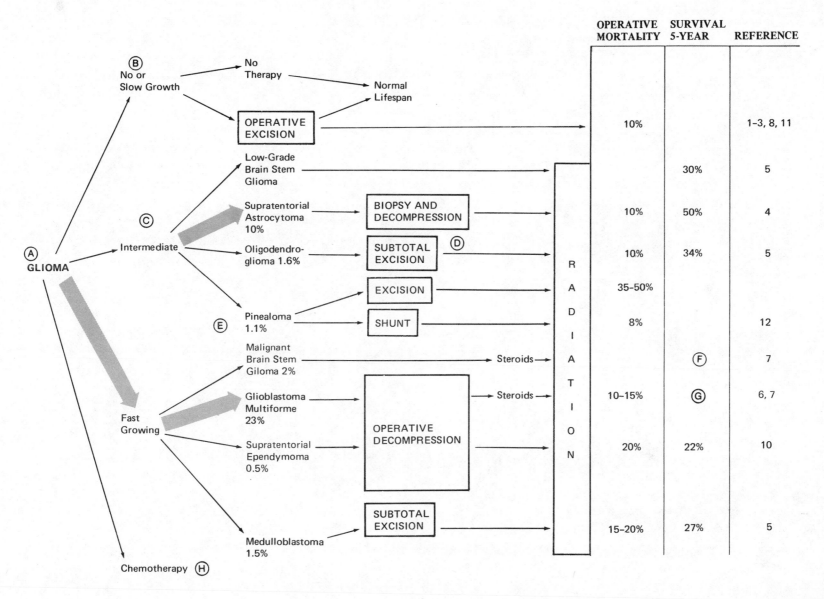

	OPERATIVE MORTALITY	SURVIVAL 5-YEAR	REFERENCE
OPERATIVE EXCISION	10%		1–3, 8, 11
Low-Grade Brain Stem Glioma		30%	5
BIOPSY AND DECOMPRESSION	10%	50%	4
SUBTOTAL EXCISION	10%	34%	5
EXCISION	35–50%		
SHUNT	8%		12
Malignant Brain Stem Glioma — Steroids		Ⓕ	7
Glioblastoma Multiforme — Steroids	10–15%	Ⓖ	6, 7
OPERATIVE DECOMPRESSION	20%	22%	10
SUBTOTAL EXCISION	15–20%	27%	5

25

Section B

Head and Neck

HYPERTHYROIDISM BY R. D. LIECHTY, M.D.

Comments

A. Because the symptoms of thyrotoxicosis are so distressing, virtually all patients receive some treatment today. About 25 per cent of patients will have a spontaneous permanent remission within a year of onset.[1]

B. Thiocarbamides, the most frequently used antithyroid drugs, produce remissions in about 25 per cent of toxic patients. Complications (dose-related) include pruritus, granulocytopenia, urticaria, arthralgias, jaundice, lymphadenopathy, and polyserositis. Remissions produced by thiocarbamides occur less frequently in children than in adults.[2]

C. With thiocarbamide treatment, the rate of sustained remissions has dropped from 50 per cent to 25 per cent over the past 15 years, possibly because of increasing iodine content in the diet.[3]

D. Propranolol, a beta blocker, controls symptoms (cardiac overactivity, sweating, tremulousness, agitation) while serum levels of T_3 and T_4 (thyroid hormones) remain elevated. It is the most rapid method of preparing patients for operation and is especially useful during pregnancy or when intervening disease (such as acute cholecystitis) necessitates urgent operation. Propranolol is available for both oral and parenteral use and must be given before, during, and after operative procedures. Some patients require up to 720 mg. daily in divided doses. Contraindications include congestive heart failure and asthma. Atropine is the antidote for propranolol. Propranolol markedly decreases thyroid vascularity and thus reduces bleeding during thyroidectomy.[4, 5]

E. Most clinics have abandoned iodine as the sole treatment of thyrotoxicosis because compared with the carbamides it is less reliable for producing euthyroidism, especially in males, older patients, and patients with toxic nodules. In some patients, inorganic iodine may exacerbate symptoms (jodbasedow). As an adjunct to the carbamides, iodine given for 7 to 10 days immediately prior to operation reduces thyroid vascularity.[2]

F. Single doses of radioactive iodine have induced remissions in 86 per cent of thyrotoxic patients treated with [131]I. Myxedema occurs in 15 per cent of these patients within one year, with an annual increment of 2 to 3 per cent becoming myxedematous as long as records are kept. Myxedema occurs even more frequently in those patients treated with multiple doses of [131]I. Although the incidences of thyroid cancer and leukemia apparently have not increased following ^{131}I treatment, that of genetic damage may be slightly elevated, rising from a normal risk of 4.0 per cent to a calculated risk of 4.025 per cent.[2, 6, 7]

G. Myxedema rates after thyroidectomy vary from 6 to more than 40 per cent.[2] However, leaving 8 to 16 gm. of tissue resulted in a rate of only 9 per cent in studies averaging 5.1 years.[8] In children, the thyroid remnant should be small (about 2 to 4 gm.). Some physicians advise total thyroidectomy to avoid the hazards of reoperation (or of ^{131}I) should the disease recur.[9]

H. In a series of 261 patients with thyrotoxicosis, surgical complications were as follows:[10]

Recurrent nerve injury	
Transient bilateral	0.38%
Transient unilateral	0.38%
Permanent bilateral	0%
Permanent unilateral	0%
Tetany	
Transient	8.4 %
Permanent	0.0 %
Wound	
Disruption	0.38%
Infection	1.5 %
Bleeding	3.4 %
Laryngeal edema requiring tracheostomy	0.38%
Deaths in 1246 operations	0%

References

1. Sattler, H.: Basedow's Disease. New York, Grune and Stratton, 1952.
2. DeGroot, L. J., and Stanbury, J. B.: The Thyroid and Its Diseases. New York, John Wiley & Sons, 1975.
3. Wartofsky, L.: Low remission after therapy for Graves' disease. Possible relations of dietary iodine with antithyroid therapy results. JAMA, 226:1083, 1973.
4. Lee, T. C., et al.: The use of propranolol in the surgical treatment of thyrotoxic patients. Ann. Surg., 177:643, 1973.
5. Starling, J. R., and Thomas, C. G.: Experience with the use of propranolol in the surgical management of thyrotoxicosis. World J. Surg., 1:251, 1977.
6. Chapman, E. M., and Maloof, F.: The use of radioiodine in the diagnosis and treatment of hyperthyroidism: ten years' experience. Medicine, 34:261, 1955.
7. Goldsmith, R. E.: Radioisotope therapy for Graves' disease. Mayo Clin. Proc., 47:953, 1972.
8. Gough, A. L., and Neill, R. W.: Partial thyroidectomy for thyrotoxicosis. Br. J. Surg., 61:939, 1974.
9. Perzik, S. L.: Total thyroidectomy in Graves' disease in children. J. Pediatr. Surg., 11:191, 1976.
10. Colcock, B. P., and King, M. L.: The mortality and morbidity of thyroid surgery. Surg. Gynecol. Obstet., 114:131, 1962.

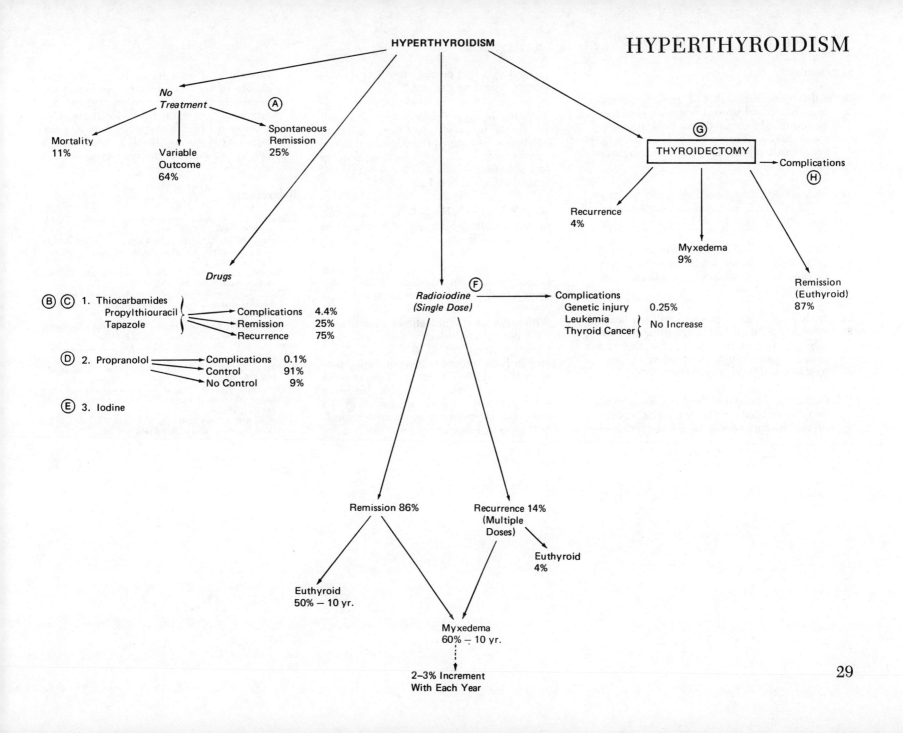

HYPERTHYROIDISM

No Treatment Ⓐ

Mortality 11%

Variable Outcome 64%

Spontaneous Remission 25%

Drugs

Ⓑ Ⓒ 1. Thiocarbamides
Propylthiouracil
Tapazole
→ Complications 4.4%
→ Remission 25%
→ Recurrence 75%

Ⓓ 2. Propranolol
→ Complications 0.1%
→ Control 91%
→ No Control 9%

Ⓔ 3. Iodine

Radioiodine (Single Dose) Ⓕ

→ Complications
Genetic injury 0.25%
Leukemia
Thyroid Cancer } No Increase

Remission 86%

Recurrence 14% (Multiple Doses)

Euthyroid 4%

Euthyroid 50% − 10 yr.

Myxedema 60% − 10 yr.

2−3% Increment With Each Year

Ⓖ THYROIDECTOMY

→ Complications Ⓗ

Recurrence 4%

Myxedema 9%

Remission (Euthyroid) 87%

29

THYROID NODULES BY R. D. LIECHTY, M.D.

Comments

A. Solitary nodules should be considered malignant until proved benign. Conversely, multinodular glands are benign unless some finding (firmness, sudden growth, vocal cord paralysis) suggests malignancy.[1]

B. At least 50 per cent of "clinically solitary nodules" are in fact one dominant nodule in a multinodular gland.[2, 6]

C. Soft nodules and those arising during pregnancy warrant a trial of suppression therapy for 3 to 6 months (Synthroid, 200 micrograms daily).[3-7]

D. Nodules that are cold on scintiscan, arise in males or in children, are firm, are rapidly growing, or are associated with voice change, local lymphadenopathy, or prior irradiation should arouse suspicion.

E. Palpation, ultrasound, and needle aspiration discriminate cysts. Aspiration results in the disappearance of 94 per cent of cysts.[4] Cysts that persist after 2 or 3 aspirations should be excised.

F. Mortality of thyroid lobectomy for a nodule should be only that of the anesthesia. Morbidity includes recurrent nerve injury (permanent) (<0.1 per cent), myxedema (<1 per cent), tetany (<0.1 per cent), and wound infection (<0.1 per cent).[8]

G. Incidence in females is 6 to 9 times that in men. Multinodular goiter increases in frequency with age.[2, 8]

H. Lacking suspicious characteristics (see Comment D), multinodular glands deserve a trial of suppression therapy.[1, 5, 7]

I. With subtotal thyroidectomy mortality is <0.1 per cent. Morbidity includes single recurrent nerve injury (0.4 per cent), injury to both nerves (<0.1 per cent), permanent tetany (<0.1 per cent), myxedema (5 per cent), reoperation for bleeding (<0.1 per cent), and wound infection (0.5 per cent). Hospitalization characteristically is for 3 to 4 days.[8]

J. Incidence of malignancy in multinodular glands varies from 4 to 17 per cent.[3] Patient selection for operation and the benign course of many thyroid malignancies account for the discrepancy between the high incidence and the low death rate (6 deaths per year per million persons).[9]

References

1. Welch, C.: Therapy for multinodular goiter. JAMA, 195:339, 1966.
2. Liechty, R. D., Graham, J., and Greemeyer, P.: Benign solitary thyroid nodules. Surg. Gynecol. Obstet., 121:511, 1965.
3. Thomas, C. G., et al.: Evaluation of dominant thyroid masses. Ann. Surg., 183:463, 1976.
4. Crile, G., Jr., and Hawks, W. A.: Aspiration biopsy of thyroid nodules. Surg. Gynecol. Obstet., 126:241, 1973.
5. Cole, W.: The treatment of non-toxic nodular goiter with desiccated thyroid. Surgery, 58:621, 1965.
6. Brooks, J. R.: The solitary nodule. Am. J. Surg., 125:477, 1973.
7. Hill, L. D., et al.: Thyroid suppression. Arch. Surg., 108:403, 1974.
8. Colcock, B. P., and King, M. L.: The mortality and morbidity of thyroid surgery. Surg. Gynecol. Obstet., 144:313, 1962.
9. DeGroot, L. J., and Stanbury, J. B.: The Thyroid and Its Diseases. New York, John Wiley & Sons, 1975.

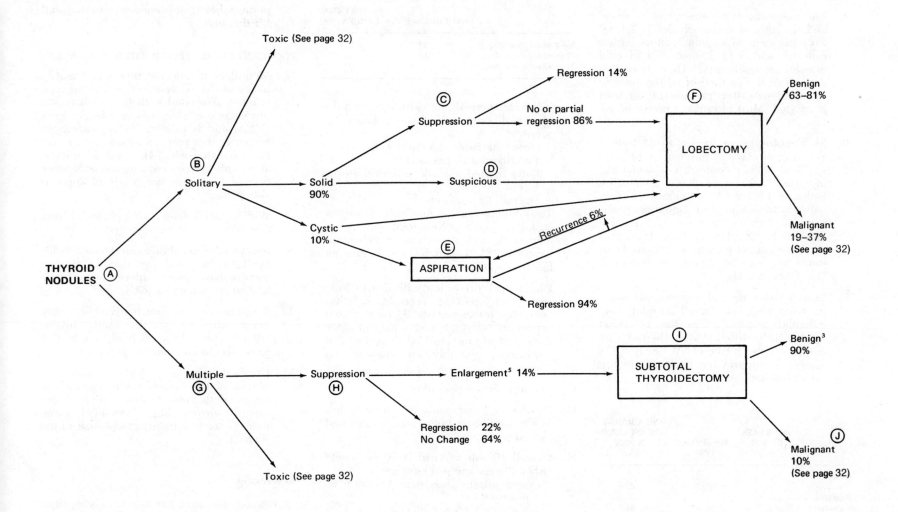

THYROID CANCER BY WILLIAM R. NELSON, M.D.

Comments

WELL DIFFERENTIATED THYROID CANCER

A. The mean age of occurrence is 43 years, and the ratio of females:males is 2:1.[14, 22] Five per cent of nodular goiters harbor cancer,[23] and 8 to 20 per cent of cold nodules are malignant.[24] There is no evidence that the method of biopsy (needle vs. excisional) alters prognosis if the tract is excised. Most physicians prefer lobectomy.[16, 17]

B. Multicentric cancer occurs in 38 to 87.5 per cent of cases.[8, 9] Survival at 10 years is 59 to 90 per cent.[5, 19] The mean age of onset is 32 years. Ratio of females: males is 1.6:1.[13] Chemotherapy is of no value in treatment. Radiation therapy has been used after surgery for extensive disease but is difficult to evaluate. It controls the bone pain of metastases. Thyroid hormone suppression therapy is important (see Comment H).

C. Postoperative thyroid suppression therapy must be given for all papillary and follicular tumors.[12] This has no effect upon poorly differentiated thyroid cancer. The same is true of ^{131}I therapy. The results of suppressive hormone therapy are as follows:[15, 21]

	DECREASE IN SIZE (%)	DISAPPEAR (%)	NO CHANGE OR INCREASE IN SIZE (%)
Benign nodule[15]	27	27	45
Papillary cancer[21]	12.5	0	86
Follicular cancer[21]	33	0	66

Results of postoperative medical therapy (thyroid hormone and/or ^{131}I therapy):[13]

	RECURRENCE (%)	DEATH FROM CANCER (%)
No medical treatment	37.4	12.5
Thyroid hormone alone	11	0
Thyroid hormone plus [131]I	2.6	0

D. Ten-year survival rate correlates with the size and extension of the primary tumor:[1, 6, 7]
   Occult (less than 1.5 cm.): 97 per cent
   Intrathyroid: 73 per cent
   Extra thyroid (outside capsule): 46 per cent
   Overall: 82 per cent
   Total lobectomy on one side produces analogous cure.[1] Near-total thyroidectomy with neck dissection (if indicated) improves ^{131}I pickup by any remaining functioning tumor.

E. Partial neck dissection will also include some "berry picking" procedures. It has been shown that metastatic differentiated carcinoma in lymph nodes may produce some type of protective effect against dissemination (possibly an immune response).[7]

F. See page 50 for morbidity.

G. Hürthle cell carcinoma is similar to follicular carcinoma both in cure rates and natural history.[2]

H. Overall 10-year survival is 70 per cent.[9] Other 10-year survival rates are:
   Occult lesions (less than 1.5 cm.): 83 per cent
   Intrathyroid: 95 per cent
   Extrathyroid (capsule breached): 65 per cent[6]

As with papillary and mixed tumors (see Comment C), lobectomy alone gives equivalent results, but near-total excision permits better subsequent scanning and ^{131}I therapy.

POORLY DIFFERENTIATED THYROID CANCER

I. Medullary thyroid carcinoma is a malignancy of the "C cells." The familial type is often associated with type II-B multiple endocrine neoplasia or adenomatosis (MEA) and is bilateral in approximately 80 per cent of cases. Sporadic tumors are not associated with MEA and are bilateral in only 30 per cent of cases. Neither thyroid hormones nor ^{131}I is of appreciable value.[3, 4, 10]

J. With bilateral disease, lymph nodes from carotid to carotid are removed.

K. Survivors of anaplastic carcinoma are difficult to find, and any that do survive usually have more differentiated forms with areas of anaplastic change.[3]

L. Radiotherapy is noncurative but may temporarily contain the tumor in involved nodes. It is relatively ineffective in poorly differentiated thyroid tumors.

M. Chemotherapy is of little value. Lymphoma of the thyroid often responds to radiation therapy. Systemic disease frequently ensues. Most "small-cell carcinomas" are in actuality lymphomas of the thyroid.[4]

References

1. Tollefsen, H. R., Shah, J. P., and Huvos, A. G.: Papillary carcinoma of the thyroid. Recurrence in the thyroid gland after initial surgical treatment. Am. J. Surg., 124:468–472, 1972.

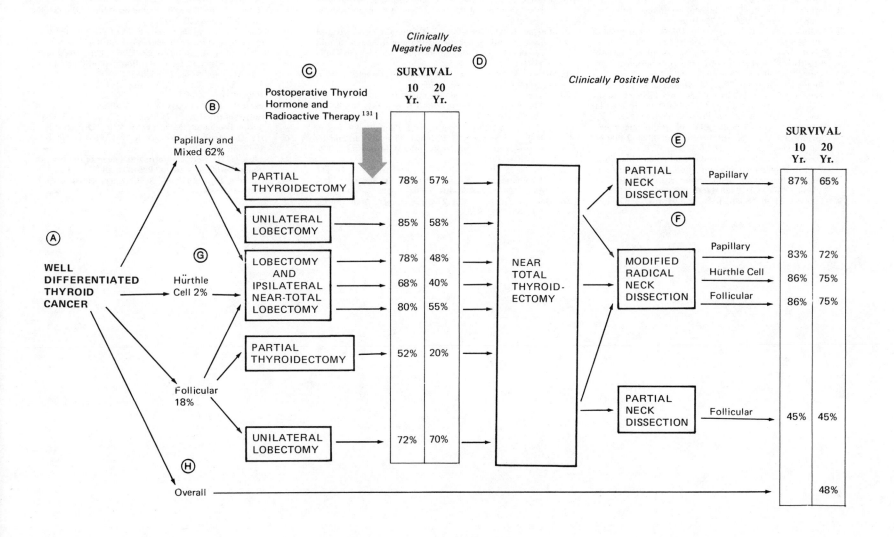

2. Tollefsen, H. R., Huvos, A. G., and Shah, J. P.: Hürthle cell carcinoma of the thyroid. Am. J. Surg., *130*:390–394, 1975.

3. Aldinger, K. A., et al.: Anaplastic carcinoma of the thyroid. Cancer, *41*:2267–2275, 1978.

4. Woolner, L. B., et al.: Primary malignant lymphoma of the thyroid. Am. J. Surg., *111*:502–523, 1966.

5. Frazell, E. L., and Foote, F. W., Jr.: Papillary cancer of the thyroid. A review of 25 years of experience. Cancer, *11*:895–922, 1958.

6. Woolner, L. B., et al.: Thyroid carcinoma: General considerations and follow-up data on 1181 cases. *In* Young, S., and Inman, D. R. (eds.): Thyroid Neoplasia. New York, Academic Press, 1968, pp. 51–77.

7. Cady, B., et al.: Changing clinical, pathologic, therapeutic, and survival patterns in differentiated thyroid carcinoma. Ann. Surg., *184*:541–552, 1976.

8. Russell, W. O., et al.: Thyroid carcinoma: Classification, intraglandular dissemination, and clinicopathological study based upon whole organ sections of 80 glands. Cancer, *16*:1425–1460, 1963.

9. Tollefsen, H. R., Shah, J. P., and Huvos, A. G.: Follicular carcinoma of the thyroid. Am. J. Surg., *126*:523–526, 1973.

10. Gordon, P. R., Huvos, A. G., and Strong, E. W.: Medullary carcinoma of the thyroid gland. Cancer, *31*:915–924, 1973.

11. Leeper, R. D.: The effect of ^{131}I therapy on survival of patients with metastatic papillary or follicular thyroid carcinoma. J. Clin. Endocrinol. Metab., *36*:1143–1152, 1973.

12. Varma, V. M., et al.: Treatment of thyroid cancer. JAMA, *214*:1437–1442, 1970.

13. Mazzaferri, E. L., et al.: Papillary thyroid carcinoma: The impact of therapy in 576 patients. Medicine, *56*:171–196, 1977.

14. Taylor, S.: Surgery of the thyroid gland. *In* De Groot, L. J., and Stanbury, J. B. (eds.): The Thyroid and Its Diseases, 4th ed. New York, John Wiley & Sons, 1975, pp. 797–798.

15. Astwood, E. B., Cassidy, C. E., and Aurbach, G. D.: Treatment of goitre and thyroid nodules with thyroid. JAMA, *174*:459–464, 1960.

16. DeCosse, J. J., et al.: Thyroid cancer. Arch. Surg., *110*:783–789, 1975.

17. Wang, C. A., Vickery, A. L., Jr., and Maloof, F.: Needle biopsy of the thyroid. Surg. Gynecol. Obstet., *143*:365–368, 1976.

18. DeGroot, L. J.: Thyroid carcinoma. Med. Clin. North Am., *59*:1233–1246, 1975.

19. Beahrs, O. H., and Pasternak, B. M.: Cancer of the thyroid gland. Curr. Probl. Surg., *3*:1–38, 1969.

20. Buckwalter, J. A., and Thomas, C. G.: The selection of surgical treatment for well-differentiated thyroid carcinomas. Ann. Surg., *176*:565–577, 1972.

21. Hill, L. D., et al.: Thyroid suppression. Arch. Surg., *108*:403–405, 1974.

22. Frazell, E. L.: The classification and clinical course of cancer of the thyroid. *In* Pack, G. T., and Ariel, I. M. (eds.): Treatment of Cancer and Allied Diseases. Vol. III. The Head and Neck. New York, Paul B. Hoeber, 1959, pp. 685–691.

23. Beahrs, O. H.: Nodular goitre and cancer of the thyroid gland. Postgrad. Med., *36*:229–233, 1964.

24. Silverberg, E., and Holleb, A. I.: Cancer statistics 1971. Cancer, *21*:13–31, 1971.

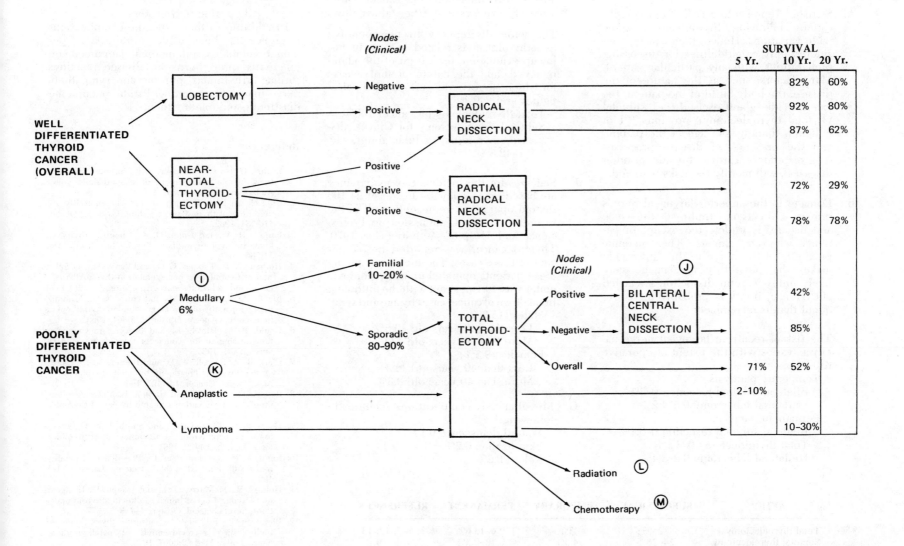

THYROIDECTOMY BY MORDANT E. PECK, M.D.

Comments

A. Statistics representing risks from complications following thyroidectomy show wide variations. Hence, they can be considered only as guidelines for discussing probabilities with any particular patient. Many factors, such as the nature of the disease, the body build of the patient, the extent of the gland excised (i.e., subtotal vs. total thyroidectomy), previous ^{131}I or radiation therapy, the age of the patient, and the presence of disease processes (i.e., respiratory, cardiac, hepatic, or other diseases), will modify the risks involved.

B. Damage to the superior laryngeal nerves primarily affects the timbre of the voice and usually is undetected except in patients who are singers. The anatomic proximity of the nerve to the upper pole makes the possibility of damage very likely unless careful dissection is carried out. Hence, injury is probably more frequent than is recognized.

C. The risk of recurrent laryngeal nerve paralysis varies with the extent of operative resection:
   Temporary paralysis
   Bilateral subtotal resection 0–2%
   Unilateral lobectomy 0.5–4.2%
   Permanent paralysis
   Bilateral subtotal resection 0–0.1%
   Total thyroidectomy 0–3.1%
   Unilateral lobectomy 0.2–3.4%

D. The incidence of hypoparathyroidism following thyroidectomy for cancer varies from 2 to 33 per cent.[19, 20] (See table below.)

E. The wide discrepancy in postoperative hypothyroidism is related to care in followup evaluation, the extent of the gland removed, and the nature of the disease for which surgery was performed. Typical figures are:[1-3, 13, 16]
   Total thyroidectomy for cancer 100%
   Subtotal thyroidectomy for Graves' disease, thyroiditis, nodular goiter, etc. 0.7–42.8%

F. Statistics for the incidence of malignancy are based on a review by Foster of 24,108 thyroid operations, representing all of the records from the Commission on Professional and Hospital Activities for 1970. Thyroid cancer was reported in 7.7 per cent of these cases. The incidence among those patients operated upon for nontoxic goiter was 10.1 per cent with the following breakdown of cancer cases by age and sex:[14]
   Males (15.3%)
   Less than 40 years old 19.5%
   More than 40 years old 13.6%
   Females (9.3%)
   Less than 40 years old 11%
   More than 40 years old 8.3%

G. Miscellaneous complications include the following:[2, 6, 14]
   Wound dehiscence 0.1%
   Skin fixation 0.2%
   Keloid 0.2%
   Thyroid crises 0.5%
   Laryngeal edema 0.2%
   Requiring tracheostomy 0.1%
   In addition to these specific complications, reference has been made to atelectasis, pulmonary embolus, pneumonia, jaundice, conjunctivitis, prep burns or allergic reactions, cardiac arrhythmias, phrenic and sympathetic nerve injury, thoracic duct fistula, pneumomediastinum, and pneumothorax.

References

1. Beahrs, O. H., and Sakulsky, S. B.: Surgical thyroidectomy in the management of exophthalmic goiter. Arch. Surg., 96:512, 1968.
2. Colcock, B. P., and King, M. L.: The mortality and morbidity of thyroid surgery. Sug. Gynecol. Obstet., 114:131, 1962.
3. Barnes, H. V., and Gann, D. S.: Choosing thyroidectomy in hyperthyroidism. Surg. Clin. North Am., 54:289, 1974.
4. Hothem, A. L., Thomas, C. G., and VanWyk, J. J.: Selection of treatment in management of thyrotoxicosis in childhood and adolescence. Ann. Surg., 187:593, 1978.
5. Block, M. A., Miller, J. M., and Horn, R. C.: Minimizing hypoparathyroidism after extended thyroid operations. Surg. Gynecol. Obstet., 123:501, 1966.
6. Gould, E. A., Hirsch, E., and Brecher, I.: Complications arising in the course of thyroidectomy. Arch. Surg., 90:81, 1965.
7. Clark, B. P., Russell, W. D., and Ibenez, M. L.: Cancer of the thyroid: Treatment by total thyroidectomy. Acta Un. Int. Cancer, 16:1425, 1960.
8. Roy, A. D., Allan, J., and Harden, R. McG.: A followup of thyrotoxic patients treated by partial thyroidectomy. Lancet, 2:684, 1967.
9. Davis, R. H., Fourman, P., and Smith, J. W. G.: Prevalence of parathyroid insufficiency after thyroidectomy. Lancet, 2:1432, 1961.
10. Jones, K. H., and Fourman, P.: Prevalence of parathyroid insufficiency after thyroidectomy. Lancet, 2:121, 1963.
11. Holt, G. R., McMurry, G. I., and Joseph, D. J.: Recurrent laryngeal nerve injuries following thyroid operations. Surg. Gynecol. Obstet., 144:567, 1977.
12. Blondeau, P.: Editorial: La chirurgie thyroidienne actuelle. Risques récurrentiels et parathyroidiens. Nouv. Presse Med., 2:3007, 1973.
13. Barraclough, B. H., and Reeve, T. S.: Postoperative

AFTER	SUBCLINICAL	TEMPORARY	PERMANENT	REFERENCES
Total thyroidectomy	25%	3%	0.6–13.6%	3, 5–7, 12, 13
Subtotal thyroidectomy	24–28%	4.5%	0.12–0.3%	1, 9, 10

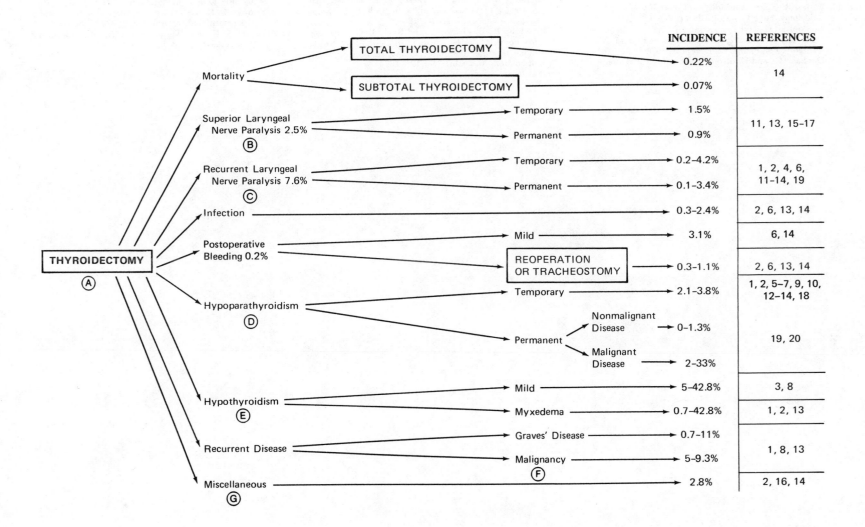

		INCIDENCE	REFERENCES
TOTAL THYROIDECTOMY		0.22%	14
SUBTOTAL THYROIDECTOMY		0.07%	
Superior Laryngeal Nerve Paralysis 2.5% ⒷB	Temporary	1.5%	11, 13, 15–17
	Permanent	0.9%	
Recurrent Laryngeal Nerve Paralysis 7.6% ⒸC	Temporary	0.2–4.2%	1, 2, 4, 6, 11–14, 19
	Permanent	0.1–3.4%	
Infection		0.3–2.4%	2, 6, 13, 14
Postoperative Bleeding 0.2%	Mild	3.1%	6, 14
	REOPERATION OR TRACHEOSTOMY	0.3–1.1%	2, 6, 13, 14
Hypoparathyroidism ⒹD	Temporary	2.1–3.8%	1, 2, 5–7, 9, 10, 12–14, 18
	Permanent → Nonmalignant Disease	0–1.3%	19, 20
	Permanent → Malignant Disease	2–33%	
Hypothyroidism ⒺE	Mild	5–42.8%	3, 8
	Myxedema	0.7–42.8%	1, 2, 13
Recurrent Disease	Graves' Disease	0.7–11%	1, 8, 13
	Malignancy	5–9.3%	
Miscellaneous ⒼG		2.8%	2, 16, 14

THYROIDECTOMY ⒶA

ⒻF

THYROIDECTOMY *Continued*

complications of thyroidectomy: A comparison of two series at an interval of 10 years. Aust. N.Z. J. Surg., *45*:21, 1975.

14. Foster, R. S., Jr.: Morbidity and mortality after thyroidectomy. Surg. Gynecol. Obstet., *146*:423, 1978.

15. Zwykielski, G., and Tyszkiewicz, T.: Injury of the superior laryngeal nerve in the course of thyroid gland surgery. Pol. Przegl. Chir., *48*:421, 1976.

16. Dunham, C., and Harrison, T.: The surgical anatomy of the superior laryngeal nerve. Surg. Gynecol. Obstet., *118*:38, 1964.

17. Moosman, D. A., and De Weese, M. S.: The external laryngeal nerve as related to thyroidectomy. Surg. Gynecol. Obstet., *127*:1011, 1968.

18. Blondeau, P., Brochard, M., and Rene, L.: Les risques fonctionnels de la chirurgie thyroidienne: Étude d'une série de 1000 interventions. II. Le riske parathyroidien. Ann. Chir., *27*:1121, 1973.

19. Thompson, N. W., Olsen, W. R., and Hoffman, G. L.: The continuing development of the technique of thyroidectomy. Surgery, *73*:913, 1973.

20. Harrold, C. C., and Wright, J.: Management of surgical hypoparathyroidism. Am. J. Surg., *112*:482, 1966.

21. Ingbar, S. H., and Werner, S. C.: The thyroid, 3rd ed. New York, Harper & Row, 1971.

HYPERPARATHYROIDISM

HYPERPARATHYROIDISM BY JOEL SIGDESTAD, M.D.

Comments

A. Other causes of hypercalcemia include malignancy, sarcoidosis, milk alkali syndrome, thiazide diuretics, multiple myeloma, and hypervitaminosis D.[1, 2] Approximately 0.6 per cent of the population is hypercalcemic, and 0.1 per cent are said to have hyperparathyroidism.[1]

B. The routine use of automatic blood chemistry determinations has altered the clinical diagnosis of hyperparathyroidism since 1970. Renal stones have decreased from 62 to 29 per cent, and "asymptomatic" hypercalcemia has increased from 5 to 40 per cent.[3]

C. Twenty per cent of asymptomatic patients will develop symptoms of increased calcium levels requiring surgery within five years.[4]

D. Parathyroid carcinoma is a rare (1 to 2 per cent) cause of hyperparathyroidism. It is treated by parathyroidectomy, with neck dissection only if nodes are involved. Five-year survival is over 50 per cent. Local tumor recurrence occurs in 30 per cent of cases, and 30 per cent will develop distant metastases.[5]

E. Average recurrence rate is 1 per cent,[7] but with familial hyperparathyroidism or multiple endocrine adenomas the recurrence rate is up to 33 per cent.[10]

F. With recent awareness that the adenoma is usually single (93 to 98 per cent of cases), excision of the single gland is deemed adequate.[3, 6, 12] Morbidity (recurrent nerve damage) is 0 to 1 per cent.[10-14]

G. Accuracy of preoperative localization varies with the test used:[11-13] (1) selective venous catheterization with parathyroid hormone assay (60 to 88 per cent), (2) arteriography (65 to 73 per cent), (3) C.T. scan (useful in mediastinal tumors) (19 per cent), or (4) esophagram (3 to 23 per cent)

H. Pathologic conditions found at re-exploration include:[13] adenoma (58 per cent), hyperplasia (26 per cent), and carcinoma (6 per cent). In 10 per cent of cases no pathology is found.

I. Tumors occur more often in the neck (81 per cent of cases) than in the mediastinum (19 per cent).[13] Of the mediastinal tumors, 67 per cent can be removed through a neck incision.

J. Complications include:[13] transient hypocalcemia (42 per cent), permanent hypocalcemia (3 per cent), and recurrent nerve injury (transient) (3 per cent).

References

1. Christensson, T., Hellstrom, K., and Wengle, B.: Hypercalcemia and primary hyperparathyroidism. Arch. Intern. Med., 137:1138–1142, 1977.
2. Purnell, D. C., Scholz, D. A., and Smith, L. H.: Diagnosis of hyperparathyroidism. Surg. Clin. North Am., 57:557–563, 1977.
3. Coffey, R. J., Lee, T. C., and Canary, J. J.: The surgical treatment of primary hyperparathyroidism. Ann. Surg., 185:518–523, 1977.
4. Purnell, D. C., et al.: Treatment of primary hyperparathyroidism. Am. J. Med., 56:800–809, 1974.
5. Schanz, A., and Castleman, B.: Parathyroid carcinoma: A study of 70 cases. Cancer, 31:600–605, 1973.
6. Purnell, D. C., Scholz, D. A., and Beahrs, O. H.: Hyperparathyroidism due to a single gland involvement. Arch. Surg., 113:369–372, 1977.
7. Paloyan, E., Paloyan, D., and Pickleman, J. R.: Hyperparathyroidism today. Surg. Clin. North Am., 53:211–220, 1973.
8. Schweitzer, V. G., et al.: Management of severe hypercalcemia caused by primary hyperparathyroidism. Arch. Surg., 113:373–381, 1978.
9. Satava, R. M., et al.: Success rate for cervical exploration for hyperparathyroidism. Arch. Surg., 110:625–628, 1975.
10. Clark, O. H., Way, L. W., and Hunt, T. K.: Recurrent hyperparathyroidism. Ann. Surg., 184:391–402, 1976.
11. Brennan, M. F., et al.: Reoperative parathyroid surgery for persistant hyperparathyroidism. Surgery, 83:669–676, 1978.
12. vanHeerden, J. A., et al.: The pathology and surgical management of primary hyperparathyroidism. Surg. Clin. North Am., 57:558–563, 1977.
13. Wang, C.: Parathyroid re-exploration. Ann. Surg., 186:140–145, 1977.
14. Cooke, T. J., et al.: Parathyroidectomy: Extent of resection and late results. Br. J. Surg., 64:153–157, 1977.

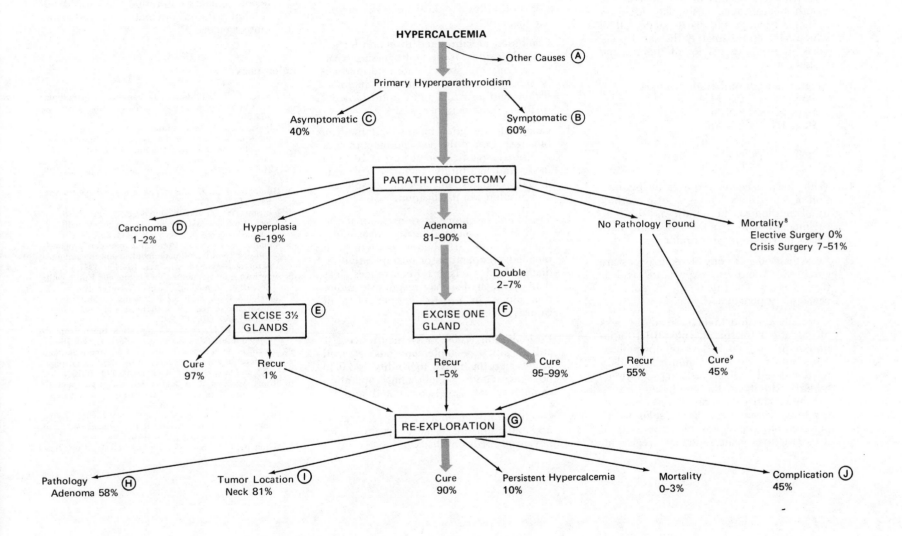

CARCINOMA OF THE ORAL CAVITY BY R. M. HIRATA, M.D., AND S. R. COLEN, M.D., D.D.S.

Comments

A. This includes lesions of the floor of the mouth, buccal mucosa, alveolar ridge, retromolar trigone, and hard palate, all of which have approximately the same prognosis. It excludes cancer of the lip and tongue.

B. Staging is as described on page 54.

Stage I	$T_1N_0M_0$
Stage II	$T_2N_0M_0$
Stage III	$T_3N_0M_0$
	$T_{1-3}N_1M_0$
Stage IV	$T_{1-3}N_{2-3}$
	T_4

C. Wide local excision requires hospitalization of 5 to 7 days. There is little morbidity of the floor of the mouth and the buccal mucosa. The alveolar ridge and hard palate may require prosthodontics.

D. Less than 50 per cent of recurrences are curable,[3, 8, 9] and life expectancy is less than 5 years. Quality of life is poor because of dysphagia and pain.

E. External radiation involves 6 to 7 weeks of outpatient treatment. Interstitial radiation requires 5 to 7 days of hospitalization. Both produce dry mouth secondary to decreased salivary gland secretions, hypersensitivity of the irradiated skin to sunshine, and osteoradionecrosis and ulceration. Tissue necrosis is seen in 15 per cent of patients and may appear from 2 months to 6 years following treatment; 80 per cent of these cases will become manifest within 2 years.[20]

F. For morbidity of radical neck dissection, see page 50.

G. Combined radiation and resection for advanced lesions is a controversial treatment. Only one study[10] had used randomly selected controls. Morbidity includes fistula, flap necrosis, and carotid blowout in 10 to 35 per cent of cases.[21, 22]

H. Composite resection means combined en bloc resection of the jaw and neck in continuity. Hospitalization at best is 10 to 14 days, and morbidity includes cosmetic deficit, changes in speech, dysphagia, and problems in mastication.

I. Treatment of choice is re-excision if the recurrence remains locally resectable. Large lesions are better treated with planned preoperative or postoperative radiation and excision. Recurrences less than 3 cm. in size may respond to radiation alone in up to 90 per cent of cases.[23, 24]

J. Postradiation (7000 rads) recurrences, if still locally resectable, are best excised widely. Postoperative morbidity is 20 to 60 per cent[12, 13] following operation through an extensively irradiated field.

K. Combinations of chemotherapy, surgery, and radiation are usually employed for advanced recurrent disease.[14, 15]

L. Approximately 15 per cent of patients will die of distant metastases when the local lesion remains controlled;[16] 15 to 33 per cent of patients develop a second squamous cancer.[17-19]

References

1. Flynn, M. B.: Morbidity and mortality of mandibular resection for malignant disease. Am. J. Surg., 134:510, 1977.
2. Gluckman, J. L., and Shumrick, D. A.: Synchronous multiple primaries of the upper aero-digestive system. Presented at Joint Meeting of the American Society for Head and Neck Surgery and the Society of Head and Neck Surgeons. Toronto, Ontario, May 29, 1978.
3. Hirata, R. M., et al.: Carcinoma of the oral cavity. Ann. Surg., 182:98, 1975.
4. Johnston, W. D., and Ballantyne, A. J.: Prognostic effect of tobacco and alcohol use in patients with oral tongue cancer. Am. J. Surg., 134:444, 1977.
5. Kalmins, I. K., et al.: Correlation between prognosis and degree of lymph node involvement in carcinoma of the oral cavity. Am. J. Surg., 134:450, 1977.
6. American Joint Committee for Staging and End-Results Reporting: Manual for Staging of Cancer, 1977.
7. Marchetta, F. C., Sako, K., and Camp, F.: Multiple malignancies in patients with head and neck cancer. Am. J. Surg., 110:537, 1965.
8. Randolph, V. L., et al.: Combination therapy of advanced head and neck cancer. Cancer, 41:460, 1978.
9. Roswit, B., et al.: Planned preoperative irradiation and surgery for advanced cancer of the oral cavity, pharynx, and larynx. Am. J. Roentgenol., 114:50, 1972.
10. Strong, M. S., et al.: A randomized trial of preoperative radiotherapy in cancer of the oropharynx and hypopharynx. Am. J. Surg., 136:494, 1978.
11. Shah, J. P., et al.: Carcinoma of the oral cavity. Factors affecting treatment failure at the primary site and neck. Am. J. Surg., 132:504, 1976.
12. Marchetta, F. C., Sako, K., and Maxwell, W.: Complica-

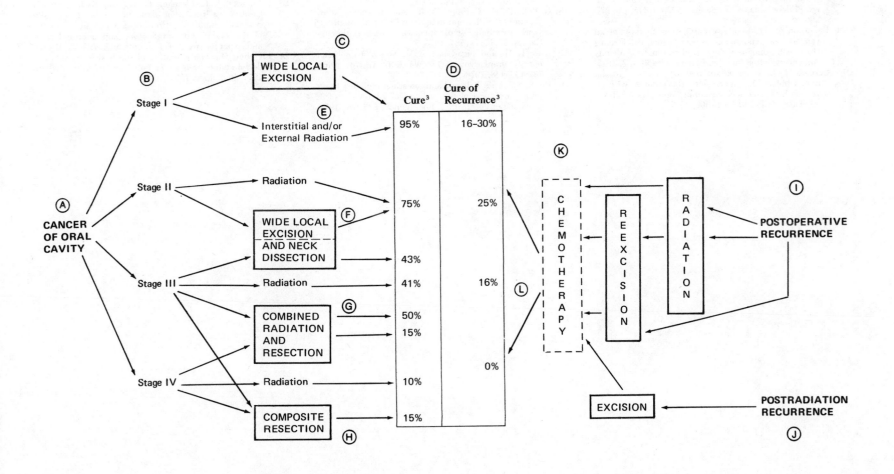

tion after radical head and neck surgery performed through previously irradiated tissues. Am. J. Surg., *114*:835–838, 1967.

13. Beahrs, O. H.: Complications of surgery for cancer of the head and neck. *In* Artz, C. P., and Hardy, J. D. (eds.): Management of Surgical Complications, 3rd ed. Philadelphia, W. B. Saunders Co., 1975, pp. 277–290.

14. Randolph V. L., et al.: Combination therapy of advanced head and neck cancer. Induction of remissions with diamminedichloroplatinum (II), bleomycin, and radiation therapy. Cancer, *41*:460–467, 1978.

15. Lerner, H. J.: Concomitant hydroxyurea and irradiation. Clinical experience with 100 patients with advanced head and neck cancer at Pennsylvania Hospital. Am. J. Surg., *134*:505–509, 1977.

16. Probert, J. C., Thompson, R. W., and Bagshaw, M. A.: Pattern of spread of distant metastases in head and neck cancer. Cancer, *33*:127–133, 1974.

17. Flynn, M. B., Mullius, F. X., and Moore, C.: Selection of treatment in squamous carcinoma of the floor of the mouth. Am. J. Surg., *126*:478–481, 1973.

18. Gilbert, E. H., Goffmet, D. R., and Bagshaw, M. A.: Carcinoma of the oral tongue and floor of mouth: 15 years' experience with linear acceleration therapy. Cancer, *35*:1517–1524, 1975.

19. Jesse, R. H., and Sugarbaker, E. V.: Squamous cell cancer of oropharynx: Why we fail. Am. J. Surg., *132*:435–438, 1976.

20. Fu, K. K., et al.: External and intestinal radiation therapy of carcinoma of the oral tongue. A review of 32 years' experience. Am. J. Roentgenol., *126*:107, 1976.

21. Yarington, C. T. Jr., Yonkers, A. J., and Beddoe, G. M.: Radical neck dissection. Arch. Otolaryngol., *97*:306, 1973.

22. Parnell, F. W.: Complications of radical neck dissection. Arch. Otolaryngol., *88*:180, 1968.

23. Schneider, J. J., Fletcher, G. H., and Barkely, H. J.: Control by irradiation alone of non-fixed clinically positive lymph nodes from squamous cell carcinoma of the oral cavity, oropharynx, supraglottic larynx, and hypopharynx. Am. J. Roentgenol., *123*:43, 1975.

24. Fletcher, H.: The evolution of the basic concepts underlying the practice of radiotherapy from 1949 to 1977. Radiology, *127*:3, 1978.

CERVICAL METASTASES IN HEAD AND NECK CANCER

CERVICAL METASTASES IN HEAD AND NECK CANCER

BY STEPHEN R. COLEN, M.D., D.D.S.

Comments

A. These data pertain to squamous cancer of the oral cavity, oropharynx, hypopharynx, and supraglottic larynx.

B. Primary control can be obtained by wide excision, radiation, or a combination of both.[7-15]

C. The decision concerning prophylactic neck dissection is based on the benefit of removing clinically occult disease (controversial[1, 17]) versus the detriment of neck dissection.
   1. The probability of occult disease depends upon the site of the primary, and its size and histologic grade.[16]
   2. Removal of the primary may involve entering the neck, which compromises the detection of future cervical node metastases and subsequent neck dissection.

D. Immediate complications of neck dissection include mortality rates of 1.5 per cent for unilateral and 2.5 per cent for bilateral procedures.[18, 19] A composite one-stage operation has a 3 per cent mortality.[20] Immediate postoperative complications are (1) lymph and chylous fistula, (2) infection, (3) skin flap necrosis, (4) hematoma-seroma, and (5) carotid artery leak. These complications occur in 10 to 35 per cent of cases.[21, 22]

   Long-term morbidity includes (1) cosmetic deformity, (2) weakness in complete arm abduction and dropped shoulder due to sacrifice of XI cranial nerve and weakness of the trapezius muscle, and (3) anesthesia of the posterior aspect of the scalp, neck, and shoulder owing to sacrifice of sensory nerve roots C_2 to C_4.

E. The per cent of positive nodes is related to the size of the primary lesion:[15, 16, 23]
   T_1: 18 to 20 per cent positive nodes
   T_2: 30 to 40 per cent positive nodes
   T_3: 40 to 65 per cent positive nodes
   For the "T" classification of each anatomic site, refer to reference 24.

F. Prophylactic radiation of the neck consists of 5000 to 6000 rads over a 5 to 6 week period. This regimen produces no detectable fibrosis of the neck skin but will produce some dryness of the oral mucosa when *both* subdigastric areas are treated.[28, 29]

G. The high cure rates presumably include the 68 per cent of patients who had no tumors in the neck to begin with.

H. The probability of another primary squamous cancer in this region is 15 to 35 per cent, broken down as follows:[14, 26, 27] head and neck, 10 to 20 per cent; esophagus, 2 to 10 per cent; bronchogenic, 3 to 10 per cent.

I. Tumor subsequently appears in the cervical nodes in the following time sequence:[25] less than 3 months, 44 per cent of cases; 3 to 6 months, 26 per cent; 6 months to 1 year, 14 per cent; more than 1 year, 16 per cent. Approximately 85 per cent of patients will manifest their disease within 1 year and more than 95 per cent will do so within 2 years.

J. With properly administered radiation (2000 rads in 5 equal daily treatments) preoperatively, no increase in operative morbidity is seen.[29] Preoperative and postoperative radiation are of equivalent value in controlling disease. A dose of 5000 to 6000 rads spread over 5 weeks preoperatively doubles the postoperative complication rate.[22, 30, 31]

K. Nodes larger than 6 cm. previously termed "fixed" are generally considered to be incurable by standard current therapy. Combinations of surgery, radiation, and chemotherapy may prove beneficial.[32-34]

References

1. Jesse, R. H., et al.: Cancer of the oral cavity. Is elective neck dissection beneficial? Am. J. Surg., *120*:505–508, 1970.
2. Fletcher, G. H., et al.: Textbook of Radiotherapy, 2nd ed. Philadelphia, Lea & Febiger, 1973, pp. 174–197.
3. Lindberg, R. D., et al.: Evolution of the clinically negative neck in patients with squamous cell carcinoma of the facial arch. Am. J. Roentgenol., *111*:60–65, 1971.
4. Berger, D. S., et al.: Elective irradiation of the neck lymphatics for squamous cell carcinomas of the nasopharynx and oropharynx. Am. J. Roentgenol., *111*:66–72, 1971.
5. Jesse, R. H., and Fletcher, G. H.: Treatment of the neck in patients with squamous cell carcinoma of the head and neck. Cancer, *39*:868–872, 1977 (Feb. Suppl.).
6. Schneider, J. J., Fletcher, G. H., and Barkley, H. T.: Control by irradiation alone of non-fixed, clinically positive lymph nodes from squamous cell carcinoma of the oral cavity, oropharynx, supraglottic larynx, and hypopharynx. Am. J. Roentgenol., *123*:42–48, 1975.
7. DeSanto, L. W., Lillie, J. C., and Devine, K. D.: Cancers of the larynx: Supraglottic cancer. Surg. Clin. North Am., 57:505–514, 1977.
8. Wilkins, S. A.: Carcinoma of the posterior pharyngeal wall. Am. J. Surg., *122*:477–481, 1971.
9. Ratzer, E. R., Schweitzer, R. J., and Frazell, E. L.: Epidermoid carcinoma of the palate. Am. J. Surg., *119*:294–297, 1970.
10. Whicker, J. H., DeSanto, L. W., and Devine, K. D.: Surgical treatment of squamous cell carcinoma of the base of the tongue. Laryngoscope, 82:1853–1860, 1972.
11. Healy, G. B., et al.: Carcinoma of the palatine arch. Am. J. Surg., *132*:498–503, 1976.

LYMPH NODE METASTASES OF SQUAMOUS CANCER OF THE HEAD AND NECK

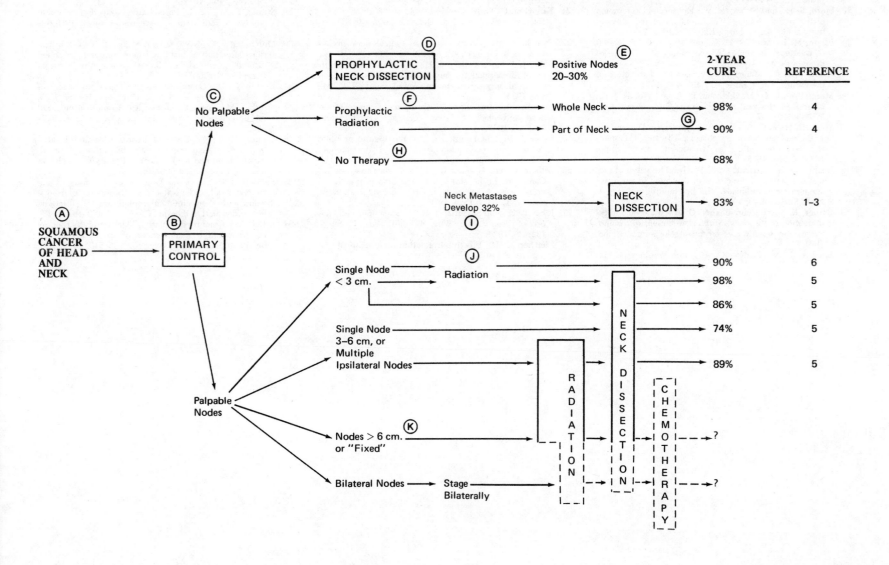

12. Shah, J. P., et al.: Carcinoma of the hypopharynx. Am. J. Surg., *132*:439–443, 1976.
13. Spiro, R. H., and Strong, E. W.: Epidermoid carcinoma of the mobile tongue: Treatment by partial glossectomy alone. Am. J. Surg., *122*:707–710, 1971.
14. Flynn, M. B., Mullins, F. X., and Moore, C.: Selection of treatment in squamous carcinoma of the floor of the mouth. Am. J. Surg., *126*:478–481, 1973.
15. Harrold, C. C.: Management of cancer of the floor of the mouth. Am. J. Surg., *122*:487–493, 1971.
16. Mendelson, B. C., Hodgkinson, D. J., and Woods, J. E.: Cancer of the oral cavity. Surg. Clin. North Am., *57*:585–596, 1977.
17. Spiro, R. H., and Strong, E. W.: Epidermoid carcinoma of the oral cavity and oropharynx: Elective, therapeutic neck dissection as treatment. Arch. Surg., *107*:382–384, 1973.
18. Beahrs, O. H., and Barber, K. W., Jr.: The value of radical dissection of structures of the neck in the management of carcinoma of the lip, mouth, and larynx. Arch. Surg., *85*:49, 1962.
19. Barber, K. W., Jr., and Beahrs, O. H.: Bilateral radical dissection of the neck: Surgical treatment of carcinoma of the mouth and larynx. Arch. Surg., *83*:388, 1961.
20. Simons, J. N., Beahrs, O. H., and Woolner, L. B.: Tumors of the submaxillary gland. Am. J. Surg., *108*:485, 1964.
21. Yarington, C. T., Jr., Yonkers, A. J., and Beddoe, G. M.: Radical neck dissection. Arch. Otolaryngol., *97*:306–308, 1973.
22. Parnell, F. W.: Complications of radical neck dissection. Arch. Otolaryngol., *88*:180–183, 1968.
23. Shah, J. P., and Tollefsen, H. R.: Epidermoid carcinoma of the supraglottic larynx: Role of neck dissection in initial surgical treatment. Am. J. Surg., *128*:494–499, 1974.
24. Chandler, J. R., et al.: Clinical staging of cancer of the head and neck: A "new" system. Am. J. Surg., *132*:525, 1976.
25. Fayos, J. V., and Lampe, I.: The therapeutic problem of metastatic neck adenopathy. Am. J. Roentgenol., *114*:65–75, 1972.
26. Gilbert, E. H., Goffinet, D. R., and Bagshaw, M. A.: Carcinoma of the oral tongue and floor of mouth: 15 years' experience with linear accelerator therapy. Cancer, *35*:1517–1524, 1975.
27. Jesse, R. H., and Sugarbaker, E. V.: Squamous cell cancer of oropharynx: Why we fail. Am. J. Surg., *132*:435, 1976.
28. Fletcher, G. H.: Elective irradiation of subclinical disease in cancers of the head and neck. Cancer, *29*:1450–1454, 1972.
29. Strong, E. W., et al.: Preoperative x-ray therapy as an adjunct to radical neck dissection. Cancer, *19*:1509–1515, 1966.
30. Marchetta, F. C., Sako, K., and Maxwell, W.: Complications after radical head and neck surgery performed through previously irradiated tissues. Am. J. Surg., *114*:835–838, 1967.
31. Beahrs, O. H.: Complications of surgery for cancer of the head and neck. *In* Artz, C. P., and Hardy, J. D. (eds.): Management of Surgical Complications, 3rd ed. Philadelphia, W. B. Saunders Co., 1975, pp. 277–290.
32. Lerner, H. J.: Concomitant hydroxyurea and irradiation: Clinical experience with 100 patients with advanced head and neck cancer at Pennsylvania Hospital. Am. J. Surg., *134*:505–509, 1977.
33. Randolph, V. L., et al.: Combination therapy of advanced head and neck cancer. Induction of remissions with diamminedichloroplatinum (II), bleomycin, and radiation therapy. Cancer, *41*:460–467, 1978.
34. Arlen, M.: Combined radiation: Methotrexate therapy in preoperative management of carcinoma of the head and neck. Am. J. Surg., *132*:536–540, 1976.

RADICAL NECK DISSECTION

RADICAL NECK DISSECTION BY ARLEN D. MEYERS, M.D.

Comments

A. The classic operation removes the lymphatic tissue and veins between the superficial and deep layers of the cervical fascia, along with the jugular vein, sternocleidomastoid muscle, XI cranial nerve, and submandibular gland. There are many modifications.[8]

B. Death is usually due to aspiration or pharyngocutaneous fistula with carotid artery erosion. Mortality is usually associated with removal of the primary tumor (of the larynx, for example) rather than with the lymph node excision.

C. This is more common on the left side, presenting as a subcutaneous or thoracic chylous effusion. Reoperative ligation of the thoracic duct is required if chyle leak persists.

D. Air embolism may occur with laceration of the internal jugular vein.

E. Factors associated with wound breakdown include prior radiation, inadequate hemostasis, poor nutrition, persistent tumor, and inadequate drainage.

F. A fistula usually will heal spontaneously if there is no persistent tumor at its origin.[11]

G. Contributing factors include postoperative radiation, orocutaneous fistula, excision of the carotid fascia, and infection. Following ligation of the common carotid artery, 25 per cent of patients die, 25 per cent are unaffected, and 50 per cent have neurologic deficits. These probabilities are age-related.[9]

H. Excision of the XI cranial nerve (accessory nerve) interferes with shoulder abduction beyond 90 degrees in one third of patients. Physical therapy minimizes adhesive capsulitis of the sternoclavicular or acromioclavicular joint following trapezius muscle atrophy.

References

1. Kirth, J. D., Sisson, G., and Becker, G.: Radical neck dissection in carcinomas of the head and neck. Surg. Clin. North Am., 53:179, 1973.
2. Yarington, C. T., Yonkers, A. S., and Beddoe, G. M.: Radical neck dissection. Arch. Otolaryngol., 97:306–308, 1973.
3. Kravse, L. G., Moreno-Torres, A., and Rodrigo, C.: Radical neck dissection. Arch. Otolaryngol., 94:153–157, 1971.
4. Parnell, F.: Complications of radical neck dissection. Arch. Otolaryngol., 88:180–183, 1968.
5. Johnson, J. T., and Cummings, C. W.: Hematoma after head and neck surgery. Otolaryngology, 86:171–175, 1978.
6. Mehra, Y. N., Arora, N. M., and Dwavedi, G. J.: Internal carotid artery thrombsois following head and neck surgery. J. Laryngol. Otol., 91:985–988, 1977.
7. Fitz-Hugh, G. J., and Cowgill, R.: Chylous fistula — complication of neck dissection. Arch. Otolaryngol., 91:543–547, 1970.
8. Lingeman, R. E., et al.: Neck dissection: Radical or conservative. Ann. Otol., 86:737–744, 1977.
9. Leikensohn, J., Milko, D., and Cotton, R.: Carotid artery rupture. Arch Otolaryngol., 104:307–310, 1978.
10. Cantrell, R.: Pharyngeal fistula: Prevention and treatment. Laryngoscope, 88:1204–1208, 1978.
11. Myers, E. N.: The management of pharyngocutaneous fistula. Arch. Otolaryngol., 95:10–17, 1972.

	NO RADIATION	FOLLOWING RADIATION	REFERENCES
Mortality Ⓑ	1%	6%	1
Intraoperative Complications			
Thoracic Duct Injury Ⓒ	1%	1%	7
Air Embolism Ⓓ	1%	1%	
Immediate Postoperative Complication			
Bleeding Requiring Second Operation	4.2%	4.2%	5
Delayed Complications			
Wound Infection and Breakdown Ⓔ	8%	50%	4
Pharyngeal Cutaneous Fistula Ⓕ	33%	50%	4
Loss of Skin Flap	0%	25%	4
Carotid Artery Blowout Ⓖ	0%	8%	4
Late Complications			
Dropped Shoulder Ⓗ	30%	30%	1

Ⓐ **RADICAL NECK DISSECTION**

51

LIP CANCER BY DAVID M. CHARLES, M.D.

Comments

A. Contrasted with 30 years ago, patients (1) seek treatment earlier (15 months vs. 18.9 months), (2) are older by 3 years, (3) have positive nodes less frequently (1 per cent vs. 4 per cent), and (4) have lower-grade lesions.[8] This presumably is due to better patient education and availability of medical care.

B. It remains controversial whether leukoplakia is a premalignant condition,[1, 12] but the evidence is in favor. It is associated with cancer in 75 per cent of cases,[8] and vermilionectomy appears to decrease the incidence of recurrent squamous cancer from 9 per cent to 3 per cent.

C. This type is a rarity,[15] and frozen section control of excised borders is curative when there are no metastases.

D. The TNM classification for lip cancer is:[10]
   Tumor size
   T_1 = less than 2 cm.
   T_2 = 2–4 cm.
   T_3 = greater than 4 cm.
   Nodes
   N_0 = none
   N_1 = single homolateral, less than 3 cm.
   N_{2a} = single homolateral, 3–6 cm.
   N_{2b} = multiple homolateral, less than 6 cm.
   N_3 = homolateral, greater than 6 cm bilateral or contralateral
   Broders' histologic classification, on percentage of cells differentiated,[4] is as follows:
   Grade 1: 75–100 per cent
   Grade 2: 50–75 per cent
   Grade 3: 25–50 per cent
   Grade 4: 0–25 per cent

Frequency of recurrence and nodal metastases correlate to higher T grades and to the less differentiated histology.[9, 16]

E. The most common clinical situation is a small, low-grade lower lip squamous cancer without nodes. With V-excision and lip shave, 98 per cent of patients will be cured in 10 years.[3, 8] Surgery and irradiation have similar cure rates.[2]

F. Nodes are clinically positive in 6 per cent of cases. Twenty per cent of these will prove to be histologically positive. Cure rates then drop to 40 to 50 per cent.[3, 8, 13]

G. Recurrences kill by (1) spread along the inferior dental nerve to the base of the skull and (2) extensive neck disease.[5] Most occur in the first 2 years.[6, 11] Recurrence to the neck only occurs in 43 per cent of cases; to the lip only in 43 per cent of cases; and to both lip and neck in 14 per cent of cases. The mean survival of those not cured is 2 to 3 years.[8] Twelve per cent of patients develop a second cancer, usually of the mouth or pharynx.[15]

Survival of those not cured:[8] 17 per cent of patients with recurrences in the lip died after a mean survival of 7.1 years. Forty-eight per cent of patients with recurrences in the neck died after a mean survival of 2.3 years. Once lymph node metastases are confirmed, 51 per cent of patients are alive at 5 years,[7] and 73 per cent have a 2-year recurrence-free interval after re-excision of the lip lesion.[5]

H. Distant metastasizes are rare,[7] usually involve the lungs, and are rapidly fatal.

I. Lymph nodes are involved in 50 per cent of upper lip cancers.[14] About 50 per cent of these patients are cured, and 27 to 42 per cent are dead in 5 years.[8, 11]

References

1. Ackerman, L. V. and Rosai, J.: Surgical Pathology, 5th ed. St. Louis, C. V. Mosby Co., 1974, p. 144.
2. Ashley, F. L., et al.: Carcinoma of the lip. A comparison of five-year results after irradiation and surgical therapy. Am. J. Surg., 110:549, 1965.
3. Bailey, B. J.: Management of carcinoma of the lip. Laryngoscope, 87:250, 1977.
4. Broders, A. C.: The microscopic grading of cancer. Surg. Clin. North Am., 21:947, 1941.
5. Brown, R. G., et al.: Advanced and recurrent squamous carcinoma of the lower lip. Am. J. Surg., 132:492, 1976.
6. Dickie, W. R., Colville, J., and Graham, W. J. H.: Recurrent carcinoma of the lip. Oral Surg., 24:449, 1967.
7. Jørgenson, K., Elbrønd, O., and Andersen, A. P.: Carcinoma of the lip. A series of 869 cases. Acta Radiol. [Ther.] (Stockh.), 12:177, 1973.
8. Hendricks, J. L., Mendelson, B. C., and Woods, J. E.: Invasive carcinoma of the lower lip. Surg. Clin. North Am., 57:837, 1977.
9. Lund, C., et al.: Epidermoid carcinoma of the lip. Histological grading in the clinical evaluation. Acta Radiol. [Ther.] (Stockh.), 14:465, 1975.
10. American Joint Committee for Cancer Staging and End-results Reporting: Manual for Staging of Cancer 1977. Chicago, American Joint Committee, 1977.
11. Molnár, L., Rónay, P., and Tapolcsányi, L.: Carcinoma of the lip. Analysis of the material of 25 years. Oncology, 29:101, 1974.
12. Shafer, W. G., Hine, M. K., and Levy, B. M.: Textbook of Oral Pathology, 3rd ed. Philadelphia, W. B. Saunders Co. 1974, p. 87.
13. Stoddart, T. G.: Conference on cancer of the lip. Based on a series of 3166 cases. Can. Med. Assoc. J., 90:666, 1964.
14. Taylor, G. W., and Nathanson, I. T.: Evaluation of neck dissection in carcinoma of the lip. Surg. Gynecol. Obstet., 69:484, 1939.
15. Weitzner, S.: Basal cell carcinoma of the vermilion mucosa and skin of the lip. Oral Surg., 39:634, 1975.
16. Wurman, L. H., Adams, G. L., and Meyerhoff, W. L.: Carcinoma of the lip. Am. J. Surg., 130:470, 1975.

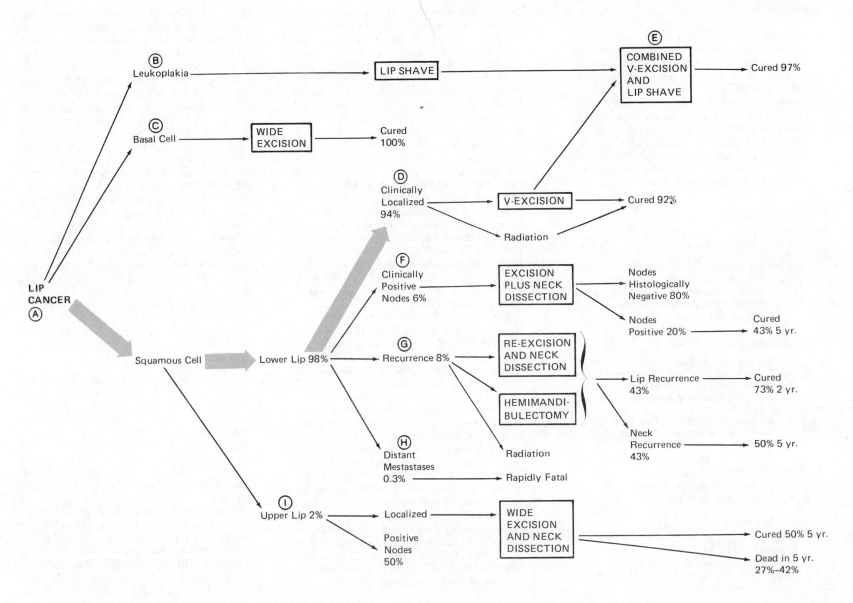

Ⓑ Leukoplakia → LIP SHAVE → Ⓔ COMBINED V-EXCISION AND LIP SHAVE → Cured 97%

Ⓒ Basal Cell → WIDE EXCISION → Cured 100%

Ⓓ Clinically Localized 94% → V-EXCISION → Cured 92%
Radiation

Ⓐ LIP CANCER → Squamous Cell → Lower Lip 98%

Ⓕ Clinically Positive Nodes 6% → EXCISION PLUS NECK DISSECTION → Nodes Histologically Negative 80%
Nodes Positive 20% → Cured 43% 5 yr.

Ⓖ Recurrence 8% → RE-EXCISION AND NECK DISSECTION / HEMIMANDI-BULECTOMY / Radiation
Lip Recurrence 43% → Cured 73% 2 yr.
Neck Recurrence 43% → 50% 5 yr.

Ⓗ Distant Mestastases 0.3% → Rapidly Fatal

Ⓘ Upper Lip 2% → Localized → WIDE EXCISION AND NECK DISSECTION
Positive Nodes 50%
→ Cured 50% 5 yr.
→ Dead in 5 yr. 27%–42%

CANCER OF THE TONGUE BY NATHAN W. PEARLMAN, M.D.

Comments

A. Ninety per cent of tongue cancers are squamous.[2] Seventy per cent originate in the anterior two-thirds (mobile/oral tongue) and 30 per cent in the base, or posterior third.[5, 30, 31] Prognosis in each location is about the same for a given stage of disease.[12, 31] Tumors of the base tend to have a worse overall prognosis than do anterior lesions, because more of the former are advanced (stage III or IV) when diagnosed.[17, 23, 30] The staging system[19] used at present is shown below:

Primary Tumor

T_0 Occult
TIS   Carcinoma *in situ*
T_1 0–2 cm. diameter
T_2 2–4 cm. diameter
T_3 >4 cm. diameter
T_4 >4 cm. diameter and invading root of tongue, bone, pterygoid muscles, or skin of neck

Neck Nodes

N_0 No clinically suspicious nodes
N_1 Single homolateral node smaller than 3 cm.
N_2 Single homolateral node 3–6 cm. or multiple homolateral nodes, none greater than 3 cm.
N_3 Single homolateral node over 6 cm. or fixed; contralateral or bilateral nodes of any size

Distant Metastases:

M_0 No distant metastases evident
M_1 Distant metastases present

Stages of Disease:

Stage I $T_1 N_0 M_0$
Stage II $T_2 N_0 M_0$
Stage III $T_3 N_0 M_0$, or $T_{1-3} N_1 M_0$
Stage IV $T_4 N_0 M_0$, or $T_{1-4} N_{2-3} M_0$, or any T, any N, M_1

B. Surgery for stage I or II disease consists of partial glossectomy with or without an elective neck dissection. Mortality for neck dissection alone is 1 to 2 per cent,[21, 33] and that of glossectomy plus neck dissection is 2 to 3 per cent.[21, 24] By subtraction, a mortality of 1 to 2 per cent for the glossectomy alone is arrived at. The morbidity of a neck dissection in 25 per cent;[33] that of glossectomy plus neck dissection, 30 to 35 per cent.[18, 20] Subtraction gives a morbidity of 5 to 10 per cent for glossectomy alone. The potential causes of morbidity and mortality are cardiac arrhythmia, pulmonary embolus, GI bleeding, pneumonia, wound hematomaseroma, flap necrosis, chylous or salivary fistula, carotid exposure or rupture, and difficulty in swallowing. Most are temporary problems, and the majority of stage I and II patients have healed wounds with near normal speech and swallowing 4 weeks postoperatively.

Initial control rates with surgery for T_{1-2} tongue lesions are 80 to 100 per cent; another 5 to 7 per cent of patients are salvageable after recurrence.[5, 6, 12, 28, 32] Twenty to 40 per cent of N_0 necks will develop neck metastases if observed, and 35 to 40 per cent of such patients will be cured by subsequent therapeutic neck dissections.[5, 22, 28, 32] Elective, or "prophylactic," neck dissections for $T_{1-2} N_0$ disease will uncover positive nodes in 25 to 30 per cent of patients, who then will be cured in 25 to 30 per cent of instances.[22, 29] Recurrence in the dissected neck (when dissection is elective) will occur in 4 to 8 per cent of all patients with $T_{1-2} N_0$ disease.[29] If the primary tumor and ipsilateral neck nodes remain controlled, 2 to 3 per cent of patients will develop contralateral neck disease and 2 to 4 per cent will develop distant metastases.[5, 28, 29, 32]

C. The mortality of radiation therapy for stage I and II disease is not mentioned in the literature but probably is less than 1 per cent. The major potential side effect is osteoradionecrosis of the mandible, occurring in 8 to 20 per cent of patients and at any time after treatment.[3, 10, 15, 26, 31] Three quarters of these heal spontaneously, while 25 per cent require sequestrectomy. Initial control of T_{1-2} lesions with radiotherapy is achieved in 70 to 90 per cent of cases; another 3 to 4 per cent are salvaged after recurrence.[3, 10, 12, 15, 26, 31] Observed N_0 necks will develop metastases in 20 to 35 per cent of instances, and subsequent neck dissections will cure 35 to 45 per cent of patients.[8, 13] Electively radiated N_0 necks will develop metastases in 2 to 5 per cent of instances.[1, 4] Salvage rates for the latter patients are not available. Distant metastases are not mentioned in the radiotherapy literature on this stage of disease but probably claim 2 to 4 per cent of patients. Figures for contralateral neck disease in these patients also are not available.

D. Surgery for stage III and IV disease (large primary tumor or palpable neck nodes) usually entails partial or total glossectomy, removal of a portion of the mandible, and neck dissection (Commando procedure). Mortality increases to 4 to 8 per cent and morbidity to 35 to 40 per cent[18, 20, 27] for the same reasons listed under stage I and II disease (see Comment B).

The control rate for T_3 primary tumors treated by surgery alone is 50 to 75 per cent; that for N_1-N_2 nodes, 70 to 80 per cent.[1, 14, 28, 32] Essentially none of these patients will be salvaged after local or neck recurrence.[12] T_4 primary tumors and N_3 neck nodes that are larger than 6 cm.

CANCER OF THE TONGUE

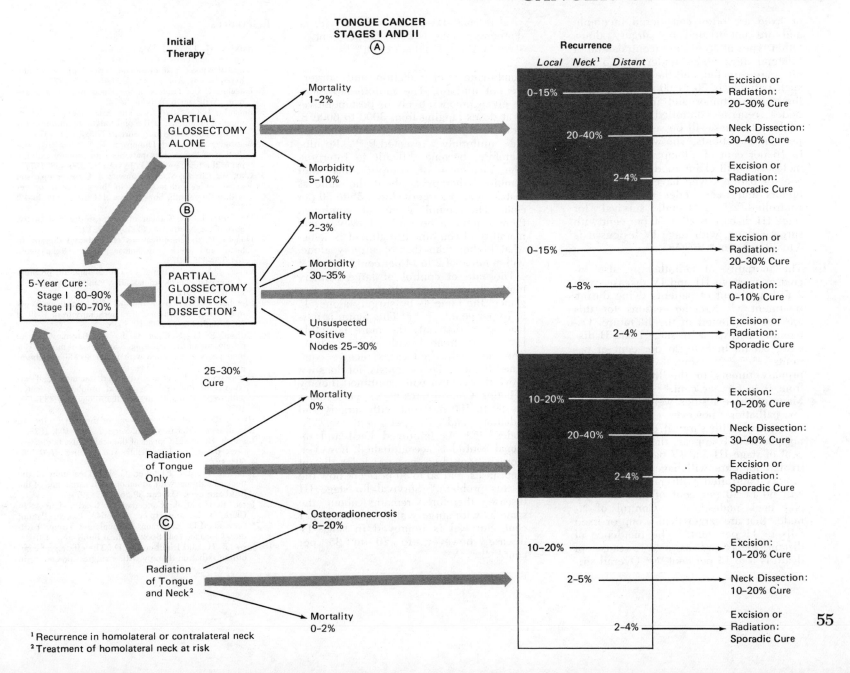

Initial Therapy

TONGUE CANCER STAGES I AND II (A)

Recurrence

Local Neck[1] Distant

PARTIAL GLOSSECTOMY ALONE
- Mortality 1-2%
- Morbidity 5-10%

(B)

PARTIAL GLOSSECTOMY PLUS NECK DISSECTION[2]
- Mortality 2-3%
- Morbidity 30-35%
- Unsuspected Positive Nodes 25-30%

25-30% Cure

(C)

Radiation of Tongue Only
- Mortality 0%
- Osteoradionecrosis 8-20%

Radiation of Tongue and Neck[2]
- Mortality 0-2%

5-Year Cure:
Stage I 80-90%
Stage II 60-70%

Recurrence values:
- 0-15% → Excision or Radiation: 20-30% Cure
- 20-40% → Neck Dissection: 30-40% Cure
- 2-4% → Excision or Radiation: Sporadic Cure
- 0-15% → Excision or Radiation: 20-30% Cure
- 4-8% → Radiation: 0-10% Cure
- 2-4% → Excision or Radiation: Sporadic Cure
- 10-20% → Excision: 10-20% Cure
- 20-40% → Neck Dissection: 30-40% Cure
- 2-4% → Excision or Radiation: Sporadic Cure
- 10-20% → Excision: 10-20% Cure
- 2-5% → Neck Dissection: 10-20% Cure
- 2-4% → Excision or Radiation: Sporadic Cure

[1] Recurrence in homolateral or contralateral neck
[2] Treatment of homolateral neck at risk

55

or fixed are often considered incurable and are not treated by surgery alone. Other types of N_3 disease (contralateral or bilateral neck nodes under 4 to 5 cm.) often are resected, and the control rate in such patients is 50 to 60 per cent.[1, 14] If the primary tumor and ipsilateral neck nodes remain controlled, contralateral neck metastases will be seen in 15 to 30 per cent of patients, who will be salvaged in 16 per cent of attempts.[1, 23, 27] Distant metastases will claim another 5 to 10 per cent of patients who have their primary tumors and neck nodes on both sides controlled.[17, 27, 29] Overall survival for stage III disease is 40 to 50 per cent with surgery alone; with stage IV lesions it is 5 to 30 per cent.[6, 12, 21, 27, 29, 32]

E. The mortality of radiotherapy also increases in stage III and IV disease, with 2 to 6 per cent of patients dying during treatment.[16, 31] Specific reasons for this are not mentioned in the literature. Osteoradionecrosis, as in stage I and II disease, occurs in 8 to 20 per cent of patients.[3, 10, 15, 26, 31] Control rates of T_{3-4} primary tumors in the literature range from 0 to 65 per cent.[3, 5, 9, 10, 12, 15-17, 26, 31] Many of these lesions were treated only for palliation, however, so that direct comparison with surgical control rates is not possible. It appears that 40 to 50 per cent of stage III and IV patients who are treated for cure will have their primary tumors controlled with radiotherapy, as will 60 to 80 per cent of patients with N_{1-2} neck nodes.[1, 4, 10, 31] Control of N_3 nodes that are larger than 6 cm. or fixed falls to 11 per cent.[10] The incidence of distant metastases as a sole cause of death is 5 to 15 per cent.[10, 16] Overall survival in stage III disease treated with radiotherapy alone is 25 to 50 per cent; in stage IV it is 0 to 20 per cent.[10, 12, 16, 17, 31]

F. Combinations of radiation and surgery are not uniform. The radiotherapy may be given preoperatively or postoperatively at doses ranging from 3000 to 6000 R. In addition, not all areas being irradiated are uniformly resected.[15, 23] Results, therefore, become difficult to interpret. The incidence of complications after combined therapy is about the same as that seen after surgery alone: 35 to 50 per cent. The complications of combined therapy tend to be worse, however, and mortality of combined treatment is somewhat higher than that of surgery alone, with a range of 2 to 14 per cent.[7, 11, 16, 23, 24]

The rate of control of large primary tumors by combined therapy is, at first glance, the same as by surgery alone: 45 to 75 per cent.[11, 12, 16, 23] This figure is misleading in that only the more favorable lesions are treated with surgery alone. The more advanced cases receive combined therapy. This suggests but does not prove that control with combined therapy is better. Control rates of N_{1-2} neck nodes are 80 to 100 per cent with surgery and radiation and 75 per cent for N_3 nodes.[1, 23, 25] As improved local and regional control is accomplished, however, more patients become at risk for distant metastases, and 20 to 30 per cent now die of this problem.[16] Survival for stage III disease, therefore, remains about the same as with surgery alone: 40 to 50 per cent. Survival is improved in stage IV disease, however, to 20 to 35 per cent.[11, 12, 16, 23, 24]

References

1. Barkley, H. T., et al.: Management of cervical lymph nodes metastases in squamous cell carcinoma of the tonsillar fossa, base of tongue, supraglottic larynx and hypopharynx. Am. J. Surg., *124*:462–467, 1972.
2. Batsakis, J. G.: Tumors of the Head and Neck. Baltimore, Williams & Wilkins, 1974.
3. Botstein, J. G., Silver, G., and Ariaratnam, L.: Treatment of carcinoma of the oral tongue by radium needle implantation. Am. J. Surg., *132*:523–524, 1976.
4. Bagshaw, M. A., and Thompson, R. W.: Elective irradiation of the neck in patients with primary carcinoma of the head and neck. JAMA, *217*:456–458, 1971.
5. Chu, W., Litwin, S., and Strawitz, J. G.: A comparison of resection and radiation in the control of cancer within the mouth. Surg. Gynecol. Obstet., *146*:38–42, 1978.
6. De Santo, L. W.: Cancer of the posterior oral cavity. Surg. Clin. North Am., *57*:597–609, 1977.
7. Donald, P. J.: Complications of combined therapy in head and neck carcinomas. Arch. Otolaryngol., *104*:329–332, 1978.
8. Fayos, J. V., and Lampe, I.: The therapeutic problem of metastatic neck adenopathy. Am. J. Roentgenol., *114*:65–75, 1972.
9. Fletcher, G. H.: The evolution of the basic concepts underlying the practice of radiotherapy from 1949 to 1977. Radiology, *127*:3–19, 1978.
10. Gilbert, E. H., Goffinet, D. R., and Bagshaw, M. A.: Carcinoma of the oral tongue and floor of mouth: Fifteen years' experience with linear accelerator therapy. Cancer, *35*:1517–1524, 1975.
11. Hamberger, A. D., et al.: Advanced squamous cell carcinoma of the oral cavity and oropharynx treated with irradiation and surgery. Radiology, *119*:433–438, 1976.
12. Hirata, R. M., et al.: Carcinoma of the oral cavity. An analysis of 478 cases. Ann. Surg., *182*:98–103, 1975.
13. Jesse, R. H., et al.: Cancer of the oral cavity. Is elective neck dissection beneficial? Am. J. Surg., *120*:505–508, 1975.
14. Jesse, R. H., and Fletcher, G. H.: Treatment of the neck in patients with squamous cell carcinoma of the head and neck. Cancer, *39*:868–872, 1977.
15. Jesse, R. H., et al.: Cancer of the head and neck. *In* Clark, R. L., and Howe, C. (eds.): Cancer Patient Care at M.D. Anderson Hospital and Tumor Institute. Chicago, Year Book Medical Publishers, 1976.
16. Jesse, R. H., and Lindberg, R. D.: The efficacy of combining radiation therapy with a surgical procedure in

**TONGUE CANCER
STAGES III AND IV**

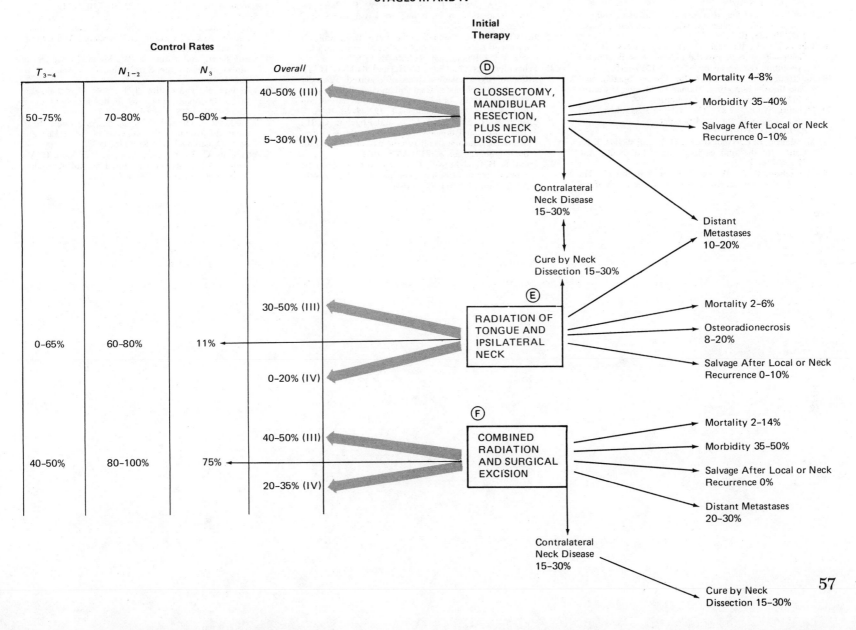

Control Rates

Initial Therapy

T_{3-4}	N_{1-2}	N_3	*Overall*

50-75% | 70-80% | 50-60% ← | 40-50% (III)

5-30% (IV)

D GLOSSECTOMY, MANDIBULAR RESECTION, PLUS NECK DISSECTION

Mortality 4-8%

Morbidity 35-40%

Salvage After Local or Neck Recurrence 0-10%

Contralateral Neck Disease 15-30%

Cure by Neck Dissection 15-30%

Distant Metastases 10-20%

0-65% | 60-80% | 11% ← | 30-50% (III)

0-20% (IV)

E RADIATION OF TONGUE AND IPSILATERAL NECK

Mortality 2-6%

Osteoradionecrosis 8-20%

Salvage After Local or Neck Recurrence 0-10%

40-50% | 80-100% | 75% ← | 40-50% (III)

20-35% (IV)

F COMBINED RADIATION AND SURGICAL EXCISION

Mortality 2-14%

Morbidity 35-50%

Salvage After Local or Neck Recurrence 0%

Distant Metastases 20-30%

Contralateral Neck Disease 15-30%

Cure by Neck Dissection 15-30%

57

CANCER OF THE TONGUE *Continued*

patients with cervical metastases from squamous cancer of the oropharynx and hypopharynx. Cancer, 35:1163–1166, 1975.

17. Jesse, R. H., and Sugarbaker, E. V.: Squamous cell carcinoma of the oropharynx: Why we fail. Am. J. Surg., 132:435–438, 1976.

18. Johnson, J. T., Rabuzzi, D. D., and Tucker, H. M.: Composite resection in the elderly: A well-tolerated procedure. Laryngoscope, 87:1509–1515, 1977.

19. American Joint Committee for Cancer Staging and End-Results Reporting: Manual for Staging of Cancer 1977. Chicago, Am. Joint Committee, 1977.

20. McGuirt, W. F., et al.: The risks of major head and neck surgery in the aged population. Laryngoscope, 87:1378–1382, 1977.

21. Mendelson, B. C., Hodgkinson, D. J., and Woods, J. E.: Cancer of the oral cavity. Surg. Clin. North Am. 57:585–596, 1977.

22. Mendelson, B. C., Woods, J. E., and Beahrs, O. H.: Neck dissection in the treatment of carcinoma of the anterior two-thirds of the tongue. Surg. Gynecol. Obstet., 143:75–80, 1976.

23. Perez, C. A., Marks, J., and Powers, W. E.: Preoperative irradiation in head and neck cancer. Semin. Oncol., 4:387–297, 1977.

24. Roswit, B., et al.: Planned preoperative irradiation for advanced cancer of the oral cavity, pharynx, and larynx. Am. J. Roentgenol., 114:59–62, 1972.

25. Schneider, J. J., Fletcher, G. H., and Barkley, H. T.: Control by irradiation alone of nonfixed clinically positive lymph nodes from squamous cell carcinoma of the oral cavity, oropharynx, supraglottic larynx and hypopharynx. Am. J. Roentgenol., 123:42–48, 1975.

26. Spanos, W. J., Shukovsky, L. J., and Fletcher, G. H.: Time, dose, and tumor volume relationships in irradiation of squamous cell carcinomas of the base of the tongue. Cancer, 37:2591–2599, 1976.

27. Spiro, R. H., and Frazell, E. L.: Evaluation of radical surgical treatment of advanced cancer of the mouth. Am. J. Surg., 116:571–577, 1968.

28. Spiro, R. H., and Strong, E. W.: Epidermoid carcinoma of the mobile tongue. Treatment by partial glossectomy alone. Am. J. Surg., 122:707–710, 1971.

29. Spiro, R. H., and Strong, E. W.: Epidermoid carcinoma of the oral cavity and oropharynx. Elective vs. therapeutic neck dissection as treatment. Arch. Surg., 107:382–384, 1973.

30. Spiro, R. H., and Strong, E. W.: Surgical treatment of cancer of the tongue. Surg. Clin. North Am. 54:759–765, 1974.

31. Vermund, H., and Gollin, F. F.: Role of radiotherapy in the treatment of cancer of the tongue. Cancer, 32:333–345, 1973.

32. Whitehurst, J. O., and Droulias, C. A.: Surgical treatment of squamous cell carcinoma of the oral tongue. Arch. Otolaryngol., 103:212–215, 1977.

33. Yarington, C. T., Yonkers, A. J., and Beddoe, G. M.: Radical neck dissection: Mortality and morbidity. Arch. Otolaryngol., 97:306–308, 1973.

TUMORS OF THE SALIVARY GLAND

TUMORS OF THE SALIVARY GLAND BY JOHN A. GROSSMAN, M.D.

Comments

A. Location and frequency of salivary gland tumors are as follows:[1, 2, 8, 11, 14, 25]
   - parotid: 75 to 85 per cent
   - submaxillary: 20 per cent
   - sublingual and minor salivary glands: rare

B. Cell types in salivary gland tumors may be:
   - mixed: 65 to 80 per cent of cases
   - Warthin's: 20 per cent
   - oncocytoma (Hürthle cell): 1 per cent
   - miscellaneous (basal cell, sebaceous cell): approximately 1 to 2 per cent

   Six to 10 per cent of all parotid tumors are Warthin's tumors; of these, 10 per cent occur bilaterally, and 80 per cent occur in men. In oncocytoma bilaterality and multinodularity are conspicuous features.

C. Eighty-four per cent of mixed-cell tumors occur in the parotid gland, 8 per cent in the submandibular, 0.5 per cent in the sublingual, and 6.5 per cent in the minor salivary glands. In the parotid gland, 80 per cent occur in the superficial lobe, 15 per cent in the deep lobe, and 5 per cent in both lobes. Incidence peaks in the fifth decade; 60 per cent of these tumors occur in women. Mixed tumors rarely are bilateral or multicentric.

D. Because there is a high probability of recurrence after enucleation, (greater than 50 per cent),[1] superficial lobectomy is the treatment of choice for all benign mixed tumors except those located in the deep lobe or in both lobes, when total conservative parotidectomy is indicated.[1, 2, 14, 25]

E. Morbidity of re-excision includes:[15, 25]
   - VIII cranial nerve weakness
     - temporary: 41 per cent
     - permanent: 3 per cent
   - fistula: 0.4 per cent
   - infection: 0.6 per cent
   - hematoma-seroma: 6.5 per cent
   - Frey's syndrome: 8–30 per cent

F. Incidence of recurrence variously is cited to be from 2 to 50 per cent.[1, 13, 25] Recurrence presumably is due to tumor cell spillage or incomplete excision. Recurrences may be widespread throughout the remaining gland and this, as well as fibrotic distortion, may require sacrifice of the VII cranial nerve while carrying out total parotidectomy.[13, 24, 25]

G. Malignant tumors may not differ in size from benign ones but may demonstrate VII cranial nerve involvement (pain, weakness) and grow quickly.[10, 14, 18-20] Seventy per cent occur in the superficial lobe 5 per cent in the deep lobe and 25 per cent in both lobes. Moderately malignant types are (1) acinous cell tumors, which are multicentric and occur twice as often in women as in men; (2) adenoid cystic tumors, which are locally very invasive — 40 per cent have metastases when first diagnosed; and (3) mucoepidermoid tumors, 90 per cent of which are low grade with only local spread. Highly malignant tumors include (1) adenocarcinoma; which may occur between the second and seventh decades and may act as high or low grade. Metastases are frequent in the high grade; (2) undifferentiated, which occurs between the seventh and eighth decade; (3) squamous, characterized by rapid growth and occurring between the fifth and sixth decade; (4) malignant mixed, occurring in the sixth decade. Its metastasis rate is 43 to 70 per cent, with metastasis most commonly in the regional nodes and lungs.

H. If the VII cranial nerve appears to be involved, it should be sacrificed.[2-4, 6, 10, 14, 18-21] Morbidity is the same as for benign lesions, but the incidence differs.[25]
   - VII cranial nerve weakness
     - temporary: 57 per cent
     - permanent: 36 per cent
   - fistula: 0.9 per cent
   - infection: 0.1 per cent
   - hematoma-seroma: 6 per cent
   - Frey's syndrome: 12 per cent

   Palsy of the VII cranial nerve produces a significant cosmetic and functional deformity. Reconstructive techniques are available running the gamut from facelift to static and dynamic slings to microscopic fascicular nerve grafting.

I. Indications for radical neck dissection include (1) clinically positive nodes and (2) undifferentiated cell type. Since 50 per cent of clinically negative necks have pathologically positive nodes, some physicians advocate routine prophylactic neck dissection.[1, 7, 14, 17-19, 21]

J. Radiation is indicated for unresectable tumors and deep tumors with fixation, skin involvement, highly anaplastic cell type, or incomplete surgical removal. It decreases the tumor bulk temporarily.

K. Five-year survival does not equate with permanent cure. For adenoid cystic tumors, 5-year survival is 75 per cent, while 20-year survival is only 13 per cent. For adenocarcinoma, 5-year survival is 78 per cent and 20-year survival is 41 per cent.

L. Retreatment may involve any of several modalities, depending upon cell type, location, and the presence of widespread disease. Treatment may include further

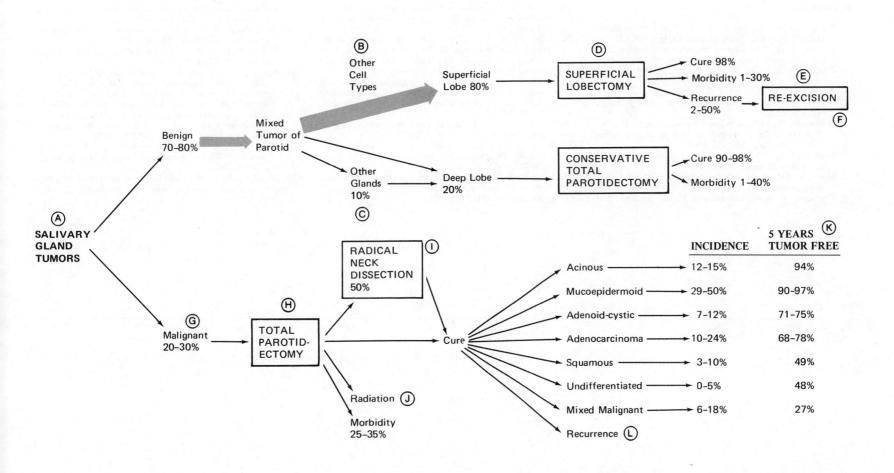

(A) SALIVARY GLAND TUMORS

Benign 70–80%

(B) Other Cell Types

Mixed Tumor of Parotid

(C) Other Glands 10%

Superficial Lobe 80%

Deep Lobe 20%

(D) SUPERFICIAL LOBECTOMY

Cure 98%
Morbidity 1–30%
Recurrence 2–50%

(E) RE-EXCISION (F)

CONSERVATIVE TOTAL PAROTIDECTOMY

Cure 90–98%
Morbidity 1–40%

(G) Malignant 20–30%

(H) TOTAL PAROTID-ECTOMY

(I) RADICAL NECK DISSECTION 50%

(J) Radiation

Morbidity 25–35%

Cure

	INCIDENCE	5 YEARS (K) TUMOR FREE
Acinous	12–15%	94%
Mucoepidermoid	29–50%	90–97%
Adenoid-cystic	7–12%	71–75%
Adenocarcinoma	10–24%	68–78%
Squamous	3–10%	49%
Undifferentiated	0–5%	48%
Mixed Malignant	6–18%	27%
Recurrence (L)		

61

TUMORS OF THE SALIVARY GLAND *Continued*

surgical excision, radiotherapy, or chemotherapy.

References

1. Batsakis, J. G.: Tumors of the Head and Neck. Baltimore, Williams & Wilkins Co., 1974, pp. 1–51.
2. Beahrs, O. H.: The surgical anatomy and technique of parotidectomy. Surg. Clin. North Am., 57:477, 1977.
3. Beahrs, O. H.: The facial nerve in parotid surgery. Surg. Clin. North Am., 43:973, 1963.
4. Beahrs, O. H., and Chong, G. C.: Management of the facial nerve in parotid gland surgery. Am. J. Surg., 142:473, 1972.
5. Beahrs, O. H., Judd, E. S., and Woodington, G. F.: Use of nerve grafts for repair of defects in the facial nerve. Ann. Surg., 153:433, 1961.
6. Beahrs, O. H., et al.: Surgical management of parotid lesions. Arch. Surg., 80:890, 1960.
7. Byers, R. M., et al.: Malignant tumors of the submaxillary gland. Am. J. Surg., 126:458, 1973.
8. Converse, J. M.: Reconstructive Plastic Surgery. 2nd ed., vols. 3 and 5. Philadelphia, W. B. Saunders Co., 1977, pp. 1794–1840, 2521–2546, 1884–1867.
9. Elkon, J., Colman, M., and Hendrickson, F. R.: Radiation therapy in the treatment of malignant salivary gland tumors. Cancer, 41:502, 1978.
10. Eneroth, C. M.: Facial nerve paralysis — A criterion for malignancy in parotid tumors. Arch. Otolaryngol. 95:300, 1972.
11. Foote, F. W., Jr., and Frazell, E. L.: Tumors of the major salivary glands. *In* Atlas of Tumor Pathology, section IV, fascicle 11. Washington, D.C., Armed Forces Institute of Pathology, 1954.
12. Guillamondegui, O. M., et al.: Aggressive surgery in treatment for parotid cancer. The role of adjunctive postoperative radiotherapy. Am. J. Roentgenol., 123:49, 1975.
13. Hanna, D. C., et al.: Management of recurrent salivary gland tumors. Am. J. Surg., 132:453, 1976.
14. Hanna, D. C., and Gaisford, J. C.: Parotid gland tumors: Diagnosis and treatment. Am. J. Surg., 104:737, 1962.
15. Laage-Hellman, J. E.: Gustatory sweating and flushing after conservative parotidectomy. Acta Otolaryngol. (Stockh.), 48:234, 1957.
16. Nanson, E. M.: Surgery of the deep lobe of the parotid gland. Surg. Gynecol. Obstet., 122:811, 1966.
17. Perzik, S. L., and Fisher, B.: The place of neck dissection in the management of parotid tumors. Am. J. Surg., 120:355, 1970.
18. Rafla, S.: Malignant parotid tumors: Natural history and treatment. Cancer, 40:136, 1977.
19. Richardson, G. S., et al.: Tumors of salivary glands. Plast. Reconstr. Surg., 55:131, 1975.
20. Robins, R. E., et al.: Carcinoma of the parotid gland. Am. J. Surg., 134:120, 1977.
21. Spiro, R. H., Huvos, A. G., and Strong, E. W.: Cancer of the parotid gland. Am. J. Surg., 130:452, 1975.
22. Spiro, R. H., Hajdu, S., and Strong, E. W.: Tumors of the submaxillary gland. Am. J. Surg., 132:463, 1976.
23. Woods, J. E., and Beahrs, O. H.: A technique for the performance of rapid parotidectomy with minimal risk. Surg. Gynecol. Obstet. 142:87, 1976.
24. Woods, J. E., Chong, G. C., and Beahrs, O. H.: Experience with 1360 primary parotid tumors. Am. J. Surg., 130:460, 1975.
25. Woods, J. E., et al.: Pathology and surgery of primary tumors of the parotid. Surg. Clin. North Am., 57:565, 1977

CANCER OF THE VOCAL CORDS

CANCER OF THE VOCAL CORDS BY ARLEN D. MEYERS, M.D.

Comments

A. Sixty per cent of laryngeal cancers involve the glottis, and 98 per cent are squamous.

B. Synchronous and metachronous tumors are usually squamous also and related to smoking and alcohol abuse.

C. Carcinoma *in situ* is an intraepithelial malignancy with full-thickness epithelial dysplasia but without basement membrane invasion. Radiation and operative excision have approximately the same cure rate.[13]

D. A T_1 lesion may involve one commissure, but the cords are mobile. The probability of cervical metastasis is 0.5 to 2 per cent with mid-cord lesions and 4 to 8 per cent if the arytenoid cartilages, anterior commissure, or supraglottic or subglottic structures are involved.

E. Following radiotherapy of a T_1 lesion, 80 per cent of patients have normal voice.

F. Laryngofissure and cordectomy involve preoperative tracheostomy, followed by subperichondral removal of the vocal cords with immediate reconstruction. Hospitalization is usually for 5 to 7 days. Hoarseness is universal postoperatively.

G. Vertical hemilaryngectomy removes the false vocal cords and arytenoid cartilage. Reconstruction to achieve glottic competence uses muscle, cartilages, or fat grafts. Hospitalization is for 5 to 7 days. Hoarseness is universal, and about 20 per cent of patients have aspiration difficulties postoperatively.

H. Indications for total laryngectomy include:[11]
   Tumor fixation of one or both cords
   Subglottic tumor extension greater than 1 cm
   Extralaryngeal tumor spread
   Interarytenoid cancer
   Extension to cricopharyngeus, pre-epiglottic space, or other areas.
Total laryngectomy involves en bloc excision with the thyroid cartilage and surrounding soft tissue. Hospitalization is for 7 to 10 days. Complications include pharyngocutaneous fistula (30 per cent of cases) and wound infection (20 per cent of cases). Patients' postoperative speech is as follows:[15] 64 per cent can use esophageal voice, 5 per cent use esophageal voice plus an artificial device, 10 per cent use an artificial device alone, and 12 per cent have no speech at all.

I. Dose of preoperative radiotherapy varies from 3000 to 7000 rads. Postoperative complication rates are high following radiation[7] and include mortality (4 per cent), pharyngocutaneous fistula (50 per cent), loss of flap from infection (25 per cent), and carotid blowout (10 per cent).

References

1. American Joint Committee for Cancer Staging and End Results Reporting: Clinical Staging Symptoms for Cancer of the Larynx. Chicago, Am. Joint Committee, 1962, pp. 1–11.
2. Wang, C. C., and Shultz, M. D.: Treatment of cancer of the larynx by irradiation. Ann. Otolaryngol., 72:635–646, 1963.
3. McGavron, M. H., Bauer, W. C., and Ogura, J. H.: The incidence of cervical lymph node metastases from epidermal carcinoma of the larynx and their relationship to certain characteristics of the primary tumor. Cancer, *14*:56–66, 1961.
4. Sessions, D. G., Marress, C. M., and McSwain, B.: Laryngofissure in the treatment of carcinoma of the vocal cord. A report of forty cases and a review of the literature. Laryngoscope, 75:490, 1965.
5. Leroux-Robert, J. L.: A statistical study of 620 laryngeal carcinomas of the glottic region personally operated upon more than five years ago. Laryngoscope, 85:1440, 1975.
6. Vermund, H.: Role of radiotherapy in cancer of the larynx as related to the TNM system of staging. Cancer, 25:485, 1970.
7. Goldman, J. L., et al.: Combined radiation and surgical therapy for cancer of the larynx and laryngopharynx. Laryngoscope, 74:1111–1134, 1964.

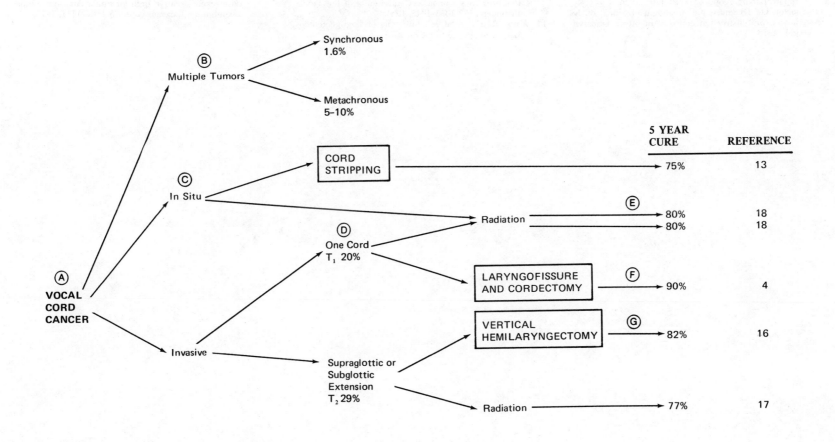

CANCER OF THE VOCAL CORDS *Continued*

8. Holinger, P. H., and Schild, J. A.: Carcinoma *in situ* of the larynx. Can. J. Otolaryngol., 3:549–50, 1974.
9. Skolnik, E. M., et al.: Carcinoma of the laryngeal glottis: Therapy and end results. Laryngoscope, 85:1453–1466, 1975.
10. Ogura, J. H., et al.: Long term therapeutic results — cancer of the larynx and hypopharynx: Preliminary report. Laryngoscope, 85:1746–1761, 1976.
11. Spector, G.: Diagnosis and treatment of cancer of the larynx: Self-instruction course. Am. Acad. Otolaryngol., 1978.
12. Som, M. L.: Hemilaryngectomy: a modified technique for cordal carcinoma with extension posteriorly. Arch. Otolaryngol., 54:524–533, 1951.
13. Doyle, P. J., Florex, A., and Douglas, G. S.: Carcinoma *in situ* of the larynx. Laryngoscope, 87:310–316, 1977.
14. Fletcher, G. H., and Klein, R.: Dose-time-volume relationships in squamous-cell carcinoma of the larynx. Radiology, 182:1032–1042, 1964.
15. Watts, R. F.: Total rehabilitation of laryngectomees. Laryngoscope, 85:671–673, 1975.
16. Ogura, J. H., Sessions, D. G., and Spector, G. J.: Analysis of surgical therapy for epidermoid carcinoma of the laryngeal glottis. Laryngoscope, 85:1522–1530, 1975.
17. Perez, C. A., et al.: Radiation therapy of early carcinoma of the true vocal cords. Cancer, 21:764–771, 1968.
18. Stewart, J. G., and Jackson, A. W.: The steepness of the dose response curve both for tumor cure and normal tissue injury. Laryngoscope, 85:1107–1111, 1975.

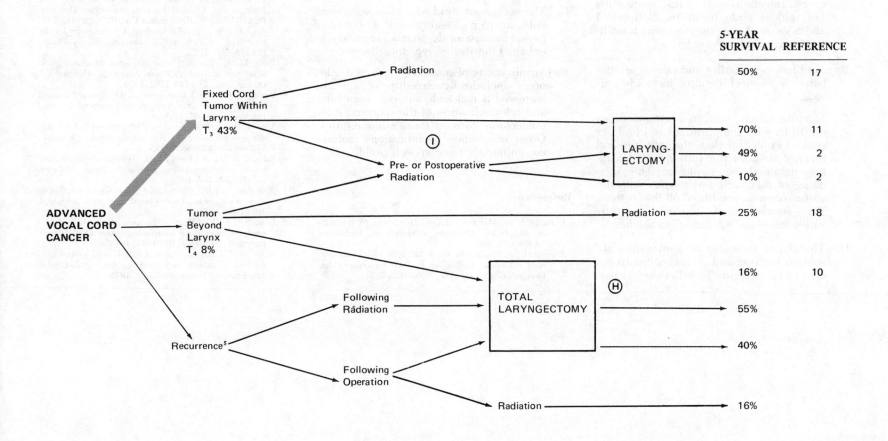

5-YEAR
SURVIVAL   REFERENCE

Fixed Cord
Tumor Within
Larynx
T₃ 43%

Radiation — 50%   17

LARYNG-
ECTOMY

70%   11

Pre- or Postoperative
Radiation

49%   2

10%   2

ADVANCED
VOCAL CORD
CANCER

Tumor
Beyond
Larynx
T₄ 8%

Radiation — 25%   18

TOTAL
LARYNGECTOMY

16%   10

Following
Radiation

55%

Recurrence⁵

40%

Following
Operation

Radiation — 16%

ACUTE EXUDATIVE TONSILLITIS/ADENOID HYPERTROPHY BY JERRY TEMPLER, M.D.

Comments

A. Streptococcus is the responsible organism in 40 per cent of cases. The first attack characteristically occurs between 3 and 4 years of age. Prior to that time, streptococcus infections might cause acute otitis but seldom acute tonsillitis. Between 4 and 8 years of age, streptococcus tonsillitis is particularly severe.[1, 2]

B. Antibiotics (penicillin and others) are the basis of medical therapy for each episode.

C. Mortality from untreated streptococcus tonsillitis with complications is 1 to 3 per cent.[3, 4] Penicillin stops the infection and therapy obviates the subsequent damaging immunologic sequelae. The incidence of rheumatic fever varies with the socioeconomic condition of the patient. The incidence of glomerulonephritis varies from one "epidemic" to another.[5]

D. The classic treatment of peritonsillar abscess is incision and drainage, but 10 per cent of cases recur. Tonsillectomy is performed electively about 6 weeks later. Early tonsillectomy with good antibiotic coverage has no more risk than interval operation and completely opens the tonsillar fossa, thus avoiding possible future abscess.[6]

E. The occasional child who loses weight or fails to gain weight over a 6-month period because of dysphagia secondary to enlarged tonsils deserves tonsillectomy.[8]

F. Complications of massively enlarged adenoids include hyponasality of speech, narrowed dental arch, anterior open bite, and retroinclination of the incisors. Adenoidectomy corrects these abnormalities. Other uncommon complications include cor pulmonale[10] and speech problems.[9]

References

1. Rantz, L. A., Maroney, M., and Di Caprio, J.: Hemolytic streptoccal infections in childhood. Pediatrics, 12:498–515, 1953.
2. Sprinkle, P. M., and Veltri, R. W.: The tonsil and adenoid dilemma: medical or surgical treatment. Otolaryngol. Clin. North Am., 7:909–925, 1974.
3. McCammon, R. W.: Natural history of respiratory tract infection patterns in basically healthy individuals. Am. J. Dis. Child., 122:232–236, 1971.
4. Vosti, K. L.: Streptococcal diseases. In Hoeprich, P. D. Infectious Diseases, 2nd ed. New York, Harper and Row, 1977, pp. 235–245.
5. Earle, D. P.: Acute glomerulonephritis. In Youmans, G. P., Paterson, P. Y., and Sommers, H. M. (eds.): The Biologic and Clinical Basis of Infectious Diseases. Philadelphia, W. B. Saunders Co., 1975, pp. 212–216.
6. Templer, J. W., et al.: Immediate tonsillectomy for the treatment of peritonsillar abscess. Am. J. Surg., 134:596–598, 1977.
7. Pratt, L. W.: Tonsillectomy and adenoidectomy: mortality and morbidity. Trans. Am. Acad. Ophthalmol. Otolaryngol., 74:1146–1152, 1970.
8. Paradise, J. L., and Bluestone, C. D.: Toward rational indications for tonsil and adenoid surgery. Hospital Practice, 11:79–87, 1976.
9. Morris, H. L.: The speech pathologist looks at the tonsils and the adenoids. Ann. Otol. Rhinol. Laryngol., 84(Suppl. 19):63–66, 1975.
10. Edison, B. D., and Kerth, J. D.: Tonsilloadenoid hypertrophy resulting in cor pulmonale. Arch. Otolaryngol., 98:205–207, 1973.
11. Bluestone, C. D.: Obstructive adenoids in relation to otitis media. Ann. Otol. Rhinol. Laryngol., 84(Suppl. 19):44–48, 1975.
12. Subtelny, J. D.: Effect of diseases of tonsils and adenoids on dentofacial morphology. Ann. Otol. Rhinol. Laryngol., 84(Suppl. 19):50–54, 1975.
13. Stool, S. E.: Diseases of the tonsils and adenoids in relation to rhinitis and sinusitis. Ann. Otol. Rhinol. Laryngol., 84(Suppl. 19):73–74, 1975.

ACUTE EXUDATIVE TONSILLITIS AND HYPERTROPHY OF THE ADENOIDS

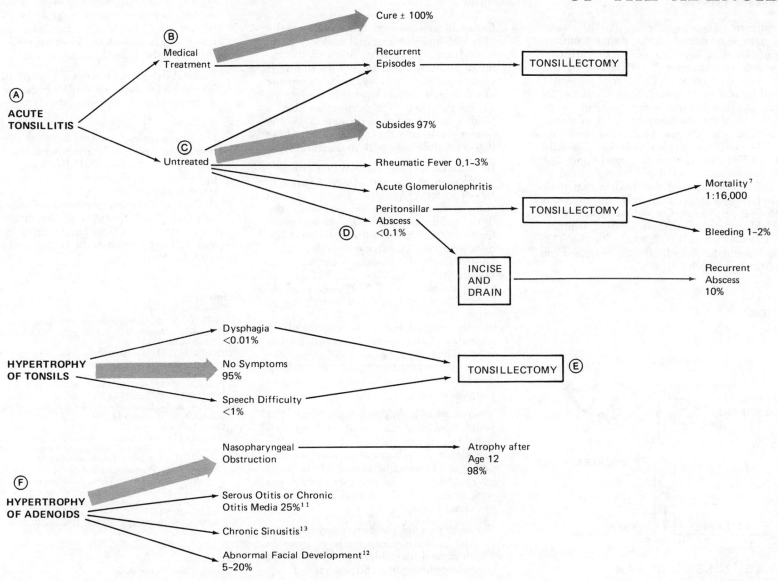

Cure ± 100%

Ⓑ
Medical
Treatment

Recurrent
Episodes → TONSILLECTOMY

Ⓐ
**ACUTE
TONSILLITIS**

Subsides 97%

Ⓒ
Untreated

Rheumatic Fever 0.1–3%

Acute Glomerulonephritis

Peritonsillar → TONSILLECTOMY → Mortality[7]
Abscess   1:16,000
<0.1%
Ⓓ   Bleeding 1–2%

INCISE
AND
DRAIN → Recurrent
         Abscess
         10%

Dysphagia
<0.01%

**HYPERTROPHY
OF TONSILS** → No Symptoms
                95% → TONSILLECTOMY **Ⓔ**

Speech Difficulty
<1%

Nasopharyngeal → Atrophy after
Obstruction   Age 12
                   98%

Ⓕ
**HYPERTROPHY
OF ADENOIDS** → Serous Otitis or Chronic
                 Otitis Media 25%[11]

Chronic Sinusitis[13]

Abnormal Facial Development[12]
5–20%

CONDUCTIVE HEARING LOSS BY BRUCE W. JAFEK, M.D., AND THOMAS J. BALKANY, M.D.

Preliminary Concepts

Conductive hearing losses (CHL) occur from pathology lateral to the stapes footplate *(arrow)*. Hearing losses medial to this are *sensorineural* in character. CHL lateral to the tympanic membrane (TM) are generally caused by obstruction (e.g., from cerumen, an insect, or other foreign body), the removal of which will allow transmission of a vibrating air column (sound wave) to the TM. Between the TM and the stapes footplate (middle zone), CHL are caused by conditions that limit free vibration of the TM (e.g., fluid in the area, perforation of the TM) or that limit transmission of that vibration by the ossicular chain (e.g., fracture). Correction requires the re-establishment of a freely mobile, continuous ossicular chain in contact with the TM, laterally, and an intact, mobile footplate (or substitute), medially.

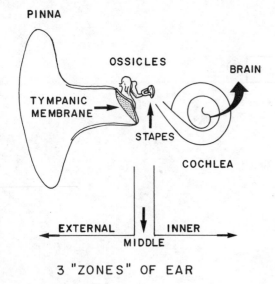

PINNA

OSSICLES

BRAIN

TYMPANIC MEMBRANE

STAPES

COCHLEA

EXTERNAL   INNER

MIDDLE

3 "ZONES" OF EAR

Comments

A. Cerumen and foreign bodies should be removed from the external auditory canal under direct vision. Irrigation of the external auditory canal to remove debris is contraindicated unless the tympanic membrane is intact. Irrigation performed in the presence of a perforation that is hidden by a foreign body may force the foreign body into the middle ear, where it is accessible only with major surgery.

B. In bilateral atresia, correction is usually undertaken on one ear at age 4 (prior to school entry). Operation on the second side, or in unilateral cases, is often deferred until age 16 to 18, when the patient can participate in the decision. Children with one good ear develop fairly normally, and the operation carries a significant risk (13 to 30 per cent) of damage to the facial nerve.[9-11] The degree of abnormality of the sound-conducting mechanism of the external and middle ears is usually proportional to the degree of abnormality of the pinna. Prognosis for improving hearing is worse with greater degrees of abnormality, and the risk of damage to the facial nerve is proportionately greater.

C. Tympanostomy (myringotomy and TM ventilation tube placement) is least successful in allergic patients. The morbidity includes infected draining ears in 15.1 per cent of cases, occlusion of the tube by clotted serum or cerumen in 2.4 per cent of cases, and external otitis in 1.0 per cent of cases.[7, 8]

D. Removal of cholesteatoma may cause a decline in hearing, especially in cases in which radical mastoidectomy (removal of tympanic membrane and ossicles) is required. Reconstruction following removal of the cholesteatoma is possible in 75 to 90 per cent of selected cases, but recurrence of cholesteatoma is more common than with the radical mastoidectomy.[5]

E. Re-establishment of normal hearing (0 to 30 dB SRT[a]) depends on the presence of a normal inner ear preoperatively.

F. Stapedectomy produces excellent hearing in approximately 90 per cent of operations. Worsening of hearing occurs in 1 to 3 per cent of cases and dizziness in 17 per cent of cases. The dizziness is usually transient; however, in 1 to 2 per cent of patients the dizziness persists for 6 months or more. Total deafness of the operated ear occurs in less than 1 per cent of cases and is more common in revision stapedectomy.[18]

References

1. Cody, D. T. R., and Taylor, W. F.: Tympanoplasty: Long-term results with incus grafts. Laryngoscope, 83:852–864, 1973.
2. Hough, J. V. D.: Tympanoplasty with the interior fascial graft technique and ossicular reconstruction. Laryngoscope, 83:1385–1413, 1970.
3. Paparella, M. M., and Shumrick, D. A.: Otolaryngology. Vol. 2: Ear. Philadelphia, W. B. Saunders, 1973.
4. Shambaugh, G. E.: Surgery of the Ear, 2nd ed. Philadelphia, W. B. Saunders, 1967, pp. 429–524.
5. Cody, D. T. R., and Taylor, W. F.: Mastoidectomy for acquired active chronic suppurative otitis media. Parts I and II: Chronic infection. J. Contin. Ed. Otorhinolaryngol. Allergy, July-September 1978.
6. Crabtree, J. A.: Tympanoplastic techniques in congenital atresia. Arch. Otolaryngol., 88:89–96, 1968.
7. Birck, H. G., and Mravel, J. J.: Myringotomy for middle ear effusions. Ann. Otol. Rhinol. Laryngol., 85:263–269, 1977.
8. Hughs, L. A., Warden, F. R., and Hudson, W. R.: Com-

---

[a]Speech reception threshold

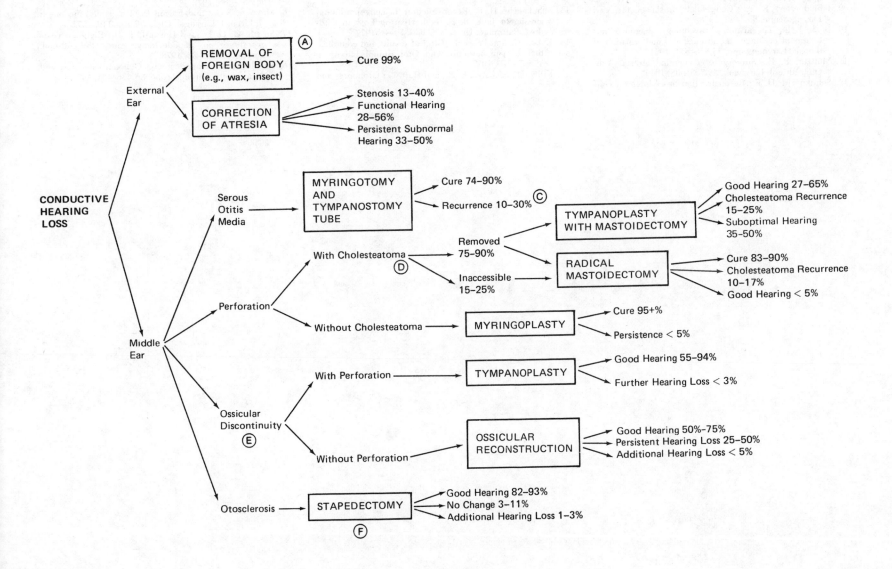

plications of tympanostomy tubes. Arch. Otolaryngol., *100*:151–154, 1974.

9. Jahrsdoerfer, R. A.: Congenital atresia of the ear. Laryngoscope, *88*:1–48, 1978.

10. Beck, J. L.: The anatomy, psychology, diagnosis and treatment of congenital absence and malformation of the ear. Laryngoscope, *35*:813–831, 1921.

11. Meltzer, P. E.: Surgery for congenital atresia. Ann. Otol. Rhinol. Laryngol., *58*:798–808, 1949.

12. Schuknecht, H. F.: Reconstruction procedures for congenital aural atresia. Arch. Otolaryngol., *101*:170–172, 1975.

13. Schuknecht, H. F.: Reconstruction for congenital aural atresia. *In* Jaffe, B. F. (ed.): Hearing Loss in Children. Baltimore, University Park Press, 1977.

14. Kokko, E., and Palva, T.: Clinical results and complications of tympanostomy. Ann. Otol. Rhinol. Laryngol., *85*:277–279, 1977.

15. Kilby, D., Richards, S. H., and Hart, G.: Grommets and glue ears: two-year results. J. Laryngol., Otol., *86*:881–888, 1972.

16. Mawson, S. K., and Fagan, P.: Tympanic effusions in children. J. Laryngol. Otol., *86*:105–119, 1972.

17. Smyth, G. D. L., and Hassard, T. H.: Eighteen years' experience in stapedectomy. Ann. Otol. Rhinol., Laryngol., *87*:1–36, 1978.

18. Sheehy, J. L.: Stapedectomy: Gelfoam compared with tissue grafts. Laryngoscope, *86*:436–444, 1976.

Vascular

CEREBROVASCULAR INSUFFICIENCY BY ROBERT G. SCRIBNER, M.D.

Comments

A. Transient ischemic attack (TIA) is defined as a focal hemispheric symptom or monocular blindness lasting less than 24 hours. Reversible ischemic neurologic deficit (RIND) lasts longer than 24 hours and also is completely reversible. Both are produced by cerebral hypoperfusion or, more commonly, by embolization.

B. The history of untreated TIAs is frightening: 17 to 47 per cent of patients have recurrent TIAs, 7 to 48 per cent develop strokes within 3 to 5 years, and 17 to 32 per cent are dead within 4 years.[1]

C. Oral anticoagulants and antiplatelet drugs decrease the incidence of TIA and stroke but do not affect survival.

D. These studies, which visualize both carotid arteries, the vertebral arteries, and intracranial vessels, have mortality and morbidity rates about equivalent to those of carotid thromboendarterectomies.[2, 3]

E. Incidence of postoperative neurologic deficit is 8 per cent for ulcerating plaque and 2 to 3 per cent for stenotic lesions.[4]

F. Carotid thromboendarterectomy (TEA) does not significantly affect longevity.

Death is usually due to myocardial infarct or other manifestations of generalized atherosclerosis.

G. Totally occluded internal carotid arteries cannot be reopened and must be bypassed if operation is indicated. There is only one report[7] of a significant number of cases. Most surgeons have much higher morbidity and mortality rates and a lower cure rate in avoiding subsequent TIAs.

H. Indications for operative repair of an asymptomatic carotid bruit are controversial. They depend on the degree of stenosis and the likelihood of future stroke. Seventeen per cent of patients have stroke as a first subsequent symptom.[8] Angiographically significant progression of stenosis occurs in 62 per cent of cases.[9] Following TEA on one carotid artery, a bruit on the other will rarely (1 in 111) first become manifest as a stroke.[10]

I. Carotid thromboendarterectomy is contraindicated (mortality up to 60 per cent[5]) following a fresh stroke. Some physicians claim that interval TEA (more than 6 weeks) improves neurologic status. Carotid TEA diminishes the probability of recurrent strokes as it does following TIAs.

J. The rarity of these lesions provides no statistically valid data.

K. Resection and graft replacement is indicated for those patients whose dissected segment is totally accessible.[11]

L. Sixteen per cent of routine carotid angiograms demonstrate tortuosity, but most of these are clinically unimportant.[12]

M. Ninety per cent of these cases are females. In one series of 40 carotid operations, only one transient postoperative neurologic deficit occurred. There were no late strokes.[13]

References

1. Toole, J.F., et al.: Transient ischemic attacks due to atherosclerosis. Arch. Neurol., 32:5, 1975.
2. Haas, W.K., et al.: Joint study of extracranial arterial occlusion. II. Arteriography. Techniques, Sites, and Complications. JAMA, 203:159, 1968.
3. Pessin, M.S., et al.: Clinical and angiographic features of carotid transient ischemic attacks. N. Engl. J. Med., 296:358, 1977.
4. Hertzer, N.R., et al.: Internal carotid back pressure, intraoperative shunting, ulcerated atheromata, and the incidence of stroke during carotid endarterectomy. Surgery, 83:306, 1978.
5. Thompson, J.E., and Talkington, C.M.: Carotid endarterectomy. Ann. Surg., 184:1, 1976.

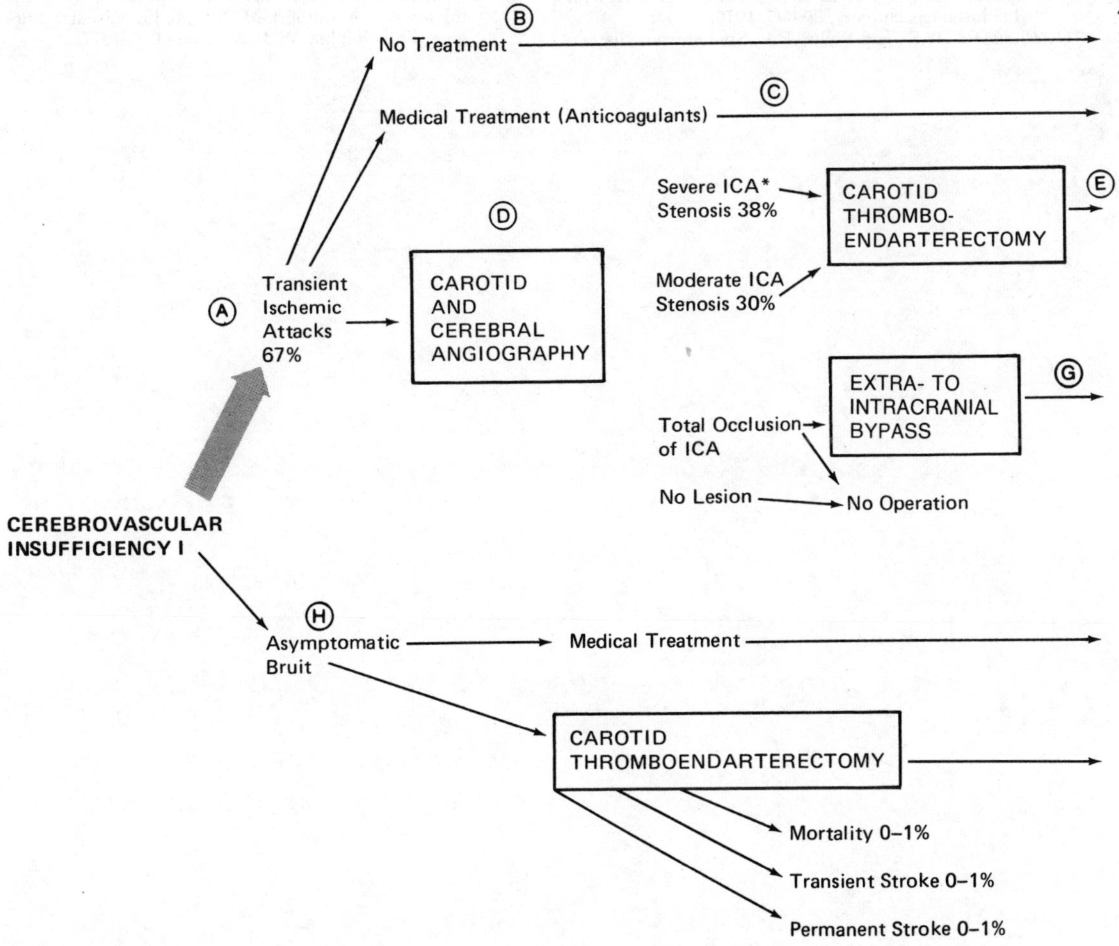

4-YEAR RESULTS (%)

	Cure	Recurrent TIA	Stroke	Alive	Ref.
Ⓑ No Treatment	45	24	26	79	1
Ⓒ Medical Treatment (Anticoagulants)	51	19	17	78	1
Ⓔ CAROTID THROMBO-ENDARTERECTOMY	93	5	5	80 Ⓕ	4–6
Ⓖ EXTRA- TO INTRACRANIAL BYPASS	90	5	4	90	7
Ⓗ Medical Treatment	56	27	17	75	8
CAROTID THROMBOENDARTERECTOMY	94	4	2	67	8,10

Ⓐ Transient Ischemic Attacks 67%

Ⓓ CAROTID AND CEREBRAL ANGIOGRAPHY

Severe ICA* Stenosis 38%

Moderate ICA Stenosis 30%

Total Occlusion of ICA

No Lesion → No Operation

CEREBROVASCULAR INSUFFICIENCY I

Asymptomatic Bruit

Mortality 0–1%

Transient Stroke 0–1%

Permanent Stroke 0–1%

*ICA = Internal carotid artery.

6. Stoney, R.J., and String, S.T.: Recurrent carotid stenosis. Surgery, *80:*705, 1976.

7. Popp, A.J., and Chater, N.: Extracranial-to-intracranial vascular anastomosis for occlusive cerebrovascular disease: Experience in 110 patients. Surgery, 82:648, 1977.

8. Thompson, J.E., Patman, R.D., and Talkington, C.M.: Asymptomatic carotid bruit — Long term outcome of patients having endarterectomy compared with unoperated controls. Ann. Surg., *188:*308, 1978.

9. Javid, H., et al.: Natural history of carotid bifurcation atheroma. Surgery, *67:*80, 1970.

10. Humphries, A.W., et al.: Unoperated asymptomatic significant internal carotid artery stenosis: A review of 182 instances. Surgery, *80:*695, 1976.

11. Ehrenfeld, W.K., and Wylie, E.J.: Spontaneous dissection of the internal carotid artery. Arch. Surg., *111:*1294, 1976.

12. Vannix, R.S., Joergenson, E.J., and Carter, R.: Kinking of the internal carotid artery. Am. J. Surg., *134:*82, 1977.

13. Ehrenfeld, W.K.: Fibromuscular dysplasia of the carotid artery. *In* Rutherford, R.B. (ed.): Vascular Surgery. Philadelphia, W. B. Saunders Co., 1977.

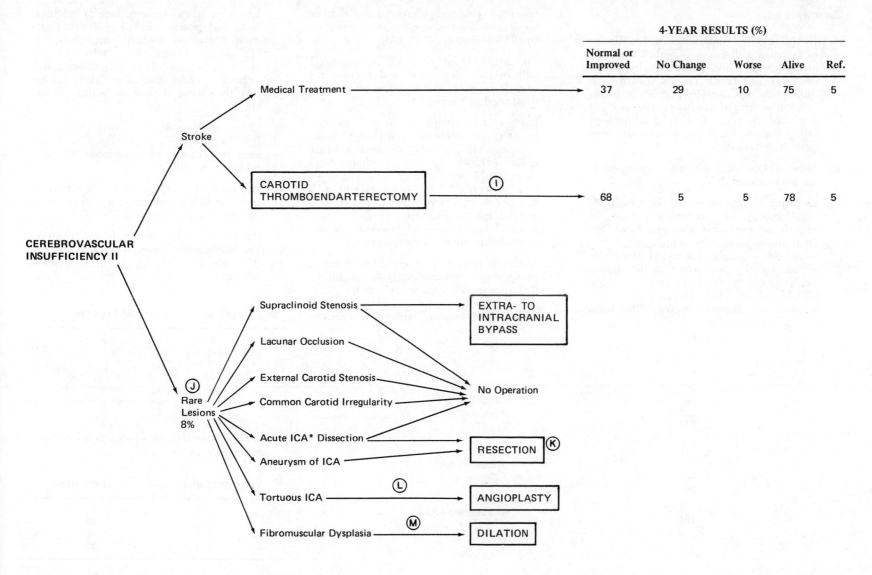

	4-YEAR RESULTS (%)				
	Normal or Improved	No Change	Worse	Alive	Ref.
Medical Treatment	37	29	10	75	5
CAROTID THROMBOENDARTERECTOMY	68	5	5	78	5

Stroke

CEREBROVASCULAR INSUFFICIENCY II

Ⓘ

Ⓙ
Rare Lesions 8%

Supraclinoid Stenosis → EXTRA- TO INTRACRANIAL BYPASS

Lacunar Occlusion

External Carotid Stenosis

Common Carotid Irregularity → No Operation

Acute ICA* Dissection

Aneurysm of ICA → RESECTION Ⓚ

Tortuous ICA ——Ⓛ——→ ANGIOPLASTY

Fibromuscular Dysplasia ——Ⓜ——→ DILATION

*ICA = Internal carotid artery.

ABDOMINAL AORTIC ANEURYSM BY RICHARD F. KEMPCZINSKI, M.D.

Comments

A. In this elderly population the incidence of associated diseases is high:[26] coronary arteriosclerosis (56 per cent), hypertension (54 per cent), chronic obstructive pulmonary disease (49 per cent), lower extremity arterial occlusive disease (13 per cent), peripheral arterial aneurysms (10 per cent),[3] and cerebrovascular disease (6 per cent).

B. Most abdominal aortic aneurysms (AAA) are asymptomatic.[22]

C. Decision for operation is individualized. Small aneurysms (less than 3 or 4 cm.) in elderly patients who otherwise have limited life expectancies should simply be observed. A similar aneurysm in an otherwise healthy person with a life expectancy longer than 5 to 10 years probably should be resected. Increasing size or symptoms of rupture are compelling indications for operation.

D. Objective evidence of increasing diameter is an indication for resection even in small (less than 6 cm.) AAAs.

E. The diameter of an AAA is measured with B-mode ultrasound, and most are resected electively.[11, 22] Relative survival is illustrated in Figure 1.[22]

F. Postoperative complications still are frequent[26] and include: pulmonary complications (40 per cent), congestive heart failure (37 per cent), myocardial infarction (2 to 15 per cent),[25, 26] renal failure (4 to 7 per cent),[25, 26] left colon ischemia (1 to 2 per cent),[16] amputation (2 per cent),[26] and paraplegia (0.25 per cent).[23] Impotence developed in 13 per cent of patients following elective resection.[14]

G. Although infection in an AAA is rare,[1] preoperative recognition is important so that appropriate antibiotics can be given and the graft placed in an uninfected bed. Indications of infection include fever, vertebral erosion, lack of calcification, and positive blood cultures. Common organisms include staphylococcus (41 per cent) and salmonella (18 per cent). AAAs infected by gram-negative organisms are 8 times more likely to rupture than those with gram-positive bacteria.[12]

H. Complete thrombosis of an AAA is rare[13] but occasionally occurs in small aneurysms (3 to 4 cm.) associated with distal occlusive disease.

I. A rapidly enlarging AAA mimicks rupture.[5] It is the indication for 10 per cent of urgent aortic resections.[22, 26]

J. Although small aneurysms can rupture, the probability varies with diameter. In 473 nonresected AAAs rupture[7] rates were:

SIZE (cm.)	% RUPTURED
<4	9.5
4–5	23
5–7	25
7–10	45
>10	60

The interval from diagnosis to rupture in 36 patients[21] was:

TIME INTERVAL (yr.)	% RUPTURED
< 1	39
1–2	69
1–3	80
1–4	92

FIGURE 1

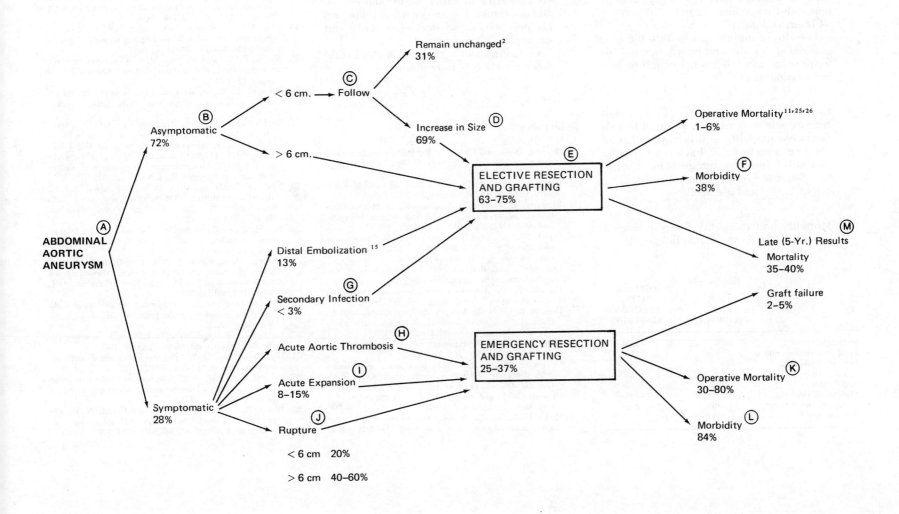

Remain unchanged[2]
31%

(C) < 6 cm. → Follow

(B) Asymptomatic
72%

Increase in Size (D)
69%

> 6 cm.

(E) ELECTIVE RESECTION
AND GRAFTING
63–75%

Operative Mortality[11,25,26]
1–6%

Morbidity (F)
38%

(M) Late (5-Yr.) Results
Mortality
35–40%

(A) ABDOMINAL
AORTIC
ANEURYSM

Distal Embolization[15]
13%

Secondary Infection (G)
< 3%

Acute Aortic Thrombosis (H)

Acute Expansion (I)
8–15%

Rupture (J)

EMERGENCY RESECTION
AND GRAFTING
25–37%

Graft failure
2–5%

Operative Mortality (K)
30–80%

Morbidity (L)
84%

Symptomatic
28%

< 6 cm   20%

> 6 cm   40–60%

Although sudden death may be the first indication of rupture, more than 50 per cent of patients survive longer than 6 hours and more than 40 per cent survive 24 hours or longer.[7]

The site of rupture can be into the free peritoneal cavity, retroperitoneum, inferior vena cava,[18] left renal vein,[20] or gastrointestinal tract.[10, 17]

K. Urgent resection because of suspected rupture when no rupture is found has an operative mortality equivalent to that of elective resection.[11, 26] Factors increasing mortality include intraperitoneal rupture,[6] anuria,[4] shock,[6] generalized atherosclerosis,[11, 24] and old age.[11]

L. Mortality and morbidity for resection of ruptured AAAs[11] are shown below:

	INCIDENCE (%)	COMPARISON WITH ELECTIVE RESECTION
Mortality		10×
Total complication rate		2×
Left colon ischemia		2×[16]
Spinal cord injury		10×[23]
Renal failure	26[9]	3–6×
Myocardial infarction	23[11]	2–10×
Congestive heart failure	30[24]	± same
Pneumonia	48[24]	

M. Patients surviving resection of AAAs have a 5-year mortality rate that is related primarily to other manifestations of atherosclerosis (i.e., myocardial infarction [41 per cent] or stroke [2 per cent]) and carcinoma (23 per cent).[11]

Graft infection with anastomotic breakdown or sepsis is infrequent.[11]

References

1. Bennett, D. E., and Cherry, J. K.: Bacterial infection of aortic aneurysms: A clinicopathologic study. Am. J. Surg., *113*:321, 1967.
2. Bernstein, E. F., et al.: Growth rates of small abdominal aortic aneurysms. Surgery, *80*:765, 1976.
3. Brewster, D. C., et al.: Angiography in the management of aneurysms of the abdominal aorta: Its value and safety. N. Engl. J. Med., *292*:822, 1975.
4. Couch, N. P., Lane, F. C., and Crane, C.: Management and mortality in resection of abdominal aortic aneurysms. Am. J. Surg., *119*:408, 1970.
5. Crisler, C., and Bahnson, H. T.: Aneurysms of the aorta. Curr. Probl. Surg., December 1972.
6. Darling, R. C.: Ruptured arteriosclerotic abdominal aortic aneurysms. Am. J. Surg., *119*:397, 1970.
7. Darling, R. C., et al.: Autopsy study of unoperated abdominal aortic aneurysms: The case for early resection. Circulation, *56* (Suppl. II):161, 1977.
8. Dent, T. L., et al.: Multiple arteriosclerotic arterial aneurysms. Arch. Surg., *105*:338, 1972.
9. DiGiovanni, R., et al.: Twenty-one years' experience with ruptured abdominal aortic aneurysms. Surg. Gynecol. Obstet., *141*:859, 1975.
10. Donovan, T. J., and Bucknam, C. A.: Aorto-enteric fistula. Arch. Surg., *95*:810, 1967.
11. Hicks, G. L., et al.: Survival improvement following aortic aneurysm resection. Ann. Surg., *181*:863, 1975.
12. Jarrett, F., et al.: Experience with infected aneurysms of the abdominal aorta. Arch. Surg., *110*:1281, 1975.
13. Jannetta, P. J., and Roberts, B.: Sudden complete thrombosis of an aneurysm of the abdominal aorta. N. Engl. J. Med., *264*:434, 1961.
14. May, A. G., DeWeese, J. A., and Rob, C. G.: Changes in sexual function following operation on the abdominal aorta. Surgery, *65*:41, 1969.
15. Nemir, P., Jr., and Micozzi, M. S.: Combined aneurysmal and occlusive arterial disease. Circulation, *56* (Suppl. II):169, 1977.
16. Ottinger, L. W., et al.: Left colon ischemia complicating aortoiliac reconstruction. Arch. Surg., *105*:841, 1972.
17. Reckless, J. P. D., McColl, I., and Taylor, G. W.: Aortoenteric fistulae: An uncommon complication of abdominal aortic aneurysms. Br. J. Surg., *59*:458, 1972.
18. Reckless, J. P. D., McColl, I., and Taylor, G. W.: Aortocaval fistulae: An uncommon complication of abdominal aortic aneurysms. Br. J. Surg., *59*:461, 1972.
19. Sommerville, R. L., Allen, E. V., and Edwards, J. E.: Bland and infected arteriosclerotic abdominal aortic aneurysms: A clinicopathologic study. Medicine, *38*:207, 1959.
20. Suzuki, M., et al.: Aorta–left renal vein fistula: An unusual complication of abdominal aortic aneurysm. Ann. Surg., *184*:31, 1976.
21. Szilagyi, D. E., Elliott, J. P., and Smith, R. F.: Clinical fate of the patient with asymptomatic abdominal aortic aneurysm and unfit for surgical treatment. Arch. Surg., *104*:600, 1972.
22. Szilagyi, D. E., et al.: Contribution of abdominal aortic aneurysmectomy to prolongation of life. Ann. Surg., *164*:678, 1966.
23. Szilagyi, D. E., et al.: Spinal cord damage in surgery of the abdominal aorta. Surgery, *83*:38, 1978.
24. Van Heeckeren, D. W.: Ruptured abdominal aortic aneurysms. Am. J. Surg., *119*:402, 1970.
25. Volpetti, G., et al.: A 22-year review of elective resection of abdominal aortic aneurysms. Surg. Gynecol. Obstet., *142*:321, 1976.
26. Young, A. E., Sandberg, G. W., and Couch, N. P.: The reduction of mortality of abdominal aortic aneurysm resection. Am. J. Surg., *134*:585, 1977.

LOWER EXTREMITY CLAUDICATION

LOWER EXTREMITY CLAUDICATION BY RICHARD F. KEMPCZINSKI, M.D.

Comments

A. Pain or cramping in the muscles precipitated by exercise and relieved by rest is usually diagnostic of arterial insufficiency.[12] Rest pain, invariably in the foot, and gangrene represent more advanced degrees of ischemia.

B. The prognosis for survival of patients who have claudication is distinctly worse than that of control patients, with cardiovascular disease accounting for 85 per cent of such deaths.[20] It is adversely affected by the association of symptomatic coronary artery disease (CAD), stroke (CVA), hypertension ($\uparrow$BP), and diabetes mellitus (DM).

	SURVIVAL (%)	
	5 Years[20]	10 Years[6]
Controls (same mean age)	90	
Claudicators (overall)	73	52
with associated conditions:		
CAD	55	9
CVA	61	
$\uparrow$BP	69	17
DM		8
DM and CAD	0[6]	

C. The majority of claudicators will remain stable or improve.[1, 10, 17] Proximal location of disease, cessation of smoking, continued exercise, weight reduction, control of hyperlipidemia, and meticulous attention to proper foot hygiene all affect prognosis favorably.[20]

D. Symptomatic progression usually occurs in patients who initially present with "severe" claudication (occurring in less than 300 feet walking distance),[10] associated diabetes mellitus (a 4 times greater risk of amputation),[20] or isolated femoropopliteal disease on angiography.[14]

E. With proper management most patients with claudication (64 per cent) will experience significant improvement or will adapt to their disability without the need for arterial reconstruction.[10]

F. Persistent, disabling symptoms force some patients to proceed with arterial revascularization even when there is no progression.

G. Even with symptomatic progression, 45 per cent of such patients will decide against vascular reconstruction and still will not progress to tissue loss.[10]

H. Most of the 6 to 7 per cent of patients with claudication who come to amputation[1, 10, 17] have "severe" claudication[10] or associated diabetes mellitus[20] or have continued smoking.[20]

I. Aortoiliac endarterectomy (AIE) is generally reserved for the younger patient (less than 55 years old) whose disease is confined to the distal aorta and the proximal common iliac arteries. Technically it is a more difficult procedure, but when indicated its results are excellent.[7] When patients with aortoiliofemoral disease were assigned preoperatively at random to either an endarterectomy or a bypass group, endarterectomy had to be abandoned in 27 per cent of cases intraoperatively because of technical considerations.[9]

J. Aortofemoral grafting (AFG) is more universally applicable than AIE. Although graft limb patency at 5 years is less (75 to 85 per cent)[7, 15] than that for AIE, patients selected for AFG characteristically have more generalized disease. Increased use of profunda femoris angioplasty at the distal anastomosis has improved 5-year limb patency to 90 per cent.[15] Continued smoking significantly reduces long-term patency.[19]

K. Axillofemoral grafting (AxFG) is a compromise procedure usually performed (88 per cent of cases) for limb salvage[8] when more conventional intra-abdominal procedures are contraindicated or when life expectancy is limited. In this elderly, high risk group, operative mortality is understandably high (2 to 8 per cent).[8-11] Rate of relief of claudication (75 per cent) parallels that of graft patency.[8] Unilateral grafts have the same patency as axillobifemoral grafts.[8] Secondary operative revision (usually thrombectomy) is required in 70 per cent of patients to maintain limb patency.[8]

L. Femorofemoral grafts (FFG) are generally reserved for poor risk patients with unilateral iliac arterial disease. Although used more liberally than AxFG, the procedure is still only rarely indicated for simple claudication (24 per cent of cases).[8] Operative mortality (5 to 15 per cent) is high in these poor risk patients requiring limb salvage.[2, 8] When performed for claudication, symptomatic relief is excellent. Five-year patency rates reflect the progression of distal arterial occlusive disease.[2, 8]

M. Profunda femoris angioplasty (PFA) is indicated for superficial femoral artery occlusion resulting in disabling claudication. It can be performed under local anesthesia when necessary. Complete relief of claudication is achieved in 40 to 50 per cent of patients, with significant improvement in 60 per cent.[16] Diabetes mellitus and occlusion of the popliteal artery both adversely affect the outcome.[4] Seventy-five per cent of patients with an

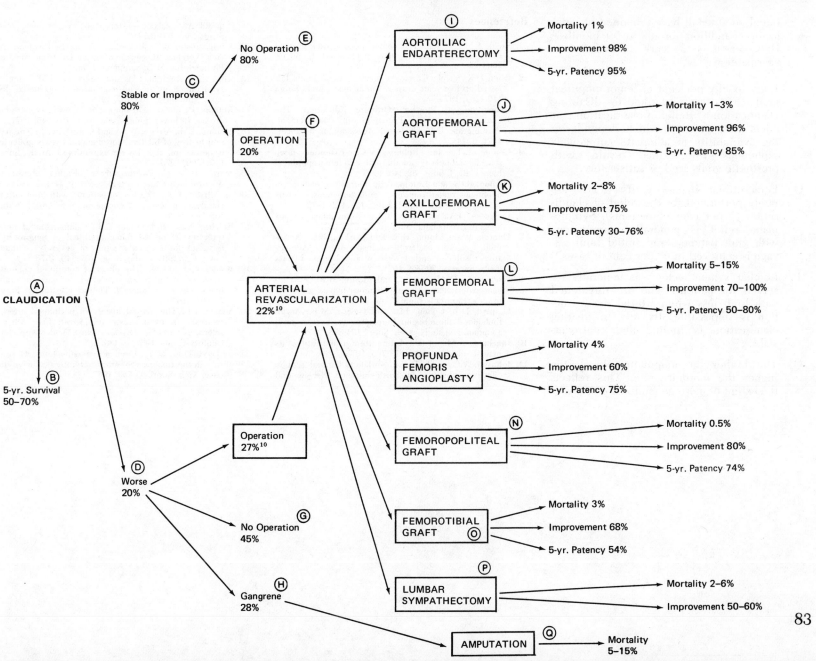

initial good result have remained in satisfactory condition for up to 39 months.[4] However, it is too early to evaluate 5-year patency.

N. Forty to fifty per cent of femoropopliteal grafts (FPG) are performed for disabling claudication.[5, 6] Relief of claudication parallels graft patency, which depends on the availability of adequate autogenous saphenous vein, since results with prosthetic grafts are less satisfactory.

O. Femorotibial bypass grafts (FTG) are rarely performed for the relief of claudication (7 per cent of patients). Symptomatic relief is generally synonymous with graft patency, and initial limb salvage is achieved in 68 per cent of cases.[18]

P. Lumbar sympathectomy is generally reserved for patients who are threatened with limb loss when arterial reconstruction is impossible. Its role in treating claudication is limited and controversial.[13, 21]

Q. The higher the amputation level, the higher the mortality rate. This reflects the extent of more generalized disease.[3]

References

1. Boyd, A.M.: The natural course of arteriosclerosis of the lower extremities. Proc. R. Soc. Med., 55:10, 1962.
2. Brief, D.K., et al.: Crossover femorofemoral grafts followed up five years or more: an analysis. Arch. Surg., 110:1294, 1975.
3. Committee on Prosthetic-Orthotic Education: The Geriatric Amputee: Principles of Management. Washington, D.C., National Academy of Sciences, 1971, p. 74.
4. Cotton, L.T., and Roberts, V.C.: Extended deep femoral angioplasty: an alternative to femoropopliteal bypass. Br. J. Surg., 62:340, 1975.
5. Darling, R.C., and Linton, R.R.: Durability of femoropopliteal reconstructions: endarterectomy versus vein bypass grafts. Am. J. Surg., 123:472, 1972.
6. DeWeese, J.A., and Rob, C.G.: Autogenous venous grafts ten years later. Surgery, 82:775, 1977.
7. Duncan, W.C., Linton, R.R., and Darling, R.C.: Aorto-iliofemoral atherosclerotic occlusive disease: comparative results of endarterectomy and Dacron bypass grafts. Surgery, 70:974, 1971.
8. Eugene, J., Goldstone, J., and Moore, W.S.: Fifteen-year experience with subcutaneous bypass grafts for lower extremity ischemia. Ann. Surg., 186:177, 1977.
9. Gaspard, D.J., Cohen, J.L., and Gaspar, M.R.: Aorto-iliofemoral thromboendarterectomy vs. bypass graft: a randomized study. Arch. Surg., 105:898, 1972.
10. Imparato, A.M., et al.: Intermittent claudication: its natural course. Surgery, 78:795, 1975.
11. Johnson, W.C., et al.: Is axillo–bilateral femoral graft an effective substitute for aortic–bilateral iliac–femoral graft? An analysis of ten years' experience. Ann. Surg., 186:123, 1977.
12. Kempczinski, R.F.: Leg claudication. In Eiseman, B., and Wotkyns, R. (eds.): Surgical Decision Making. Philadelphia, W.B. Saunders, 1978.
13. Kim, G.E., Ibrahim, I.M., and Imparato, A.M.: Lumbar sympathectomy in end-stage arterial occlusive disease. Ann. Surg., 183:157, 1976.
14. Kuthan, F., et al.: Development of occlusive arterial disease in lower limbs. Arch. Surg., 103:545, 1971.
15. Malone, J.M., Moore, W.S., and Goldstone, J.: The natural history of bilateral aortofemoral bypass grafts for ischemia of the lower extremities. Arch. Surg., 110:1300, 1975.
16. Martin, P., et al.: On the surgery of atherosclerosis of the profunda femoris artery. Surgery, 71:182, 1972.
17. McAllister, F.F.: The fate of patients with intermittent claudication managed nonoperatively. Am. J. Surg., 132:593, 1976.
18. Reichle, F.A., and Tyson, R.R.: Comparison of long-term results of 364 femoropopliteal or femorotibial bypasses for revascularization of severely ischemic lower extremities. Ann. Surg., 182:449, 1975.
19. Robicsek, F., et al.: The effect of continued cigarette smoking on the patency of synthetic vascular grafts in Leriche's syndrome. J. Thorac. Cardiovasc. Surg., 70:107, 1975.
20. Schatz, I.J.: The natural history of peripheral arteriosclerosis. In Brest, A.N., and Moyer, J.H.: Atherosclerotic Vascular Disease. New York, Appleton-Century-Crofts, 1967, p. 480.
21. Szilagyi, D.E., et al.: Lumbar sympathectomy: Current role in the treatment of arteriosclerotic occlusive disease. Arch. Surg., 95:753, 1967.

LUMBAR SYMPATHECTOMY

LUMBAR SYMPATHECTOMY BY R. TAWES, M.D., AND ROBERT G. SCRIBNER, M.D.

Comments

A. Lumbar sympathectomy is usually an adjuvant procedure to primary arterial reconstruction for ischemia of the lower extremity; it may be the sole procedure for (1) severe claudication with extensive lesions or (2) rest pain or ischemic ulcers in unreconstructible situations. Following sympathectomy, the temperature of the skin is permanently elevated but not to the degree noticed immediately following operation.[1] Responsible physiologic factors may be (a) increase in skin blood flow, (b) enhancement of arteriovenous shunts, or (c) decrease in peripheral vascular resistance. Muscle capillary flow probably is not increased.

B. Postsympathectomy neuralgia occurs in 8 to 35 per cent of patients. The pain usually begins one to two weeks after sympathectomy and remits gradually after a few weeks. It is often nocturnal, localized to the thigh, deep, and boring.[2, 3]

C. Women are not affected. In a large series of 1344 lumbar sympathectomies, 10 per cent of male patients experienced loss of ejaculation.[2] Nerve fibers serving ejaculation stem mainly from L1, with a few from L2. Vasomotor activity depends on L2, L3, and L4. The best compromise is resection of two ganglia at the L3-L4 level.

D. Orthostatic hypotension occurs only after simultaneous bilateral lumbar sympathectomy. It is related to the decrease in peripheral resistance and usually recedes in 10 to 14 days.[4] Postoperative retroperitoneal hemorrhage can cause hypotension but rarely requires reoperation. Rare complications are ureteral injury, prolonged ileus, and pulmonary embolism.

E. Patients who have disease limited to the femoropopliteal segments and who have no tissue necrosis may have an increased exercise tolerance.[2]

F. Pain relief may be related to decreasing vasoconstriction and norepinephrine at terminal sensory receptors. Most physicians do not believe that afferent sensory fibers exist in the sympathetic nervous system of the lower extremities.[4-6]

G. Healing of skin ulcers reflects the increase in skin blood flow. In one series of 29 patients, 62 per cent did not require amputation.[5]

H. Postoperative mortality is usually cardiac in origin. Long-term mortality (1 to 10 years) may be as low as 15 per cent, but for patients with limbs threatened by tissue loss, long-term survival reflects the malignant nature of severe arteriosclerosis — only 50 per cent are still alive at five years.[6, 7]

References

1. Delaney, J., and Scarpino, J.: Limb arteriovenous shunting following sympathetic denervation. Surgery, 73:202, 1973.
2. Callow, A. D., and Simeone, F. A.: The Grimonster symposium on the occasion of the 50th anniversary of the first lumbar sympathectomy. Arch. Surg., 113:295, 1978.
3. Raskin, N. H., et al.: Postsympathectomy neuralgia. Am. J. Surg., 128:75, 1974.
4. De Takats, G.: Sympathectomy revisited: Dodo or phoenix? Surgery, 78:644, 1975.
5. Kim, G. E., Ibrahim, I. M., and Imparato, A. M.: Lumbar sympathectomy in end-stage arterial occlusive disease. Ann. Surg., 183:157, 1976.
6. Berardi, R. S., and Siroospour, D.: Lumbar sympathectomy in the treatment of peripheral vascular occlusive disease. Am. J. Surg., 130:309, 1975.
7. Warren, R.: Sympathectomism. Arch. Surg., 111:928, 1976.

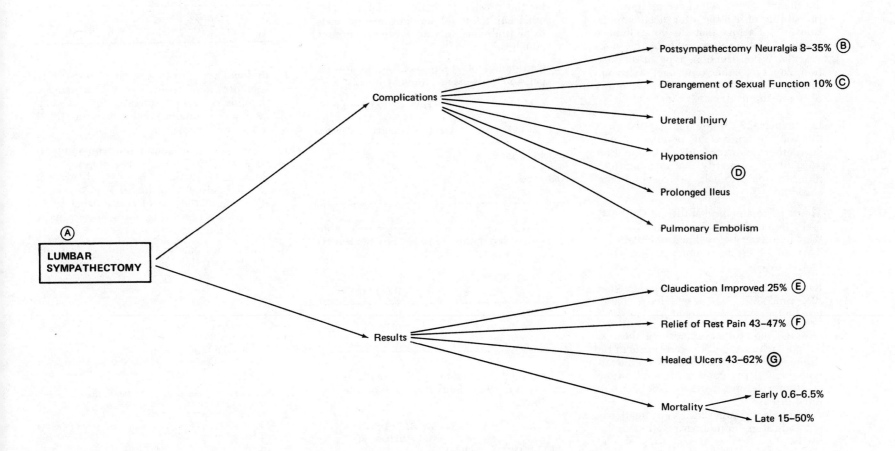

AMPUTATION FOR ARTERIAL DISEASE BY FRANK YAMAMOTO, M.D.

Comments

A. Sixty-nine to 87 per cent of all lower extremity amputations are for atherosclerosis.[1, 4] Thirteen per cent of these patients are diabetics[2, 3, 5-7] who have an improved probability of healing after distal amputations.[5, 8, 9] Factors that do not influence healing probabilities include previous vascular reconstruction, type of amputation, flap, sympathectomy, age, sex, symptoms, and immediate postoperative fitting of a prosthetic device.[2, 4, 6, 7, 9, 12, 13]

B. Life expectancy following amputation is that of an equivalent population who have atherosclerosis with no amputation. Mortality is primarily that of atherosclerotic, cardiac, renal, or cerebral disease.[2, 4, 6, 9, 13]

C. There is greater probability of contralateral amputation following above-knee than following below-knee amputations.[6] This merely reflects more severe obliterative disease.

D. Ratio of above-knee (AK) to below-knee (BK) procedures varies widely. A characteristic figure is 59 per cent AK.[2, 8, 9, 14]

E. Hospital mortality rates, except those of patients who have untreated sepsis in the stump, are largely a result of pulmonary embolus (±1 per cent) and complications of atherosclerotic, cardiac, cerebral, and renal disease.

Prophylactic superficial vein ligation is not indicated; miniheparinization probably is.

The relationship between hospital mortality and level of amputation is not certain.[4, 6, 9] Including the mortality of reoperation, the rate for BK procedures is probably higher.

F. Ten to 53 per cent of above-knee amputees ever want or get a prosthetic device. A permanent prosthesis cannot be used for approximately 4 weeks after amputation. About half of those who are fitted for the prosthesis discard it later.[14] The other half (56 to 60 per cent) use the artificial limb for walking with or without crutches.[3, 4, 6, 8, 9, 14]

G. Correlation of stump healing to lowest palpable pulse is as follows:[8]

LEVEL	LOWEST PALPABLE PULSE (%)		
	Aortic	Femoral	Popliteal
Distal Leg and Foot	0	43	48
Below-knee	77	72	88
Above-knee	79	92	44

H. Correlation between Doppler detectible pulse and below-knee stump healing is as follows:[8, 10, 13]

FEMORAL BP	% HEALED
Undetectable	17
<70 mm Hg	73
>70 mm Hg	100

I. Correlation of stump healing with degree of stump bleeding at operation is as follows:

LEVEL OF AMPUTATION	STUMP BLEEDING AT AMPUTATION (%)		
	Little or None	Diminished	Normal
Distal	36	54	70
Below-knee	69	77	93

J. Correlation of xenon flow and below-knee stump healing is as follows:[13]

SKIN BLOOD FLOW (ml./100 gm./min.)	% HEALED
2.63	74
2.70	100

K. Below-knee prostheses characteristically can be fitted within two weeks using a temporary pylon suitable for walking, and a permanent device can be fitted after eight weeks.

L. Transmetatarsal amputations for obliterative arterial disease may require prolonged hospitalization (4 to 6 weeks) while healing is in doubt. The benefit of this amputation is, of course, that it requires no prosthesis and allows almost normal leg activity.

M. Little hard data are available concerning prognosis following toe amputation.

References

1. McKittrick, J. B.: Amputation of lower extremities. GP, 13:104–113, 1956.
2. Tillgren, C.: Obliterative arterial disease of the lower limbs: A study of the course of the disease. Acta Med. Scand., 178:10–3119, 1965.
3. Watkins, A. L., and Liao, S. J.: Rehabilitation of persons with bilateral amputation of lower extremities. JAMA, 166:1584–1586, 1958.
4. Chapman, C. E., et al.: Follow-up study on a group of older amputees. JAMA, 170:1396–1402, 1959. (Reprinted in Orthopedic and Prosthetic Appliance Journal, 13:62–73, 1959.)
5. Clarke-Williams, M. J.: The elderly lower limb amputee. Gerontol. Clin. (Basel), 10:321–333, 1968.
6. Kihn, R. B., Warren, R., and Beebe, C. W.: The geriatric amputee. Ann. Surg., 176:305–313, 1972.
7. Barnes, R. W., Shanik, C. D., and Slaymaker, E. E.: An

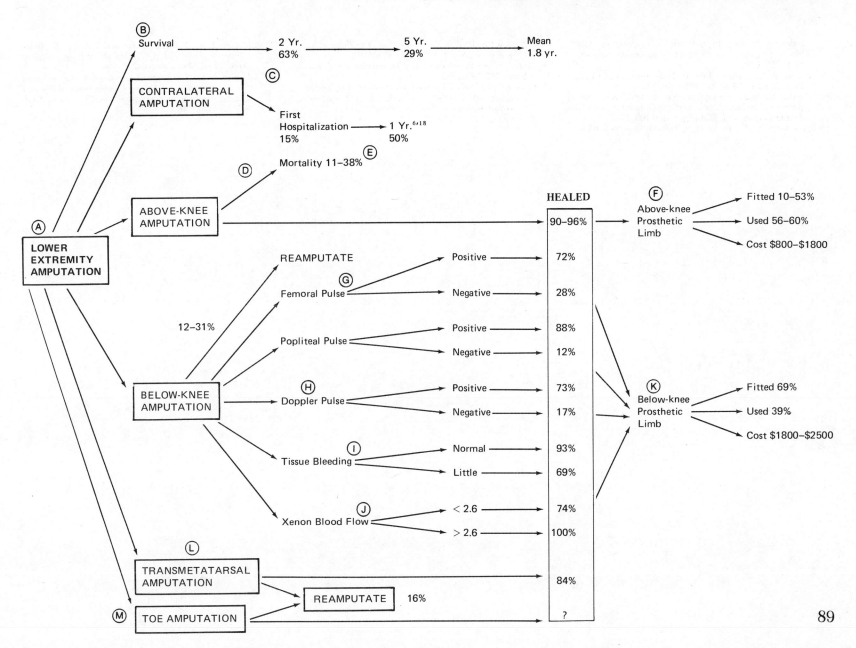

index of healing in below-knee amputation: Leg blood pressure by Doppler ultrasound, Surgery, 79:13–20, 1976.

8. Wilson, A. L.: Survey of the diabetic amputee. Orthop. Pros. Appl. J., 20:58–60, 1966.

9. Vankka, E.: Study on arteriosclerotics undergoing amputations, including pre- and postoperative periods. Acta Orthop. Scand. [Suppl.], 104:1–108, 1967.

10. Strandness, D. E., Jr., et al.: Ultrasonic flow detection:

A useful technic in the evaluation of peripheral vascular disease, Am. J. Surg., 113:311, 1967.

11. Moore, W. S.: Determination of amputation level. Arch. Surg., 107:798, 1973.

12. Cohen, S. I., et al.: The deleterious effect of immediate postoperative prosthesis in below-knee amputation for ischemic disease. Surgery, 76:992, 1974.

13. Lowenthal, M., Posniak, A. O., and Tobis, J. S.: Rehabilitation of the elderly double above-knee amputee. Arch. Phys. Med., 39:290–295, 1968.

14. Olejniczak, S.: Summary of leg amputations and prosthetic replacement at Wayne County General Hospital during the five year period 1961–1965. Mich. Med., 66:723–726, 1967.

PERIPHERAL ARTERIAL
EMBOLISM

PERIPHERAL ARTERIAL EMBOLISM BY ROBERT B. RUTHERFORD, M.D.

Comments

A. Etiology of peripheral arterial embolism may be:

ETIOLOGY	INCIDENCE (%)	SITE
Ulcerated plaque	6 (4–12)[a]	Proximal artery
Aneurysm	2 (1–3)	10% (6–23%)
Cardiovascular procedures	2 (1–7)	
Arteriosclerotic heart disease (ASHD)		
With infarction	30 (26–36)	Heart 90%
With fibrillation	30 (26–38)	(77–94%)
Rheumatic heart disease (RHD)		
With fibrillation	20 (16–38)	
Miscellaneous	10 (7–21)	

[a] Figures in parentheses indicate range.

Among patients whose emboli are of cardiac origin, 75 per cent have ASHD.[4, 6, 10] At one time, one-half to two-thirds had RHD; now that figure is about one-fifth. About 50 per cent have fibrillation and one-third have myocardial infarct. Ulcerated plaques increasingly are becoming recognized as a common origin of arterial emboli. Etiology markedly affects mortality rate,[5, 6, 13] localization of embolus,[13] probability of recurrence,[4] and success of embolectomy.[5]

B. Excluding pulmonary arterial and cerebral emboli arising from ulcerating plaques, common sites of lodgment are:

LOCATION	FREQUENCY
Peripheral	84%
Arm	9% (5–16%)
Subclavian	1%
Axillary	2%
Brachial	6%
Leg	75%
Aortoiliac	25%
Femoral	37%
Popliteal and distal	13%
Visceral	16%
Brain	7% (1–21%)
Kidney	4% (2–7%)
Gut	4% (3–6%)
Spleen	1%

Site of lodgment affects prognosis of both life and limb.[6, 4]

C. Introduction of the balloon catheter for clot extraction has improved limb salvage rates[10, 13] more than mortality rates. The increasing frequency of emboli due to ASHD myocardial infarcts has largely obscured improvement in operative and postoperative cure.

D. Effect of treatment delay:

OUTCOME	LESS THAN 24 HOURS	MORE THAN 24 HOURS
Mortality[2]	20%	25%
Amputation		
Study 1[6]	4%	19%
Study 2[7]	6%	14%
Study 3[13]	18%	34%
Study 4[10]	13%	23%
Distal pulses present[10]	71%	39%

Data in the algorithm do not involve differences in treatment delay.

E. Mortality depends primarily on the nature of the underlying disease.[6]

CAUSES OF DEATH AFTER EMBOLECTOMY[10]	% OF PATIENTS
Myocardial infarction	49
Pulmonary embolism	11
Recurrent or synchronous embolism	27
Operative procedure	5
Other (sepsis, pneumonia)	8

F. Postembolectomy complications include: leg edema (15 per cent), neurologic deficit (11 per cent), wound hematoma or in-

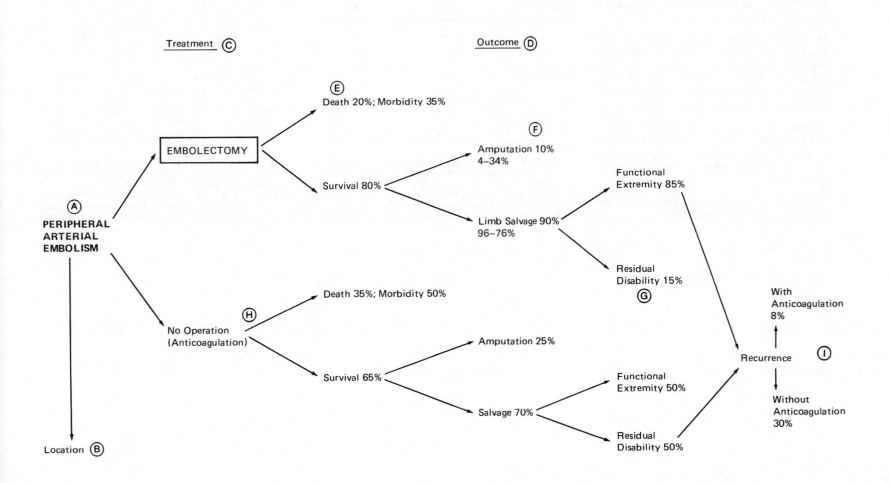

fection (9 per cent), subintimal dissection (1 per cent), and arteriovenous fistula (1 per cent).[10] Overall morbidity, including general complications such as congestive heart failure, atelectasis, and others, varies from 27 to 40 per cent.[6, 7, 10]

G. Residual disability relates mainly to delayed or incomplete embolectomy leading to amputation, residual ischemic symptoms, ischemic neuropathy, and ischemic necrosis or fibrosis of muscles encompassed by fascial compartments.

H. Nonoperative therapy is seldom risked until the patient is moribund or ischemia marginal,[4] so comparable statistics must be interpolated from pre-embolectomy experience.

I. Although heparin reduces recurrence, its use carries its own morbidity.[10]

TREATMENT	EMBOLIC RECURRENCE	WOUND COMPLICATION
No anticoagulation	31%	4%
Heparin	8%	33%
Warfarin	8%	7%

References

1. Satiani, B., Gross, W. S., and Evans, W. E.: Improved limb salvage after arterial embolectomy. Ann. Surg., *188*:153, 1978.
2. Greep, J. M., et al.: A combined technique for peripheral arterial embolectomy. Arch. Surg., *105*:869, 1972.
3. Barker, C. F., Francis, E. R., and Roberts, B.: Peripheral arterial embolism. Surg. Gynecol. Obstet., *123*:22, 1966.
4. Darling, R. C., Austen, W. G., and Linton, R. R.: Arterial embolism. Surg. Gynecol. Obstet. *144*:106, 1977.
5. Freund, U., Romanoff, H., and Floman, Y.: Mortality rate following lower limb arterial embolectomy: Causative factors. Surgery, 77:201, 1975.
6. Thompson, J. E., et al.: Arterial embolectomy: A 20-year experience with 163 cases. Surgery, 67:212, 1970.
7. Levy, J. F., and Butcher, H. R., Jr.: Arterial emboli: An analysis of 125 patients. Surgery, 68:968, 1970.
8. Haimovici, H., Moss, C. M., and Vieth, F. J.: Arterial embolectomy revisited. Surgery, 78:409, 1975.
9. Haimovici, H.: Arterial embolism. *In* Haimovici, H. (ed.): Vascular Diseases. Philadelphia, J. B. Lippincott Co., 1970.
10. Green, R. M., DeWeese, J. A., and Rob, C. G.: Arterial embolectomy before and after the Fogarty catheter. Surgery, 77:24, 1975.
11. Stallone, R. J., et al.: Analysis of morbidity and mortality from arterial embolectomy. Surgery, 65:207, 1969.
12. Fogarty, T. J., et al.: A method for extraction of arterial emboli and thrombi. Surg. Gynecol. Obstet., *116*:241, 1963.
13. Hight, D. W., Tilney, N. L., and Couch, N. P.: Changing clinical trends in patients with peripheral arterial emboli. Surgery, 79:172, 1976.
14. Fogarty, T. J.: Arterial embolism. *In* Dale, W. A. (ed.): Management of Arterial Occlusive Disease. Chicago, Year Book Medical Publishers, 1971.

ANGIOGRAPHY

ANGIOGRAPHY

ANGIOGRAPHY BY ROBERT LATTES, M.D.

Comments

A minor complication is one that is temporary, resulting in complete recovery without surgical intervention. A major complication has permanent sequelae or is transiently severe, requiring intensive therapy and additional hospitalization.

Angiography requires a 24-hour hospitalization. Its duration is generally from half an hour to 4 hours, depending on the number of vessels studied and the number of injections required. Radiation surface dose is 1 to 4 rads per standard filming sequence, with multiple sequences frequently being performed.

Factors affecting reported complication rates include:

1. Definition of complication.
2. Date of report and use of newer techniques and equipment, particularly improved catheter and guide wire materials,[3, 4, 7] and less toxic contrast agents.
3. Patient populations that have unique factors predisposing to complications, such as arteriosclerotic disease, both extremes of age,[14] aortic valvular incompetence,[14] subarachnoid hemorrhage,[16] decreased cardiac output, anemia, hypotension, hypertension, migraine, intracerebral neoplasm,[22] and other problems. The complication rate of patients with cerebral vascular disease is approximately 4 times that in patients without ischemic lesions.[16, 20] Children under 10 have approximately twice the complications of those over 10 years of age.[14]

Neurologic complications are usually related to pre-existing cerebrovascular disease and are rare in the absence of it.[12, 16] Complications of the primary disease may be impossible to distinguish from complications of angiography. The rate of major complications before and after angiography have been found to be almost identical.[2] Eighty to 90 per cent of complications of cerebral angiography are minor, occurring at the puncture site.

CEREBRAL ANGIOGRAPHY

A. Transfemoral cerebral angiography is the preferred method of cerebral angiography because all cerebral vessels can be studied selectively with a single arteriotomy. The femoral artery is large and accessible, so this technique results in fewer complications than when alternative methods are used. The greatest risk is femoral artery thrombosis, because collateral circulation to the leg is poor.[8-11, 14, 15, 20, 21]

B. The technique of percutaneous carotid artery puncture is relatively simple and does not require fluoroscopy. It offers excellent visualization of the intracerebral carotid circulation and of the carotid bifurcation; however, the posterior fossa is not seen. Optimal visualization of both carotid circulations requires two punctures, thereby doubling the complication rate.[8, 10, 12, 14]

C. Transaxillary catheter cerebral angiography is the alternative to femoral catheterization in the presence of severe femoral arteriosclerosis. There is a high complication rate owing to the small caliber of the artery, its proximity to the brachial plexus, and the tight compartment formed by the axillary fascia. The incidence of arteriospasm and thrombosis is 3 times that for femoral artery puncture; however, the rich collateral supply to the arm makes loss of limb rare.[1, 5, 11, 13-15, 19, 20, 22]

Neurologic deficit related to compression of the brachial plexus by hematoma is the most frequent serious complication. Permanent deficit can be prevented by prompt exploration and decompression of the neurovascular sheath after paresis develops.[1, 13, 19]

Due to the greater severity of a smaller hematoma, anticoagulation is a greater risk factor than with femoral arteriography.

D. Retrograde brachial cerebral angiography is not used frequently because of the limited quality of these examinations and the unreliable opacification of the left carotid distribution.[8, 10, 11, 14, 17, 19, 20] The local complication rate is 3 to 5 times that of femoral puncture, and in some series approaches 100 per cent;[10] however, these complications are seldom severe. It is considered by some to be the preferred technique in patients with severe arteriosclerosis,[20] the complication rate being equal in arteriosclerotic people and those with normal vessels.[12]

ABDOMINAL AND LOWER EXTREMITY ARTERIOGRAPHY

E. Translumbar aortography currently is used less frequently than in the past, despite a lower complication rate than that of transfemoral aortography.[6, 11, 14, 17] There is normally hemorrhage of approximately 50 cc. into the retroperitoneum. This may cause transient peritoneal signs clinically. Higher complication rates in older literature are a result of subintimal injections and dissections obtained with rigid translumbar needles. These complications are rare with the flexible Teflon sheaths now in use. Paraplegia and renal failure were occasional complications of

Complications

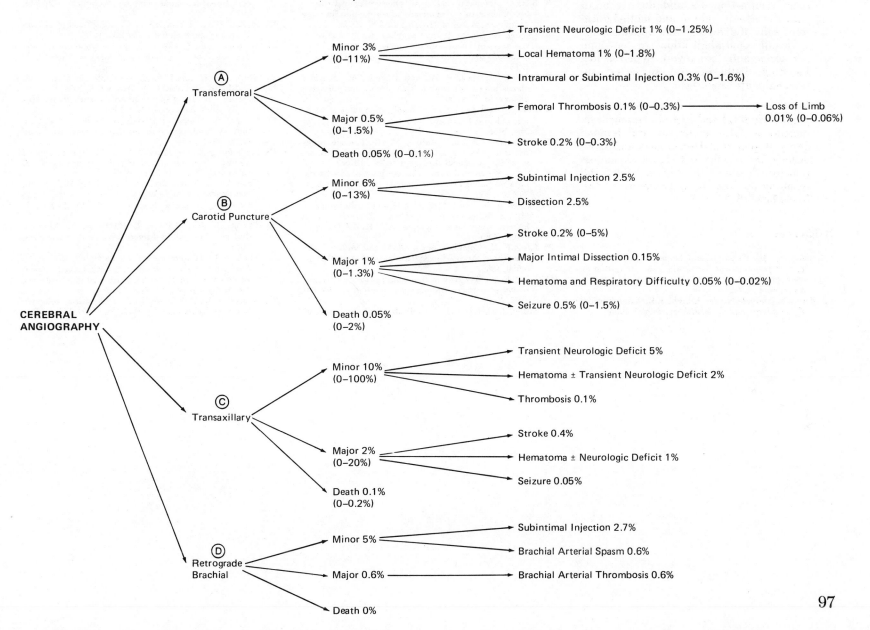

older contrast media and do not occur with the newer sodium and methylglucamine salts of diatrizoate and iothalamate.

Specific contraindications to translumbar aortography are severe hypertension, bleeding diathesis, and suspected suprarenal aortic aneurysm.

F. Most complications of transfemoral aortography are local and include hemorrhage, hematoma, false aneurysm, and femoral artery thrombosis. Hematomas and hemorrhage are usually not significant unless puncture is above the inguinal ligament, resulting in loss of containment by the fascia lata.[9-11, 14, 17, 18, 26]

References

1. Antonovic, R., Rosch, J., and Dotter, C.T.: Complications of percutaneous transaxillary catheterization for arteriography and selective chemotherapy. Am. J. Roentgenol., *126*:386, 1976.
2. Baum, S., Stein, G.N., and Kuroda, K.K.: Complications of "no arteriography." Radiology, 86:835, 1966.
3. Björk, L.: Heparin coating of catheters against thromboembolism in percutaneous catheterization for angiography. Acta Radiol. [Diagn.], *12*:576, 1972.
4. Cramer, R., Moore, R., and Amplatz, K.: Reduction of the surgical complication rate by the use of a hypothrombogenic catheter coating. Radiology, *109*:585, 1973.
5. Dudrick, S., Masland, W., and Mishkin, M.; Brachial plexus injury following axillary artery puncture. Radiology, *88*:271, 1967.
6. Haut, G., and Amplatz, K.: Complication rates of transfemoral and transaortic catheterization. Surgery, *63*: 594, 1968.
7. Hawkins, I. F., and Kelley, M. J.: Benzalkonium-heparin coated angiographic catheters. Experience with 563 patients. Radiology, *109*:589, 1973.
8. Hilal, S. K.: Hemodynamic changes associated with the intra-arterial injection of contrast media. Radiology, *80*:615, 1966.
9. Jacobsson, B., and Schlossman, D.: Thromboembolism of leg following percutaneous catheterization of femoral artery for angiography. Acta Radiol. [Diagn.], 8:109, 1969.
10. Lang, E. K.: Complications of direct and indirect angiography of the brachiocephalic vessels. Acta Radiol., 5:296, 1966.
11. Lang, E. K.: A survey of the complications of percutaneous retrograde arteriography. Radiology, *88*:950, 1967.
12. Miller, J. D. R., et al.: Complications of cerebral angiography and pneumography. Radiology, *124*:741, 1977.
13. Molnar, W., and Paul, D. J.: Complications of axillary arteriotomies. Radiology, *104*:269, 1972.
14. Mortensen, J. D.: Clinical sequelae from arterial needle puncture, cannulation and incision. Circulation, 35:1118, 1967.
15. Newton, T. H., and Potts, D. G.: Radiology of the Skull and Brain. St. Louis, C. V. Mosby Co., 1974.
16. Patterson, R. H.: Complications of carotid arteriography. Arch. Neurol., *10*:513, 1964.
17. Ross, R. S.: Cooperative study on cardiac catheterization. Arterial complications. Circulation, 37(Suppl. III)37:39–41, 1968.
18. Seidenberg, B., and Hurwitt, E. S.: Retrograde femoral (Seldinger) aortography: Surgical complications in 26 cases. Ann. Surg., *163*:221, 1966.
19. Staal, A., van Voorthuisen, A. E., and van Dijk, L. M.: Neurological complications following arterial catheterisation by the axillary approach. Br. J. Radiol., *39*:115, 1966.
20. Taveras, J. M., and Wood, E. H.: Diagnostic Neuroradiology, 2nd ed. Baltimore, Williams & Wilkins, 1976.
21. Vitek, J. J.: Femorocerebral angiography: Analysis of 2000 consecutive examinations, with special emphasis on carotid artery catheterization in older patients. Am. J. Roentgenol., *118*:633, 1973.
22. Wescott, J. L., and Taylor, P. T.: Transaxillary selective four-vessel arteriography. Radiology, *104*:277, 1972.

Complications

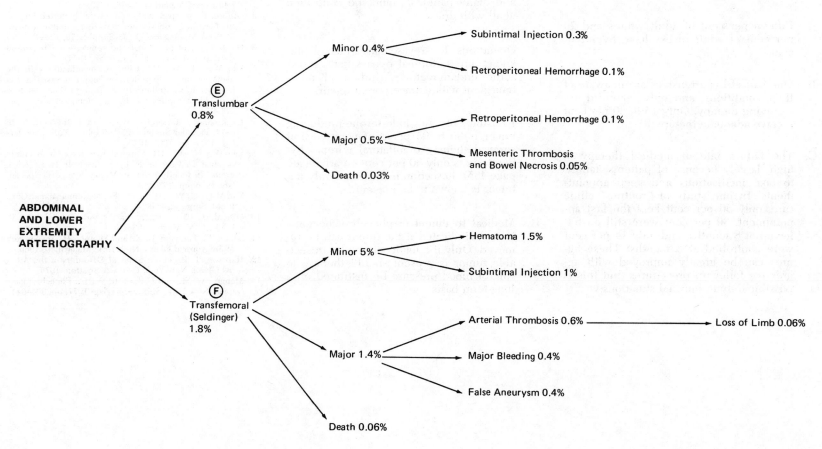

ABDOMINAL
AND LOWER
EXTREMITY
ARTERIOGRAPHY

Ⓔ Translumbar 0.8%

Minor 0.4%
→ Subintimal Injection 0.3%
→ Retroperitoneal Hemorrhage 0.1%

Major 0.5%
→ Retroperitoneal Hemorrhage 0.1%
→ Mesenteric Thrombosis and Bowel Necrosis 0.05%

Death 0.03%

Ⓕ Transfemoral (Seldinger) 1.8%

Minor 5%
→ Hematoma 1.5%
→ Subintimal Injection 1%

Major 1.4%
→ Arterial Thrombosis 0.6% ——————— Loss of Limb 0.06%
→ Major Bleeding 0.4%
→ False Aneurysm 0.4%

Death 0.06%

HYPERTENSION BY CHARLES W. VAN WAY, III, M.D.

Comments

A. The following blood pressure readings indicate hypertension:

Men under 45	130/90
Men over 45	140/95
Women	160/95

Fifteen per cent of adult whites and 20 per cent of adult blacks have hypertension.[1]

B. One-half of hypertensives are unaware of their conditions, and only one-third are receiving therapy. Only 15 to 20 per cent receive adequate therapy.[1, 2]

C. The failure rate of medical therapy is high, largely because of patients' failure to take medications and keep appointments. In one study of "routine" clinic care, only 50 per cent kept the first appointment, 30 per cent were still on followup at 8 months, and only 14 per cent were controlled at 8 months. These figures can be greatly improved with aggressive followup procedures, but this is possible only in unusual situations.[1-3]

D. Incidence figures for surgically correctable hypertension are inaccurate.[1, 4, 8]

E. Drug therapy for renovascular hypertension, according to the study of Hunt, is much less effective than surgical therapy, and many patients cannot be controlled at all with drugs.

F. Operations for revascularization of the kidney are aortorenal bypass graft, transaortic endarterectomy, and renal autotransplant with extracorporeal repair.

G. Excision of an aldosterone-producing tumor is 90 to 95 per cent curative, but surgical therapy of bilateral adrenal hyperplasia is only 30 per cent curative (see page 455). Resection is indicated only if a tumor is known to be present.

H. Medical treatment of pheochromocytoma is contraindicated if the tumor can be removed. Only if a malignant and unresectable tumor is present should therapy to control blood pressure be instituted on a long-term basis.

References

1. Kaplan, N. M.: Clinical Hypertension. New York, Medcom Press, 1973, pp. 1–33.
2. Wilber, J. A., and Darvon, J. G.: Hypertension: A community problem. Am. J. Med., 52:653, 1972.
3. Finnerty, F. A., Mattie, E. C., and Finnerty, F. A., III: Hypertension in the inner city. II. Detection and followup. Circulation, 47:76, 1973.
4. Gifford, R. W., Jr.: Evaluation of the hypertensive patient with emphasis on detecting curable causes. Milbank Mem. Fund Q., 47(Suppl.):170, 1969.
5. Hunt, J. C., et al.: Renal and renovascular hypertension. Arch. Intern. Med., 133:988, 1974.
6. Van Way, C. W., III: Clinical considerations in the management of hypertension and renovascular hypertension. In Rutherford, R. B. (ed.): Vascular Surgery. Philadelphia, W. B. Saunders Co., 1977, pp. 971–978.
7. Dean, R. H.: Aortorenal bypass. In Rutherford, R. B. (ed.): Vascular Surgery. Philadelphia, W. B. Saunders Co., 1977, pp. 1007–1013.
8. Van Way, C. W., III: Surgical hypertension in family practice. In Cozetto, F. J., and Brettell, H. R. (eds.): Topics in Family Practice. Miami, Symposia Specialists, 1976, pp. 367–389.
9. Van Way, C. W., III, et al.: Pheochromocytoma. Curr. Probl. Surg., June 1974.
10. O'Neal, L. W.: Surgery of the Adrenal Glands. St. Louis, C. V. Mosby, 1968.
11. Glenn, F., Peterson, R. E., and Mannix, H., Jr.: Surgery of the Adrenal Gland. New York, MacMillan, 1966.
12. Harrison, T. B., et al.: Surgical Disorders of the Adrenal Gland. New York, Grune & Stratton, 1975.
13. Manger, W. M., and Gifford, R. W., Jr.: Pheochromocytoma. New York, Springer-Verlag, 1977, pp. 304–344.

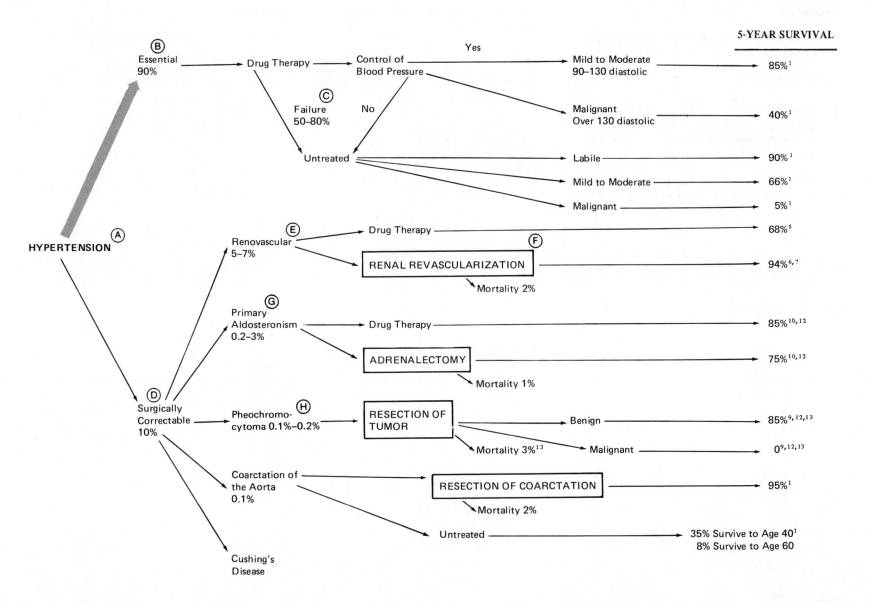

5-YEAR SURVIVAL

Ⓑ Essential 90%
→ Drug Therapy → Control of Blood Pressure
— Yes → Mild to Moderate 90–130 diastolic → 85%[1]
— No → Malignant Over 130 diastolic → 40%[1]

Ⓒ Failure 50–80% → Untreated
→ Labile → 90%[1]
→ Mild to Moderate → 66%[1]
→ Malignant → 5%[1]

Ⓐ HYPERTENSION

Ⓔ Renovascular 5–7%
→ Drug Therapy → 68%[5]
→ Ⓕ RENAL REVASCULARIZATION → 94%[6,7]
Mortality 2%

Ⓖ Primary Aldosteronism 0.2–3%
→ Drug Therapy → 85%[10,12]
→ ADRENALECTOMY → 75%[10,12]
Mortality 1%

Ⓓ Surgically Correctable 10%

Ⓗ Pheochromocytoma 0.1%–0.2%
→ RESECTION OF TUMOR
→ Benign → 85%[9,12,13]
Mortality 3%[13] → Malignant → 0[9,12,13]

Coarctation of the Aorta 0.1%
→ RESECTION OF COARCTATION → 95%[1]
Mortality 2%
→ Untreated → 35% Survive to Age 40[1]
8% Survive to Age 60

Cushing's Disease

MAJOR VASCULAR LIGATIONS BY EDWARD EHRICHS, M.D.

Comments

A. Central nervous system ischemia is significantly reduced if ligation is not performed when carotid stump pressure is less than 60 mm. Hg.[13]

B. Complete division of the innominate artery has been shown to be the most effective and safest therapy for tracheo–innominate artery erosion.[4]

C. Ultrasound evaluation of the palmar circulation indicates that 4.8 to 12.8 per 1000 patients will show acute ischemia with radial artery ligation.[14]

D. In their review of the literature Kim and associates have shown an overall mortality rate of 3.7 per cent secondary to hepatic failure in 345 patients.[6]

E. Bilateral ligation of the internal jugular vein appears to be safest if staged 3 to 6 weeks apart. If not staged, it should be accompanied by tracheostomy to protect the airway and may require drainage of cerebrospinal fluid.[15]

References

1. Nishioka, H.: Report on the cooperative study of intracranial aneurysms and subarachnoid hemorrhage. J. Neurosurg., 25:660, 1066.
2. Vijay, K. K., Taylor, A., and Derek, S. G.: Proximal carotid ligation for internal carotid aneurysms. J. Neurosurg., 39:503, 1973.
3. Shintani, A., and Zervas, N. T.: Consequence of ligation of the vertebral artery. J. Neurosurg., 36:447, 1972.
4. Jones, J. W., et al.: Tracheo–innominate artery erosion. Ann. Surg., 184:194, 1976.
5. DeBakey, M. E., and Simeone, F. A.: Battle injuries of the arteries in World War II. Ann. Surg., 123:534, 1946.
6. Kim, D. K., Kinne, D. W., and Fortner, J. G.: Occlusion of the hepatic artery in man. Surg. Gynecol. Obstet., 136:966, 1973.

LIGATION OF MAJOR ARTERIES

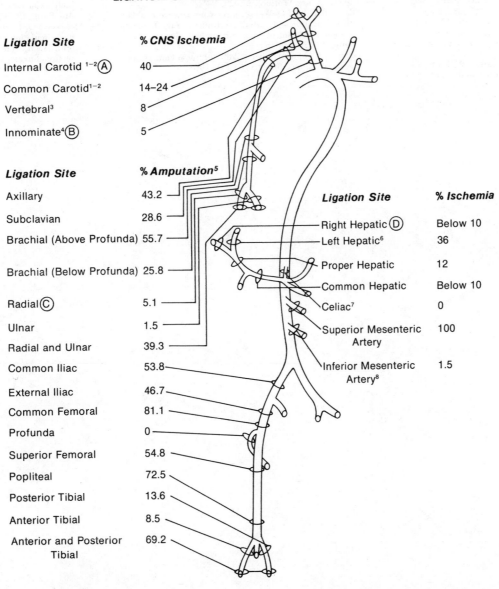

Ligation Site	% CNS Ischemia
Internal Carotid [1-2] (A)	40
Common Carotid [1-2]	14–24
Vertebral [3]	8
Innominate [4] (B)	5

Ligation Site	% Amputation [5]
Axillary	43.2
Subclavian	28.6
Brachial (Above Profunda)	55.7
Brachial (Below Profunda)	25.8
Radial (C)	5.1
Ulnar	1.5
Radial and Ulnar	39.3
Common Iliac	53.8
External Iliac	46.7
Common Femoral	81.1
Profunda	0
Superior Femoral	54.8
Popliteal	72.5
Posterior Tibial	13.6
Anterior Tibial	8.5
Anterior and Posterior Tibial	69.2

Ligation Site	% Ischemia
Right Hepatic (D)	Below 10
Left Hepatic [6]	36
Proper Hepatic	12
Common Hepatic	Below 10
Celiac [7]	0
Superior Mesenteric Artery	100
Inferior Mesenteric Artery [8]	1.5

MAJOR VASCULAR LIGATIONS *Continued*

7. Appleby, L. H.: The coeliac axis in the expansion of the operation for gastric carcinoma. Cancer, 6:704, 1953.
8. Johnson, W. C., and Nabseth, D. C.: Visceral infarction following aortic surgery. Ann. Surg., 180:312, 1974.
9. Nesbit, R. M., and Wear, J. B.: Ligation of the inferior vena cava above the renal veins. Ann. Surg., 154:332, 1961.
10. Pollak, E. W., Sparks, F. C., and Barker, W. F.: Inferior vena cava interruption: Indications and results with caval ligation, clips, and intracaval devices. J. Cardiovasc. Surg. (Torino), 15:629, 1974.
11. Adams, J. T., and DeWeese, J. A.: Comparative evaluation of ligation and partial interruption of the femoral vein in the treatment of thromboembolic disease. Ann. Surg., 172:795, 1970.
12. James, E. C., et al.: Division of the left renal vein: A safe surgical adjunct. Surgery, 83:151, 1978.
13. Oller, D. W., Gee, W., and Kingsley, J. R.: Treatment for high extracranial internal carotid artery aneurysms. Am. Surg., 42:311, 1976.
14. Mozersky, D. J., et al.: Ultrasonic evaluation of the palmar circulation. Am. J. Surg., 126:810, 1973.
15. Morfit, H. M.: Simultaneous bilateral radical neck dissection. Surgery, 31:216, 1952.

LIGATION OF MAJOR VEINS

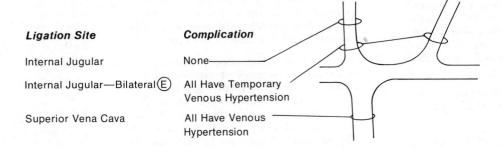

Ligation Site	Complication
Internal Jugular	None
Internal Jugular—Bilateral (E)	All Have Temporary Venous Hypertension
Superior Vena Cava	All Have Venous Hypertension

Ligation Site	% Mortality	% Leg Edema
Inferior Vena Cava		
Above Adrenal[9]	50	43
Above Renal[9]	55	43
Below Renal[10]	15	43
Femoral[11]	15	75

Ligation Site	Loss of Function
Right Renal	100%
Left Renal[12]	None

VARICOSE VEINS BY LEWIS MOLOGNE, M.D.

Comments

A. Geographic variation in incidence is great. In the U.S., Europe, and Russia the incidence is 10 to 15 per cent in people over 20, 19 per cent in men over 30, and 40 per cent in women over 30.[3-5] Despite this frequency, reliable data about prognosis are notoriously lacking. The cited probabilities are a composite of quoted sources.

B. Total disappearance occasionally occurs following childbirth or removal of a pelvic mass.

C. Anti-inflammatory agents are the primary nonoperative treatment.

D. The probability of significant bleeding is unknown, but in 1971 23 people in England died of bleeding leg varicosities.[9]

E. Of all patients with significant varicosities, 14 per cent will develop leg ulcers.[23] Of all venous ulcers, 40 per cent are due to superficial varicosities and 60 per cent to postphlebitic deep venous insufficiency.[22]

F. Recurrence is usually due to incomplete removal of the collateral veins at the saphenofemoral junction.[16]

G. Morbidity includes[18] hematoma (2 per cent incidence), deep venous thrombosis (3 per cent), injury to femoral artery or vein (0.02 per cent), pulmonary emboli (1 per cent), and infection (1 per cent).

H. The number of injections required depends on the number of varicosities, but characteristically it involves 2 to 3 outpatient sessions over several weeks. Severe side effects occur once per 1000 injections or at a rate of ± 1 per cent per patient with 10 injections.[22] The rate of pulmonary embolus as a complication is ± 0.1 per cent.[19]

References

1. Agrifoglio, G.: The surgical treatment of varicose veins: A method practised in Italy. *In* Hobbs, J. T. (ed.): The Treatment of Venous Disorders. Philadelphia, J. B. Lippincott Co., 1977, p. 138.
2. Beresford, S. A. A., et al.: Varicose veins: A comparison of surgery and injection—compression sclerotherapy. Lancet, 1:921, 1978.
3. Bezzouni, F.: The management of varicose veins: A method practised in Russia. *In* Hobbs, J. T. (ed.): The Treatment of Venous Disorders. Philadelphia, J. B. Lippincott Co., 1977, p. 174.
4. Borschberg, E.: The Prevalence of Varicose Veins in the Lower Extremities. Basel, S. Karger, 1967, p. 126.
5. Burkitt, D. P.: Varicose veins. Arch. Surg., 111:1327, 1976.
6. Burnand, K. G., et al.: The relative importance of incompetent communicating veins in the production of varicose veins and varicose ulcers. Surgery, 82:9–14, 1977.
7. Dee, R., and Finkelstein, J. E.: Treatment of varicose veins: Sclerotherapy with compression or stripping with multiple ligations? Angiology, 28:223, 1977.
8. Dejode, L. R.: Injection-compression treatment of varicose veins. Br. J. Surg., 57:285, 1970.
9. Evans, G. A., et al.: Spontaneous fatal hemorrhage caused by varicose veins. Lancet, 2:1359, 1973.
10. Fegan, W. G.: Varicose Veins. London, Heinemann, 1967.
11. Hobbs, J. T.: Superficial thrombophlebitis. *In* Hobbs, J. T. (ed.): The Treatment of Venous Disorders. Philadelphia, J. B. Lippincott Co., 1977, p. 414.
12. Hobbs, J. T.: A random trial of the treatment of varicose veins by surgery and sclerotherapy. *In* Hobbs, J. T. (ed.): The Treatment of Venous Disorders. Philadelphia, J. B. Lippincott Co., 1977, p. 195.
13. Kwoan, J. H., Jones, R. N., and Connally, J. E.: Simpli-

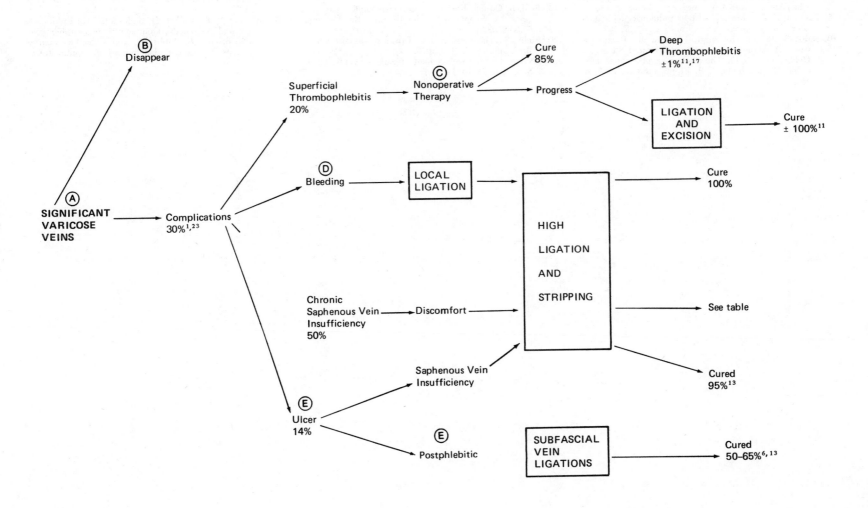

fied technique for the management of refractory varicose ulcer. Surgery, *80*:743, 1976.

14. Leu, H. J.: Therapie der Saphena-magna Varikosis: Chirugie oder Sklerosierung? Proxis Schweiz Rundschau Med, 57:491–494, 1968.

15. Lofgren, E. P.: Clinically suspect pulmonary embolism after vein stripping. Mayo Clin. Proc., *51*:77, 1976.

16. Nabatoff, R. A.: The surgical treatment of varicose veins: A method practised in the United States. *In* Hobbs, J. T. (ed.): The Treatment of Venous Disorders. Philadelphia, J. B. Lippincott Co., 1977, p. 155.

17. McNamara, M. F., et al.: Venous disease. Surg. Clin. North Am., 57:1201, 1977.

18. Natali, J.: Surgical treatment of varices. J. Cardiovasc. Surg., 5:713, 1964.

19. Reid, R. G., and Rothne, N. G.: Treatment of varicose veins by compression sclerotherapy. Br. J. Surg., 55:889, 1968.

20. Rinlin, S.: The surgical cure of primary varicose veins. Br. J. Surgery, 62:913, 1975.

21. Seddon, J.: The management of varicose veins. Br. J. Surg., 60:345, 1973.

22. Sigg, K.: Treatment of varicose veins by injection sclerotherapy: A method practised in Switzerland. *In* Hobbs, J. T. (ed.): The Treatment of Venous Disorders. Philadelphia, J. B. Lippincott Co., 1977, p. 113.

23. Widmer, L. K., Mall, T. H., and Martin, H.: Epidemiology and sociomedical importance of peripheral venous disease. *In* Hobbs, J. T. (ed.): The Treatment of Venous Disorders. Philadelphia, J. B. Lippincott Co., 1977, p. 3.

HIGH LIGATION AND EXCISION OF SAPHENOUS VEINS	EXCELLENT TO GOOD RESULTS	RECURRENCE	MORBIDITY	MORTALITY	CURED OR IMPROVED AT 6 YEARS[12]			References
					Dilated Superficial Veins	Lower Leg Perforators	Long or Short Saphenous Vein	
	80–85%	5–30% Ⓕ	7% Ⓖ	0.02%	45%	43%	86%	1, 2, 14–16 18, 20–22

Ⓗ

INJECTION	80–95%	15–100%	2%	0.01%	79%	100%	29%	2, 3, 7, 8, 10 14, 19, 21, 22

POSTOPERATIVE DEEP VEIN THROMBOSIS BY GLENN KELLY, M.D.

Comments

A. Factors increasing the incidence of post-operative deep vein thrombosis (DVT) include previous DVT, varicose veins, age (over 40 years), congestive heart failure, malignancy, and type of operation. Surgery of the lower extremity (especially hip replacement) is associated with up to 54 per cent DVT and 4 per cent pulmonary emboli.[1,2] Special prophylactic measures (i.e., low-dose heparin plus dihydroergotamine) are required in these patients.[3]

B. The wide variance in reported incidence is due largely to different methods of detection. Venography, the standard against which other methods are compared, occasionally fails to demonstrate small calf veins and is subject to differences in interpretation. Noninvasive tests include Doppler ultrasound and impedance plethysmography. ^{125}I scans ignore proximal thigh and pelvic thrombi while detecting all calf valve thrombi that are not yet clinically significant. Numbers are averaged from several sources.

METHOD	ACCURACY (%)	REFERENCES
Clinical	40–50	4, 8
Noninvasive		
laboratory studies	75–95	5, 6
^{125}I fibrinogen scan	92	7, 8
Contrast venogram	90–100	9

C. The effectiveness of other prophylactic measures can be compared by calling low-dose heparin 100 per cent effective and no prophylaxis 0 per cent effective. Results vary in patients with hip surgery.

TREATMENT	EFFECTIVENESS (%)	REFERENCES
Pulsating boot	100	10
Dextran	50–80	11, 12
Coumadin	25	13
Elastic stockings	25?	14

D. Tibial and soleal veins are the site of most postoperative DVT. However, only 6 per cent (controls) or 0.6 per cent (low-dose heparin group) progress to clinically significant popliteal-femoral or iliac DVT.[3]

E. Full-dose heparin usually is administered with an intravenous loading dose of 100 to 150 U. per kg. followed by continuous-drip intravenous heparin to maintain the whole blood clotting time, activated clotting time, or partial thromboplastin time at 2 to 2½ times normal.[15]

F. See page 114.

G. Complications of full-dose heparin therapy occur especially in the elderly and despite careful laboratory control.[16] Numbers are an average from several sources.

COMPLICATIONS	INCIDENCE (%)
Minor hemorrhage	6
Major hemorrhage	3
Intracranial bleeding	1

H. Low-dose heparin prophylaxis consists of subcutaneous administration of 5000 units 2 hours preoperatively and every 8 to 12 hours postoperatively until the patient is fully mobile.[3]

I. Complications of low-dose heparin prophylaxis:[17]

COMPLICATION	INCIDENCE (%)
Operative blood loss	0.4
Postoperative wound hematoma	1.2
Postoperative blood loss	1.0

J. The incidence of chronic venous insufficiency (CVI) following isotopic DVT of minor soleal veins is unknown but must be quite small, unless subsequent propagation into the femoral-popliteal or perforating veins is extensive. DVT (studied prior to the heparin era) leads to CVI in 45 per cent of patients within 5 years, 72 per cent within 10 years, and 91 per cent within 15 years.[18] Similar followup in patients treated with heparin is not available.

References

1. Sigel, B., Ipsen, J., and Felix, R.: The epidemiology of lower extremity deep venous thrombosis in surgical patients. Ann. Surg., *174*:278, 1974.
2. Evarts, M.: Thromboembolic disease in orthopedic patients. Contemp. Surg., 6:65, 1975.
3. Kakkar, V.V.: The current status of low-dose heparin in the prophylaxis of thrombophlebitis and pulmonary embolism. World J. Surg., 2:3, 1978.
4. Cranley, J., Canos, A., and Sull, W.: The diagnosis of deep venous thrombosis: Fallibility of clinical symptoms and signs. Arch. Surg., *111*:34, 1976.
5. Yao, J., Henkin, R., and Bergan, J.: Venous thromboembolic disease: Evaluation of new methodology in treatment. Arch. Surg., *104*:664, 1974.
6. Alexander, R., et al.: Thrombophlebitis and thromboembolism: Results of a prospective study. Ann. Surg., *180*:883, 1974.
7. Kakkar, V.: The diagnosis of deep vein thrombosis using ^{125}I fibrinogen test. Arch. Surg., *104*:152, 1972.

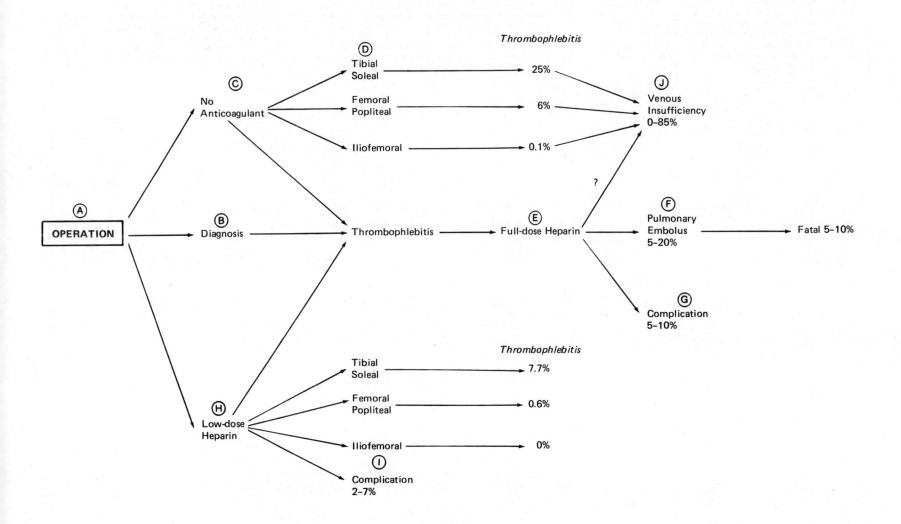

POSTOPERATIVE DEEP VEIN THROMBOSIS *Continued*

8. Milne, R., et al.: Postoperative deep venous thrombosis: A comparison of diagnostic techniques. Lancet, 2:445, 1971.
9. Thomas, M.: Phlebography. Arch. Surg., *104*:145, 1972.
10. Cotton, L., and Roberts, V.: The prevention of deep vein thrombosis with particular reference to mechanical methods of prevention. Surgery, *81*:228, 1977.
11. A multi-unit controlled trial of heparin versus dextran in the prevention of deep vein thrombosis. Lancet, 2:118, 1974.

12. Evarts, M.: Thromboembolic disease in orthopedic patients: Prophylaxis and treatment. Contemp. Surg., 6:57, 1975.
13. Vroonhoven, T., Zijl, J., and Muller, H.: Low-dose subcutaneous heparin versus oral anticoagulants in the prevention of postoperative deep venous thrombosis. Lancet, *1*:375, 1974.
14. Wilkins, R., and Stanton, J.: Elastic stockings in the prevention of pulmonary embolism. N. Engl. J. Med., *248*:1087, 1953.

15. Genton, E.: Guidelines for heparin therapy. Ann. Intern. Med., *80*:77, 1974.
16. Pitney, W., Pettit, J., and Armstrong, L.: Control of heparin therapy. Br. Med. J., *4*:139, 1970.
17. An international, multi-center trial: Prevention of fatal postoperative pulmonary embolism by low doses of heparin. Lancet, 2:7924, 1975.
18. Bauer, G.: A roentgenological and clinical study of the sequels of thrombosis. Acta Chir. Scand., *86*:1, 1942.

POSTOPERATIVE PULMONARY EMBOLUS

POSTOPERATIVE PULMONARY EMBOLUS BY GLENN KELLY, M.D.

Comments

A. Contributing factors are previous thromboembolism, predisposing drugs, varicose veins, lengthy immobilization, advanced age, malignancy, and type of surgery. Procedures to the lower extremity, especially hip surgery, afford the greatest risk.[1]

B. The incidence of pulmonary embolus (PE) depends upon whether standard clinical and x-ray techniques, isotope scanning, arteriography, or autopsy findings are used for diagnosis. The average incidence for major general surgery patients over 40 years old is 0.5 to 1.0 per cent, half of which are fatal. Use of low-dose heparin prophylaxis decreases this incidence to 0.2 per cent, half of which are fatal.

LOCATION	% FATAL[2,3]	% NONFATAL[4]
Tibial-soleal		26
Femoral-popliteal	"majority"	23
Iliofemoral	73	13
Undetermined		37

C. Fifty-eight per cent of massive acute pulmonary emboli occur in patients with previously unrecognized deep vein thrombosis (DVT).[7]

D. Accuracy of diagnostic tests including false negatives and false positives is shown in the following table.

TEST	% ACCURACY[c]	REFERENCES
Clinical evaluation[a]	50	5, 6, 9
Isotope lung scan[b]	80	7, 8
Pulmonary arteriogram	90–100	5, 9, 10

[a]Includes chest x-ray, EKG, and enzyme tests.
[b]Uses ^{99m}Tc macroaggregated albumin flow scan and ^{113}Xe ventilation scan performed sequentially. Few false negatives, frequent false positives.
[c]These are averages based on several series.

E. It is difficult to distinguish recurrent embolism from propagation of existing thrombus and pulmonary infarction. Mortality rates vary in recurrent PE according to treatment:

TREATMENT	% RECURRENT FATAL PE	REFERENCES
None	26	11
Heparin	1	11
Urokinase	17	12
Caval ligation	11	13
Caval plication	8	14
Umbrella	0.8	15

F. On occasion patients will have contraindications to (4 per cent) or complications from (8 per cent) anticoagulation and will require caval interruption.[16]

G. Techniques of caval interruption and their prognosis are shown in the table below.[17]

TECHNIQUE	% RECURRENT PE	% CHRONIC VENOUS INSUFFICIENCY	REFERENCE
Ligation	5–50	45	17
Plication	3–9	16	17
Clip	4–14	30	17
Umbrella	3	5[a]	16

[a]Recent experience suggests a much higher caval occlusion rate (50 per cent), implying later increased insufficiency. Results depend on whether patients receive anticoagulation therapy following umbrella insertion.

References

1. Kiil, J., et al.: Prophylaxis against postoperative pulmonary embolism and deep vein thrombosis by low-dose heparin. Lancet, 1:1115, 1978.
2. Sevitt, S., and Gallagher, N.: Venous thrombosis and pulmonary embolism: A clinicopathlogical study in injured and burned patients. Br. J. Surg., 48:475, 1961.
3. Coon, W., and Coller, F.: Some epidemiologic considerations in thromboembolism. Surg. Gynecol. Obstet., 109:487, 1959.
4. Browse, N., and Thomas, M.: Source of nonlethal pulmonary emboli. Lancet, 1:258, 1974.
5. Trujillo, M., Castillo, A., and Espana, J.: Bedside pulmonary angiography in the critically ill patient. Crit. Care Med., 4:151, 1976.
6. Wenger, N., Stein, P., and Willis, P.: Massive acute pulmonary embolism. The deceivingly nonspecific manifestations. JAMA, 220:843, 1972.
7. AMA archives symposium on diagnostic techniques in phlebothrombosis. Arch. Surg., 104:132, 1972.

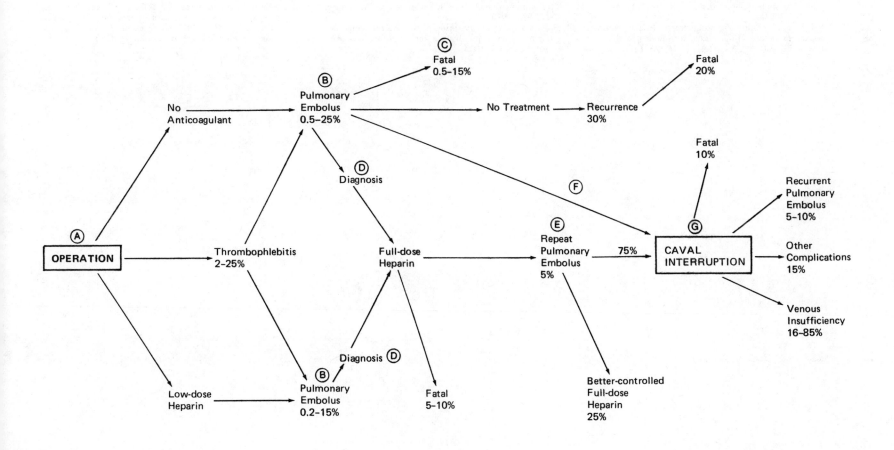

8. Moses, D., Silver, T., and Bookstein, J.: The complementary roles of chest radiography, lung scanning, and selective pulmonary angiography in the diagnosis of pulmonary embolism. Circulation, *49*:174, 1974.

9. Sasahara, A., et al.: Pulmonary angiography in the diagnosis of thromboembolic disease. N. Engl. J. Med., *270*:1075, 1964.

10. Dalen, J., et al.: Pulmonary angiography in acute pulmonary embolism: Indications, techniques, and results in 367 patients. Am. Heart J., *81*:175, 1971.

11. Barritt, D., and Jordan, S.: Anticoagulant drugs in the treatment of pulmonary embolism: A controlled trial. Lancet, *1*:1309, 1960.

12. Urokinase — pulmonary embolism trial. Circulation, *47* and *48* (Suppl. II):II-7, 1973.

13. Ochsner, A., Ochsner, J., and Sanders, H.: Prevention of pulmonary embolism by caval ligation. Ann. Surg., *171*:923, 1970.

14. Spencer, F., et al.: Plication of the inferior vena cava for pulmonary embolism. A report of 20 cases. Ann. Surg., *155*:827, 1962.

15. Bohling, C., Auer, A., and Hershey, F.: The Mobin-Uddin caval filter for prevention of pulmonary emboli. Am. J. surg., *128*:809, 1974.

16. Fullen, W., McDonough, J., and Altmeier, W.: Clinical experience with vena caval filters. Arch. Surg., *106*:582, 1973.

17. Moretz, W., and Wray, C.: Pulmonary embolism and complications of vena cava interruption procedures. *In* Beebe, H. (ed.): Complications in Vascular Surgery. Philadelphia, J. B. Lippincott, 1973.

ACUTE ILIOFEMORAL
VENOUS THROMBOSIS

ACUTE ILIOFEMORAL VENOUS THROMBOSIS BY E. EINARSSON, M.D., AND B. EKLÖF, M.D.

Comments

A. Iliofemoral venous thrombosis is a unilateral thrombosis that extends above the inguinal ligament but not into the inferior vena cava. Final diagnosis is confirmed by phlebography, employing low osmolar contrast medium. Acute iliofemoral venous thrombosis is surgically important because of the risk for pulmonary embolus (greater than 50 per cent), venous gangrene, and severe post-thrombotic syndrome. Mean age of patients is 54 years[1] and sex distribution is equal.[2] The ratio between the left iliac vein and the right iliac vein is 3:1.[3] The risk for women taking oral contraceptives of developing thrombosis is 1:1,500.[4] Trauma (operation) is responsible for 42 per cent of cases.[3] Thirty per cent of patients have a malignant disease.[5]

B. In the no-treatment group, data are collected from Browse's prospective study,[6] from Havig's postmortem study,[7] and from Bauer's untreated patients.[8]

C. Anticoagulant treatment means intravenous heparin alone or in combination with peroral anticoagulants.

D. Thrombolytic treatment includes the use of plasminogen activators such as streptokinase and urokinase.

E. Thrombectomy is performed using the Fogarty catheter under local or general anesthesia. Some surgeons use continuous local heparin infusion postoperatively.

F. Thrombectomy with a temporary fistula is performed under general anesthesia. (See reference 24.) The AV fistula is usually closed in a second operation after 6 to 8 weeks. The rather low incidence of the post-thrombotic syndrome is explained by the fact that there are no long-term followup studies reported yet using this method.

References

1. Haller, J. A., and Abrams, B. L.: Use of thrombectomy in the treatment of acute iliofemoral venous thrombosis in forty-five patients. Ann. Surg., 158:561, 1963.
2. Mahoner, H.: Results of surgical operations for venous thrombosis. Surg. Gynecol. Obstet., 129:66, 1969.
3. Mavor, G. E., and Galloway, J. M. D.: Iliofemoral venous thrombosis. Br. J. Surg., 56:45, 1969.
4. Boston Collaborative Drug Surveillance Program: Oral contraceptives and venous thromboembolic disease, surgically confirmed gallbladder disease, and breast tumours. Lancet, 1:1399, 1973.
5. Mavor, G. E., and Galloway, J. M. D.: Collaterals of the deep venous circulation of the lower limb. Surg. Gynecol. Obstet., 125:561, 1967.
6. Browse, N. L., Clemenson, G., and Croft, D. N.: Fibrinogen-detectable thrombosis in the legs and pulmonary embolism. Br. Med. J., 1:603, 1974.
7. Havig, Ö.: Deep vein thrombosis and pulmonary embolism. An autopsy study with multiple regression analysis of possible risk factors. Acta Chir. Scand. [Suppl.], 478, 1977.
8. Bauer, G.: Thrombosis. Early diagnosis and abortive treatment with heparin. Lancet, 1:447, 1946.
9. Duckert, F., et al.: Treatment of deep vein thrombosis with streptokinase. Br. Med. J., 1:479, 1975.
10. Bauer, G.: Clinical experiences of a surgeon in the use of heparin. Am. J. Cardiol., 14:29–35, 1964.
11. Matsubara, J., et al.: Long-term followup results of the iliofemoral venous thrombosis. J. Cardiovasc. Surg., 17:234, 1976.
12. Basu, D., et al.: A prospective study of the value of monitoring heparin treatment with the activated partial thromboplastin time. N. Engl. J. Med., 287:324, 1972.
13. Bauer, G.: Thirteen years' experience of heparin therapy. Thrombosis and embolism. I. International conference, Basel, 1954.
14. Widmer, L. K., et al.: Heparin oder Thrombolyse in der Behandlung der tiefen Beinvenenthrombose. Vasa, 3:422, 1974.
15. Mavor, G. E., et al.: Streptokinase therapy in deep vein thrombosis. Br. J. Surg., 60:468, 1973.
16. Eklöf, B., et al.: Spontaneous rupture of liver and spleen with severe intra-abdominal bleeding during streptokinase treatment of deep venous thrombosis. Vasa, 6:369, 1977.
17. Kriessmann, A., et al.: Fibrinolytic therapy in deep venous thrombosis of the upper and lower extremity. Fortschr. Med., 95:858, 1977.
18. Johansson, E., Ericson, K., and Zetterquist, S.: Streptokinase treatment of deep venous thrombosis of the lower extremity. Acta Med. Scand., 199:89, 1976.
19. Albrechtson, U., et al.: Post-thrombotic syndrome after streptokinase treatment in 35 patients with deep venous thrombosis of the leg. (To be published.)
20. Lansing, A. M., and Davis, W. M.: Five-year followup study of iliofemoral venous thrombectomy. Ann. Surg., 168:620, 1968.
21. Lindhagen, J., et al.: Iliofemoral venous thrombectomy. J. Cardiovasc. Surg., 19:319, 1978.
22. Fogarty, T. J.: Surgical concepts of iliofemoral venous thrombosis. Surg. Digest., June 27, 1968.
23. Karp, R. B., and Wylie, E. J.: Recurrent thrombosis after iliofemoral venous thrombectomy. Surg. Forum, 17:147, 1966.
24. Vollmar, J.: Reconstruction of the iliac veins and inferior vena cava. In Hobbs, J. T. (ed.): The Treatment of Venous Disorders. Lancaster, England, MTP Press Ltd., 1977.
25. Albrechtson, U., Einarsson, E., and Eklöf, B.: Thrombectomy with a temporary AV fistula in 50 patients with iliofemoral venous thrombosis. (To be published.)
26. Christenson, J., Einarsson, E. and Eklöf, B.: Infection complications after thrombectomy in deep venous thrombosis. Acta Chir. Scand., 143:431, 1977.

ACUTE ILIOFEMORAL VENOUS THROMBOSIS

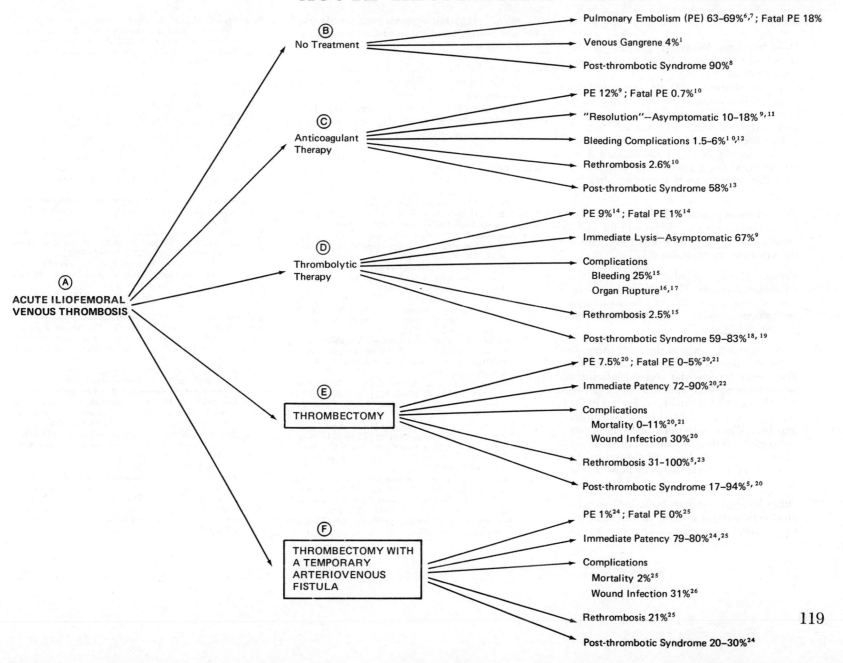

(A) **ACUTE ILIOFEMORAL VENOUS THROMBOSIS**

(B) No Treatment
- Pulmonary Embolism (PE) 63–69%[6,7]; Fatal PE 18%
- Venous Gangrene 4%[1]
- Post-thrombotic Syndrome 90%[8]

(C) Anticoagulant Therapy
- PE 12%[9]; Fatal PE 0.7%[10]
- "Resolution"—Asymptomatic 10–18%[9,11]
- Bleeding Complications 1.5–6%[10,12]
- Rethrombosis 2.6%[10]
- Post-thrombotic Syndrome 58%[13]

(D) Thrombolytic Therapy
- PE 9%[14]; Fatal PE 1%[14]
- Immediate Lysis—Asymptomatic 67%[9]
- Complications
  Bleeding 25%[15]
  Organ Rupture[16,17]
- Rethrombosis 2.5%[15]
- Post-thrombotic Syndrome 59–83%[18,19]

(E) THROMBECTOMY
- PE 7.5%[20]; Fatal PE 0–5%[20,21]
- Immediate Patency 72–90%[20,22]
- Complications
  Mortality 0–11%[20,21]
  Wound Infection 30%[20]
- Rethrombosis 31–100%[5,23]
- Post-thrombotic Syndrome 17–94%[5,20]

(F) THROMBECTOMY WITH A TEMPORARY ARTERIOVENOUS FISTULA
- PE 1%[24]; Fatal PE 0%[25]
- Immediate Patency 79–80%[24,25]
- Complications
  Mortality 2%[25]
  Wound Infection 31%[26]
- Rethrombosis 21%[25]
- Post-thrombotic Syndrome 20–30%[24]

119

VASCULAR ACCESS FOR DIALYSIS BY MELVIN M. NEWMAN, M.D.

Comments

A. One hundred thousand people in the world (32,000 in the U.S.) are kept alive by hemodialysis.[1]

    A flow of 200 to 300 ml. per minute is required to maintain patency.[2] This is seldom a cause of heart failure, even with flows up to 1000 ml. per minute.[3]

    The first choice for access is an arteriovenous fistula in the nondominant arm. However, if the patient lives sufficiently long the surgeon must use other sites for access.

B. Percutaneous puncture of the femoral vein is used for emergency dialysis or for a predictably limited number of dialyses, since the vessels may thrombose.[4]

C. Various plastic cannulas have been used for external shunts. These have the advantage of easy access, but the disadvantages are infection, clotting, discomfort, and the danger of bleeding.[5]

D. A direct anastomosis of the cephalic vein to the radial artery at the wrist remains the first choice for vascular access.[6] When the veins draining the fistula have been thrombosed by repeated puncture, fistulas to the basilic vein or fistulas in the upper arm are feasible.[7] When both upper extremities are no longer suitable for fistulas, then the saphenous vein can be anastomosed to the anterior or posterior tibial artery at the ankle.

E. Other biologic conduits include (1) autologous vein graft (obsolete),[8] (2) modified bovine carotid artery,[9] (3) cadaveric artery or vein,[10] (4) mandril-grown graft (rarely used any more),[11] and (5) modified human umbilical vein.[12]

F. Other internal conduits include (1) expanded polytetrafluoroethylene,[13] which is becoming increasingly popular, and (2) Dacron velour tubes, which have been used in a few instances but are more difficult for routine dialysis.[14]

References

1. Kolff, W. J.: Exponential growth and future of artificial organs. Artificial Organs, 1:8–18, 1977.
2. Butt, K. M. H., Friedman, E. A., and Kountz, S. L.: Angioaccess. Curr. Probl. Surg., 13:1–74, 1976.
3. a. Anderson, C. B., et al.: Cardiac failure and upper extremity arteriovenous dialysis fistulas. Arch. Intern. Med., 136:292–297, 1976.
   b. Fee, H. J., et al.: High-output congestive failure from femoral arteriovenous shunts for vascular access. Ann. Surg., 183:321–323, 1976.
4. a. Shaldon, S., Chiandussi, L., and Higgs, B.: Hemodialysis by percutaneous catheterization of the femoral artery and vein with regional heparinization. Lancet, 2:857–859, 1961.
   b. Shaldon, S., et al.: Refrigerated femoral venousvenous hemodialysis with coil preservation for rehabilitation of terminal uremic patients. Br. Med. J., 1:1716–1717, 1963.
5. a. Quinton, W., Gillard, D., and Scribner, B. H.: Cannulation of blood vessels for prolonged hemodialysis. Trans. Am. Soc. Artif. Intern. Organs, 6:104–109, 1960.
   b. Ramirez, O., et al.: The winged in-line shunt. Trans. Am. Soc. Artif. Intern. Organs, 12:220–221, 1966.
   c. Thomas, G. I.: A large vessel applique A-V shunt for hemodialysis. Trans. Am. Soc. Artif. Intern. Organs, 15:288–292, 1969.
   d. Buselmeier, T. J., et al.: A new subcutaneous arteriovenous shunt: Applicable in cases where the standard Quinton-Scribner shunt and arteriovenous fistula have failed. Surgery, 73:512–520, 1973.
   e. Newman, M. M.: Personal experience with 155 shunt operations, 1968–1971.
6. a. Brescia, M. J., et al.: Chronic hemodialysis using venipuncture and a surgically created arteriovenous fistula. N. Engl. J. Med., 275:1089–1092, 1966.
   b. Butt, K. M. H.: Blood access. Clin. Nephrol., 9:138–143, 1978.
7. Crockett, R. E.: Blood access for haemodialysis. Nephron, 12:338–354, 1974.
8. May, J., et al.: Saphenous vein arteriovenous fistula in regular dialysis treatment. N. Engl. J. Med., 280:770, 1969.
9. a. Hutchin, P., et al.: Bovine graft arteriovenous fistulas for maintenance hemodialysis. Surg. Gynecol. Obstet., 141:255–258, 1975.
   b. VanderWerf, B. A., et al.: Three-year experience with bovine graft arteriovenous (A-V) fistulas in 100 patients. Trans. Am. Soc. Artif. Intern. Organs, 21:296–299, 1975.
   c. Merickel, J. H., et al.: Bovine carotid artery shunts in vascular access surgery. Arch. Surg., 109:245–249, 1974.
10. a. Tice, D. A., and Zerbino, V.: Clinical experience with preserved human allografts for vascular reconstruction. Surgery, 72:260–267, 1972.
   b. Abu-dalu, J., et al.: Hemodialysis treatment by means of a cadaver arterioallograft. Arch. Surg., 105:798–801, 1972.
11. Sparks, C. H.: Silicone mandril method for growing reinforced autogenous femoro-popliteal artery grafts in situ. Ann. Surg., 177:293–300, 1973.
12. a. Dardik, I. J., and Dardik, H.: The fate of umbilical cord vessels used as interposition arteriografts in the baboon. Surg. Gynecol. Obstet., 140:567–571, 1975.
   b. Mindich, B. P., et al.: Umbilical cord vein fistula for vascular access in hemodialysis. Trans. Am. Soc. Artif. Intern. Organs, 21:273–279, 1975.
13. a. Campbell, C. D., et al.: Expanded polytetrafluoroethylene as a small artery substitute. Trans. Am. Soc. Artif. Intern. Organs, 20:86–90, 1974.
   b. Butler, H. G., Baker, L. D., and Johnson, J. M.: Vascular access for chronic hemodialysis: polytetrafluoroethylene (PTFE) versus bovine heterograft. Am. J. Surg., 134:791–793, 1977.
   c. Haimov, M.: Clinical experience with the expanded polytetrafluoroethylene vascular prosthesis. Angiology, 29:1–6, 1978.
14. Levowitz, B. S., et al.: Prosthetic arteriovenous fistula for vascular access in hemodialysis. Am. J. Surg., 132:368–372, 1976.

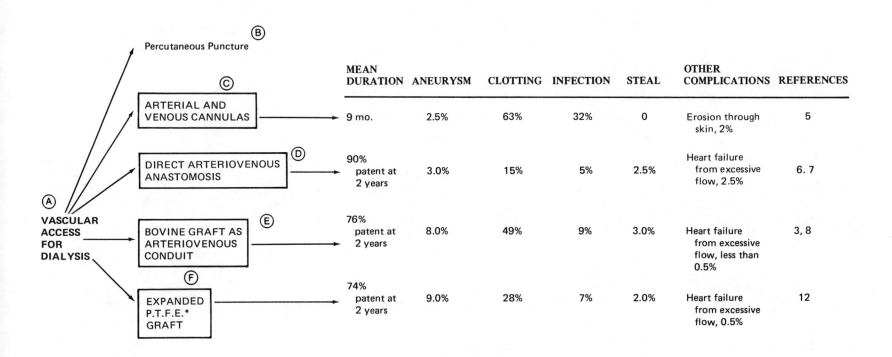

	MEAN DURATION	ANEURYSM	CLOTTING	INFECTION	STEAL	OTHER COMPLICATIONS	REFERENCES
ARTERIAL AND VENOUS CANNULAS	9 mo.	2.5%	63%	32%	0	Erosion through skin, 2%	5
DIRECT ARTERIOVENOUS ANASTOMOSIS	90% patent at 2 years	3.0%	15%	5%	2.5%	Heart failure from excessive flow, 2.5%	6. 7
BOVINE GRAFT AS ARTERIOVENOUS CONDUIT	76% patent at 2 years	8.0%	49%	9%	3.0%	Heart failure from excessive flow, less than 0.5%	3, 8
EXPANDED P.T.F.E.* GRAFT	74% patent at 2 years	9.0%	28%	7%	2.0%	Heart failure from excessive flow, 0.5%	12

Percutaneous Puncture

VASCULAR ACCESS FOR DIALYSIS

*Polytetrafluoroethylene (Gore-Tex)

121

Section D

Thoracic

CHEST INJURY BY G. E. ARAGON, M.D., AND BEN EISEMAN, M.D.

Comments

PENETRATING CHEST INJURY

A. The 15 to 25 per cent of penetrating chest wall injuries that do not respond to tube drainage[1-3] usually are due to (1) penetration of the lung by tube, (2) placement of tube below the diaphragm, (3) failure to evacuate all air or blood, (4) subcutaneous emphysema, or (5) empyema (0.5 to 2 per cent), all of which are failures in tube technique. In addition, injury to an intercostal artery will cause uncontrolled bleeding to the outside or into the chest unless the artery is ligated.

B. Hemothorax or hemopneumothorax occurs in 75 per cent of penetrating stab wounds and almost routinely in gunshot wounds. Isolated pneumothorax occurs in only 21 per cent of cases, and there are no intrathoracic findings in 10 per cent of penetrating stab wounds.[1]

C. In less than 5 per cent of civilian chest wounds in which treatment is prompt and unevacuated hemothorax unlikely will decortication be required to free a trapped lung following chest injury.[4]

Mortality from the operation is less than 5 per cent and morbidity is 10 per cent, consisting primarily of temporary air leaks and a rare empyema if the lung does not expand fully.

D. All penetrating chest wounds are suspect for penetrating the diaphragm. Ten to 15 per cent of stab wounds and 40 per cent of bullet wounds do so. Mortality of unrecognized associated abdominal injury is 8 to 10 per cent and is related to the number of abdominal organs involved and to delay in the recognition of these injuries. Peritoneal lavage is helpful in establishing diagnosis.[3, 5]

E. Ten to 15 per cent of penetrating chest injuries involve the heart. Hospital mortality of 15 to 30 per cent varies depending on how promptly the patient is taken to an organized trauma center capable of emergency care. In 5 to 7 per cent of cases, major vessels are injured. The right ventricle is most at risk for penetration (46 per cent), followed by the left ventricle (35 per cent) and the right atrium (26 per cent).[1, 3, 6]

F. Paracentesis relief of tamponade is an acceptable holding maneuver, but with gunshot wounds and 20 per cent of stab wounds tamponade will recur and early thoracotomy will be required following penetrating injuries involving the heart.[3] For patients seen soon after penetrating injury occurs, thoracotomy is the safest course if there is a high suspicion of cardiac penetration. Depending on the screening process before a patient comes to operation, survival can be up to 80 per cent. When chests are opened in the Emergency Department, the yield will be lower.

G. Post-traumatic respiratory distress syndrome (RDS) may occur following either blunt or penetrating trauma. Early onset RDS occurring within 2 to 5 days following injury,[29] if treated by standard means such as fluid restriction following resuscitation and positive end expiratory pressure (PEEP) on a mechanical respirator, can be almost totally cured (90 per cent of cases) after 5 to 7 days of careful treatment. Conversely, late onset RDS, usually associated with bacterial sepsis and multiple organ failure, has a correspondingly bad prognosis (15 per cent survival).[8]

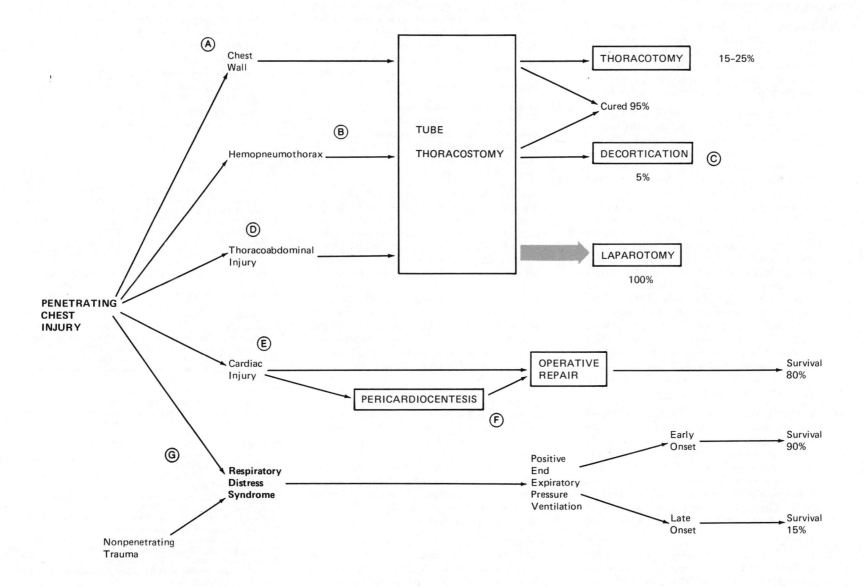

CHEST INJURY *Continued*

BLUNT CHEST INJURY

A. Fractured ribs, though painful for several days, are not life-threatening unless a sufficient number are broken to cause instability of the chest wall (flail chest). Even with obvious flail segments many young people will get along without difficulty.

B. Although some degree of flail occurs in 10 to 12 per cent of patients with severe blunt chest trauma,[2] only about 35 per cent will require mechanical ventilation, and these primarily will be because of the underlying lung contusion and not chest wall instability.[9] Associated sternal fracture significantly worsens instability.

   When mechanical ventilation is required it usually must be continued for 14 to 22 days and has a mortality of 20 to 35 per cent.[9, 10] Morbidity is 100 per cent and includes difficulty in weaning, inability to remove chest tubes while the patient is on the ventilator because of the danger of tension pneumothorax, and infection. Intermittent mechanical ventilation with PEEP has decreased mean ventilation time to 5 days,[11] as has internal stabilization of fractured ribs and sternum in selected cases.[12, 13] The latter should be undertaken when the two coincide.

C. Eighty to 83 per cent of blunt chest trauma cases are managed satisfactorily with tube thoracostomy and suction alone; 14 per cent need observation alone, and 3 to 6 per cent require early thoracotomy. The high incidence (73 per cent) of associated injuries accounts for most of the mortality.[2, 4] Thirty to 35 per cent of patients have coincidental abdominal injuries.

D. Rupture of the bronchus or trachea is rare (2 to 8 per cent) in those patients dying of trauma.[14] It is manifest by voluminous persistent air leak in 70 per cent of cases and deep pneumomediastinum in 30 per cent.[15] Most of these cases die before they reach the hospital, but of the remainder, 60 per cent are not diagnosed until after the first week following injury.[16] The overall mortality for ruptured bronchus is 30 per cent.[16, 17]

E. Rupture of the diaphragm by blunt trauma requires a severe injury. In 95 per cent of such patients, rupture is on the left side.[18] Mortality is 18 per cent; 11 per cent succumb from other injuries soon after operation.[19, 20]

F. Sudden deceleration or severe blows to the chest can rupture the aorta; 23 per cent occur at the root, 8 per cent at the arch, and 69 per cent immediately below the left subclavian artery.[21] Ten to 15 per cent of these patients reach the hospital alive,[22] and of these, two thirds are potentially curable.[23] Twenty per cent survive only one hour. Thereafter, 30 per cent die within 6 hours, 40 per cent within 24 hours, 72 per cent by 8 days, and 90 per cent by 10 weeks if not operated upon.[25] If the operation is performed within 24 hours, survival is 65 per cent.[23, 24]

G. A blow severe enough to sever the subclavian artery as it leaves the chest usually fractures the first rib, which is a good indication of this condition.[26] Peripheral pulses are still present via collateral vessels or because of incomplete rupture in 50 per cent of cases.[26] The artery can be repaired in 60 per cent of patients; 15 per cent require ligation.[27] The arm is almost always saved. Mortality is usually from associated head injuries.

H. Blunt cardiac injuries are treated in much the same way as penetrating trauma, except that operative exploration is pursued less vigorously and tamponade is treated at least once by needle aspiration. The exact frequency of cure (±30 per cent) by willingness to persist with multiple aspirations depends on case selection. So does the survival (±80 per cent) of those patients that require early open thoracotomy. If operation is solely for tamponade, all patients should survive, but if it is for traumatic rupture of the heart or the base of the aorta, few will survive.

References

1. Oparah, S. S., and Mandal, A. K.: Penetrating stab wounds of the chest: experience with 200 consecutive cases. J. Trauma, 16:868, 1976.
2. Dougall, A. M., et al.: Chest trauma — current morbidity and mortality. J. Trauma, 17:547, 1977.
3. Siemens, R., et al.: Indications for thoracotomy following penetrating thoracic injury. J. Trauma, 17:493, 1977.
4. Sturm, J. T., Points, B. J., and Perry, J. F.: Hemopneumothorax following blunt trauma to the thorax. Surg. Gynecol. Obstet., 141:539, 1975.
5. Sandiasagra, F. A.: Penetrating thoracoabdominal injuries. Br. J. Surg., 64:638, 1977.
6. Mattox, K. L., et al.: Logistic and technical considerations in the treatment of the wounded heart. Circulation, 51 and 52 (Suppl. 1):1210, 1975.
7. Eiseman, B., and Walker, L.: The changing pattern of post-traumatic respiratory distress syndrome. Ann. Surg., 181:693, 1975.
8. Eiseman, B., Beart, R., and Norton, L.: Multiple organ failure. Surg. Gynecol. Obstet., 144:323, 1977.
9. Trinkle, J. K., et al.: Management of flail chest without mechanical ventilation. Ann. Thorac. Surg., 19:355, 1975.
10. Lewis, F., Thomas A. N., and Schlobohm, R. M.: Control of respiratory therapy in flail chest. Ann. Thorac. Surg., 20:170, 1975.
11. Cullen, P. et al.: Treatment of flail chest. Arch. Surg., 110:1099, 1975.
12. Paris, F., et al.: Surgical stabilization of traumatic flail chest. Thorax, 30:521, 1975.
13. Powers, S. R.: Editorial: Management of flail chest. Ann. Thorac. Surg., 19:480, 1975.
14. Bertelsen, S., and Howitz, P.: Injuries to the trachea and bronchi. Thorax, 27:188, 1972.
15. Eijgelaar, A., and Homan van der Hyde, J. N.: A reliable early symptom of bronchial or tracheal rupture. Thorax, 25:120, 1970.

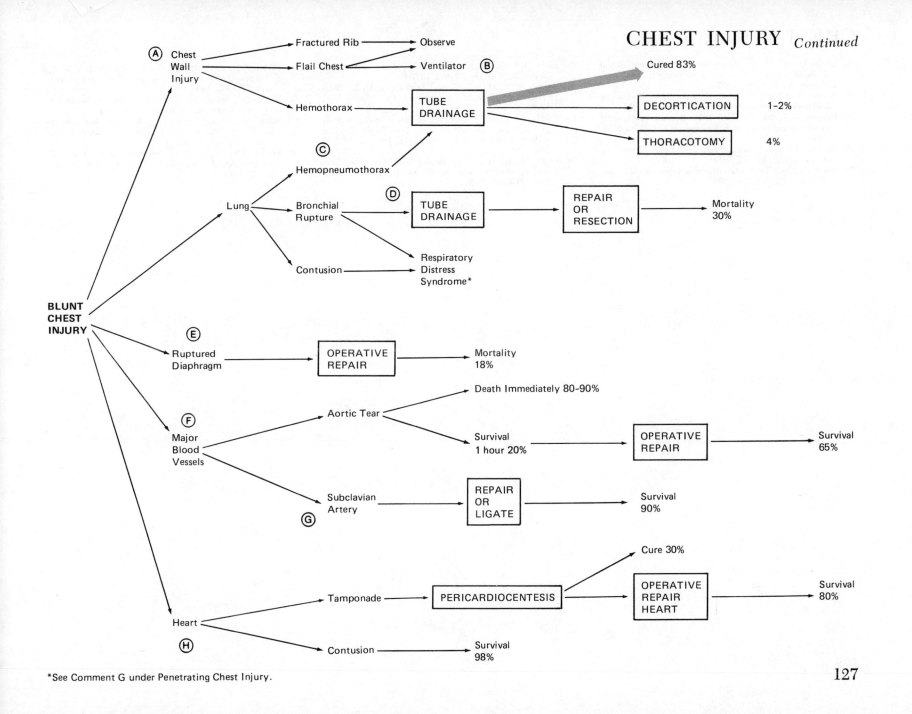

Ⓐ Chest Wall Injury

Fractured Rib ──→ Observe

Flail Chest ──→ Ventilator Ⓑ

Cured 83%

Hemothorax ──→ TUBE DRAINAGE

DECORTICATION   1-2%

THORACOTOMY   4%

Ⓒ Lung

Hemopneumothorax

Bronchial Rupture ──→ Ⓓ TUBE DRAINAGE ──→ REPAIR OR RESECTION ──→ Mortality 30%

Contusion ──→ Respiratory Distress Syndrome*

BLUNT CHEST INJURY

Ⓔ Ruptured Diaphragm ──→ OPERATIVE REPAIR ──→ Mortality 18%

Ⓕ Major Blood Vessels

Aortic Tear ──→ Death Immediately 80-90%

Survival 1 hour 20% ──→ OPERATIVE REPAIR ──→ Survival 65%

Subclavian Artery ──→ REPAIR OR LIGATE ──→ Survival 90%

Ⓖ

Heart

Tamponade ──→ PERICARDIOCENTESIS ──→ Cure 30%

──→ OPERATIVE REPAIR HEART ──→ Survival 80%

Contusion ──→ Survival 98%

Ⓗ

*See Comment G under Penetrating Chest Injury.

16. Kirsh, M. M., et al.: Management of tracheobronchial disruption secondary to nonpenetrating trauma. Ann. Thorac. Surg., 22:93, 1977.
17. Payne, W. S., and DeRemu, R.: Injuries of the trachea and major bronchi. Postgrad. Med., 49:152, 1971.
18. Epstein, L. I., and Lempke, R. E.: Rupture of the right hemidiaphragm due to blunt trauma. J. Trauma, 8:19, 1968.
19. Grimes, O. F.: Traumatic injuries of the diaphragm. Am. J. Surg., 128:175, 1974.
20. Hood, R. M.: Traumatic diaphragmatic hernia. Ann. Thorac. Surg., 12:311, 1971.
21. Vasko, J. S., et al.: Nonpenetrating trauma to the thoracic aorta. Surgery, 82:400, 1977.
22. Wilson, R. F., Murray, C., and Antonenko, D. R.: Nonpenetrating thoracic injuries. Surg. Clin. North Am., 57:17, 1977.
23. Bodily, K., et al.: The salvageability of patients with post-traumatic rupture of the descending thoracic aorta in a primary trauma center. J. Trauma, 17:754, 1977.
24. Keich, M. M., et al.: The treatment of acute traumatic rupture of the aorta: A 10-year experience. Ann. Surg., 184:308, 1976.
25. Parmley, L. F., Mattingly, T. W., and Manion, W. C.: Nonpenetrating traumatic injury to the aorta. Circulation, 17:1086, 1958.
26. Sturm, J. T., et al.: Blunt trauma to the subclavian artery. Surg. Gynecol. Obstet., 138:915, 1974.
27. Schaff, H. V., and Brawley, R. K.: Operative management of penetrating vascular injuries of the thoracic outlet. Surgery, 82:182, 1977.
28. Markovchick, V. J., et al.: Traumatic acute pericardial tamponade. J. Am. Coll. Emergency Physicians, 6:562, 1977.

EMPYEMA

EMPYEMA BY JOSEPH KOVARIK, M.D.

Comments

A. Organisms that cause empyema include Staphylococcus (45 per cent of cases), Streptococcus (15 per cent), and gram-negative bacilli (40 per cent). Mixed organisms are responsible for 50 per cent of empyema cases.[1-3]

B. In children, thoracentesis and antibiotics cure 85 per cent of cases.[4] In adults, postpneumonic empyema is cured by thoracentesis and antibiotics in about 20 per cent of instances.[1-3] Needle thoracentesis is used for diagnosis and identification of the organism as well as for therapeutic purposes.

C. Postoperative pleural effusion, whether sterile or containing pus, is usually sympathetic to subdiaphragmatic collection, and its prognosis depends in part on draining the subdiaphragmatic abscess as well as caring for the empyema.

D. Tube thoracostomy is performed if fluid persists. Its purpose is to remove fluid and obliterate the infected cavity. As with any abscess, it must be drained. This procedure is curative in about 25 per cent of cases.[1-3]

E. Only in established empyema with a localized cavity is rib resection and open drainage used. It is curative for about 35 per cent of patients, but many weeks may be required for the cavity to heal even with completely dependent drainage.

F. Decortication for postpneumonic empyema is often more difficult technically than when performed for clotted hemothorax following trauma; therefore, it has a higher morbidity rate.

G. This category includes infection following spontaneous pneumothorax, needle thoracentesis, and esophageal fistula.[1-3]

H. Empyema following lobectomy usually connotes inadequate expansion of the remaining lung to fill the hemithorax. Treatment and prognosis involve obliterating the dead space. Following pneumonectomy, empyema usually implies a bronchial stump leak (bronchopleural fistula). Empyema following pneumonectomy has an overall mortality of 4 per cent if those dying of cancer are excluded. Of course, most of these patients die of cancer, not empyema.

I. If life expectancy from cancer is limited and the fistula is tolerable, no other treatment may be needed.

J. Bronchoplasty is reclosure of the leaking bronchus by direct closure or reinforcement with muscle.

K. Often used in the past, thoracoplasty is now a relatively rare operation but may be curative in persistent empyema.

L. Reoperative closure of a stump blowout following pneumonectomy is rarely successful after more than 24 to 48 hours. (See page 150).

References

1. Snider, G.L., and Saleh, S.S.: Empyema of the thorax in adults: Review of 105 cases. Dis. Chest, 54:410, 1968.
2. Yeh, T.J., Hall, D.P., and Ellison, R.G.: Empyema thoracis: A review of 110 cases. Am. Rev. Respir. Dis., 88:785, 1963.
3. Geha, A.S.: Pleural empyema. J. Thorac. Cardiovasc. Surg., 61:626, 1971.
4. Stiles, Q.R., et al.: Pleural empyema in children. Ann. Thorac. Surg., 10:37, 1970.
5. Arom, K.V., et al.: Post-traumatic empyema. Ann. Thorac. Surg., 23:254, 1977.
6. Langston, H.T.: Empyema thoracis. Ann. Thorac. Surg., 2:766, 1966.
7. Barker, W.L., et al.: Management of persistent bronchopleural fistulas. J. Thorac. Cardiovasc. Surg., 62:393, 1971.
8. Clagett, O.T.: Changing aspects of the etiology and treatment of pleural empyema. Surg. Clin. North Am., 53:863, 1973.
9. Stafford, E.G., and Clagett, O.T.: Postpneumonectomy empyema. J. Thorac. Cardiovasc. Surg., 63:771, 1972.
10. Sensening, D.M., Rossi, N.P., and Ehrenhaft, J.L.: Decortication for chronic nontuberculous empyema. Surg. Gynecol. Obstet., 117:443, 1963.

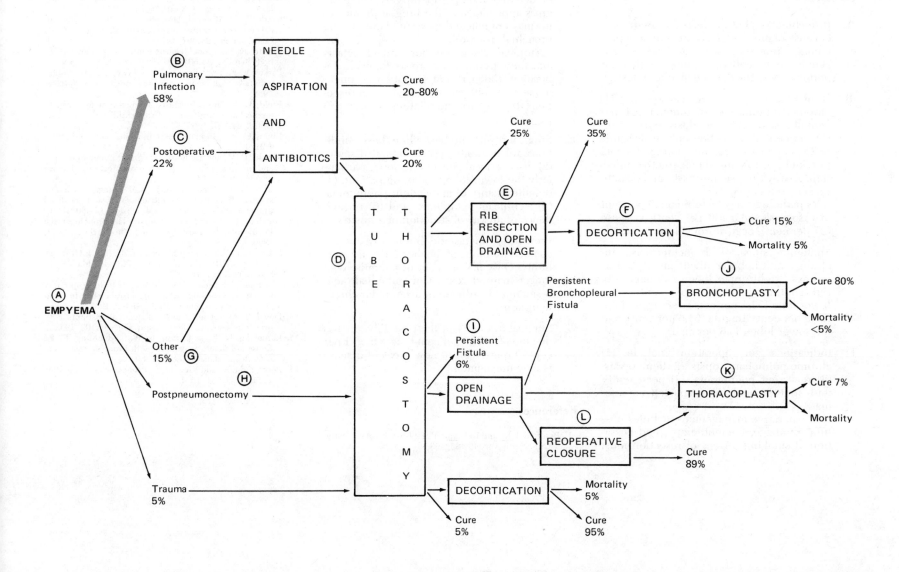

BRONCHIECTASIS BY WILLIAM HAMAKER, M.D.

Comments

A. Bronchiectasis has decreased in frequency because of more effective treatment of pulmonary infection with antibiotics and avoidance of collapse, immunization for pertussis, and the decline of tuberculosis.[1-3]

B. Bronchiectasis may be caused by (1) chronic suppurative pneumonia (24 per cent of cases), (2) tuberculosis (6 per cent), (3) congenital bronchoesophageal fistula (1.25 per cent), (4) retained foreign body (2 per cent), or (5) chronic obstructive infection, airway disease, pertussis, and exanthemata (±66 per cent).[4]

   Its pathology may be tubular (35 per cent of cases), saccular (30 per cent), varicose (27 per cent), or fusiform (11 per cent).[6]

C. Anatomic sites of bronchiectasis, including multilobular involvement, are as follows:[7] right upper lobe (30.0 per cent), right middle lobe (62.5 per cent), right lower lobe (54.4 per cent), left upper lobe (21.9 per cent), lingula (65.6 per cent), and left lower lobe (85.6 per cent).

D. Indications for operation include (1) chronic pulmonary sepsis, (2) hemoptysis, (3) recurrent pneumonia, (4) persistently foul sputum, and (5) suspected carcinoma.

   Preoperative management includes postural drainage, chemotherapy, and cessation of smoking.[3] Areas of resection must be decided upon preoperatively, since the gross appearance of the lung at thoracotomy may not reflect the extent of underlying bronchial disease.[1]

   Surgical resections for bronchiectasis and their frequencies are as follows:[8] lobectomy (50 per cent of patients), pneumonectomy (40 per cent), segmental resection (10 per cent), and bilateral resection (6 per cent).

E. Surgical results are best when these conditions are present:[11] (1) unilateral disease, (2) disease localized to one lobe, particularly the lower lobe, (3) young patient, (4) definite history of antecedent pneumonia, (5) significant symptoms, and (6) no evidence of airway obstruction or sinusitis.

F. Previously, metastatic brain abscess accounted for much of the mortality and morbidity. Only 9.4 per cent of patients lived longer than 30 years. Cor pulmonale and respiratory insufficiency account for chronic disability.[12-15]

G. Surgical mortality in the past 35 years has declined from 10 per cent to less than 1 per cent.[3] Progression of new areas of disease is now uncommon.[9]

References

1. Bradford, J. K., and DeCamp, P. T.: Bronchiectasis. Surg. Clin. North Am., *46*:485, 1966.
2. Ochsner, A.: Bronchiectasis — disappearing pulmonary lesion. N.Y. State J. Med., 75:1683, 1975.
3. Sanderson, J. M., et al.: Bronchiectasis: Results of surgical and conservative management. A review of 393 cases. Thorax, 29:407, 1974.
4. Kürklü, E. V.: Bronchiectasis consequent upon foreign body. Thorax, 28:601, 1973.
5. Parker, E. F., Brailsford, L. E., and Gregg, D. B.: Tuberculous bronchiectasis. Am. Rev. Respir. Dis., 98:240, 1968.
6. Field, C. E.: Bronchiectasis: A long-term followup of medical and surgical cases from childhood. Arch. Dis. Child., *44*:587, 1969.
7. Field, C. E.: Bronchiectasis in childhood. Pediatrics, *4*:21, 1949.
8. Kürklü, E. V., and Le Roux, B. T.: Left pneumonectomy and middle lobectomy for bronchiectasis. Thorax, 28:535, 1973.
9. Sealey, W. C., Bradham, R. R., and Young, W. G.: The surgical treatment of multisegmental and localized bronchiectasis. Surg. Gynecol. Obstet., *123*:80, 1966.
10. Hewlett, T. H., and Ziperman, H. H.: Bronchiectasis: Results of pulmonary resection. J. Thorac. Surg., *40*:71, 1960.
11. Sabiston, D. C., Jr., and Spencer, F. C. (eds.): Gibbon's Surgery of the Chest, 3rd ed. Philadelphia, W. B. Saunders Co., 1976.
12. Cherniak, N. S., et al.: The role of acute lower respiratory infection in causing pulmonary insufficiency in bronchiectasis. Ann. Intern. Med., *66*:489, 1967.
13. Dowd, J. M., et al.: Cause of death in patients with bronchiectasis. Am. Rev. Respir. Dis., 88:103, 1963.
14. Konietzko, N. F. J., Carton, R. W., and LeRoy, E. P.: Causes of death in patients with bronchiectasis. Am. Rev. Respir. Dis., *100*:852, 1969.
15. Perry, K. M. A., and King, D. S.: Bronchiectasis. Am. Rev. Tuberc., *41*:531, 1941.

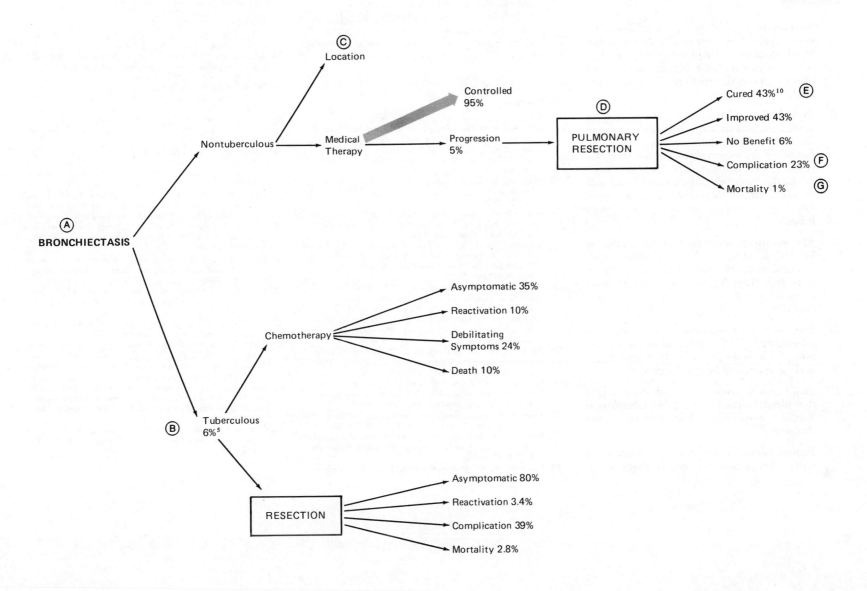

LUNG ABSCESS BY GEORGE STARKEY, M.D.

Comments

A. Seventy-five to 90 per cent of cases involve anaerobic bacteria (*Bacteroides melaninogenicus, Fusobacterium nucleatum*, microaerophilic Streptococcus, and others).[1] Overall mortality is 1 to 2 per cent.[1, 8]

B. Bronchial aspiration when the patient is semiconscious or unconscious (because of alcohol or stroke, following anesthesia, or for other reasons) initiates most lung abscesses. Characteristically, they are located in the dependent lobes and lung segments (axillary segment of right upper lobe or superior segments of lower lobes.)[1, 2]

C. The entire management of lung abscess has been changed by antibiotics. Previously, mortality was 34 per cent;[4, 5] now it is less than 5 per cent,[5] and medical therapy alone is satisfactory in most cases.[1, 8]

D. Indications for operation are (1) suspected cancer,[6, 17-20] (2) nonresponse to antibiotics,[15] (3) hemoptysis,[16] (4) empyema,[9-14] and (5) recurrent lung infection.[15]

E. Empyema follows rupture of abscess into the pleural space with a bronchopleural fistula, requiring thoracostomy tube drainage.[9-14]

F. Bronchoscopic removal of a foreign body early after aspiration avoids abscess formation and is essential for cure of an established abscess. Aspiration usually accompanies unconsciousness from alcohol, brain injury, anesthesia, or other conditions.

References

1. Feingold, S. M.: Necrotizing pneumonias and lung abscess. *In* Hoeprich, P. D. (ed.): Infectious Diseases, 2nd ed. N.Y., Harper and Row, 1977.
2. Brock, R. C.: Lung Abscess. Springfield, Ill., Charles C Thomas, 1952.
3. Bernhard, W. F., Malcolm, J. A., and Wylie, R. N.: A study of 148 cases due to aspiration. Dis. Chest, 43:620, 1963.
4. Sweet, R. H.: Lung abscess: Analysis of Massachusetts General Hospital cases from 1933–1937. Surg. Gynecol. Obstet., 70:1011–21, 1960.
5. Schweppe, H. I., Knowles, J. H., and Kane, L.: Lung abscess: An analysis of the Massachusetts General Hospital cases from 1943–1956. N. Engl. J. Med., 265:1039–1043, 1961.
6. Chidi, S. C., and Mendelsohn, H. J.: A study of the results of treatment based on 90 consecutive cases. J. Thorac. Cardiovasc. Surg., 68:168–172, 1974.
7. Sabiston, B. P., and Spencer, F. C., (eds.): Gibbon's Surgery of the Chest, 3rd ed. Philadelphia, W. B. Saunders, 1976.
8. Bartlett, J. G., and Gorback, S. L.: Treatment of aspiration pneumonia and primary lung abscess. Penicillin G vs. clindamycin. JAMA, 234:935, 1975.
9. Perlman, L. V., Lerner, E., and D'Esopo, N.: Clinical classification and analysis of 97 cases of lung abscess. Am. Rev. Respir. Dis., 99:390, 1969.
10. Vainrub, B., et al.: Percutaneous drainage of lung abscess. Am. Rev. Respir. Dis., 117:153–160, 1978.
11. Groff, D. B., and Marquis, J.: Treatment of lung abscess by transbronchial catheter drainage. Radiology, 107:61–62, 1973.
12. Cameron, E. W. J., and Whitton, I. D.: Percutaneous drainage in treatment of *Klebsiella pneumoniae* lung abscess. Thorax, 32:673–676, 1977.
13. Connors, J. P., Roper, C. L., and Ferguson, T. B.: Transbronchial catheterization of pulmonary abscess. Ann. Thorac. Surg., 19:254, 1975.
14. Sandler, B. P.: Prevention of cerebral abscess secondary to pulmonary suppuration. Dis. Chest, 48:32, 1965.
15. Weiss, W.: Cavitary behavior in acute primary nonspecific lung abscess. Am. Rev. Respir. Dis., 108:1273–1275, 1975.
16. Thoms, N. W., et al.: Life-threatening hemoptysis in primary lung abscess. Ann. Thorac. Surg., 14:347, 1972.
17. Glenn, W. W. L., Liebow, A. A., and Lindskog, G. E.: Thoracic and Cardiovascular Surgery with Related Pathology, 3rd ed. New York, Appleton-Century-Crofts, 1976.
18. Block, A. J., Wagley, P. F., and Fisher, A. M.: Lung abscess: A re-evaluation of the indications for surgery. Johns Hopkins Med. J., 125:19, 1969.
19. Glover, R. P., and Clagett, O. J.: Pulmonary resection for abscess of the lung. Surg. Gynecol. Obstet., 86:385, 1948.
20. Shaw, R. R., and Paulson, D. L.: Pulmonary resection for chronic abscess of the lung. J. Thorac. Surg., 17:514, 1948.
21. Griffith, G. L., Maull, K. I., and Sachatello, C. R.: Septic pulmonary embolization. Surg. Gynecol. Obstet., 144:105, 1977.
22. Collins, C. G.: Suppurative pelvic thrombophlebitis. Am. J. Obstet. Gynecol., 108:681, 1970.
23. Stein, J. M., and Pruitt, B. A.: Suppurative thrombophlebitis. N. Engl. J. Med., 282:1452, 1970.
24. Vidal, E., et al.: Lung abscess secondary to pulmonary infarction. Ann. Thorac. Surg., 11:557, 1971.
25. Goodwin, N. J., Castronuovo, J. J., and Friedman, E. A.: Recurrent septic pulmonary embolization complicating maintenance hemodialysis. Ann. Intern. Med., 71:29, 1969.
26. Mattox, K. L., and Guinn, G. A.: Emergency resection for massive hemoptysis. Ann. Thorac. Surg., 17:377, 1974.

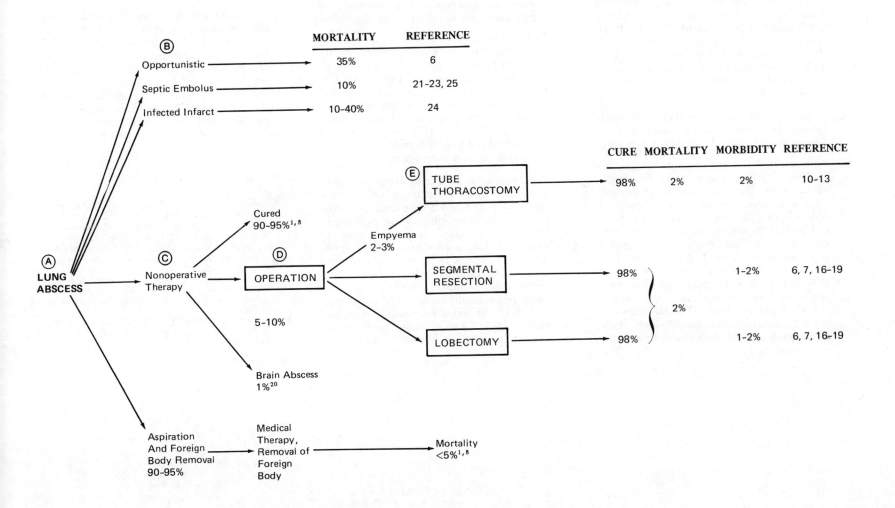

PULMONARY TUBERCULOSIS BY ROBERT K. BROWN, M.D.

Comments

A. Indications for surgery and prognosis in the pre-1972 era were entirely different from those of today. Collapse procedures predominated from about 1925 to 1950. After more effective antituberculosis drugs became available (beginning about 1945), resections became the usual surgical procedure, particularly from 1950 to 1970. (See page 139.)

B. At the present time, drug therapy for pulmonary tuberculosis has become so effective as to eliminate the need for surgery.

C. As a result of the use of drug therapy, definitive elective operations for tuberculosis are rare. The few cases done are salvage procedures for late complications of old collapse therapy and occasionally of old resections. Empyema may recur 40 to 50 years after the original unexpanded pneumothorax. A cold abscess may present as a soft fluctuant nontender mass in the chest wall, extracostal but often having a sinus communication to the old calcified empyema space. Osteomyelitis of a rib is possible but rarely seen. Late bronchopleural or bronchopleurocutaneous fistula may appear, and occasionally there is a sudden massive hemorrhage from an old, unhealed thick-walled cavity. Present-day management and prognosis of tuberculosis are detailed in the algorithm.

D. Differential diagnosis with lung cancer is also a thing of the past. A suspicious lesion that turns out not to be cancer is almost never tuberculosis but usually is hamartoma, fungal granuloma, healed pneumonia, or cyst. Scar carcinoma is a peripheral small adenocarcinoma shown histologically to be adjacent to a healed or calcified but not bacteriologically identified scar in lung parenchyma.

E. Bronchopleural fistula is always a tough problem but often is correctable. Dorman and associates[10] had 5 long-term survivors out of 6 patients after doing permanent open chest drainage. In certain cases of persistent fistula after dependent drainage or thoracoplasty, or both, Barker and co-workers[9] used pedicled muscle grafts (intercostal, serratus anterior, latissimus dorsi, or pectoralis major). The sinus tract is widely excised down to the bronchial stump; the stump is closed with catgut sutures, and the muscle is sutured to the bronchus and all interstices of the pleural space. Fifteen of 18 such closures were successful, and there was one death.

F. A related problem, not tuberculous but often requring surgery, is mycobacterial infection. The so-called atypical mycobacteria (*M. kansasii* , *M. intracellulare*, *M. fortuitum*) are highly resistant to drugs and produce lung disease that usually progresses to cavity formation. If the cavity remains open, with persistent positive sputum, surgical excision, usually by lobectomy, is indicated.[12]

References

1. Alexander, J.: Surgery of Pulmonary Tuberculosis. Philadelphia, Lea & Febiger, 1925.
2. Steele, J. D.: The surgical treatment of pulmonary tuberculosis. Ann. Thorac. Surg., 6:484–502, 1968.
3. McLaughlin, J. S. and Hankins, J. R.: Current aspects of surgery for pulmonary tuberculosis. Ann. Thorac. Surg., 17:513–525, 1974.
4. Prytz, S., Hansen, J. L.: A followup examination of patients with pulmonary tuberculosis resected on suspicion of tumour. Scand. J. Respir. Dis.: 57:239–246, 1976.
5. Das, P. B., and David, J. G.: Role of surgery in treatment of pulmonary tuberculosis. Can J. Surg., 18:512–518, 1975.

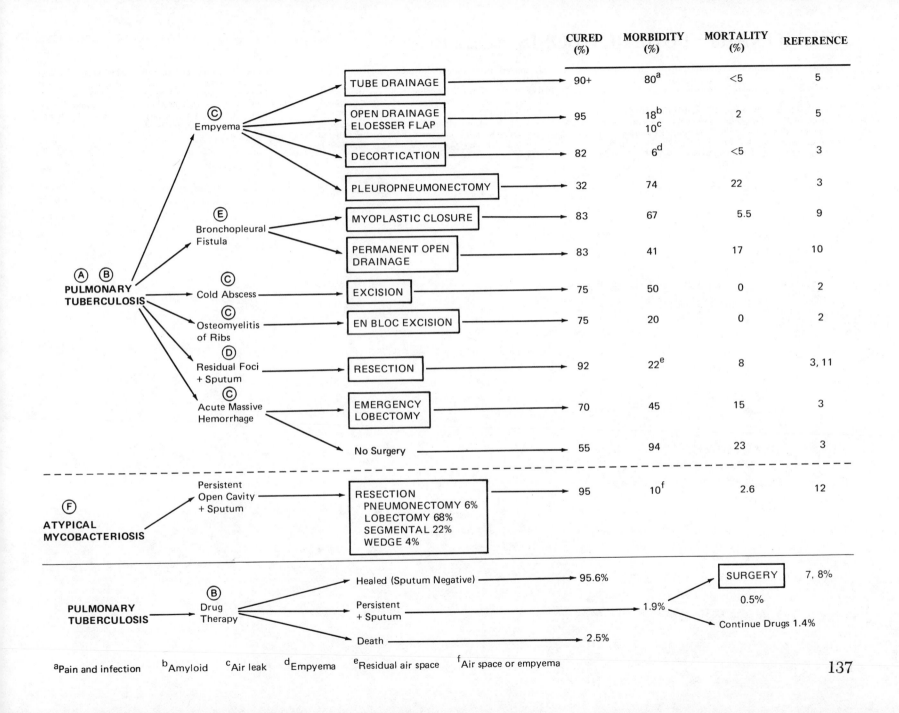

		CURED (%)	MORBIDITY (%)	MORTALITY (%)	REFERENCE
Empyema	TUBE DRAINAGE	90+	80[a]	<5	5
	OPEN DRAINAGE ELOESSER FLAP	95	18[b] 10[c]	2	5
	DECORTICATION	82	6[d]	<5	3
	PLEUROPNEUMONECTOMY	32	74	22	3
Bronchopleural Fistula	MYOPLASTIC CLOSURE	83	67	5.5	9
	PERMANENT OPEN DRAINAGE	83	41	17	10
Cold Abscess	EXCISION	75	50	0	2
Osteomyelitis of Ribs	EN BLOC EXCISION	75	20	0	2
Residual Foci + Sputum	RESECTION	92	22[e]	8	3, 11
Acute Massive Hemorrhage	EMERGENCY LOBECTOMY	70	45	15	3
	No Surgery	55	94	23	3

(A) (B) PULMONARY TUBERCULOSIS — (C) Empyema, (E) Bronchopleural Fistula, (C) Cold Abscess, (C) Osteomyelitis of Ribs, (D) Residual Foci + Sputum, (C) Acute Massive Hemorrhage

(F) ATYPICAL MYCOBACTERIOSIS

Persistent Open Cavity + Sputum → RESECTION
  PNEUMONECTOMY 6%
  LOBECTOMY 68%
  SEGMENTAL 22%
  WEDGE 4%
→ 95 | 10[f] | 2.6 | 12

PULMONARY TUBERCULOSIS → (B) Drug Therapy
  Healed (Sputum Negative) → 95.6% → SURGERY 7, 8%
  Persistent + Sputum → 1.9% → 0.5% / Continue Drugs 1.4%
  Death → 2.5%

[a]Pain and infection   [b]Amyloid   [c]Air leak   [d]Empyema   [e]Residual air space   [f]Air space or empyema

137

PULMONARY TUBERCULOSIS *Continued*

6. Dross, V. P.: Retrospective critical review and analysis of bilateral staged pulmonary resections for treatment of pulmonary tuberculosis. South. Med. J., 69:273–277, 1976.

7. British Medical Research Council: Controlled clinical trial of four short-course regimens of chemotherapy for two durations in the treatment of pulmonary tuberculosis. Am. Rev. Respir. Dis., 118:39–48, 1978.

8. Dutt, A. K. et al.: Followup of patients with tuberculo-sis treated in a general hospital program. Chest, 74:19–23, 1978.

9. Barker, W. L., et al.: Management of persistent bronchopleural fistulas. J. Thorac. Cardiovasc. Surg., 62:393–401, 1971.

10. Dorman, J. P., et al.: Open thoracostomy drainage of postpneumonectomy empyema with bronchopleural fistula. J. Thorac. Cardiovasc. Surg., 66:979–981, 1973.

11. Delarue, N. C., et al.: Experience with surgical salvage in pulmonary tuberculosis: Application to general thoracic surgery. Can J. Surg., 18:519–528, 1975.

12. Elkadi, A., Salas, R., and Almond, C. H.: Surgical treatment of atypical pulmonary tuberculosis. J. Thorac. Cardiovasc. Surg., 72:435–440, 1976.

INDICATIONS	OPERATION	CASES	CURED (%)	MOR-BIDITY (%)	MOR-TALITY (%)	REFER-ENCE
Thick-walled Cavity	Thoracoplasty		37	39	14[a] 19[b]	1
	Plombage		50	35	15	2
	Cavernostomy[c]		25+	60	50	3
	Resection					
	Pneumonectomy	330	68	35+	12	2
	Lobectomy	2362	74	40	2.7	2
	Segmental lobectomy	2775	64	68	0.9	2
	Wedge	794	91	37	0	2
	TOTAL	6261				
Residual Caseous Focus (Suspected Cancer)	Resection					
	Pneumonectomy	6%	80	31	20[d]	4
	Lobectomy	20%	81	19	0	4
	Segmental	19%	87	13	0	4
	Wedge	27%	98	25	0	4
	Enucleation	28%	87	21	0	4
Destroyed Lung Tissue	Thoracoplasty		12	65	58	5
	Resection		38	52	15	5
Bronchiectasis	Resection		91	40	3	2
Bronchostenosis	Thoracoplasty		11	70	31	2
	Resection		68	45	8	2
Empyema						
Mixed	Drainage		15	80	78	3
Pure TB	Decortication		80	38	10	3
	Drainage		68	40	4	3
Bilateral Cavitary Disease	Bilateral resection (two stages)		86	28	0	6

[a] Two-month mortality
[b] Late mortality
[c] Very few done
[d] Overall mortality 2.3% for this group

SOLITARY PULMONARY NODULE BY DANIEL L. SMITH, M.D.

Comments

A. Solitary pulmonary nodule is an asymptomatic, circumscribed, homogeneous density found in the periphery of the lung on chest x-ray; calcification and cavitation may be present.

B. The miscellaneous category includes bronchogenic cysts, arteriovenous malformations, pulmonary infarcts, pulmonary sequestrations, and pleural or chest wall tumors.[1]

C. The ratio of granuloma to primary malignancy increases in areas where histoplasmosis and coccidioidomycosis are endemic.[5]

D. Incidence of primary malignancy is related to age.[2,5] In people under 35, it is 1 per cent; in those 35 to 45, 14 per cent; and in those over 45, 50 per cent.

E. In bronchogenic carcinoma appearing as a peripheral nodule, calcium is present in 4 per cent of cases[2]; 4 per cent are cavitary.[2] Cytology is positive in 35 per cent of cases.[3,4] Needle aspiration is positive in 85 per cent of cases.[3] The mortality of this procedure is less than one per cent, and morbidity (pneumothorax, hemothorax) is 10 per cent. Mediastinoscopy is positive in 35 per cent of patients.[3] The mortality of mediastinoscopy is 0.08 per cent and morbidity is 1.6 per cent.

There is no difference in survival among various cell types, but there is increased survival with smaller tumors.[1,6]

Two-thirds of peripheral primary tumors are adenocarcinoma or of the undifferentiated large-cell type.[1,6] The prognosis for peripheral bronchogenic carcinoma is five times better than for the equivalent cell type at the hilum.[1,3]

F. Eighteen per cent of suspected solitary metastatic pulmonary nodules are primary bronchogenic carcinoma at thoracotomy.[8,9] The prognosis improves the longer the latent period between control of the primary and visualization of the pulmonary metastasis.[7,9-11]

G. Five-year survival varies with site of primary tumor.[8,9,11] In tumors of the uterus, cervix, colorectum, or testis, 5-year survival is 50 per cent. In tumors of the breast or kidney, 5-year survival is 30 per cent.

References

1. Steele, J. D.: The solitary pulmonary nodule. J. Thorac. Cardiovasc. Surg., 46:21, 1963.
2. Higgins, G. A., Shields, T. W., and Keehn, R. J.: The solitary pulmonary nodule. Arch. Surg., 110:570, 1975.
3. Lillington, G. A.: The solitary pulmonary nodule —1974. Am. Rev. Respir. Dis., 110:699, 1974.
4. Bains, M. S., Martini, N., and Beattie, E. J., Jr.: Treatment of primary malignant "coin lesions" of the lung. Surg. Clin. North Am., 54:825, 1974.
5. Trunk, G., Gracey, D. R., and Byrd, R. B.: The management and evaluation of the solitary pulmonary nodule. Chest, 66:236, 1974.
6. Jackman, R. J., et al.: Survival rates in peripheral bronchogenic carcinomas up to four centimeters in diameter presenting as solitary pulmonary nodules. J. Thorac. Cardiovasc. Surg., 57:1, 1969.
7. Feldman, P. S., and Kyriakos, M.: Pulmonary resection for metastatic sarcoma. J. Thorac. Cardiovasc. Surg., 64:784, 1972.
8. Choksi, L. B., Takita, H., and Vincent, R. G.: The surgical management of solitary pulmonary metastasis. Surg. Gynecol. Obstet., 134:479, 1972.
9. Cline, R. E., and Young, W. G.: Long-term results following surgical treatment of metastatic pulmonary tumors. Am. Surg., 36:61, 1970.
10. Turney, S. Z., and Haight, C.: Pulmonary resection for metastatic neoplasms. J. Thorac. Cardiovasc. Surg., 61:784, 1971.
11. Wheatley, A., and Howard, N.: The surgical treatment of lung metastasis. Br. J. Surg., 54:364, 1967.

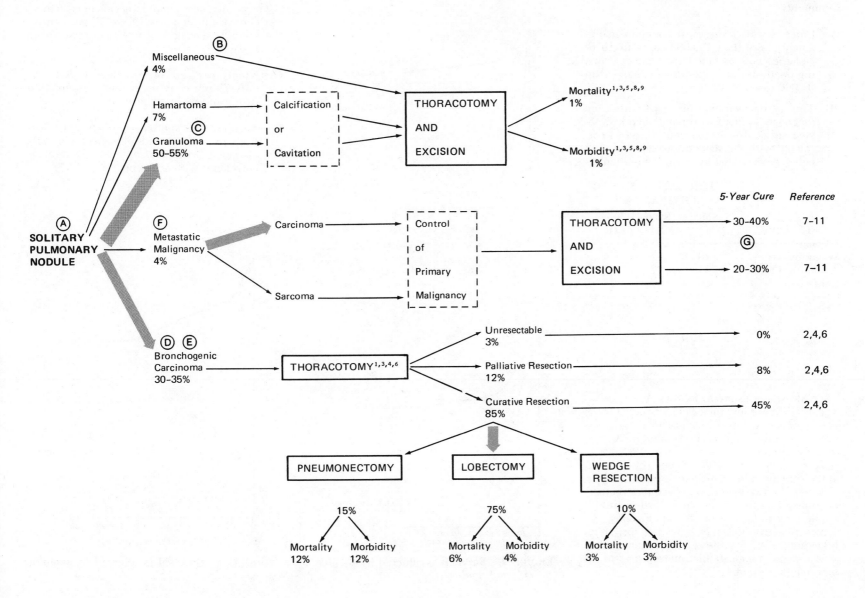

LUNG CANCER BY FRANK MANART, M.D., AND SYLVAN BAER, M.D.

Comments

A. Lung cancer is the most common malignancy (more than 100,000 cases in 1976) and the most common malignancy causing death in the United States (more than 93,000 cases in 1976).[25]

B. The median survival of all patients from diagnosis to death is 6 months and the 5-year survival is 10 per cent. Survival correlated with the stage of disease and with cell type is shown in the following table:

CELL TYPE	CUMULATIVE 5-YEAR SURVIVAL (%)[15]		
	Stage I[a]	Stage II[b]	Stage III[c]
Squamous	40	17	14
Adenocarcinoma	31	7	7
Large cell	30	7	11

[a]Stage I = $T_1N_0M_0$
$T_1N_1M_0$
$T_2N_0M_0$
[b]Stage II = T_2N_1
[c]Stage III = T_1 any N or M
N_2 any T or M
M_1 any T or N

TNM categories are as follows:[20]

T_1 = (1) tumor less than 3 cm. in diameter; (2) no evidence of invasion proximal to lobar bronchus; and (3) tumor surrounded by lung or visceral pleura.

T_2 = (1) tumor more than 3 cm. in diameter, and (2) tumor more than 2 cm. from carina.

T_3 = (1) extension to adjacent structure; (2) tumor less than 2 cm. from carina; and (3) whole lung atelectasis or pleural effusions.

N_0 = negative nodes; N_1 = positive ipsilateral hilar nodes; N_2 = positive mediastinal nodes.

M_0 = no demonstrable metastases; M_1 = metastases present.

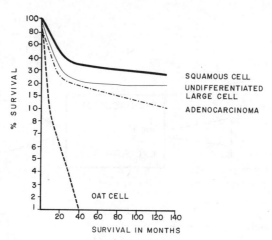

FIGURE 1. Survival as affected by cell type.[21]

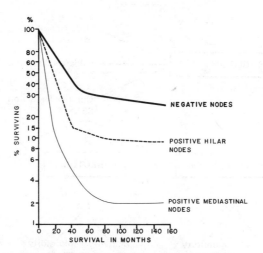

FIGURE 2. Survival as affected by involvement of lymph nodes.[21]

The recurrence rate of lung cancer is 30 to 35 per cent in the first year, 20 to 25 per cent in the second year, and 10 to 15 per cent in the third year.[21,31]

C. Ninety per cent of visualized lesions but only 75 per cent of peripheral tumors are diagnosed by bronchoscopy.[34]

D. Accuracy of sputum cytology increases from 78 per cent with one specimen to 94 per cent with 5 samples.[18] Accuracy is correlated with cell type.[17]

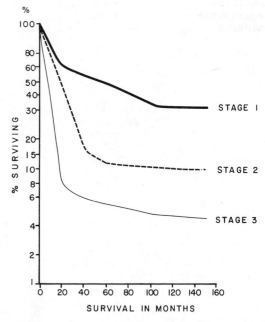

FIGURE 3. Survival as affected by stage of disease.[21]

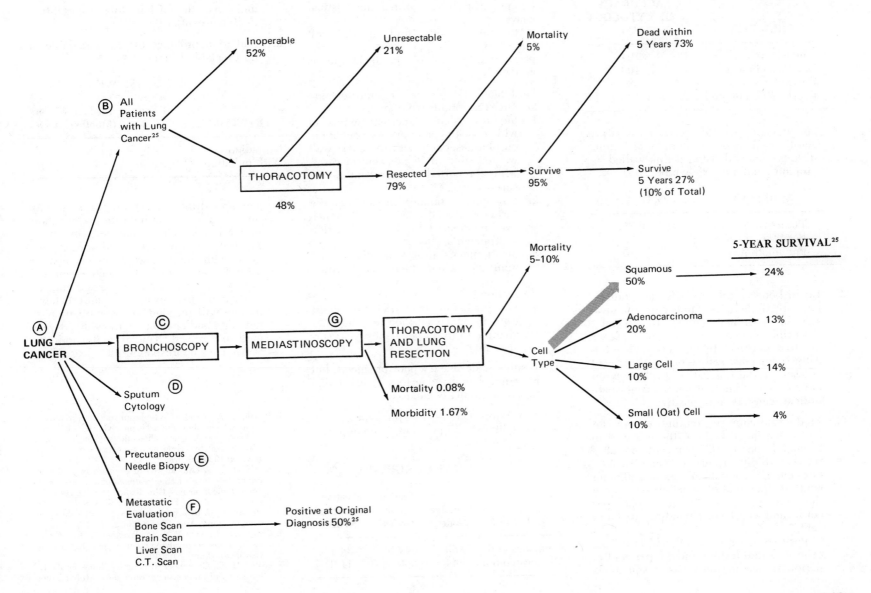

CELL TYPE	ACCURACY OF CYTOLOGY (%)
Squamous	94
Adenocarcinoma	±100
Oat cell	86
Poorly differentiated	26

E. Percutaneous needle biopsy is used primarily for diagnosis of peripheral lesions. Results obtained using a thin-walled aspiration needle are shown below:[34]

RESULT	% OF CASES
Tissue retrieved	75
Positive for cancer	90
Pneumothorax	10

F. Liver, bone, and brain scans are indicated only if there is clinical or chemical suggestion of metastases.[28] In clinically resectable patients, 1 per cent of scans are true positive. In patients with clinically suspicious evaluations, 10 per cent of scans are false negative. In those without suspicious findings, 80 per cent of abnormal scans are false positive.

G. Mediastinoscopy is routine except for small peripheral lesions (those less than 2 cm.). It has a 0.08 per cent mortality rate. Morbidity occurs at a rate of 1.67 per cent and consists of bleeding (0.6 per cent), 0.1 per cent of which cases require thoracotomy; pneumothorax (0.3 per cent), and vocal cord paralysis (0.3 per cent).[3]

   Positive nodes are found in 65 to 100 per cent of central lesions and 4.6 per cent of peripheral adenocarcinomas or squamous

lesions that have normal mediastinal x-rays.[9]

   Most false negative findings are in left lung lesions (25 per cent) where the parasternal variant of the technique is used.[3, 9]

H. Most Stage III lesions are unresectable for cure. Exceptions include:
   1. Superior sulcus (Pancoast) tumors, in which, with preoperative radiation, en bloc resection with the chest wall was possible in 67 per cent of cases, with a reported 34 per cent 5-year survival rate.[24]
   2. Low-grade tumors involving the carina or lateral tracheal wall, which may be treated by sleeve resection and pneumonectomy.[10]
   3. Small tumors near (less than 2 cm. from) the carina, which may occasionally be cured by sleeve bronchial resection.[22]
   4. Low-grade tumors involving the chest wall, in which en bloc resection has given a 16 to 32 per cent 5-year survival rate.[4, 5]

I. Positive nodes have a poor prognosis, but resection lymphadenectomy plus radiation is occasionally curative.[13]

J. The rate of cure by pneumonectomy (mortality 8 to 15 per cent) is no improvement over that of lobectomy (mortality 1 to 10 per cent).[13, 14]

5-YEAR SURVIVAL (%)

CELL TYPE	Negative Nodes	Positive Hilar Nodes	Positive Mediastinal Nodes
Squamous cell	53	47.5	34.4
Adenocarcinoma	44	0	11.8

K. Radiation prolongs life in inoperable or unresectable lesions.[2, 6, 27, 29, 30]

SURVIVAL

TREATMENT	1 Year (%)	Median (Months)	4 Years (%)
No radiation	16	6	0
With radiation	22–36	27	6

L. The only drugs used as surgical adjuvants for which hard data indicate prolongation of survival are chromomysin-A_3 and mitomycin-C. Five-year survival was 50 per cent with these two drugs, compared with 22 per cent in retrospective controls who received no adjuvant chemotherapy.[12] Forty-two per cent of unresectable tumors will respond to a combination of radiation and chemotherapy with a 1-year median survival. This is a 9-month increase over nonresponders.[1]

References

1. Bitran, J. A., et al.: Cyclophosphamide, Adriamycin, methotrexate and procarbazine (CAMP)—Effective four-drug combination chemotherapy for metastatic non–oat cell bronchogenic carcinoma. Cancer Treat. Rev., 60:1225, 1976.
2. Deely, T. J.: A clinical trial to compare two different tumor dose levels in the treatment of advanced carcinoma of the bronchus. Clin. Radiol., 17:299, 1966.
3. Foster, E. D., Munro, D. D., and Dobell, A. R. C.: Mediastinoscopy: A review of anatomical relationships and complications. Ann. Thorac. Surg., 13:273, 1972.
4. Geha, A. S., Bernatz, P. E., and Woolner, L. B.: Bronchogenic carcinoma involving the thoracic wall. J. Thorac. Cardiovasc. Surg., 54:3, 1967.
5. Grillo, H. C., Greenberg, J. J., and Wilkins, E. W., Jr.: Resection of bronchogenic carcinoma involving thor-

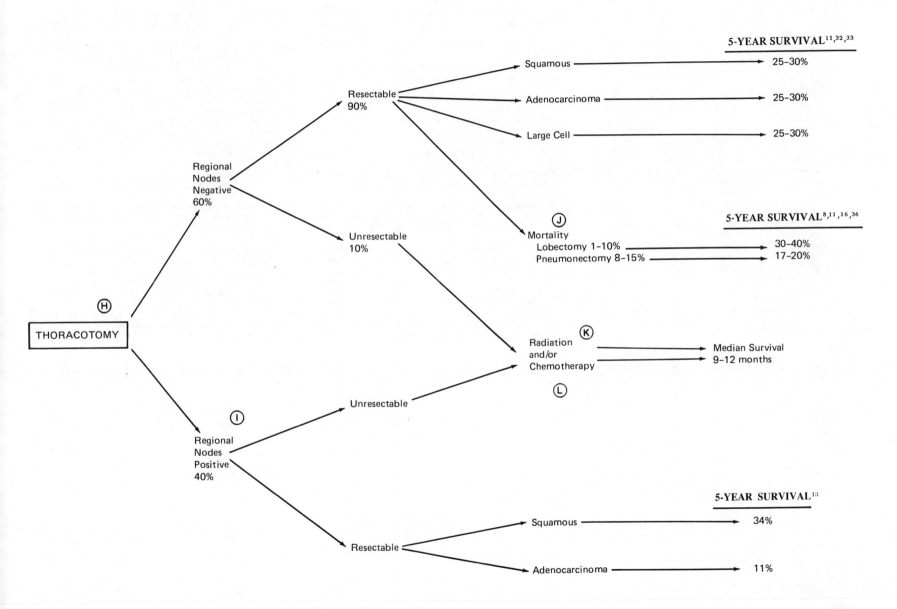

acic wall. J. Thorac. Cardiovasc. Surg., *51*:417, 1966.

6. Guttman, R.: Radical supervoltage therapy in inoperable carcinoma of the lung. *In* Deely, T. J. (ed.): *Modern Radiotherapy: Carcinoma of the Bronchus.* New York, Appleton-Century-Crofts, 1971, p. 181.

7. Hansen, H. H., et al.: Combination chemotherapy of advanced lung cancer: A randomized trial. Cancer, *38*:2201, 1976.

8. Higgins, G. A., et al.: Cytoxan as an adjuvant to surgery. Prognostic factors in lung cancer. Ann. Thorac. Surg., *7*:492, 1969.

9. Hutchinson, C. M., and Mills, N. L.: The selection of patients with bronchogenic carcinoma for mediastinoscopy. J. Thorac. Cardiovasc. Surg., *71*:768, 1976.

10. Jensik, R. J., Fahen, L. P., and Malloy, F. J.: Tracheal sleeve pneumonectomy for advanced carcinoma of the lung. Surg. Gynecol. Obstet., *134*:231, 1972.

11. Jones, J. C., et al.: Long-term survival after surgical resection for bronchogenic carcinoma. J. Thorac. Cardiovasc. Surg., *54*:383, 1967.

12. Katsuki, H., Shimada, K., and Koyama, A.: Long-term intermittent adjuvant chemotherapy for primary, resected lung cancer. J. Thorac. Cardiovasc. Surg., *70*:590, 1975.

13. Kirsh, M. K., et al.: Carcinoma of the lung: Results of treatment over ten years. Ann. Thorac. Surg., *21*:371, 1976.

14. Latarjet, M., and Bes, J.: The surgical treatment of primary bronchopulmonary cancer. *In* Saegresser, F., and Petterol, J. (eds.): Surgical Oncology. Baltimore, Williams & Wilkins, 1970.

15. Legha, S. S., Muggia, F. M., and Carter, S. K.: Adjuvant chemotherapy in lung cancer: Review and prospects. Cancer, *39*:1415, 1977.

16. LeRoux, B. T.: Bronchial carcinoma. Thorax, *23*:136, 1968.

17. Lukeman, J. M.: Reliability of cytologic diagnosis in cancer of the lung. Cancer Chemother. Rep., *4*:79, 1973.

18. Meyer, J. A., and Ymiker, W. O.: A review of problems relating to the diagnostic triad in lung cancer — Bronchoscopy, scalene lymph node biopsy, and cytopathology of bronchial secretions. Med. Clin. North Am., *41*:1233, 1961.

19. Mittman, C.: Assessment of operative risk in thoracic surgery. Ann. Rev. Resp. Dis., *84*:197, 1961.

20. Mountain, C. F.: Surgical therapy in lung cancer: Biologic, physiologic, and technical determinants. Semin. Oncol., *1*:253, 1974.

21. Mountain, C. F., Carr, D. T., and Anderson, W. A. D.: A system for the clinical staging of lung carcinoma. Am. J. Roentgenol. Radium Ther. Nucl. Med., *120*:130, 1974.

22. Naruke, T., Yoneyama, T., and Ogata, T.: Bronchoplastic procedures for lung cancer. J. Thorac. Cardiovasc. Surg., *73*:927, 1977.

23. Olsen, G. W., Block, J. J., and Swensen, E. W.: Pulmonary function — Evaluation of the lung resection candidate: A prospective study. Ann. Rev. Resp. Dis., *111*:379, 1975.

24. Paulson, D. L.: Carcinomas in the superior sulcus. J. Thorac. Cardiovasc. Surg., *70*:1095, 1975.

25. Paulson, D. L., and Reisch, J. J.: Long-term survival after resection for bronchogenic carcinoma. Ann. Surg., *184*:332, 1976.

26. Paulson, D. L., and Urschel, H. C.: Selectivity in the surgical treatment of bronchogenic carcinoma. J. Thorac. Cardiovasc. Surg., *62*:994, 1971.

27. Perez, C. A.: Radiation therapy in the management of carcinoma of the lung. Cancer, *39*:901, 1977.

28. Ramsdell, J. W., et al.: Multiorgan scans for staging lung cancer. J. Thorac. Cardiovasc. Surg., *73*:653, 1977.

29. Roswick, B., Patno, M. E., and Rapp, R.: The survival of patients with inoperable lung cancer: A large-scale randomized study of radiation versus placebo. Radiology, *90*:688, 1968.

30. Rubin, P., Ciccio, S., and Setisan, B.: The controversial status of radiation therapy in lung cancer. *In* Proceedings of the 6th National Cancer Conference. Philadelphia, J. B. Lippincott, 1970, p. 855.

31. Shields, T. W., Robinette, D., and Keehn, R. J.: Bronchial carcinoma treated by adjuvant cancer chemotherapy. Arch. Surg., *109*:329, 1974.

32. Shields, T. W., et al.: Relationship of cell type and lymph node metastasis to survival after resection of bronchial carcinoma. Ann. Thorac. Surg., *20*:501, 1975.

33. Stanford, W., et al.: Results of treatment of primary carcinoma of the lung: Analysis of 3000 cases. J. Thorac. Cardiovasc. Surg., *72*:441, 1976.

34. Zavala, D. C., and Rossi, N. P.: Nonthoracotomy diagnostic techniques for pulmonary disease. Arch. Surg., *107*:152, 1973.

PULMONARY LOBECTOMY

PULMONARY LOBECTOMY BY BENSON B. ROE, M.D.

Comments

A. Mortality reflects patient selection and indications for lobectomy. Resection for tuberculosis and infection carries higher morbidity and mortality rates than resection for tumor.[1-5] An accurate incidence of complications is impossible to document because of differences in reporting and interpretation. Incidences of complications are cited here when recent reliable reports are available; elsewhere they are estimated.

B. Bronchopleural fistula, consisting of a persistent major air leak that exceeds the characteristic minor and temporary (1 to 3 day) leak, occurs in 4 per cent of patients.[2]

C. Thoracostomy tube drainage with adequate suction should bring the remaining lung to the parietal pleura and result in symphysis. A persistent fistulous tract without a pleural space will always close spontaneously.[6]

D. Reclosure of a leaking lobectomy stump is seldom possible unless performed within 1 to 3 days after resection. More proximal bronchial transection and closure (up to pneumonectomy) is usually necessary.

E. Intercostal muscle flaps are reported to close bronchial stumps in lobectomy as in pneumonectomy.[8, 11]

F. Persistent space results from either air leak or unsuccessful pleural evacuation. It can simply be observed through gradual resolution unless (1) ventilation is impaired, (2) infection develops (empyema),[4, 7, 8] or (3) the space is expanding.

G. The incidence of empyema following lobectomy is reported to be as low as 1.8 per cent,[2] but it probably occurs in unreported experience between 10 and 15 per cent of the time. Its development is related to the failure of postoperative pleural evacuation, because empyema cannot occur in an obliterated space.[1, 5, 7, 9, 10]

H. When open drainage results in a space that is unlikely to close by granulation, that space can be obliterated by thoracoplasty to result in healing and closure.

I. Cardiac arrhythmias range in incidence between 3 and 30 per cent, correlating with age.[1, 4, 12, 13] As in the case of pneumonectomy, mortality is increased by arrhythmia, but separate figures are not available for lobectomy. Onset usually occurs on the second or third postoperative day.

J. Torsion of the remaining lobe(s) following lobectomy is a rare but grave complication of unreported incidence that is related to technical management.[14, 15]

References

1. Shields, T.W.: Pulmonary resections. *In* Shields, T.W., (ed.): General Thoracic Surgery. Philadelphia, Lea & Febiger, 1972, chapter 20.
2. Jensik, R.J., et al.: Sleeve lobectomy for carcinoma. J. Thorac. Cardiovasc. Surg., 64:400, 1972.
3. Barker, W.L., Langston, H.T., and Naffah, P.: Post-resectional thoracic spaces. Ann. Thorac. Surg., 2:299, 1966.
4. Kirsh, M.M., et al.: Complications of pulmonary resection. Ann. Thorac. Surg., 20:215, 1975.
5. Ashor, G.L., et al.: Long-term survival in bronchogenic carcinoma. J. Thorac. Cardiovasc. Surg., 70:581, 1975.
6. Roe, B.B.: The use and abuse of chest drainage. West. J. Surg., 61:706, 1953.
7. Barker, W.L., Langston, H.T., and Naffah, P.: Post-resection thoracic spaces. Ann. Thorac. Surg., 2:299, 1966.
8. Barker, W.L., et al.: Management of persistent bronchopleural fistula. J. Thorac. Cardiovasc. Surg., 62:393, 1971.
9. Yeh, T.J., Hall, D.P., and Ellison, R.G.: Empyema thoracis: A review of 110 cases. Am. Rev. Resp. Dis. 88:785, 1963.
10. Dieter, R., et al.: Empyema treated with neomycin irrigation and closed chest drainage. J. Thorac. Cardiovasc. Surg., 59:496, 1970.
11. Hankins, J.R., Miller, J.E., and McLaughlin, J.S.: The use of chest wall muscle flaps to close bronchopleural fistulas: Experience with 21 patients. Ann. Thorac. Surg., 25:491, 1975.
12. Mowry, F., and Reynolds, E.F.: Cardiac rhythm disturbances complicating resectional surgery of the lung. Ann. Intern. Med. 61:688, 1964.
13. Shields, T.W., and Yjiki, G.T.: Digitalization for prevention of arrhythmias following pulmonary surgery. Surg. Gynecol. Obstet., 126:743, 1968.
14. Mullin, M.J., et al.: Pulmonary lobar gangrene complicating lobectomy. Ann. Surg., 175:62, 1972.
15. Schuler, J.G.: Intraoperative lobar torsion producing pulmonary infarction. J. Thorac. Cardiovasc. Surg., 65:951, 1973.

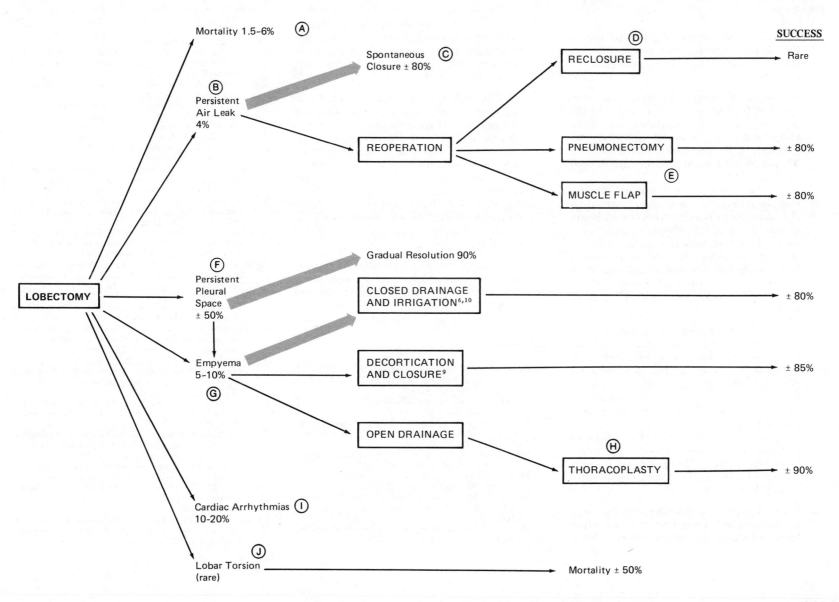

Mortality 1.5–6% (A)

SUCCESS

Spontaneous (C)
Closure ± 80%

RECLOSURE (D) → Rare

(B)
Persistent
Air Leak
4%

REOPERATION

PNEUMONECTOMY → ± 80%

MUSCLE FLAP (E) → ± 80%

LOBECTOMY

(F)
Persistent
Pleural
Space
± 50%

Gradual Resolution 90%

CLOSED DRAINAGE
AND IRRIGATION[6,10] → ± 80%

Empyema
5–10%
(G)

DECORTICATION
AND CLOSURE[9] → ± 85%

OPEN DRAINAGE

THORACOPLASTY (H) → ± 90%

Cardiac Arrhythmias (I)
10–20%

Lobar Torsion (J)
(rare) ——————————————— Mortality ± 50%

PNEUMONECTOMY BY BENSON B. ROE, M.D.

Comments

A. Mortality and morbidity primarily reflect the stage of disease, pulmonary reserve, surgical expertise, and postoperative care.[1-5]

B. Incidence of bronchial stump leak currently is 0.25 per cent, compared with 25 per cent formerly. Mortality therefrom varies with age, state of debility, and promptness of recognition and treatment. This accounts for a significant part of total mortality.[1, 5, 6]

 Spontaneous closure is rare unless the leak is minuscule, and direct operative closure seldom is effective after 48 hours unless there is an adequate uninfected residual stump, which usually will not blow out to begin with. Surgeons seldom leave such long bronchial stumps. Late closure can be effected using muscle pedicles[5, 7-9] with or without thoracoplasty.

C. Incidence of empyema is reported to be 2 to 10 per cent but now characteristically is less than 5 per cent. Although most frequent in the early postoperative period, it may appear months later. Contamination, preoperative irradiation, fistula, and residual diseases are all predisposing factors.

 Open drainage is required in 10 to 15 per cent of empyema cases with intact bronchial stump. Thoracoplasty is warranted for cure if life expectancy is sufficiently long.[13]

D. Some degree of pulmonary insufficiency is inevitable. Preoperative predictive tests include (1) forced expiratory volume in the first second (FEV-1) predicted to exceed 0.8 L postoperatively, (2) resting hyperpnea that responds to preoperative treatment, and (3) mean pulmonary artery pressure that is less than 10 mm. Hg above normal.[23, 24]

E. Cardiac arrhythmias occur in 3.4 to 30 per cent of cases and correlate with age (4.2 per cent of patients are younger than 50 and 17 per cent are over 50).[1, 5, 15, 17] There is one report of a 50 per cent incidence in patients over 70![17] Mortality is 4 per cent without and 14 per cent with arrhythmias. Onset characteristically is on the second or third postoperative day.[15] Prophylactic digitalization reduces the incidence of arrhythmias and the resulting mortality.[16]

F. Esophageal fistula is uncommon but results in empyema, requires reoperation, and carries a mortality of ± 40 per cent.[18-20]

References

1. Shields, T.W.: Pulmonary resections. In Shields, T.W., (ed.): General Thoracic Surgery. Philadelphia, Lea & Febiger, 1972, chapter 20.
2. Jensik, R.J., et al.: Sleeve lobectomy for carcinoma. J. Thorac. Cardiovasc. Surg., 64:400, 1972.
3. Gaskin, R.J., and Bergmann, M.: Pneumonectomy by "en masse" stapling of hilar vessels. Ann. Thorac. Surg., 19:242, 1975.
4. Vincent, R.G., et al.: Surgical therapy of lung cancer. J. Thorac. Cardiovasc. Surg. 71:581, 1976.
5. Kirsh, M.M., et al.: Complications of pulmonary resection. Ann. Thorac. Surg., 20:215, 1975.
6. Malove, G., et al.: Bronchopleural fistula: Present-day study of an old problem. Ann. Thorac. Surg., 11:1, 1971.
7. Barker, W.L., et al.: Management of bronchopleural fistula. J. Thorac. Cardiovasc. Surg., 62:393, 1971.
8. Demos, N.J., and Timmes, J.J.: Myoplasty for closure of tracheobronchial fistula. Ann. Thorac. Surg., 15:88, 1973.
9. Hankins, J.R., Miller, J.E., and McLaughlin, J.S.: The use of chest wall muscle flaps to close bronchopleural fistulas: Experience with 21 patients. Ann. Thorac. Surg., 25:491, 1978.
10. Zumbro, G.L., et al.: Empyema after pneumonectomy. Ann. Thorac. Surg., 15:615, 1973.
11. Clagett, O.T., and Geraci, J.E.: A procedure for management of postpneumonectomy empyema. J. Thorac. Cardiovasc. Surg., 45:141, 1963.
12. Dieter, R., et al.: Empyema treated with neomycin irrigation and closed chest drainage. J. Thorac. Cardiovasc. Surg., 59:496, 1970.
13. Dorman, J.P., et al.: Open thoracostomy drainage of postpneumonectomy empyema and bronchopleural fistula. J. Thorac. Cardiovasc. Surg., 66:979, 1973.
14. Pontoppidan, H., Geffin, B., and Lowenstein, E.: Acute respiratory failure in the adult. N. Engl. J. Med., 287:690, 743, 799; 1972.
15. Mowry, F., and Reynolds, E.F.: Cardiac rhythm disturbances complicating resectional surgery of the lung. Ann. Intern. Med., 61:688, 1964.
16. Shields, T.W., and Yjiki, G.T.: Digitalization for prevention of arrhythmias following pulmonary surgery. Surg. Gynecol. Obstet., 126:743, 1968.
17. Wheat, M.W., and Burford, T.H.: Digitalis in surgery: Extension and classical indications. J. Thorac. Cardiovasc. Surg., 41:162, 1961.
18. Benjamin, I., Olsen, A., and Ellis, E.H., Jr.: Esophagopleural fistula: A rare postpneumonectomy complication. Ann. Thorac. Surg., 7:139, 1969.
19. Engleman R.M., Spencer, E.C., and Berg, P.: Postpneumonectomy esophagopleural fistula: Successful one-stage repair. J. Thorac. Cardiovasc. Surg., 59:871, 1970.
20. Sethi, G.K., and Takaro, T.: Esophagopleural fistula following pulmonary resection. Ann. Thorac. Surg., 25:74, 1978.
21. Patel, D.R., Shrivastav, R., and Sabety, A.M.: Cardiac torsion following intrapericardial pneumonectomy. J. Thorac. Cardiovasc. Surg., 65:626, 1973.
22. Deiraniya, A.K.: Cardiac herniation following intrapericardial pneumonectomy. Thorax, 29:545, 1974.
23. Pecora, D.V., and Brook, P.R.: Evaluation of cardiopulmonary reserve in candidates for chest surgery. J. Thorac. Cardiovasc. Surg., 44:60, 1962.
24. Olsen, G. N., and Block, A. J.: Pulmonary function testing in evaluation for pneumonectomy. Hospital Practice, 8:137–144, 1973.

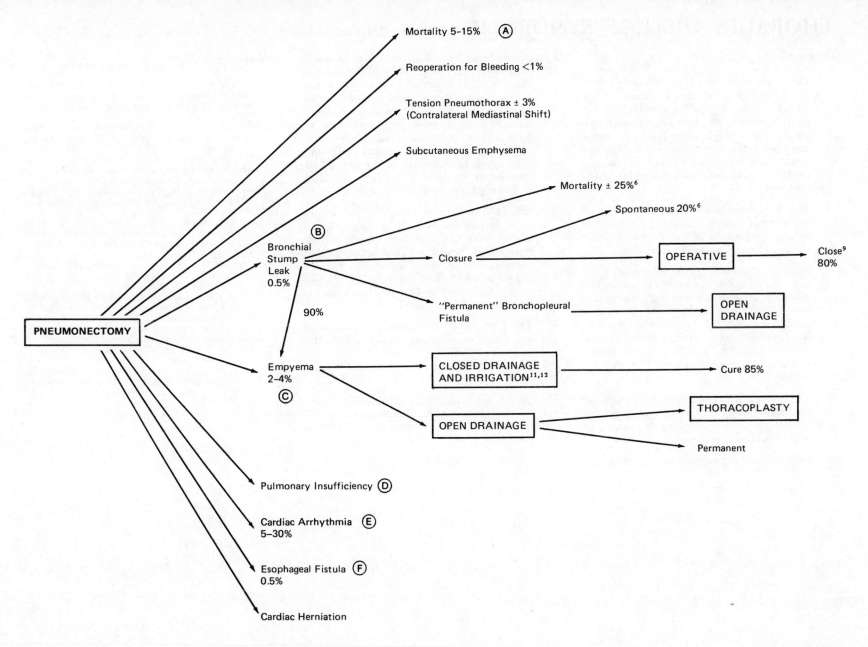

PNEUMONECTOMY

Mortality 5-15% Ⓐ

Reoperation for Bleeding <1%

Tension Pneumothorax ± 3%
(Contralateral Mediastinal Shift)

Subcutaneous Emphysema

Bronchial
Stump
Leak
0.5%
Ⓑ

Mortality ± 25%[6]

Spontaneous 20%[6]

Closure

OPERATIVE

Close[9]
80%

"Permanent" Bronchopleural
Fistula

OPEN
DRAINAGE

90%

Empyema
2-4%
Ⓒ

CLOSED DRAINAGE
AND IRRIGATION[11,12]

Cure 85%

OPEN DRAINAGE

THORACOPLASTY

Permanent

Pulmonary Insufficiency Ⓓ

Cardiac Arrhythmia Ⓔ
5-30%

Esophageal Fistula Ⓕ
0.5%

Cardiac Herniation

THORACIC OUTLET SYNDROME BY DAVID B. ROOS, M.D.

Comments

A. Incidence depends on prereferral screening. The following data are those of the author: carpal tunnel syndrome (33 per cent), cervical arthritis (33 per cent), cervical disc syndrome (4 per cent), shoulder inflammation or trauma (28 per cent), and uncommon lesions (angina pectoris, multiple sclerosis, and others) (2 per cent).

B. This is the common manifestation (± 98 per cent of cases). The mild forms afflict a large proportion of the population and obviously need no active treatment.

C. Muscle stretching, strengthening exercises to improve posture, and medications to relieve tension and discomfort may be effective in 80 to 90 per cent of moderate cases.[1] In a referral practice, most patients have already tried "conservative treatment," and 54 per cent require operative decompression of the thoracic outlet.

D. The most effective operation is transaxillary resection of the first rib and any congenital anomalies affecting the neurovascular structures in the outlet.[2]

E. Symptoms of intermittent venous obstruction (edema, cyanosis, and others) usually imply external compression of the subclavian vein. Persistence implies thrombosis. Venography is indicated even for moderate symptoms. Anticoagulants and nonoperative therapy are ineffective in 74 to 84 per cent of such patients.[3, 4]

Chronic edema secondary to vein compression or thrombosis may be helped by removal of the first rib and any anomalies to decompress collateral vessels.

F. Arterial insufficiency may be due either to an anomalous first rib or band or to an aneurysm or plaque intermittently releasing emboli. Resection, prosthetic graft, or sympathectomy may variously be required in addition to releasing the thoracic outlet obstruction that produced the arterial lesion.[5]

G. These results with minimal complications are those of surgeons familiar with the operation.[6-8] Those unfamiliar with the procedure have a far higher cost/benefit ratio.

H. Distal ischemia from plaque emboli may be so advanced that amputation is required.[10] Thoracic outlet decompression then is too late.

References

1. Rosati, L.M., and Lord, J.W.: Neurovascular Compression Syndromes of the Shoulder Girdle. (Modern Surgical Monographs). New York, Grune & Stratton, 1961.
2. Roos, D.B.: Congenital anomalies associated with thoracic outlet syndrome: anatomy, symptoms, diagnosis, and treatment. Am. J. Surg., 132:771, 1976.
3. Tilney, N.L., Griffiths, H.J.G., and Edwards, E.A.: Natural history of major venous thrombosis of the upper extremity. Arch. Surg., 101:292, 1970.
4. Swinton, N.W., Edgett, J.W., and Hall, R.J.: Primary subclavian-axillary vein thrombosis. Circulation, 38:737, 1968.
5. Roos, D.B.: Sympathectomy for the upper extremities: anatomy, indications, and techniques. In Rutherford, R.B.: Vascular Surgery. Philadelphia, W.B. Saunders Company, 1977.
6. Rainer, W.G., Vigor, W., and Newby, J.P.: Surgical treatment of thoracic outlet compression. Am. J. Surg., 116:704, 1968.
7. Urschel, H.C., Jr., and Razzuck, M.A.: Management of thoracic outlet syndrome — current concepts. N. Engl. J. Med., 286:1140, 1972.
8. Roos, D.B.: Experience with first rib resection for thoracic outlet syndrome. Ann. Surg., 173:429, 1971.
9. Lord, J.W.: Thrombosis of the subclavian artery. West. J. Surg., 68:11, 1960.
10. Judy, K.L., and Heymann, R.L.: Vascular complications of thoracic outlet syndrome. Am. J. Surg., 123:521, 1972.

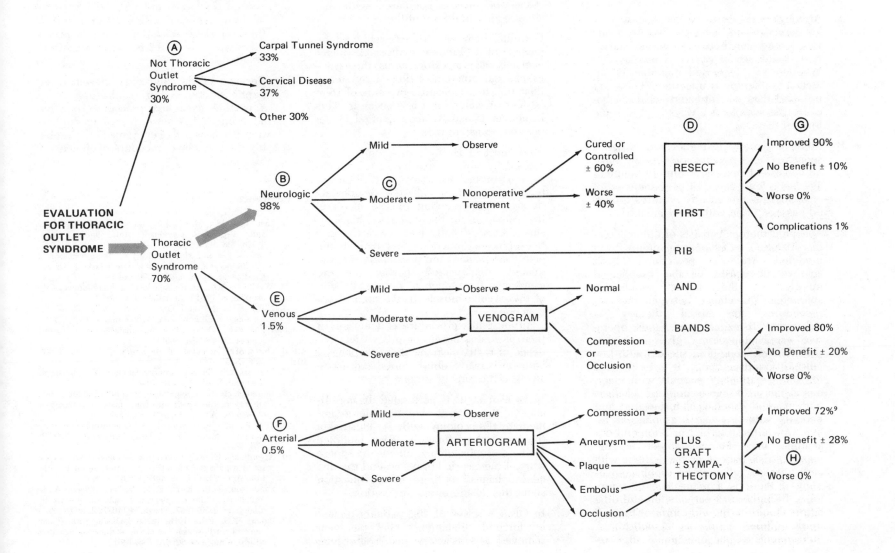

ACHALASIA OF THE ESOPHAGUS BY JAMES T. ANDERSON, M.D.

Comments

A. Although mild forms of the disease may go unrecognized, achalasia usually leads to repeated bronchopneumonia and starvation. Incidence of cancer is increased.[1-3] Whether this increased incidence is affected by therapy is uncertain. There are no solid data on untreated achalasia because the symptoms always lead to some form of therapy.

B. Medical therapy is ineffective. Nitrates, sedatives, and psychologic therapy have no consistent success.[4, 5] Simple bougienage has a low chance of permanent relief of dysphagia and usually requires repeated passage, often with every meal.[6, 7]

C. Accepted therapy consists of either forceful dilatation or esophagomyotomy by a modified Heller's procedure. Both achieve disruption of the esophageal muscle at the lower esophageal sphincter. The choice between the two procedures for initial therapy is debated.[8-11] In experienced hands, operative esophagomyotomy gives a higher probability of long-term success with low morbidity and mortality. It is to be used for young patients,[12] patients with vigorous achalasia,[13] severe forms of achalasia with marked esophageal tortuosity,[4] and patients with associated esophageal reflux.[4] An initial trial of 1 or 2 forceful dilatations may be warranted in the marginal-risk patient or the patient with early disease, followed by esophagomyotomy if there is a recurrence of symptoms. In higher-risk patients forceful dilatation should be the only form of therapy until definite failure is demonstrated. Subsequent esophagomyotomy after repeated dilatations carries a decreased chance of success compared with that done as an initial form of therapy.[14, 15]

D. Forceful dilatation is best achieved by passage of a Plummer hydrostatic dilator over a thread to a position across the gastroesophageal junction, followed by steady dilatation to a measured pressure of 18 to 20 feet of water for a few seconds. This maneuver is usually accompanied by severe but transient pain.[4, 16]

E. The modified Heller's procedure as described by Ellis[4, 17] involves a transthoracic longitudinal myotomy on the left anterolateral surface of the esophagus through the encircling muscle fibers of the esophagus to the mucosa. This incision extends distally just across the gastroesophageal junction (less than 1 cm. onto the stomach) and proximally into the dilated, thick-walled portion of the esophagus far enough to ensure division of the circular muscle in the area of obstruction.

An antireflux procedure is done only if there is hiatus hernia or preexisting evidence of reflux or if the gastroesophageal junction is inadvertently mobilized excessively at the time of surgery.[22-24]

F. If the esophagus is perforated during dilatation, the patient should undergo immediate thoracotomy with (1) closure of the mucosal perforation, (2) a modified Heller's esophagotomy, and/or (3) a loose wrap of the gastric fundus around the distal esophagus[18] if there is any question about the closure of the perforation.

G. In Olsen's series of 452 patients treated by forceful dilatation,[16] 60.2 per cent achieved a satisfactory result after one dilatation. Ninety-four patients required a second dilatation and only 38.3 per cent of these achieved a satisfactory result. If three or more dilatations were required, there was only a 19.2 per cent satisfactory result.

H. Because of the frequency of reflux and peptic strictures after esophagomyotomy, a routine antireflux procedure is often advisable.[22-24] A loose, partial fundoplication (such as a Belsey Mark IV) is probably the antireflux procedure of choice.

References

1. Just-Viera, J.O., Morris, J.D., and Haight, C.: Achalasia and esophageal carcinoma. Ann. Thorac. Surg., 3:526–538, 1967.
2. Hankins, J.R. and McLaughlin, J.S.: The association of carcinoma of the esophagus with achalasia. J. Thorac. Cardiovasc. Surg., 69:355–360, 1975.
3. Wychulis, A.R., et al.: Achalasia and carcinoma of the esophagus. JAMA, 215:1638–1641, 1971.
4. Ellis, F.H., Jr., and Olsen, A.M.: Achalasia of the Esophagus. Philadelphia, W.B. Saunders Co., 1969.
5. Field, C.E.: Octyl nitrate in achalasia of the cardia. Lancet, 2:848–851, 1944.
6. Hertz, A.F.: Achalasia of the cardia. Q. J. Med., 8:300–308, 1915.
7. Vinson, P.P.: Diagnosis and treatment of cardiospasm. Postgrad. Med., 3:13–18, 1948.
8. Benedict, E.B.: Bougienage, forceful dilatation, and surgery in the treatment of achalasia: A comparison of results. JAMA, 188:355–357, 1964.
9. Yon, J., and Christensen, J.: An uncontrolled comparison of treatments for achalasia. Ann. Surg., 182:672–676, 1975.
10. Arvanitakis, C.: Achalasia of the esophagus: A reappraisal of esophagomyotomy vs. forceful pneumatic dilation. Am. J. Dig. Dis., 20:841–846, 1975.
11. Sanderson, D.R., Ellis, F.H., Jr., and Olsen, A.M.: Achalasia of the esophagus: Results of therapy by dilatation, 1950–1967. Chest, 58:116–121, 1970.
12. Payne, W.S., Ellis, F.H., Jr., and Olsen, A.M.: Treatment of cardiospasm (achalasia of the esophagus) in children. Surgery, 50:731–735, 1961.

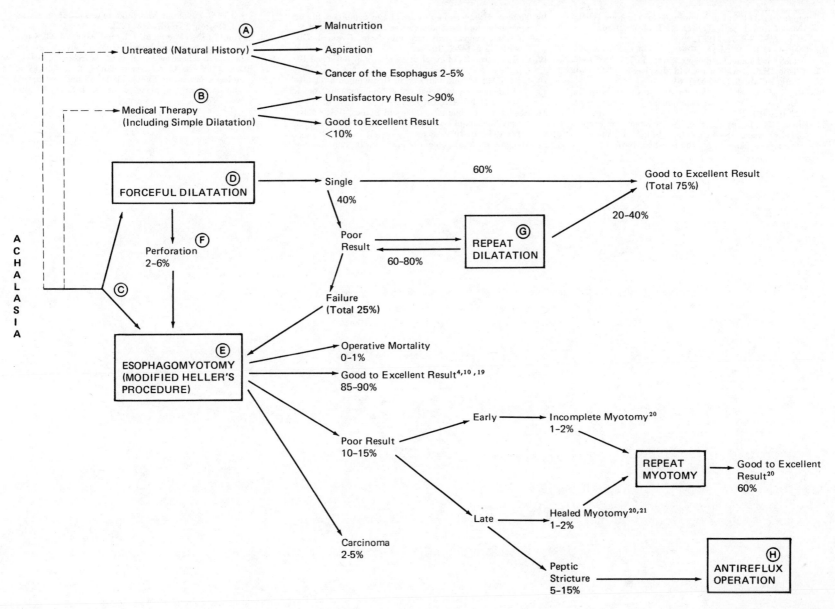

A C H A L A S I A

Untreated (Natural History)

(A)
→ Malnutrition
→ Aspiration
→ Cancer of the Esophagus 2-5%

Medical Therapy
(Including Simple Dilatation)

(B)
→ Unsatisfactory Result >90%
→ Good to Excellent Result
  <10%

FORCEFUL DILATATION (D)

(C)

Perforation
2-6% (F)

ESOPHAGOMYOTOMY
(MODIFIED HELLER'S
PROCEDURE) (E)

Single ——60%——→ Good to Excellent Result
(Total 75%)

40%

Poor
Result ——60-80%——→ REPEAT DILATATION (G) ——20-40%——→

Failure
(Total 25%)

→ Operative Mortality
  0-1%
→ Good to Excellent Result[4,10,19]
  85-90%

Poor Result
10-15%

Early ——→ Incomplete Myotomy[20]
          1-2%

Late ——→ Healed Myotomy[20,21]
         1-2%

REPEAT MYOTOMY ——→ Good to Excellent Result[20]
60%

Carcinoma
2-5%

Peptic Stricture
5-15% ——→ ANTIREFLUX OPERATION (H)

13. Sanderson, D.R., et al.: Syndrome of vigorous achalasia: Clinical and physiological observations. Dis. Chest, 52:508–517, 1967.
14. Clagett, O.T.: Achalasia: Editorial: Dilatation or myotomy? J. Thorac. Cardiovasc. Surg., 53:757–758, 1967.
15. Allison, P.R.: Swallowing and dysphagia. J. R. Coll. Surg. Edinb., 6:113–120, 1961.
16. Olsen, A.M., et al.: The treatment of cardiospasm. Analysis of a 12-year experience. J. Thorac. Surg., 22:164–187, 1951.
17. Ellis, F.H., Jr., et al.: Esophagomyotomy for esophageal achalasia: Experimental, clinical and manometric aspects. Ann. Surg., 166:640–656, 1967.

18. Thomas, H.F., et al.: Results of the combined fundic patch-fundoplication operation in the treatment of reflux esophagitis with stricture. Surg. Gynecol. Obstet., 135:241–245, 1972.
19. Collected results of esophagomyotomy in reference 10, p. 196.
20. Ellis, F.H., Jr., and Gibb, P.S.: Reoperation after esophagomyotomy for achalasia of the esophagus. Am. J. Surg., 129:407–412, 1975.
21. Rees, J.R., Thorbjarnarson, B., and Barnes, W.H.: Achalasia: Results of operation in 84 patients. Ann. Surg., 171:195–201, 1970.
22. Menguy, R.: Management of achalasia by transabdomi-

nal cardiomyotomy and fundoplication. Surg. Gynecol. Obstet., 133:482–484, 1971.
23. Peyton, M.D., Greenfield, L.J., and Elkins, R.C.: Combined myotomy and hiatal herniorrhaphy: A new approach to achalasia. Am. J. Surg., 128:786–790, 1974.
24. Black, J., Vorbach, A.N., and Collis, J.L.: Results of Heller's operation for achalasia of the esophagus. The importance of hiatal repair. Br. J. Surg., 63:949–953, 1976.

REFLUX ESOPHAGITIS

REFLUX ESOPHAGITIS BY ROSS S. DAVIES, M.D.

Comments

A. Diagnosis depends upon the patient's symptoms, radiographic visualization, endoscopic findings, and manometric determinations. Acid perfusion studies and 24-hour pH monitoring may further delineate the presence of reflux esophagitis.[1-3]

B. In a normal population, the reported incidence of hiatal hernia varies from 1.3 to 45 per cent. The association of reflux esophagitis is greater in the presence of a hiatal hernia. Approximately 55 to 70 per cent of reflux esophagitis patients have hiatal hernia.[4-6]

C. Medical therapy of reflux esophagitis consists of diet, antacid therapy (including H_2 blockers), and bed elevation. Drugs to increase gastric emptying and increase the tone of the gastroesophageal junction have also been used.[7, 8]

D. Repair of hernia alone is seldom performed. Its principal features involve reducing the hernia sac, reapproximating the crura, and keeping the stomach in the abdomen. The recurrence rate with long-term follow-up is too high.[10, 11]

E. The rationale of this procedure is to relieve any gastric outlet obstruction and to decrease acid production, thus decreasing the degree of acid esophagitis.[12]

F. The principal features of the Hill repair include reduction of the hernia, dissection of the preaortic fascia and median arcuate ligament, and suturing of the phrenoesophageal bundle to the preaortic fascia and median arcuate ligament. Imbrication of the phrenoesophageal bundle with simultaneous pressure measurements of the lower esophageal sphincter precisely defines the limits of the repair.[13]

G. The principal features of the Belsey Mark IV repair include transthoracic mobilization of the esophagus, crural approximation, and a 270-degree fundoplication of the gastric cardia around the anterolateral two-thirds of the esophagus. A second row of sutures is placed above the plication and through the tendinous portion of the diaphragm to replace the reconstructed esophagogastric junction below the diaphragm.[14]

H. The Nissen procedure consists of a 360-degree fundoplication of the greater curvature around a 4 to 5 cm. length of distal esophagus. Its success depends upon the creation of a flap-valve at the gastroesophageal junction.[15]

I. Life-threatening complications of reflux esophagitis are rare. The complications that require surgical therapy are primarily persistent esophagitis, stricture formation, and hemorrhage.[16-18]

J. Recurrent reflux esophagitis following primary repair is a difficult problem. Approximately 60 per cent of patients with recurrent reflux following surgical correction will require reoperation, and the mortality rate is almost 4 times that for primary repair.[19, 20]

References

1. Skinner, D.B., and Booth, D.J.: Assessment of distal esophageal function in patients with hiatal hernia. Ann. Surg., 172:627, 1970.
2. Bernstein, L.M., Frain, R.C., and Pacini, R.: Differentiation of esophageal pain from angina pectoris: Role of the esophageal acid perfusion test. Medicine, 41:143, 1962.
3. Johnson, L.F., and DeMester, T.R.,: 24-hour pH monitoring of the distal esophagus — A quantitative measure of gastroesophageal reflux. Am. J. Gastroenterol., 62:325, 1974.
4. Brick, I.B., and Amory, H.I.: Incidence of hiatus hernia in patients without symptoms. Arch. Surg., 60:1045, 1950.
5. Wolf, B.S., et al.: The incidence of hiatal hernia in routine barium meal examination. Mt. Sinai J. Med. N.Y., 26:598, 1959.
6. Henderson, R.D., and Godden, J.O.: Motor Disorders of the Esophagus. Baltimore, Williams & Wilkins, 1976, p. 44.
7. Higgs, R.H., Smyth, R.D., and Castell, D.O.: Gastric alkalinization: Effect on lower esophageal sphincter pressure and serum gastrin. N. Engl. J. Med., 291:486, 1974.
8. Robinson, O.P.W.: Metoclopramide — A new pharmacologic approach? Postgrad. Med. J., 49 (Suppl. 4):9, 1973.
9. Gastroesophageal reflux. A panel by correspondence. Arch. Surg., 108:16, 1974.
10. Woodward, E.R., Thomas, H.F. and McAlhany, J.C.: Comparison of crural repair and Nissen fundoplication in the treatment of esophageal hiatal hernia with peptic esophagitis. Ann. Surg., 173:783, 1971.
11. Allison, P.R.: Hiatus hernia — A 20-year retrospective survey. Ann. Surg., 178:273-276, 1973.
12. Pearson, F.G., et al.: Role of vagotomy and pyloroplasty in the therapy of symptomatic hiatus hernia. Am. J. Surg., 117:130, 1967.
13. Hill, L.D.: An effective operation for hiatus hernia: An eight-year appraisal. Ann. Surg., 166:681, 1967.
14. Skinner, D.B., and Belsey, R.H.R.: Surgical management of esophageal reflux and hiatus hernia: Long-term results with 1030 patients. J. Thorac. Cardiovasc. Surg., 53:33, 1967.
15. Polk, H.C., Jr., and Zeppa, R.: Hiatal hernia and esophagitis: A survey of indications for operations and technic and results of fundoplication. Ann. Surg., 173:775, 1971.
16. DenBesten, L.: Hiatal hernia and gastroesophageal reflux. In Varco, R.L., and Delaney, J.P. (eds.): Controversies in Surgery. Philadelphia, W.B. Saunders, 1976.
17. Smith, L.C., and Bradshaw, H.H.: Esophageal hiatal hernia. Surg. Gynecol. Obstet., 109:230, 1959.
18. Raptis, S., and Milne, D.M.: A review of the management of 100 cases of benign stricture of the esophagus. Thorax, 27:599, 1972.
19. Orringer, M., Skinner, D., and Belsey, R.: Long-term results of the Mark IV operation for hiatal hernia and analysis of recurrences and their treatment. J. Thorac. Cardiovasc. Surg., 63:25, 1972.
20. Hill, L.D.: Management of recurrent hiatal hernia. Arch. Surg., 102:394, 1971.

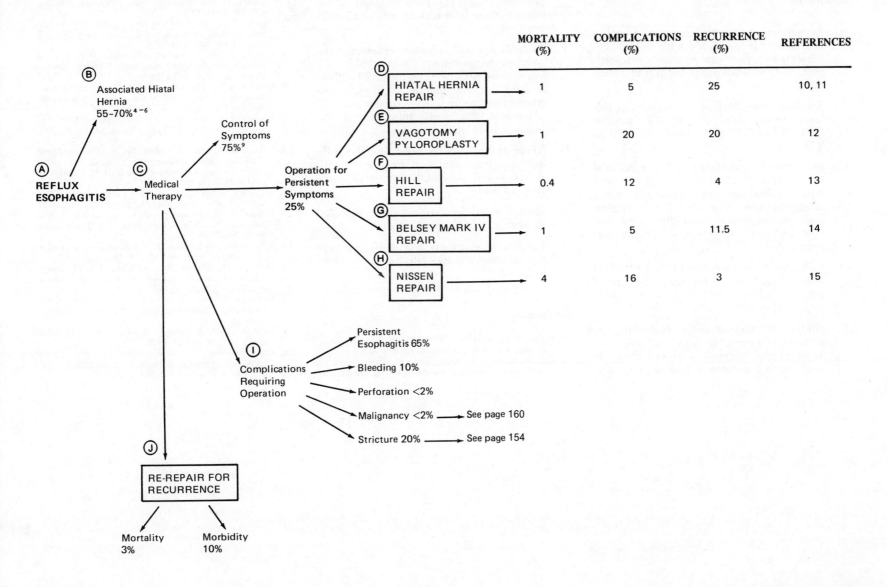

	MORTALITY (%)	COMPLICATIONS (%)	RECURRENCE (%)	REFERENCES
(D) HIATAL HERNIA REPAIR	1	5	25	10, 11
(E) VAGOTOMY PYLOROPLASTY	1	20	20	12
(F) HILL REPAIR	0.4	12	4	13
(G) BELSEY MARK IV REPAIR	1	5	11.5	14
(H) NISSEN REPAIR	4	16	3	15

(B) Associated Hiatal Hernia 55–70%[4–6]

(A) REFLUX ESOPHAGITIS

(C) Medical Therapy

Control of Symptoms 75%[9]

Operation for Persistent Symptoms 25%

(I) Complications Requiring Operation

Persistent Esophagitis 65%

Bleeding 10%

Perforation <2%

Malignancy <2% → See page 160

Stricture 20% → See page 154

(J) RE-REPAIR FOR RECURRENCE

Mortality 3%

Morbidity 10%

159

ESOPHAGEAL CANCER BY RICHARD K. PARKER, M.D.

Comments

A. Frequency is 4:1 male:female. Esophageal cancer is associated with alcoholism, tobacco use, poor oral hygiene, malnutrition, and the drinking of hot liquids, such as tea.

B. Arbitrary classification of levels is as follows: upper third (T1 to T4), middle third (T4 to T8), and lower third (T8 to T12).

C. Resection is undertaken only for hopeful cure. About half of such patients will have residual gross or microscopic tumor after resection. The operative mortality and postoperative morbidity therefore contraindicate operation for many patients.

D. Radiation characteristically is 4000–5000 rads over 4 to 6 weeks. Sixty per cent of patients achieve palliation of pain and improved swallowing.[5, 6, 11]

E. Options for reconstruction following operative resection include (1) advancement of the stomach into the chest or neck, with anastomotic leakage rate of 8 per cent,[1-4] and (2) colon or small bowel interposition, with leakage rate of 15 to 25 per cent.[1-4]

F. In addition to palliative resection and gastroesophagostomy (acceptable for lower third and perhaps for middle third lesions) options include (1) bypass gastroesophagostomy, (2) dilatation, (3) placement of a plastic tube through the lesion, and (4) gastrostomy.

G. There is controversy regarding the difficult-to-repeat results of Pearson[5, 6] with radiation and those of the operative resection of Ong.[3, 4]

H. Middle third lesions are best resected through a right thoracotomy.

I. Esophagogastrostomy has a 10 per cent anastomotic leakage rate in lower third lesions.[8, 9]

References

1. Payne, W. S., and Olsen, A. M.: The Esophagus. Philadelphia, Lea & Febiger, 1974, pp. 239–59.
2. Gunnlaugsson, C. H., et al.: Analysis of the records of 1657 patients with carcinoma of the esophagus and cardia of the stomach. Surg. Gynecol. Obstet., 130:997–1005, 1970.
3. Ong, G. B., et al.: Resection for carcinoma of the superior mediastinal segment of the esophagus. World J. Surg., 2:497–504, 1978.
4. Ong, G. B., et al.: Factors influencing morbidity and mortality in esophageal carcinoma. J. Thorac. Cardiovasc. Surg., 76:745–754, 1978.
5. Pearson, J. G.: The value of radiotherapy in the management of esophageal cancer. Am. J. Roentgenol. Radium Ther. Nucl. Med., 105:500, 1969.
6. Pearson, J. G.: Value of radiation therapy — Cancer of gastrointestinal tract. II. Esophagus. JAMA, 227:181, 1974.
7. Nakayama, K., and Kinoslita, Y.: Surgical treatment combined with preoperative concentrated radiation — Cancer of gastrointestinal tract. II. Esophagus. JAMA, 227:178, 1974.
8. O'Connor, T., et al.: Esophageal prosthesis for palliative intubation. Arch. Surg., 87:275, 1963.
9. Palmer, E. D.: Peroral prosthesis for management of incurable esophageal carcinoma. Am. J. Gastroenterol., 59:47, 1973.
10. Ellis, F. H., and Salzman, F.: Carcinoma of the esophagus. Postgrad. Med., 61:167–174, 1977.
11. Marks, R. D., Scruggs, H. J. and Wallace, K. M.: Preoperative radiation therapy for carcinoma of the esophagus. Cancer, 38:84–89, 1976.
12. Parker, F. F., and Gregorie, H. B.: Carcinoma of the esophagus — Long-term results. JAMA, 235:1018–20, 1976.
13. Skinner, D. B.: Esophageal malignancies. Surg. Clin. North Am., 56:137–47, 1976.
14. Kasai, M., Mori, S., and Watanabe, T.: Follow-up results after resection of thoracic esophageal carcinoma. World J. Surg., 2:523–551, 1978.

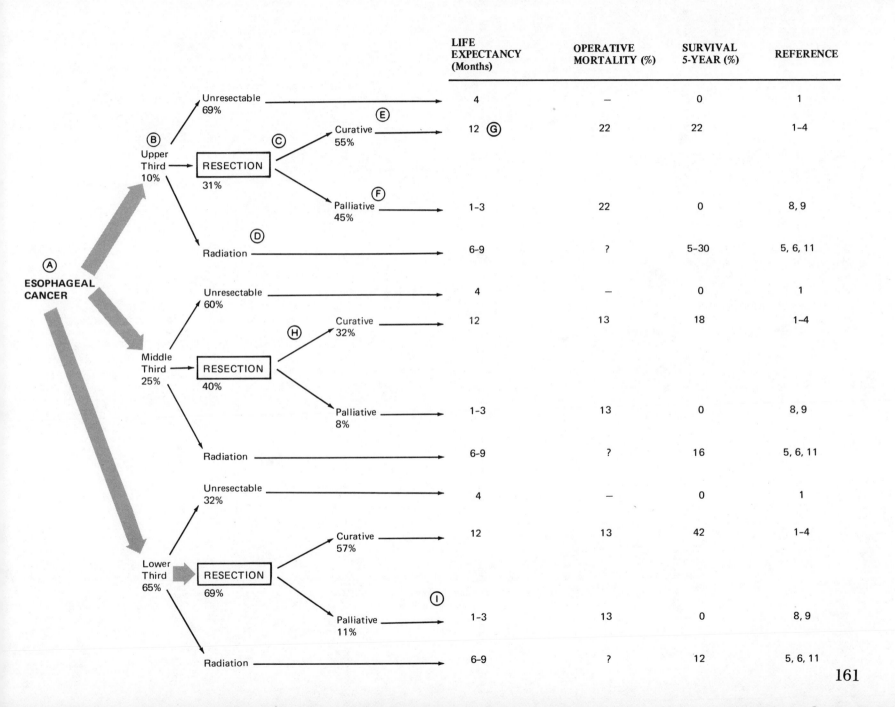

	LIFE EXPECTANCY (Months)	OPERATIVE MORTALITY (%)	SURVIVAL 5-YEAR (%)	REFERENCE
Unresectable 69%	4	—	0	1
Curative 55%	12 Ⓖ	22	22	1–4
Palliative 45%	1–3	22	0	8, 9
Radiation	6–9	?	5–30	5, 6, 11
Unresectable 60%	4	—	0	1
Curative 32%	12	13	18	1–4
Palliative 8%	1–3	13	0	8, 9
Radiation	6–9	?	16	5, 6, 11
Unresectable 32%	4	—	0	1
Curative 57%	12	13	42	1–4
Palliative 11%	1–3	13	0	8, 9
Radiation	6–9	?	12	5, 6, 11

161

Section E

Cardiac

PATENT DUCTUS ARTERIOSUS BY DANIEL L. SMITH, M.D.

Comments

A. Improved ventilatory support and better treatment of neonatal respiratory distress syndrome has increased the incidence of patent ductus arteriosus (PDA) to 80 per cent.[2-5]

B. Indication for ligation is resistant congestive heart failure as judged by (1) persistent hypercarbia (pCO_2 greater than 60) despite adequate oxygenation, (2) increasing cardiomegaly, and (3) left atrium–to–aorta ratio of greater than 1.15 to 1 on echocardiography.[3]

C. The high mortality rate is not related to the operation but is due primarily to irreversible lung disease (bronchopulmonary dysplasia) and the complications of low systemic cardiac output (necrotizing enterocolitis and CNS hemorrhage);[3-7] earlier surgery prevents many of these complications.[8,9]

D. The incidence of PDA is 20 times greater at high altitude compared with that at sea level.[10,12]

E. Once heart failure develops in an adult with PDA, it is usually intractable to therapy. The average age of death is 37.[13,14]

F. There is no difference between ligation and division in morbidity, mortality, or recurrence rates. Division is safer when (1) the ductus is greater than half the size of the aorta or greater than 6 mm in diameter or (2) the pulmonary artery pressure is greater than 30 mm. Hg.[15,16] With increasing age the ductus becomes shorter, wider, more friable, calcific, and liable to aneurysm formation; it then becomes safer to use cardiopulmonary bypass for closure.[11,17]

G. The more frequent complications include left recurrent nerve damage (1 per cent of cases) or chylous fistula (1 per cent of cases).[11]

References

1. Kostis, J. B., and Moghadam, A. N.: Patent ductus arteriosus in early infancy. Cardiovasc. Clin., 2:231, 1970.
2. Rudolph, A. M., and Heymann, M. A.: Medical treatment of the ductus arteriosus. Hospital Practice, 12:57, 1977.
3. Rittenhouse, E. A., et al.: Patent ductus arteriosus in premature infants. J. Thorac. Cardiovasc. Surg., 71:187, 1976.
4. Murphy, D. A., et al.: Management of premature infants with patent ductus arteriosus. J. Thorac. Cardiovasc. Surg., 67:221, 1974.
5. Edmunds, L. H., Jr., et al.: Surgical closure of the ductus arteriosus in premature infants. Circulation, 48:856, 1973.
6. Zachman, R. D., et al.: Incidence and treatment of the patent ductus arteriosus in the ill premature infant. Am. Heart J., 87:697, 1974.
7. Clarke, D. R., et al.: Patent ductus arteriosus ligation and respiratory distress syndrome in premature infants. Ann. Thorac. Surg., 22:138, 1976.
8. Lewis, C. E., et al.: Early surgical intervention in premature infants with respiratory distress and patent ductus arteriosus. Am. J. Surg., 128:829, 1974.
9. Levitsky, S., et al.: Interruption of patent ductus arteriosus in premature infants with respiratory distress syndrome. Ann. Thorac. Surg., 22:131, 1976.
10. Campbell, M.: Natural history of persistent ductus arteriosus. Br. Heart J., 30:4, 1968.
11. Wright, J. S., and Newman, D. C.: Ligation of the patent ductus. J. Thorac. Cardiovasc. Surg., 75:695, 1978.
12. DuBrow, I. W., Fisher, E., and Hastreiter, A.: Intermittent functional closure of patent ductus arteriosus in a 10 month old infant: Hemodynamic documentation. Chest, 68:110, 1975.
13. Fairley, G. H., and Goodwin, J. F.: Patent ductus arteriosus in adult life. Br. J. Dis. Chest, 53:263, 1959.
14. Keys, A., and Shapiro, M. J.: Patency of the ductus arteriosus in adults. Am. Heart J., 25:158, 1943.
15. Waterman, D. H., Samson, P. C., and Bailey, C. P.: Surgery of patent ductus arteriosus. Dis. Chest, 29:102, 1956.
16. Wilcox, B. R., and Peters, R. M.: Surgery of patent ductus arteriosus. Ann. Thorac. Surg., 3:126, 1967.
17. Pifarré, R., Rice, P. L., and Nemickas, R.: Surgical treatment of calcified patent ductus arteriosus. J. Thorac. Cardiovasc. Surg., 65:635, 1973.

PATENT DUCTUS ARTERIOSUS

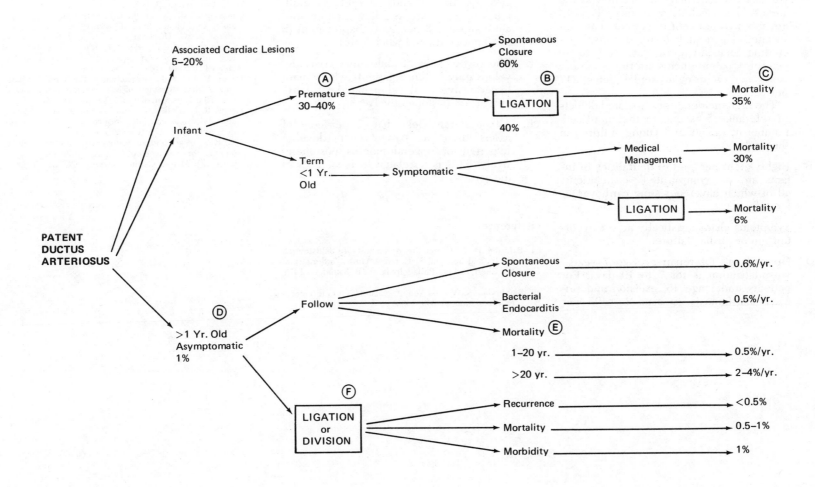

165

COARCTATION OF THE AORTA BY MARVIN POMERANTZ, M.D.

Comments

A. Six to 8 per cent of patients with congenital heart disease have coarctation of the aorta.[8][1] The male:female ratio is 4:1.[8] Seventy-five per cent of patients have associated congenital heart defects,[17] including bicuspid aortic valve (18 to 40 per cent), patent ductus arteriosus (23 per cent), and ventricular septal defect (17 per cent).

 The high incidence of associated defects in reference 5 is due to the inordinate number of infants and young children in the study.

B. Eighty-eight per cent of mortalities in infants are in "complicated" coarctations, all of which have coexisting cardiovascular defects.[5]

C. Symptoms characteristically are of hypertension or cardiac failure.

D. Optimal age for repair is 4 to 7 years.[7] Hospitalization is for 7 to 10 days. For patients under age 15, excision and primary anastomosis is used in ±95 per cent of cases. Tube graft is more commonly necessary in the older age group, in whom the aorta and intercostal vesicles are friable and sclerotic. Overall, types of repair are as follows: end-to-end anastomosis (98 per cent), flap or graft (2 to 40 per cent), and patch (rare).

E. The severe pain of abdominal crisis develops only in those patients who remain hypertensive or develop paradoxical hypertension postoperatively.[8,9]

F. Although rare (less than 1 per cent of cases), there are patients who develop hypertension several months postoperatively. This is unrelated to re-stenosis of the aorta.[1]

References

1. Bahnson, H. T.: Coarctation of the aorta. *In* Sabiston, D. C., Jr., and Spencer, F. C. (eds.): Gibbon's Surgery of the Chest, 3rd ed. Philadelphia, W. B. Saunders, 1976, p. 95.
2. Bainbridge, M. V., and Yen, A.: Coarctation in the elderly. Circulation, *31*:209, 1965.
3. Brewer, L. A., et al.: Spinal cord complications following surgery for coarctation of the aorta. A study of 66 cases. J. Thorac. Cardiovasc. Surg., *64*:368, 1972.
4. Campbell, M.: Natural history of coarctation of the aorta. Br. Heart J. 32:633, 1970.
5. Lindesmith, G. G., et al.: Coarctation of the thoracic aorta. Ann. Thorac. Surg., *11*:482, 1971.
6. Reifenstein, G. H., Levine, S. A., and Gross, R. A.: Coarctation of the aorta. A review of 104 autopsied cases of the "adult type," 2 years of age or older. Am. Heart J., 33:146, 1947.
7. Tawes, R. L., et al.: Coarctation of the aorta in infants and children. A review of 333 operative cases, including 179 infants. Circulation, 39(Suppl. I):173, 1969.
8. Tawes, R. L., Bull, J. C., and Roe, B. B.: Hypertension and abdominal pain after resection of aortic coarctation. Ann. Surg., *171*:409, 1970.
9. Will, R. J., et al.: Sodium nitroprusside and propranolol therapy for management of postcoarctectomy hypertension. J. Thorac. Cardiovasc. Surg., 75:722, 1978.

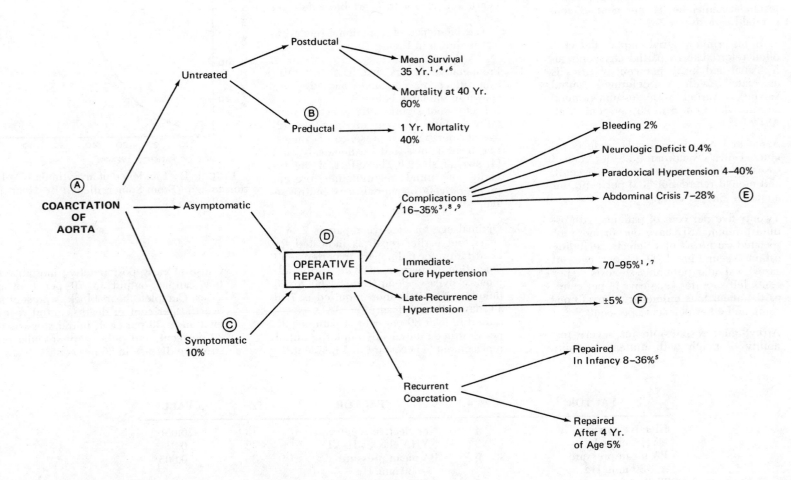

COARCTATION OF AORTA (A)

- Untreated
  - Postductal
    - Mean Survival 35 Yr.[1],[4],[6]
    - Mortality at 40 Yr. 60%
  - Preductal (B)
    - 1 Yr. Mortality 40%
- Asymptomatic
- Symptomatic 10% (C)

OPERATIVE REPAIR (D)

- Complications 16–35%[3],[8],[9] (E)
  - Bleeding 2%
  - Neurologic Deficit 0.4%
  - Paradoxical Hypertension 4–40%
  - Abdominal Crisis 7–28%
- Immediate-Cure Hypertension → 70–95%[1],[7]
- Late-Recurrence Hypertension → ±5% (F)
- Recurrent Coarctation
  - Repaired In Infancy 8–36%[5]
  - Repaired After 4 Yr. of Age 5%

ATRIAL SEPTAL DEFECT BY DAVID CLARKE, M.D.

Comments

OSTIUM PRIMUM

A. Atrial septal defect (ASD) as a primary lesion accounts for 11 per cent of congenital heart disease.[9]

B. Ostium primum atrial septal defect is often referred to as partial atrioventricular canal and in 88 per cent of cases is associated with a deformed mitral valve.[11] In various series ostium primum accounts for from 5 to 25 per cent of all ASDs.[9, 16]

C. Associated noncardiovascular defects include Down's syndrome (3.5 per cent of cases), Turner's syndrome (1.5 per cent), and mental retardation (3.0 per cent), for a total of (8.0 per cent).[18]

D. Twenty-five per cent of patients with ostium primum ASD have one or more associated cardiovascular defects, including ostium secundum ASD (9 per cent of cases), valvular pulmonic stenosis (7 per cent), left superior vena cava (4 per cent), partial anomalous pulmonary veins (3 per cent), and other defects (5 per cent).[11]

E. Arrhythmias responsible for severe disability or death with untreated ostium primum ASD can be categorized as follows: nodal bradycardia (13 per cent of patients), atrial fibrillation (40 per cent), paroxysmal ventricular tachycardia (7 per cent), and complete heart block (40 per cent).[15]

The incidence of arrhythmia related to age is shown in Figure 1.[15]

F. Preoperative factors that have a significant effect on operative mortality are shown in the table below.[11]

Factors not significantly affecting mortality include (1) year of operation, (2) age at operation, (3) presence of congestive heart failure and cardiomegaly, and (4) size of shunt.[6] The effect of the severity of mitral regurgitation present preoperatively on mortality is controversial.[10, 11]

G. Optimal age for elective repair is 2 to 5 years, but earlier repair is indicated for heart failure or pulmonary hypertension.[1] Operation is performed with cardiopulmonary bypass. Pump time is 60 to 90 minutes. Hospitalization required is 7 to 14 days. Patch closure of ASD is required in over 80 per cent of patients; 85 per cent need mitral valvuloplasty; mitral replacement is necessary in 4 per cent.[11]

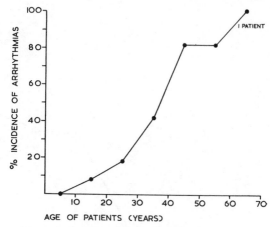

FIGURE 1. Incidence of arrhythmia in relation to age. (From Somerville, J.: Br. Heart J., 27:413, 1965.)

H. Cause of early postoperative mortality is low cardiac output in 70 per cent of cases. Complete heart block is present in over 50 per cent of deaths, mitral regurgitation in 30 per cent, mitral stenosis in 20 per cent, and pulmonary vascular obstructive disease in 20 per cent.[11]

FACTOR	%+	FACTOR	%+	p VALUE
Elective repair	4	Nonelective repair	18	<0.05
NYHA class I	3	NYHA classes II–VI	22	<0.01
PA mean pressure <30 mm. Hg	6	PA mean pressure ≥30 mm. Hg	33	<0.005
PVR < 3 mm. Hg/L./min./m²	5	PVR ≥ 3 mm. Hg/L./min./m²	44	<0.001

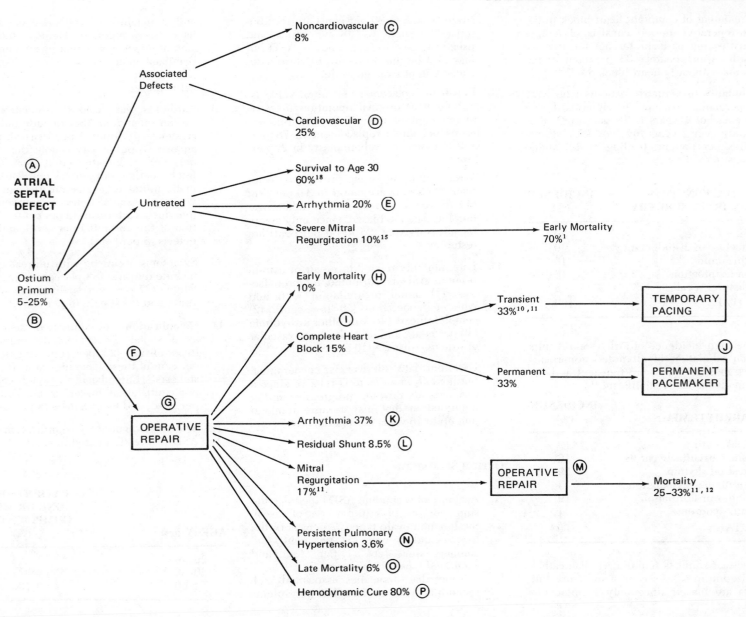

Noncardiovascular (C)
8%

Associated
Defects

Cardiovascular (D)
25%

(A)
**ATRIAL
SEPTAL
DEFECT**

Survival to Age 30
60%[18]

Untreated

Arrhythmia 20% (E)

Severe Mitral
Regurgitation 10%[15]

Early Mortality
70%[1]

Ostium
Primum
5-25%

(B)

(F)

Early Mortality (H)
10%

Transient
33%[10],[11]

TEMPORARY
PACING

(I)

Complete Heart
Block 15%

(J)

Permanent
33%

PERMANENT
PACEMAKER

(G)

**OPERATIVE
REPAIR**

Arrhythmia 37% (K)

Residual Shunt 8.5% (L)

Mitral
Regurgitation
17%[11].

(M)

OPERATIVE
REPAIR

Mortality
25-33%[11],[12]

Persistent Pulmonary
Hypertension 3.6% (N)

Late Mortality 6% (O)

Hemodynamic Cure 80% (P)

I. Treatment of complete heart block in the postoperative period consists of temporary pacing or isoproterenol infusion, or both. Approximately 33 per cent of patients with early heart block die.[10, 11]

J. Mortality in pediatric patients who have a permanent pacemaker implanted for an average of 4 years is 18 per cent.[5] Morbidity over 4 years involves 3.5 malfunctions per patient, leading to 4.8 operations per patient.[5]

MALFUNCTION REQUIRING SURGERY	INCIDENCE (%)
Generator failure	30
Lead fracture or dislodgment	40
High threshold	10
Erosion or infection	15
Manufacturer recall	5
TOTAL	100

K. The high incidence of arrhythmia results from tabulation of all noted abnormalities, most of which are transient and not hemodynamically significant.[11]

ARRHYTHMIA	INCIDENCE (%)
Junctional rhythm	19
Paroxysmal atrial tachycardia	16
Ectopic atrial rhythm	29
Atrioventricular dissociation	13
Atrial flutter or fibrillation	19
Sick sinus syndrome	4
TOTAL	100

L. Residual shunt is found at cardiac catheterization in 8.5 per cent of survivors, but data are biased since only symptomatic survivors (25 to 30 per cent) are recatheterized.[11] Shunt is always atrial and usually related to recurrence of ASD but may also be due to failure to close associated patent foramen ovale.

M. Repair or replacement of mitral valve is performed at original operation in over 80 per cent of cases.[11] Reoperation requires prosthetic replacement in 78 per cent of cases and valvuloplasty in 22 per cent.[12]

N. Mean pulmonary artery pressures greater than 30 mm Hg are found in 3.6 per cent of survivors at repeat cardiac catheterization but data are biased, since only symptomatic survivors (25 to 30 per cent) are restudied.[11]

O. Late mortality related to repair of ostium primum ASD is attributed to three factors: (1) mitral regurgitation with and without reoperation (50 per cent), (2) complete heart block or other arrhythmia (40 per cent), and (3) pulmonary vascular obstructive disease (10 per cent).[10]

P. Excellent late survival is encouraging, but hemodynamic cure is relative since a few patients develop progressive mitral regurgitation that may require reoperation up to 15 years postoperatively.[12]

Ostium Secundum

A. Anatomy of secundum ASDs includes the sinus venosus type (6 per cent of cases), the foramen ovale type (27 per cent), the low secundum type (54 per cent), the coronary sinus type (1 per cent), and combined types (12 per cent).[13]

Noncardiac anomalies associated with secundum ASD are rare, but polysplenia and anomalies of the osseous system have been reported. Genetic transmission of this lesion occurs by an autosomal dominant gene when associated osseous abnormalities or a prolonged P–R interval is present.[9]

B. Cardiovascular lesions associated with ostium secundum ASD include pulmonary stenosis (10 per cent of cases), partial anomalous pulmonary venous drainage (7 per cent), rheumatic mitral stenosis (Lutembacher's syndrome) (1 per cent), rheumatic mitral regurgitation (0.3 per cent), ventricular septal defect (5 per cent), patent ductus arteriosus (3 per cent), coarctation of the aorta (0.3 per cent), and other defects (5 per cent).[9]

C. Symptoms occurring with untreated ASD include dyspnea (83 per cent of patients), fatigue (27 per cent), palpitations (38 per cent), and chest pain (6 per cent).[3]

D. Complications of untreated secundum atrial septal defect include pulmonary hypertension (22 per cent of cases; 14 per cent of these have hypoxemia), mitral stenosis (Lutembacher's syndrome) (4 per cent), atrial flutter or fibrillation (8 per cent), and heart failure (8 per cent).[3]

E. The development of complications with ASD is directly related to age.[3]

AGE (Years)	PATIENTS WITH ONE OR MORE COMPLICATIONS (%)
20–40	14
40–60	24
>60	100

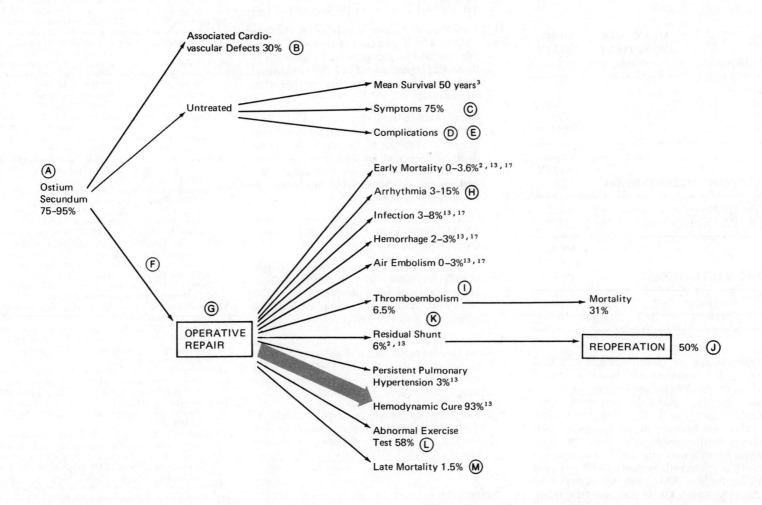

Associated Cardio-
vascular Defects 30% (B)

Untreated

Mean Survival 50 years[3]

Symptoms 75% (C)

Complications (D) (E)

(A)
Ostium
Secundum
75–95%

(F)

(G)

OPERATIVE
REPAIR

Early Mortality 0–3.6%[2],[13],[17]

Arrhythmia 3–15% (H)

Infection 3–8%[13],[17]

Hemorrhage 2–3%[13],[17]

Air Embolism 0–3%[13],[17]

(I)
Thromboembolism
6.5%

(K)
Residual Shunt
6%[2],[13]

Persistent Pulmonary
Hypertension 3%[13]

Hemodynamic Cure 93%[13]

Abnormal Exercise
Test 58% (L)

Late Mortality 1.5% (M)

Mortality
31%

REOPERATION 50% (J)

F. Preoperative factors that affect operative mortality for closure of secundum ASD are age, pulmonary hypertension, and mitral valve disease.

AUTHOR	MEAN AGE OF PATIENT (Years)	MOR-TALITY (%)
Sellers	13	3.6[13]
Hanlon	32	5.4[7]
Gault	46	12.5[6]
Yalav	62	25.0[19]

PULMONARY HYPERTENSION	MOR-TALITY (%)[13]
Systolic PA Pressure <40 mm. Hg	1.8
Systolic PA Pressure >40 mm. Hg	11.0

MITRAL VALVE DISEASE	MOR-TALITY (%)[13]
Absent	1.8
Present	16.0

G. Optimal age for elective repair is 2 to 5 years, but repair should be done earlier if heart failure or pulmonary hypertension is significant.[1] Various techniques have been used to close secundum ASDs, but because of safety, open repair using cardiopulmonary bypass or deep hypothermia and circulatory arrest in infants is preferred. Seventy to 80 per cent of secundum ASDs can be closed with direct suture.[16] Great care must be taken to evacuate all air from the heart during the repair.[17] Associated lesions, particularly mitral and tricuspid valve abnormalities, should be repaired at the time of ASD closure.[14] Usual perfusion time for closure of secundum ASD is 30 minutes, and most patients can be discharged from the hospital 5 to 7 days postoperatively.

H. Arrhythmias follow repair of secundum ASD in 3 to 15 per cent of cases.[13, 17] Complete heart block occurs in 40 per cent of these and is permanent in 7 per cent. Atrial flutter or fibrillation occurs in the other 60 per cent.

I. Thromboembolism can occur early (1.5 per cent of cases) or late (5 per cent) and has been seen up to 11 years postoperatively. Patients at greatest risk are those with atrial fibrillation or pulmonary hypertension, or both, who are over 40 years of age at operation.[8]

J. Half of residual shunts are large enough (Qp:Qs ratio greater than 1.5:1) to require reoperation.[13, 17]

K. Causes of residual shunts include failure of defect closure (50 per cent of cases), missed anomalous pulmonary vein (33 per cent), and misdirection of inferior vena caval flow (17 per cent).[13, 17]

L. Intense upright exercise results in a smaller increase in cardiac output in 58 per cent of patients who have had ASD closure than is achieved in normal subjects.[4]

M. Late mortality may be due to residual shunt (nonoperated), pulmonary hypertension, mitral valve disease, or thromboembolism.[8, 13]

References

1. Clarke, D. R.: Congenital heart disease I and II. *In* Eiseman, B., and Wotkyns, R. S. (eds.): Surgical Decision Making. Philadelphia, W. B. Saunders Company, 1978, pp. 92–95.
2. Cohn, L. H., et al.: Operative treatment of atrial septal defect: Clinical and haemodynamic assessments in 175 patients. Br. Heart J., 29:725, 1967.
3. Craig, R. J., and Selzer, A.: Natural history and prognosis of atrial septal defect. Circulation, 37:805, 1968.
4. Epstein, S. E., et al.: Hemodynamic abnormalities in response to mild and intense upright exercise following operative correction of an atrial septal defect or tetralogy of Fallot. Circulation, 47:1065, 1973.
5. Gamble, W. J., and Owens, J. P.: Pacemaker therapy for conduction defects in the pediatric population. *In* Roberts, N. K., and Gelband, H. (eds.): Cardiac Arrhythmias in the Neonate and Child. New York, Appleton-Century-Crofts, 1977, pp. 469–525.
6. Gault, J. H., et al.: Atrial septal defect in patients over the age of forty years. Circulation, 37:261, 1968.
7. Hanlon, C. R., et al.: Atrial septal defect: Results of repair in adults. Arch. Surg., 99:275, 1969.
8. Hawe, A., et al.: Embolic complications following repair of atrial septal defects. Circulation, 39 and 40 (Suppl. I):185, 1969.
9. Keith, J. D.: Atrial septal defect: Ostium secundum, ostium primum, and atrioventricularis communis (common AV canal). *In* Keith, J. D., Rowe, R. D., and Vlad, P. (eds.): Heart Disease in Infancy and Childhood. New York, Macmillan, 1978, pp. 380–404.
10. Levy, S., Blondeau, P., and Dubost, C.: Long-term followup after surgical correction of partial form of common atrioventricular canal (ostium primum). J. Thorac. Cardiovasc. Surg., 67:353, 1974.
11. Losay, J., et al.: Repair of atrial septal defect primum. J. Thorac. Cardiovasc. Surg., 75:248, 1978.
12. McMullan, M. H., et al.: Surgical treatment of partial atrioventricular canal. Arch. Surg., 107:705, 1973.
13. Sellers, R. D., et al.: Secundum type atrial septal defects: Early and late results of surgical repair using extracorporeal circulation in 275 patients. Surgery, 59:155, 1966.
14. Shigenobu, M., et al.: Surgery for mitral and tricuspid insufficiency associated with secundum atrial septal defect. J. Thorac. Cardiovasc. Surg., 78:290, 1978.
15. Somerville, J.: Ostium primum defect: Factors causing deterioriation in the natural history. Br. Heart J., 27:413, 1965.
16. Spencer, F. C.: Atrial septal defect, anomalous pulmonary veins, and atrioventricular canal. *In* Sabiston, D. C., Jr., and Spencer, F. C. (eds.): Gibbon's Surgery of the Chest. Philadelphia, W. B. Saunders Company, 1976, pp. 983–999.
17. Stansel, H. C., Jr., et al.: Surgical treatment of atrial septal defect. Am. J. Surg., 131:485, 1971.
18. Weyn, A. S., et al.: Atrial septal defect — Primum type. Circulation, 31 and 32 (Suppl. III):13, 1965.
19. Yalav, E., et al.: Surgery for atrial septal defect in patients over 60 years of age. J. Thorac. Cardiovasc. Surg., 62:788, 1971.

CYANOTIC HEART DISEASE

CYANOTIC HEART DISEASE BY GEORGE PAPPAS, M.D.

Comments

A. Dextro-transposition of the great arteries is responsible for 8 per cent of all congenital heart disease[1, 2] and 36 per cent of cyanotic heart disease.[2] Longevity without treatment is 3 months.[1] Fifty per cent of cases live only one month; 10 per cent live one year.

B. Balloon atrial septostomy in the neonate is the most commonly used palliative procedure for transposition.

C. Balloon atrial septostomy (BAS) is done as an emergency procedure in the neonate by using a balloon catheter during cardiac catheterization. Seventy-eight per cent of these patients are alive at one year; 10 per cent are alive at three years.[3] Morbidity includes cerebral vascular accident (hypoxia), which occurs in 3 to 13 per cent of cases.[4]

D. The Hanlon-Blalock procedure (closed atrial septectomy) is done when a BAS fails, usually on patients 1 to 6 months of age. Hospital mortality has been reported as 53 per cent in infants less than 3 months old and 5 per cent for those more than 3 months old.[5] Others report a mortality of 5 per cent in infants less than 9 weeks old.[6]

E. Pulmonary artery banding, for patients with a large ventricular septal defect, is done to reduce pulmonary blood flow and pressure (pulmonary pressure reduced to half its original systemic value). Hospital mortality rate is 12 per cent.[7]

F. Corrective procedures are usually performed at age 6 to 12 months. Most patients have had a balloon atrial septostomy.

G. Mustard's repair involves the construction of a pericardial or synthetic atrial baffle using standard cardiopulmonary bypass or profound hypothermia and circulatory arrest (in infants).

Atrial arrhythmias occur in 10 to 90 per cent of cases.[14] They are reduced by protecting the SA and its artery.

Systemic venous obstruction is present in 5 to 31 per cent of cases,[15] and pulmonary venous obstruction occurs in 41 per cent.[16] Late complications arise in 73 per cent of cases[17] and include caval-pulmonary venous obstruction, tricuspid insufficiency, and others. These late complications have occurred in 100 per cent of symptomatic patients and 61 per cent of asymptomatic patients.[17]

H. In the Senning repair atrial venous return is altered by using the patient's own atrial tissues. Atrial arrhythmias are rare with this technique.

I. Arterial switch is performed by transposing the great arteries and the coronary arteries.[12] It is used for patients with ventricular septal defects (VSDs) with high ventricular pressures to accommodate systemic blood flow.

J. The Rastelli repair involves closure of the VSD and creation of an external conduit from the right ventricle to the pulmonary artery.[13] It is used with transposition, VSDs and significant pulmonic stenosis. Complications associated with homograft conduits occur more frequently than when heterografts are used. Reoperation is needed in 20 per cent of cases (for stenosis and recurrent VSD).[18] Other potential complications are compression of the conduit by the sternum and tachyarrhythmias.

K. The tetralogy of Fallot occurs in 11 per cent of congenital heart disease patients and 20 per cent of those with cyanotic heart disease. Longevity is 12 years if the condition is untreated. Thirty-three per cent of patients live only 2 years.

L. These various systemic pulmonary artery shunts are usually performed during infancy, with total correction at 2 to 4 years of age. The mortality rate of the palliative procedures is low (±5 per cent?).

M. The Blalock-Taussig (B-T) shunt from the subclavian to the pulmonary artery is the preferable palliative procedure because of minimal pulmonary hypertension. The incidence of severe pulmonary vascular disease with a B-T shunt ranges from 2 per cent (less than 8 years' duration) to 30 per cent (more than 8 years' duration).[25] With the Waterston-Cooley (W-C) or Potts shunt, the incidence ranges from 3 per cent (less than 5 years' duration) to 17 to 28 per cent (more than 5 years' duration).[26]

Takedown of a B-T shunt is easier than with other types.

N. The Waterston-Cooley shunt is from the ascending aorta to the right pulmonary artery. It can be performed rapidly in critically ill infants.

O. The Potts shunt is from the descending aorta to the left pulmonary artery but is seldom used now.

P. Morbidity of complete repair of tetralogy of Fallot includes[28] residual ventricular septal defect (greater than 1.5 Qp:Qs ratio) (2 per cent), residual outflow obstruction (3 per cent), and right ventricular outflow tract aneurysm (4 per cent).

Q. In tricuspid atresia[1, 2] the incidence of congenital heart disease is 3 per cent

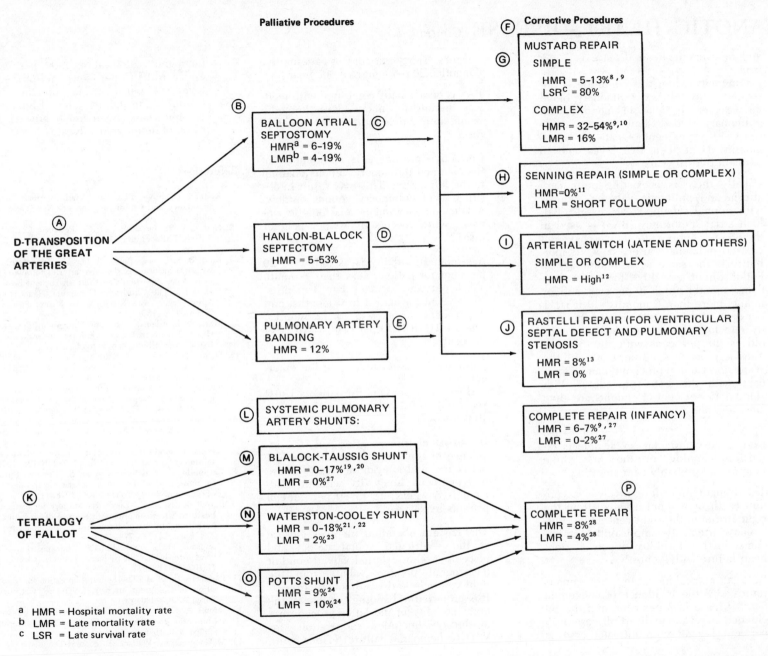

Palliative Procedures

Corrective Procedures

Ⓕ

Ⓖ MUSTARD REPAIR
   SIMPLE
   HMR = 5-13%[8],[9]
   LSR[c] = 80%

   COMPLEX
   HMR = 32-54%[9],[10]
   LMR = 16%

Ⓑ BALLOON ATRIAL
   SEPTOSTOMY Ⓒ
   HMR[a] = 6-19%
   LMR[b] = 4-19%

Ⓗ SENNING REPAIR (SIMPLE OR COMPLEX)
   HMR=0%[11]
   LMR = SHORT FOLLOWUP

Ⓐ D-TRANSPOSITION
   OF THE GREAT
   ARTERIES

HANLON-BLALOCK
SEPTECTOMY Ⓓ
   HMR = 5-53%

Ⓘ ARTERIAL SWITCH (JATENE AND OTHERS)
   SIMPLE OR COMPLEX
      HMR = High[12]

PULMONARY ARTERY
BANDING Ⓔ
   HMR = 12%

Ⓙ RASTELLI REPAIR (FOR VENTRICULAR
   SEPTAL DEFECT AND PULMONARY
   STENOSIS
      HMR = 8%[13]
      LMR = 0%

Ⓛ SYSTEMIC PULMONARY
   ARTERY SHUNTS:

COMPLETE REPAIR (INFANCY)
   HMR = 6-7%[9],[27]
   LMR = 0-2%[27]

Ⓜ BLALOCK-TAUSSIG SHUNT
   HMR = 0-17%[19],[20]
   LMR = 0%[27]

Ⓟ

Ⓚ TETRALOGY
   OF FALLOT

Ⓝ WATERSTON-COOLEY SHUNT
   HMR = 0-18%[21],[22]
   LMR = 2%[23]

COMPLETE REPAIR
   HMR = 8%[28]
   LMR = 4%[28]

Ⓞ POTTS SHUNT
   HMR = 9%[24]
   LMR = 10%[24]

a HMR = Hospital mortality rate
b LMR = Late mortality rate
c LSR = Late survival rate

and of cyanotic heart disease is 7 per cent.

Longevity when this condition is untreated is as follows: pulmonary blood flow decreased, 3 to 11 months; with pulmonary blood flow increased, 8 years. Fifty per cent of patients live 6 months, 34 per cent live 1 year and 10 per cent live 10 years.

R. Usually there is coexisting pulmonary atresia and pulmonic valvular stenosis with normal related great vessels. Balloon atrial septostomy (BAS) is used in the 85 per cent of patients who have decreased pulmonary artery flow. Its morbidity is the same as with tetralogy of Fallot. Shunt mortality[29] for infants less than 6 months old is 50 per cent, and for infants more than 6 months old it is 11 per cent. With shunts the hospital mortality rate for infants less than 12 months old is 29 per cent with the Blalock-Taussig procedure, 33 per cent with the Waterston-Cooley procedure, and 33 per cent with the Potts procedure. With shunts, 45 per cent of patients are alive after 15 years.[30]

S. These patients (15 per cent of cases) have large ventricular septal defects requiring banding in the first three months and probably later shunting.[29]

T. The Fontan procedure involves a conduit (with or without a valve) from the right atrium to the right ventricle or pulmonary artery. Its applicability is circumscribed. Morbidity involves right heart failure with ascites.[4]

U. In total anomalous pulmonary venous return,[1, 2, 32] the incidence of congenital heart disease is 2 per cent, and the incidence of cyanotic heart disease is 7 per cent. Longevity in untreated cases is 7 weeks. Thirty per cent of patients live 6 months; 20 per cent live one year.

V. BAS is occasionally combined with medical therapy in infants, with hemodynamic improvement in 65 per cent of cases.[33]

W. Corrective procedure is anastomosis of the common pulmonary venous channel to the left atrium. This may result in obstruction of pulmonary venous outflow. A late complication is anastomotic stenosis, which occurs in 10 per cent of cases.[35]

X. Age-related mortality is as follows:[34] 20 per cent for patients less than 1 month old, 9 per cent for ages 1 to 3 months, 10 per cent for ages 3 to 6 months, and 0 per cent for ages 6 to 12 months. Overall, HMR is 13 per cent, LMR is 14 per cent.

Y. Mortality is age-related, as in the emergency group.[36, 37]

HMR is 29 per cent for patients 1 to 2 years old and 2 per cent for those 2 to 10 years old.

Z. In persistent truncus arteriosus, the incidence of congenital heart disease is 1 per cent[1, 2] and of cyanotic heart disease is 4 per cent. Longevity without treatment is 5 weeks; 15 to 30 per cent of patients live 1 year.[38]

AA. The Rastelli operation involves closure of the ventricular septal defect and placement of an external valved conduit (heterograft porcine valve) from the right ventricle to the pulmonary artery.[39] It is preferred to banding because of the high mortality of the latter procedure.[40] Morbidity[41] includes reoperation (for VSD or homograft failure) (4 per cent), homograft calcification (100 per cent), endocarditis (3 per cent), and prolonged fever (24 per cent) for porcine valve conduits. The failure rates of homograft conduits have been much greater than those of heterograft valves.

References

1. Keith, J. D., Rowe, R. D., and Vlad, P.: Heart Disease in Infancy and Childhood, 2nd ed. New York, Macmillan Co., 1967.
2. Nadas, A. S., and Fyler, D. C.: Pediatric Cardiology, 3rd ed. Philadelphia, W. B. Saunders Co., 1972, pp. 438, 681.
3. Kidd, B. S. L., and Rowe, R. D.: The fate of children with transposition of the great arteries following balloon atrial septostomy. In Kidd, B. L.., and Rowe, R. D. (eds.): The Child with Congenital Heart Disease After Surgery. Mt. Kisco, N. Y., Futura Publishing Co., 1976, p. 153.
4. Moss, A. J., Adams, F. H., and Emmanouilides, G. C.: Heart Disease in Infants, Children and Adolescents. Baltimore, Williams & Wilkins Co., 1977.
5. Deverall, P. B., et al.: Palliative surgery in children with transposition of the great arteries. J. Thorac. Cardiovasc. Surg., 58:721–729, 1969.
6. Spencer, F. C.: Monitoring technique during palliative operations for transposition of the great vessels. In Barratt-Boyes, B. G., Neutze, J. M., and Harris, E. A.: Heart Disease in Infancy: Diagnosis and Surgical Treatment. New York, Longman, 1973, pp. 261–265.
7. Stark, J., et al.: Banding of the pulmonary artery for transposition of the great arteries and ventricular septal defect. Circulation, 41 (Suppl. 2):116–122, 1970.
8. Zavanella, C., and Subramanian, S.: Review: Surgery for transposition of the great arteries in the first year of life. Ann. Surg., 187:143–150, 1978.
9. Barratt-Boyes, B. G.: Corrective surgery for congenital heart disease in infants with the use of profound hypothermia and circulatory arrest techniques. Aust. N. Z. J. Surg., 47:737–774, 1977.
10. Campsaur, G. L., et al.: Repair of transposition of the great arteries in 123 pediatric patients. Circulation, 47:1032–1041, 1973.
11. Parenzan, L., et al.: The Senning operation for transposition of the great arteries. J. Thorac. Cardiovasc. Surg., 76:305–320, 1978.
12. Jatene, A. D., et al.: Anatomic correction of transposition of the great vessels. J. Thorac. Cardiovasc. Surg., 72:364–370, 1976.
13. McGoon, D. C., Wallace, R. B., and Danielson, G. K.:

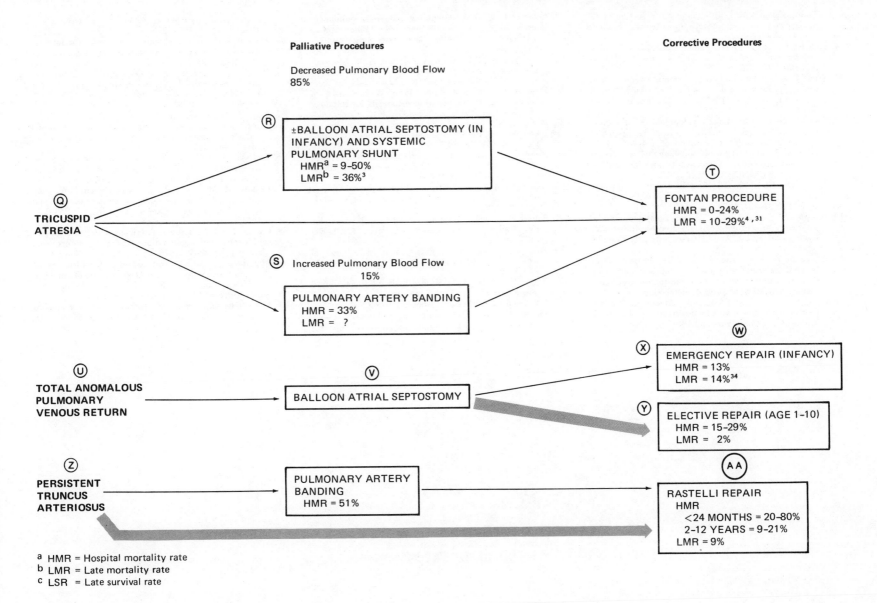

Palliative Procedures

Decreased Pulmonary Blood Flow
85%

Corrective Procedures

(R) ±BALLOON ATRIAL SEPTOSTOMY (IN INFANCY) AND SYSTEMIC PULMONARY SHUNT
HMR[a] = 9–50%
LMR[b] = 36%[3]

(Q) **TRICUSPID ATRESIA**

(T) FONTAN PROCEDURE
HMR = 0–24%
LMR = 10–29%[4],[31]

(S) Increased Pulmonary Blood Flow
15%

PULMONARY ARTERY BANDING
HMR = 33%
LMR = ?

(U) **TOTAL ANOMALOUS PULMONARY VENOUS RETURN**

(V) BALLOON ATRIAL SEPTOSTOMY

(W)
(X) EMERGENCY REPAIR (INFANCY)
HMR = 13%
LMR = 14%[34]

(Y) ELECTIVE REPAIR (AGE 1–10)
HMR = 15–29%
LMR = 2%

(Z) **PERSISTENT TRUNCUS ARTERIOSUS**

PULMONARY ARTERY BANDING
HMR = 51%

(A A) RASTELLI REPAIR
HMR
<24 MONTHS = 20–80%
2–12 YEARS = 9–21%
LMR = 9%

[a] HMR = Hospital mortality rate
[b] LMR = Late mortality rate
[c] LSR = Late survival rate

CYANOTIC HEART DISEASE *Continued*

Transposition with ventricular septal defect and pulmonary stenosis: The Rastelli operation. Isr. J. Med. Sci., *11*:82–88, 1975.

14. El-Said, G., et al.: Dysrhythmias after Mustard operation for transposition of the great arteries. Am. J. Cardiol., *30*:526, 1972.

15. Stark, J., et al.: Obstruction to systemic venous return following the Mustard operation for transposition of the great arteries. J. Thorac. Cardiovasc. Surg., *68*:742–749, 1974.

16. Driscoll, D. J., et al.: Late development of pulmonary venous obstruction following Mustard's operation using a Dacron baffle. Circulation, *55*:484–488, 1977.

17. Hagler, D. J., et al.: Clinical, angiographic and hemodynamic assessment of late results after Mustard repair. Circulation, *57*:1214–1220, 1978.

18. Marcelletti, C., et al.: The Rastelli operation for transposition of the great arteries. J. Thorac. Cardiovasc. Surg., *72*:427–434, 1976.

19. Chopra, P. S., et al.: The Blalock-Taussig operation: The procedure of choice in the hypoxic infant with tetralogy of Fallot. Ann. Thorac. Surg., *22*:235–238, 1976.

20. Barratt-Boyes, B. G., and Neutze, J. M.: Primary repair of tetralogy of Fallot in infancy using profound hypothermia with circulatory arrest and limited cardiopulmonary bypass. Ann. Surg., *178*:406–411, 1973.

21. Stewart, S., Mahoney, E. B., and Manning, J.: The Waterston anastomosis with no deaths in the neonate. J. Thorac. Cardiovasc. Surg., *72*:588–592, 1976.

22. Ortega, M. A., et al.: Ascending aorta–right pulmonary artery anastomosis in children with complex cardiac malformation. J. Thorac. Cardiovasc. Surg., *69*:927–933, 1975.

23. Waterston, D. J., Stark, J., and Ashcraft, K. W.: Ascending aorta to right pulmonary artery shunts: Experience with 100 patients. Surgery, *72*:897–904, 1972.

24. Paul, M. H., Miller, R. A., and Potts, W. J.: Long term results of aortic-pulmonary anastomosis for tetralogy of Fallot. Circulation, *23*:525–533, 1961.

25. Hofschire, P. J., et al.: Pulmonary vascular disease complicating the Blalock-Taussig anastomosis. Circulation, *56*:124–126, 1977.

26. Newfeld, E. A., et al.: Pulmonary vascular disease after systemic-pulmonary arterial shunt operations. Am. J. Cardiol., *39*:715–720, 1977.

27. Castaneda, A. R., et al.: Repair of tetralogy of Fallot in infancy. J. Thorac. Cardiovasc. Surg., *74*:372–381, 1977.

28. Poirier, R. A., et al.: Late results after repair of tetralogy of Fallot. J. Thorac. Cardiovasc. Surg., *75*:900–908, 1977.

29. Williams, W. G., et al.: Tricuspid atresia: Routes of treatment in 160 children. Am. J. Cardiol., *38*:235–240, 1976.

30. Kyger, E. R., III, et al.: Surgical palliation of tricuspid atresia. Circulation, *52*:685–690, 1975.

31. Danielson, G. K.: Personal communication.

32. Delisle, G., et al.: Total anomalous pulmonary venous connection: Report of 93 autopsied cases with emphasis on diagnostic and surgical considerations. Am. Heart J., *91*:99–122, 1976.

33. Mullins, C. E., et al.: Balloon atrial septostomy for total anomalous pulmonary venous return. Br. Heart J., *35*:752–759, 1973.

34. Whight, C. M., et al.: Total anomalous pulmonary venous connection: Long-term results following repair in infancy. J. Thorac. Cardiovasc. Surg., *75*:52–63, 1978.

35. Katz, N. M., Kirklin, J. W., and Pacifico, A. D.: Concepts and practices in surgery for total anomalous pulmonary venous connection. Ann. Thorac. Surg., *25*:479–487, 1978.

36. Wukasch, D. C., et al.: Total anomalous pulmonary venous return: Review of 125 patients treated surgically. Ann. Thorac. Surg., *19*:622–633, 1975.

37. Gomes, M. M. R., et al.: Long-term results following correction of total anomalous pulmonary venous connection. J. Thorac. Cardiovasc. Surg., *61*:253–257, 1971.

38. Calder, L., et al.: Truncus arteriosus: Clinical angiographic and pathologic findings in 100 patients. Am. Heart J., *92*:23–38, 1976.

39. Appelbaum, A., et al.: Surgical treatment of truncus arteriosus with emphasis on infants and small children. J. Thorac. Cardiovasc. Surg., *71*:436–440, 1976.

40. Barratt-Boyes, B. G.: Personal communication.

41. Marcelletti, C., et al.: Early and late results of surgical repair of truncus arteriosus. Circulation, *55*:636–641, 1977.

VENTRICULAR
SEPTAL DEFECT

VENTRICULAR SEPTAL DEFECT BY BRACK HATTLER, M.D.

Comments

A. This algorithm is limited to ventricular septal defects (VSDs) that are the patient's major cardiac malformation and in which muscular tissue separates the defect from the tricuspid valve. It excludes VSD which forms only a part of the overall problem, e.g., atrioventricular canal defects. Within this context there are three anatomic groups of VSD. Most frequent is high or membranous VSD immediately upstream to the aortic valve.[10] Less common defects are those immediately upstream to the pulmonary valve and defects in the muscular septum (10 per cent of defects), which may be multiple. Infrequent causes of VSD are trauma and myocardial infarction.

B. Up to 50 per cent of patients with VSDs have additional cardiac anomalies. Some of the more common are: patent ductus arteriosus (6 per cent of cases), atrial septal defect (9 per cent), coarctation of the aorta (26 per cent), and tetralogy of Fallot (11 per cent).[6, 24]
A common noncardiac malformation seen with ventricular septal defect is pigeon breast.

C. Five to 15 per cent of children become symptomatic in the first year and as many as 25 per cent within this subset will die.[17, 22]

D. Probability of symptoms is related to the duration and magnitude of the shunt. Shunt flow is related to pressure differentials between the two ventricles, left and right ventricular compliance, and the size of the defect.

E. Symptomatic infants with large shunts (greater than 1.4:1) across the defect often have significant pulmonary vascular disease by age 2. Severe, fixed pulmonary vascular changes leading to reversal of shunt flow precede development of the Eisenmenger complex, at which point closure of the defect is no longer feasible.

F. Patients who have multiple VSDs that may require a left ventricular approach for total closure, as well as infants with severe coarctation of the aorta, may be a subgroup of patients who do better with pulmonary artery banding as the initial procedure (i.e., at the time of coarctation repair). Simple ASD or patent ductus arteriosus should not deter consideration of primary VSD closure in infancy, since these defects can easily be repaired at the same procedure. At present some surgical teams are repairing the coarctation and the ventricular septal defect at the same operation.

G. Cardiac failure due to large shunts may necessitate pulmonary artery banding as a preliminary procedure in as many as 40 to 50 per cent of infants with multiple ventricular septal defects.[1]

H. Uncomplicated ventricular septal defect is also known as Roger's disease.[18]

I. There is increasing use of primary repair even in infants less than 1 year old because mortality of the single operation (using deep hypothermia or pump oxygenator) is less than the cumulative mortality of banding and a subsequent curative closure.[13, 16]

J. In children over 6 months old, mortality is low and associated primarily with large defects and moderate to severe pulmonary hypertension.[2] Operative repair in those under 6 months old is becoming progressively safer.

K. Bands that are too loose produce persistent heart failure;[14] those that are too tight produce obstruction of right ventricular outflow. Migration of the band distally can result in obstruction of proximal branch arteries.[7] Aortic insufficiency can result from cusp prolapse (usually the right aortic coronary cusp) through the VSD.[22] Usually this occurs with defects upstream to the pulmonic valve and is an indication for VSD closure, even though the shunt itself may not be symptomatic. Even after VSD closure there may be persistent aortic insufficiency, raising the question of the advisability of valve replacement at the time of VSD closure.[5]

L. A nonrestrictive ventricular septal defect associated with obstruction of right ventricular outflow and an overriding aorta constitute the main features of the tetralogy of Fallot. Large ventricular septal defects may produce an acquired infundibular pulmonic stenosis.

M. Even in infancy total correction can now be performed with less than 5 per cent mortality.[12, 19] Correction following a prior shunt has a cumulative mortality greater than that of initial correction.[12, 19]

N. Palliative shunt procedures at present are limited to those infants who, because of their size and severity of illness, will not tolerate a total correction. Such shunts (Potts, Blalock-Taussig, Waterston) increase pulmonary blood flow.

References

1. Breckenridge, I. M., et al.: Multiple ventricular septal defects. Ann. Thorac. Surg., 13:128, 1972.
2. Cartmill, T. B., et al.: Results of repair of ventricular septal defect. J. Thorac. Cardiovasc. Surg., 52:486, 1966.

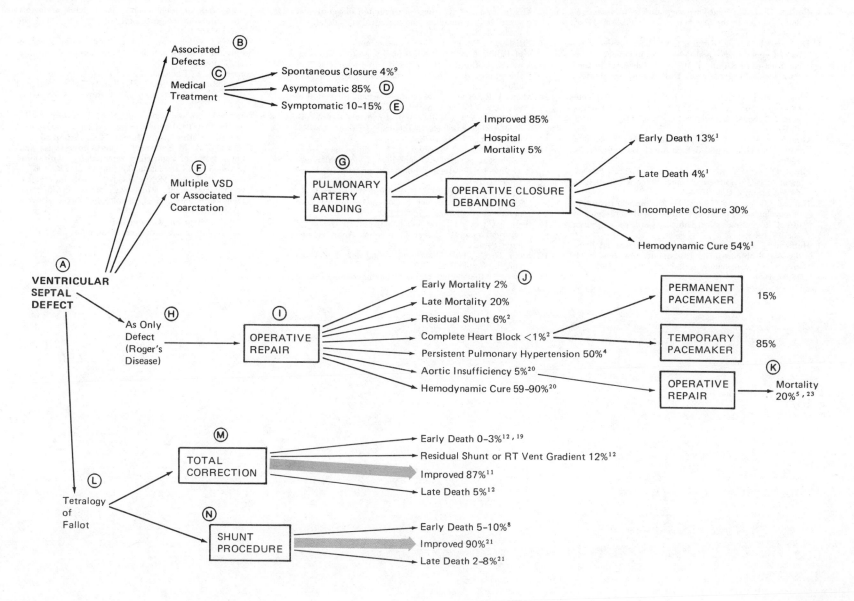

VENTRICULAR SEPTAL DEFECT *Continued*

3. Collins, G., et al.: Ventricular septal defect: Hemodynamic changes in the first five years of life. Am. Heart J., *84*:695, 1972.
4. DuShane, J. W., and Kirklin, J. W.: Late results of repair of ventricular septal defect on pulmonary vascular disease. *In* Kirklin, J. W., (ed.): Advances in Cardiovascular Surgery. New York, Grune & Stratton, 1973.
5. Ellis, F. H. Jr., Ongley, P. A., and Kirklin, J. W.: Ventricular septal defect and aortic valvular incompetence: Surgical considerations. Circulation, *27*:789, 1963.
6. Girard, D. A., et al.: Cardiac malformations associated with ventricular septal defect. Am. J. Cardiol., *17*:73, 1966.
7. Girod, D. A., et al.: Results of two-stage surgical treatment of large ventricular septal defects. Circulation, *49 & 50* (Suppl. 2):9, 1974.
8. Hallman, G. L., and Cooley, D. A.: Surgical treatment of tetralogy of Fallot: Experience with indirect and direct techniques. J. Thorac. Cardiovasc. Surg., *46*:196, 1963.
9. Hoffman, J. I. E.: Natural history of congenital heart disease. Problems in its assessment with special reference to ventricular septal defects. Circulation, *37*:97, 1968.
10. Kirklin, J. W., et al.: Surgical correction of ventricular septal defect: Anatomic and technical considerations. J. Thorac. Surg., *33*:45, 1957.
11. Lillehei, C. W., et al.: Corrective surgery for tetralogy of Fallot. Long-term followup by postoperative recatheterization in 69 cases and certain surgical considerations. J. Thorac. Cardiovasc. Surg., *48*:556, 1964.
12. Malm, J. R., et al.: An evaluation of total correction of tetralogy of Fallot. Circulation, *27*:805, 1963.
13. McNicholas, K. W., et al.: Surgical management of ventricular septal defects in infants. J. Thorac. Cardiovasc. Surg., *75*:346, 1978.
14. Menahem, S., and Venables, A. W.: Pulmonary artery banding in isolated and complicated ventricular septal defects: Results and effects on growth. Br. Heart J., *34*:87, 1972.
15. Morgan, B. C., Griffiths, S. P., and Blumenthal, S.: Ventricular septal defect. I. Congestive heart failure in infancy. Pediatrics, *25*:54, 1960.
16. Rein, J. C., et al.: Early and late results of closure of ventricular septal defect in infancy. Ann. Thorac. Surg., *24*:1, 1977.
17. Ritter, D. G., et al.: Ventricular septal defect. Circulation, *32*(Suppl. 3):42, 1965.
18. Roger, H.: Recherches cliniques sur la communication congenitale des deux coeurs, par inacclusion du septum interventriculaire. Bull. d'Acade de Med. de Paris, *8*:1074, 1879.
19. Shumway, N. E., et al.: Results of total surgical correction for Fallot's tetralogy. Circulation, 31 (Suppl. 1):57, 1965.
20. Somerville, J., Brandao, A., and Ross, D. N.: Aortic regurgitation with ventricular septal defect: Surgical management and clinical features. Circulation, *41*:317, 1970.
21. Taussig, H. B., and Bauersfeld, S. R.: Followup studies on the first 1000 patients operated on for pulmonary stenosis or atresia. Ann. Intern. Med. 38:1, 1953.
22. VanPraagh, R., McNamara, J. J., and Gross, R. E.: Anatomic types of ventricular septal defect with aortic insufficiency. Circulation, *36*: (Suppl. 2): 256, 1967.
23. VanPraagh, R., and McNamara, J. J.: Anatomic types of ventricular septal defect with aortic insufficiency: Diagnostic and surgical considerations. Am. Heart J., *75*:604, 1968.
24. Wood, P., Magidson, O., and Wilson, P. A. O.: Ventricular septal defect with note on acyanotic Fallot's tetralogy. Br. Heart J., *16*:387, 1954.

MITRAL VALVE DISEASE

MITRAL VALVE DISEASE BY WILLIAM HALSETH, M.D.

Comments

I. MITRAL STENOSIS

A. Fifty to 75 per cent of patients have a history of documented rheumatic fever; 30 per cent have had Sydenham's chorea. Congenital mitral stenosis is rare. Three times as many women as men develop mitral stenosis. Symptoms characteristically appear 20 to 30 years after the causative condition.

B.

DEGREE OF STENOSIS	VALVE AREA (cm.²)	LEFT ATRIAL PRESSURE (mm. Hg)	END-DIASTOLIC REST GRADIENT (mm. Hg)
Mild	2.1–2.5	20	<5
Moderate	1.6–2.0	25	5–10
Severe	<1.5	25–50	>10

C. More than 50 per cent of mitral valve lesions following rheumatic fever are mitral stenosis.

D. Survival of medically treated patients with mitral stenosis according to grade is shown in the following table.

AUTHOR	PATIENTS	SURVIVAL 5 Years (%)	10 Years (%)	20 Years (%)
Olesen[1]	271	—	34	14
Munoz[3]	52	45	—	—
Rowe[2]	250	—	61	—
Rowe[2]	Grade I	—	84	—
	Grade II	—	42	—
	Grade III	—	15	—
	Grade IV	—	0	—

Causes of death of medically treated patients with mitral stenosis include:[2] congestive heart failure (61 per cent), systemic embolus (19 per cent), pulmonary embolus (9 per cent), bacterial endocarditis (4 to 5 per cent), and unrelated causes (3 to 6 per cent).

E. Complications of medical treatment of mitral stenosis over 10 years of treatment include:[2] atrial fibrillation (15 per cent of cases), rheumatic heart failure (24 per cent), paroxysmal atrial fibrillation (12 per cent), hemoptysis (9 per cent), pulmonary emboli (8 per cent), bacterial endocarditis (2 per cent), ventricular dysfunction (20 to 30 per cent), and systemic emboli (9 to 25 per cent). Systemic emboli leading to cerebral emboli is a complication that has a 50 per cent mortality rate.

F. Operative mortality was about equivalent (0 to 2 per cent) for closed and open commissurotomy.[4-9] Reoperation for restenosis of the mitral valve following closed valvotomy was up to 60 per cent, vs. 0 to 3 per cent for open valvotomy.[9, 10, 32-34]

Continued on page 186

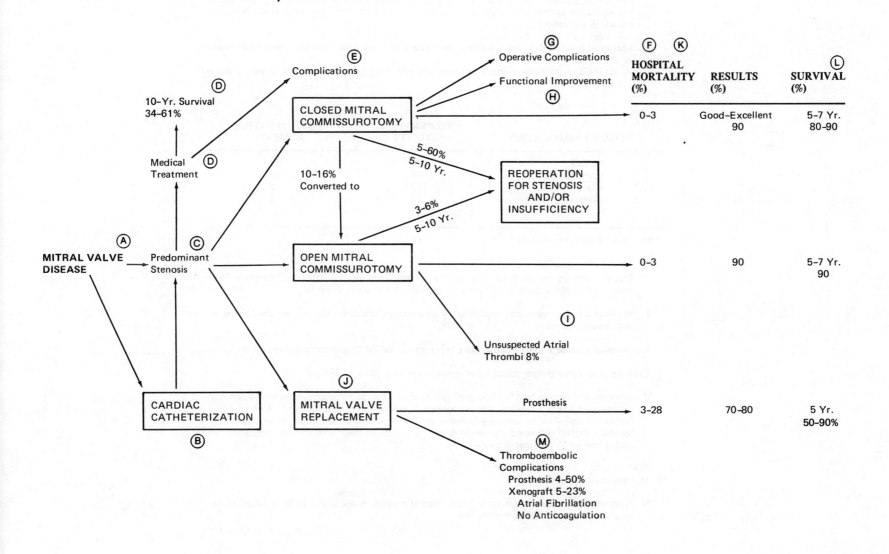

MITRAL VALVE DISEASE *Continued*

G. Complications were equivalent in the open and the closed operations: infection (1 per cent of cases),[1] reoperation bleeding (1 to 4 per cent),[4] pulmonary complications (10 per cent),[4] intraoperative emboli (2 to 6 per cent closed vs. 1 to 3 per cent open),[10] and postoperative emboli (8 per cent).[4]

H. Improved functional cardiac classification was demonstrated following closed mitral valvotomy in 192 patients.[10]
A decrease in pulmonary artery pressure and left atrial pressure occurred following mitral valvotomy.[7, 12]

NYHA[a] CLASSIFICATION	PREOPERATIVE PATIENTS	POSTOPERATIVE PATIENTS
Class I	1	99
Class II	48	88
Class III	132	4
Class IV	11	1
TOTAL	192	192

[a]New York Heart Association.

I. During open operation, 8 per cent of patients had unsuspected left atrial thrombus. With history of systemic embolus, 27 per cent of patients had atrial thrombus.[4, 10]

J. Prosthetic replacement may be necessary for a heavily calcified valve or a combined stenotic and regurgitant valve.

K. Hospital mortality rate of mitral valve replacement varied from 3 to 28 per cent.[11, 13–17]

L. Five-year survival after mitral valve replacement was 50 to 90 per cent.[11, 13, 16, 17]

M. Systemic emboli occurred in 23 per cent of patients with atrial fibrillation, large left atrium, and no anticoagulation following porcine xenograft mitral valve replacement.[18] Without atrial fibrillation and with no anticoagulation, only 5 per cent of patients had thromboemboli.[16] Systemic emboli following prosthetic mitral valve replacement without anticoagulation occurred in 4 to 50 per cent of cases.[11–13]

II. MITRAL REGURGITATION

N. Nonrheumatic causes are more common than rheumatic endocarditis in the etiology of this condition. The percentage is unknown.

Continued on page 188

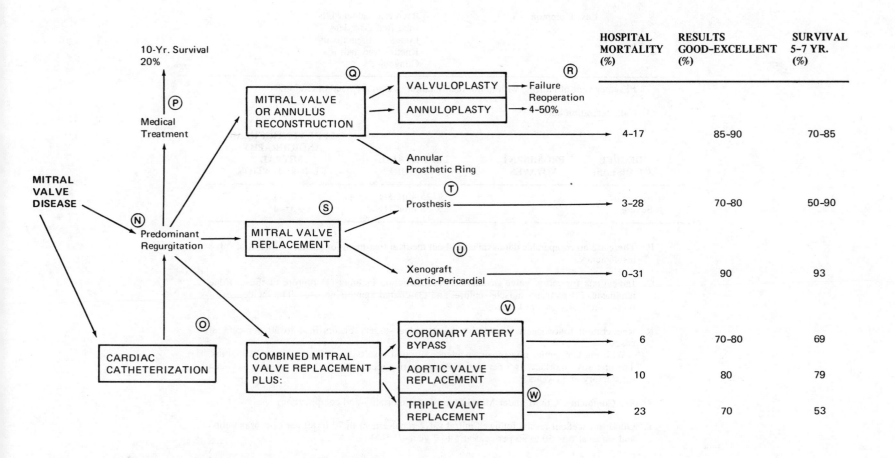

	HOSPITAL MORTALITY (%)	RESULTS GOOD–EXCELLENT (%)	SURVIVAL 5–7 YR. (%)
MITRAL VALVE OR ANNULUS RECONSTRUCTION	4–17	85–90	70–85
Prosthesis	3–28	70–80	50–90
Xenograft Aortic-Pericardial	0–31	90	93
CORONARY ARTERY BYPASS	6	70–80	69
AORTIC VALVE REPLACEMENT	10	80	79
TRIPLE VALVE REPLACEMENT	23	70	53

MITRAL VALVE DISEASE *Continued*

CAUSES

More Common	Mitral valve prolapse
	Papillary muscle dysfunction
	Chordae tendineae rupture
Less Common	Bacterial endocarditis
	Inherited disorders
	Lupus erythematosus
	Rheumatoid arthritis
	Congenital

Fifty per cent of patients with mitral regurgitation eventually need operation.[19]

O. Catheterization data:

DEGREE OF DISEASE	PROMINENT V WAVES	LEFT ATRIAL PRESSURE	LEFT VENTRICULAR ANGIOGRAPHY MITRAL REGURGITATION
Moderate	+	25 mm. Hg	2^+–3^+
Severe	+	25–50 mm. Hg	3^+–4^+

P. There are no comparable data available about medical treatment for patients with mitral valve insufficiency.

Q. Indications for mitral valve or annulus reconstruction include: (1) rupture of the chordae tendineae, (2) papillary muscle rupture, and (3) dilated annulus fibrosus. The incidences of these conditions are not known.

R. Reoperation following reconstructive mitral valve surgery occurs in 4 to 50 per cent of cases.[21-24]

   With the Carpentier ring repair, incidence of good results was 85 per cent at 33 months. The operative mortality is 5 per cent.[30] Postoperative reconstructive valve function has been satisfactory at 11 years.[20]

S. See Comments K to M under Mitral Stenosis for mortality and complications.

T. Good to excellent results followed mitral valve replacement in 70 to 80 per cent of patients, and survival was 50 to 90 per cent at 5 to 7 years.[11, 13-17]

U. Long-term (10-year) results of using porcine valves are unknown. Good results are reported at 5 to 7 years.[16, 18, 25-26]

V. Mortality rate from coronary artery bypass combined with mitral valve replacement is about equal to that of isolated mitral valve replacement—6 per cent.[27]

Tricuspid insufficiency characteristically accompanies severe, chronic mitral stenosis and prolonged pulmonary hypertension. Relief of mitral valve disease results in regression of tricuspid insufficiency.[28]

The incidence of failure with tricuspid annuloplasty is 7 per cent.[29-31]

W. Triple valve replacement has a hospital mortality of 23 per cent with 5-year survival of 53 per cent.[32] Combined aortic and mitral valve replacement has a 10 per cent operative mortality.[11]

References

1. Olesen, K. H.: The natural history of 271 patients with mitral stenosis under medical treatment. Br. Heart J. *24*:349–357, 1962.
2. Rowe, J. C., et al.: The course of mitral stenosis without surgery: Ten and twenty-year perspectives. Ann. Intern. Med., *52*:741–749, 1960.
3. Munoz, S., et al.: Influence of surgery on the natural history of rheumatic mitral and aortic valve disease. Am. J. Cardiol., *35*:234–42, 1975.
4. Finnegan, J. O., et al.: Open approach to mitral commissurotomy. J. Thorac. Cardiovasc. Surg., *67*:75–82, 1974.
5. Gerami, S., et al.: Open mitral commissurotomy: Results of 100 consecutive cases. J. Thorac. Cardiovasc. Surg., *62*:366–70, 1971.
6. Mullin, M. J., et al.: Experience with open mitral commissurotomy in 100 consecutive patients. Surgery, *76*:974–982, 1974.
7. Roe, B. B., et al.: Open mitral valvotomy. Ann. Thorac. Surg., *12*:483–491, 1971.
8. Harken, D. E., et al.: The surgical treatment of mitral stenosis: Valvuloplasty. N. Engl. J. Med., *239*:801–809, 1948.
9. Kiser, I. C., et al.: Long-term results of closed mitral commissurotomy. J. Cardiovasc. Surg., *8*:263–70, 1967.
10. Grantham, R. N., et al.: Transventricular mitral valvulotomy. Analysis of factors influencing operative and late results. Circulation, *50*(Suppl.):200, 1974.
11. Kirklin, J. W., and Pacifico, A. D.: Surgery for acquired valvular heart disease, part II. N. Engl. J. Med., *288*:194, 1973.
12. Hammermeister, K. E., et al.: Prediction of late survival in patients with mitral valve disease from clinical, hemodynamic and quantitative angiographic variables. Circulation, *57*:341, 1978.
13. Starr, A., et al.: Mitral valve replacement. An appraisal at 10 years of non–cloth-covered vs. cloth-covered caged ball prosthesis. (Abstr.) Circulation, *51* & *52*(Suppl. 2): 30, 1975.
14. Starr, A.: Mitral valve replacement with ball valve prosthesis. Br. Heart J. *33*(Suppl.):47, 1971.
15. Bonchek, L. I., and Starr, A.: Ball valve prostheses: Current appraisal of late results. Am. J. Cardiol., *35*:843, 1975.
16. Cohn, L. H., Sanders, J. H., and Collins, J.: Actuarial comparison of Hancock porcine and prosthetic disc valves for isolated mitral valve replacement. Circulation, *54*(Suppl. 3):III60–3, 1976.
17. Fishman, N. H., et al.: Five-year experience with the Smeloff-Cutter mitral prosthesis. J. Thorac. Cardiovasc. Surg., *62*:345, 1971.
18. Edmiston, W. A., et al.: Thromboembolism in mitral porcine valve recipients. Am. J. Cardiol., *41*:508, 1978.
19. Crawley, S. I., Morris, D. C., and Silverman, B. D.: Valvular heart disease. *In* Hurst, J.: The Heart, 4th ed. New York, McGraw-Hill, 1978, p. 1064.
20. Reed, G. E.: Repair of mitral regurgitation. Am. J. Cardiol., *31*:494, 1973.
21. Selzer, A., et al.: Immediate and long-range results of valvuloplasty for mitral regurgitation due to ruptured chordae tendineae. Circulation, *45*(suppl.):52, 1972.
22. West, P. N., and Weldon, C. S.: Reconstructive valve surgery. Ann. Thorac. Surg., *25*:167, 1978.
23. Reed, G. E., Clauss, R. H., and Spencer, F. C.: Controversy between replacement and repair of mitral valve. *In* Brewer, L. A., III (ed.): Prosthetic Heart Valves. Springfield, Ill., Charles C Thomas, 1969, p. 458.

24. Manhas, D. R., et al.: Reconstructive surgery for treatment of mitral incompetence: Early and late results in 91 patients. J. Thorac. Cardiovasc. Surg., 62:781, 1971.
25. Albert, H. M., Bryant, L. R., and Schechter, F. G.: Seven-year experience with mounted porcine valves. Ann. Surg., 185:717, 1977.
26. Tandon, A. P., Smith, D. R., and Ionescu, M. I.: Long-term hemodynamic behavior of Ionescu-Shiley pericardial xenograft heart valve. Paper presented at the 27th annual Scientific Session of the American College of Cardiology, Anaheim, Calif., March 1978.
27. Berger, T. J., Karep, R. B., and Kouchoukos, N. T.: Valve replacement and myocardial revascularization. Circulation, 51 & 52(suppl. 1):126, 1973.
28. Braunwald, N. S., Ross, J., and Morrow, A. G.: Conservative management of tricuspid regurgitation in patients undergoing mitral valve replacement. Circulation, 35(suppl. 1):63, 1967.
29. Grondin, P., et al.: Carpentier's annulus and DeVega's annuloplasty. J. Thorac. Cardiovasc. Surg., 70:852, 1975.
30. Chopra, P., et al.: Carpentier ring annuloplasty in severe non-calcific mitral insufficiency. Arch. Surg., 112:1469, 1977.
31. Carpentier, A., et al.: A new reconstructive operation for correction of mitral and tricuspid insufficiency. J. Thorac. Cardiovasc. Surg., 61:1, 1971.
32. Stephenson, L. W., Kouchoukos, N. T., and Kirklin, J. W.: Triple valve replacement: An analysis of eight years' experience. Ann. Thorac. Surg., 23:327, 1977.
33. Logan, A., et al.: Reoperation for mitral stenosis. Lancet, 1:443–449, 1962.
34. Author's experience: of 174 patients, 7 per cent required reoperation at 1 to 10 years.

AORTIC VALVE DISEASE

AORTIC VALVE DISEASE BY W. GERALD RAINER, M.D.

Comments

CONGENITAL AORTIC STENOSIS

A. Three to 6 per cent of all patients with congenital heart disease have this condition (1000 to 2000 infants per year in the U.S.[1]).

B. After the first year of life, mortality during the first 2 decades in patients with congenital aortic stenosis is 14 times that of the normal population.[3] (See table.)

C. Congestive heart failure occurs in 60 per cent of infants with congenital aortic stenosis. Presence of symptoms, severe pressure gradient (greater than 49 mm. Hg), and associated fibroelastosis make prognosis very poor.[1]

D. Most patients improve after valvotomy, with relief of left ventricular outflow tract obstruction. Results are poorest in those patients with small aortic root or associated left-sided hypoplasia, or both. Of all patients alive at 11 years of age, a statistically significantly larger number of those treated surgically will be alive 15 years later.[1, 3, 9]

E. Although sudden death occurs less frequently after surgery, the risk is still present. Death probably occurs secondary to arrhythmia. Aortic insufficiency occurs in 30 to 40 per cent of patients undergoing valvotomy and accounts for symptoms in about 20 per cent of cases. These usually present preoperatively in about 11 per cent of patients.[1]

F. Major causes of late postoperative death are bacterial endocarditis, arrhythmia (probable cause of sudden death), and congestive heart failure (secondary to aortic insufficiency created intraoperatively).[1, 4-11]

G. If the need for reoperation arises while the patient is still quite young (less than 10 to 12 years of age), repeat valvotomy may be appropriate. However, more often than not reoperation may be necessary at a later age (12 years or older); then, valve replacement becomes a serious consideration.[12-14] Aortic valve replacement in children 12 to 15 years of age is associated with an operative mortality of 17 per cent and a late mortality of 15 per cent.[12-15]

ACQUIRED AORTIC STENOSIS

H. Male predominance of this condition is 3:1 to 4:1.[16] The "critical" systolic orifice is 0.6 cm.[2] in an average-size adult.[17] Only one-third of patients give a history of rheumatic fever.[16] Symptomatic patients with a systolic gradient greater than 50 mm Hg should be considered for surgery without delay.

I. Congestive failure often is the first symptom in the aged.[18] Effort syncope and angina usually are early symptoms.

J. Five per cent of sudden deaths in older patients with aortic stenosis occur *without* prior symptoms.[19] In 80 per cent of patients dying from aortic stenosis, symptoms have been present for more than 4 years.[19] Average life span after onset of congestive heart failure is 1 to 3 years.[19] Average life span after onset of effort syncope or angina is 3 to 4 years.[18] Right ventricular decompensation means death within 1 year.[18]

K. Morbidity and mortality vary with operative selection of patients (failure, multivalvular disease, co-existing coronary disease and other conditions, conduct of surgical procedure (with or without coronary perfusion, hypothermia, cardioplegia, and so on), and choice of prosthetic valve for replacement. These and other factors (such as anticoagulant therapy) contribute to a wide range of reported results.

L. Incidence of thromboembolism varies with type of valve and anticoagulation

AGE (Years)[3]	MORTALITY (%/Year)	ASYMPTO-MATIC (%)	SYMPTOMS		SUDDEN DEATH[a] (%/Year)
			Mild (%)	Severe (%)	
0–10	2.1	50	20	20	0.4–0.9
10–20	1.4				
20–30	1.1				
30–40	2.4	20	29	40	
40–50	4.8				

[a]Cumulative: 0.8%/year.[1] Sudden death is usually associated with severe stenosis, left ventricular hypertrophy, and syncope, dyspnea, or chest pain.

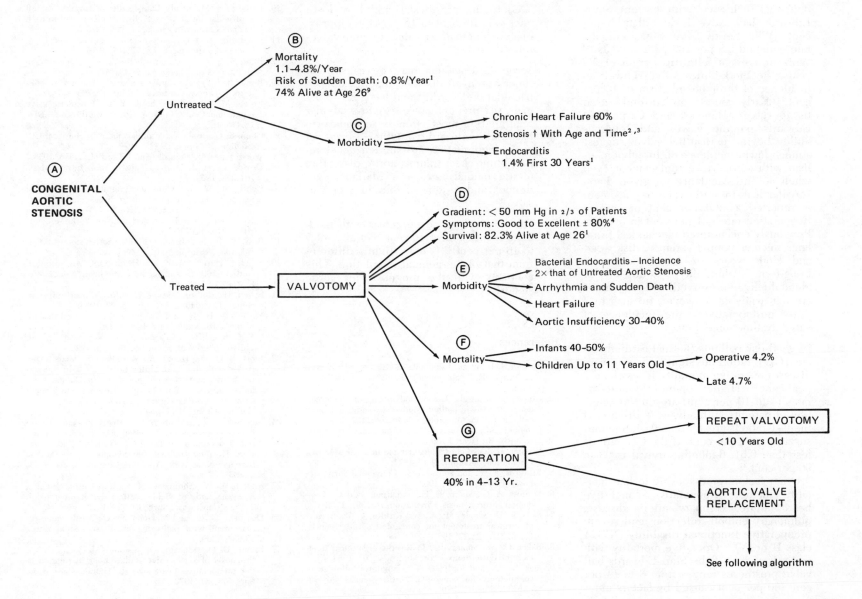

Ⓑ Mortality
1.1–4.8%/Year
Risk of Sudden Death: 0.8%/Year[1]
74% Alive at Age 26[9]

Untreated

Ⓒ Morbidity
→ Chronic Heart Failure 60%
→ Stenosis ↑ With Age and Time[2,3]
→ Endocarditis
  1.4% First 30 Years[1]

Ⓐ
**CONGENITAL
AORTIC
STENOSIS**

Ⓓ Gradient: < 50 mm Hg in 2/3 of Patients
Symptoms: Good to Excellent ± 80%[4]
Survival: 82.3% Alive at Age 26[1]

Treated → VALVOTOMY

Ⓔ Morbidity
→ Bacterial Endocarditis—Incidence
  2× that of Untreated Aortic Stenosis
→ Arrhythmia and Sudden Death
→ Heart Failure
→ Aortic Insufficiency 30–40%

Ⓕ Mortality
→ Infants 40–50%
→ Children Up to 11 Years Old → Operative 4.2%
                               → Late 4.7%

Ⓖ
REOPERATION
40% in 4–13 Yr.

→ **REPEAT VALVOTOMY**
  <10 Years Old

→ **AORTIC VALVE
REPLACEMENT**
  ↓
  See following algorithm

193

regimen. Incidence with current Starr-Edwards ball valve is less than 5 per cent. (With Series 2400 valve, embolic rate equalled 2.8 per 100 patient-years.)[24] With an average followup period of 2½ years, the Bjork-Shiley valve showed an incidence of thromboembolism of 10 per cent.[23] Early reports on currently used tissue valves (Hancock and Carpentier-Edwards porcine valves and Ionescu-Shiley bovine pericardial valve) suggest a much lower incidence of thromboembolism with aortic valve replacement even when *no* anticoagulants are given. Paravalvular leak in aortic valve replacement is reported as 2.6 per cent of cases.[22] Reoperation rate is 1 per cent in 5 years. Previously encountered mechanical problems, such as poppet variance, disk wear, and cloth wear, are now uncommon. Long-term durability studies of glutaraldehyde-preserved tissue valves are not available; however, up to 5 to 7 years postoperatively the incidence of valve dysfunction is low.

M. In good-risk patients (normal cardiothoracic [C-T] ratio, no significant coronary disease) operative mortality is less than 2 per cent.[22] Higher operative mortality rates (4 to 10 per cent) are due to selection of patients with advanced disease. If the C-T ratio is greater than 0.61, 6-month survival is 78 per cent. If the C-T ratio is less than 0.61, 6-month survival is 93 to 96 per cent.[27]

Other factors predisposing to late mortality include preoperative congestive heart failure, coronary artery disease, pulmonary emboli, infection, and severe preoperative functional disability (NYHA class II or IV).[22] Operative mortality with various models of the Starr-Edwards ball valve prostheses ranges from 8 to 14 per cent (60 per cent caused by factors unre-lated to the prosthesis), and late death rates vary from 14 to 16 per cent (approximately one-half are due to non–valve-related causes).[24]

N. Aortic insufficiency may be caused by rheumatic heart disease, hypertension, or bacterial endocarditis and has a 2:1 to 3:1 male sex predominance.[20] *Acute* valvular regurgitation most often is secondary to bacterial endocarditis. Other causes of acute regurgitation are sudden deceleration blunt chest trauma, aortic dissection (cystic medial necrosis — Marfan's syndrome), and rupture of the sinus of Valsalva.[18]

O. The relatively good prognosis with moderate insufficiency (10-year mortality of 5 to 16 per cent)[21] is only slightly different from that of the general population. This contrasts with the prognosis for aortic stenosis.

References

1. Stewart, J. R., et al.: Congenital aortic stenosis: Ten to 22 years after valvulotomy. Arch. Surg., *113*:1248, 1978.
2. Cohen, L. S., et al.: The natural history of congenital aortic stenosis in patients studied by serial left heart catheterization. Ann. Intern. Med., *68*:1152, 1968.
3. Campbell, M.: The natural history of congenital aortic stenosis. Br. Heart J., *30*:514, 1968.
4. Wagner, H. R., et al.: Clinical course in aortic stenosis. Circulation, *56*(suppl. 1):47, 1977.
5. Edwards, F. R., and Jones, R. S.: Congenital aortic stenosis. Thorax, *17*:218, 1962.
6. Morrow, A. G., Sharp, E. H., and Braunwald E.: Congenital aortic stenosis. Circulation, *18*:1091, 1958.
7. Ellis, F. H., Ongley, P. A., and Kirklin, J. W.: Results of surgical treatment for congenital aortic stenosis. Circulation, 25:29, 1962.
8. Baker, C. and Somerville, J.: Results of surgical treatment of aortic stenosis. Br. Med. J., *1*:197, 1964.
9. Jack, W. D., and Kelly, D. T.: Long-term followup of valvulotomy for congenital aortic stenosis. Am. J. Cardiol., 38:231, 1976.
10. Lawson, R. M., et al.: Late results of surgery for left ventricular outflow tract obstruction in children. J. Thorac. Cardiovasc. Surg., 71:334, 1976.
11. Chiarielli, L., et al.: Congenital aortic stenosis. J. Thorac. Cardiovasc. Surg., 72:182, 1976.
12. Blieden, L. C., et al.: Prosthetic valve replacement in children. Ann. Thorac. Surg., *14*:545, 1972.
13. Berry, B. E., et al.: Cardiac valve replacement in children. J. Thorac. Cardiovasc. Surg., 68:705, 1974.
14. Freed, M. D., and Bernhard, W. F.: Prosthetic valve replacement in children. Prog. Cardiovasc. Dis., 18:475, 1975.
15. Chen, S. C., et al.: Valve replacement in children. Circulation, 56(suppl. 2): 117, 1977.
16. Wood, P.: Aortic stenosis. Am. J. Cardiol., *1*:553, 1958.
17. Dexter, L., et al.: Aortic stenosis. Arch. Intern. Med., *101*:254, 1958.
18. Cobbs, B. W., Jr.: Clinical recognition and medical management of rheumatic heart disease and other acquired vascular disease. *In* Hurst, J. W., and Logue, R. B., (eds.): The Heart, 2nd ed. New York, McGraw-Hill, 1970, p. 773.
19. Ross, J., Jr., and Braunwald, E.: Aortic stenosis. Circulation, 38(suppl. 5): 61, 1968.
20. Segal, J., Harvey, W. P., and Hufnagel, C. A.: A clinical study of 100 cases of severe aortic insufficiency. Am. J. Med., 21:200, 1956.
21. Scheu, H., Rothlin, M. and Hegglin, R.: Aortic insufficiency. Circulation, 38(suppl. 5):77, 1968.
22. Muller, W. H., Jr., and Crosby, I. K.: Acquired disease of the aortic valve. *In* Sabiston, D. C., and Spencer, F. C. (eds.): Gibbon's Surgery of the Chest, 3rd ed. Philadelphia, W.B. Saunders, 1976, p. 1228.
23. Bjork, V. O., and Henze, A.: More than 6½ years' experience with the Bjork-Shiley heart valves in the aortic, mitral, and tricuspid positions. *In* Davila, J. C., (ed.): 2nd Henry Ford Hospital International Symposium on Cardiac Surgery. New York, Appleton-Century-Crofts, 1977, p. 454.
24. Bonchek, L. I., and Starr, A.: Valve replacement with ball-valve prosthesis: Selection of prosthesis and timing of operation. *In* Davila, J. C., (ed.): 2nd Henry Ford Hospital International Symposium in Cardiac Surgery. New York, Appleton-Century-Crofts, 1977, p. 466.
25. Angell, W. W., Shumway, N. E., and Cosek, J. C.: A five-year study of viable aortic valve homografts. J. Thorac. Cardiovasc. Surg., 64:329, 1972.
26. Duvoisin, G. E., and McGoon, D. C.: Aortic valve replacement with ball-valve prosthesis. Arch. Surg., 99:684, 1969.
27. Braun, L. O., Kincaid, O. W., and McGoon, D. C.: Prognosis of aortic valve replacement in relation to the preoperative heart size. J. Thorac. Cardiovasc. Surg., 65:381, 1973.

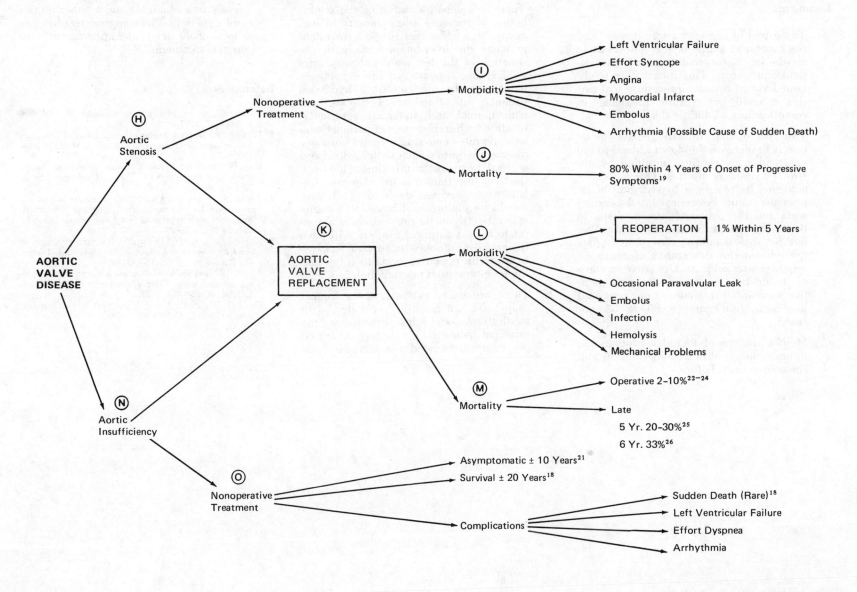

Ⓗ Aortic Stenosis

Nonoperative Treatment

Ⓘ Morbidity
- Left Ventricular Failure
- Effort Syncope
- Angina
- Myocardial Infarct
- Embolus
- Arrhythmia (Possible Cause of Sudden Death)

Ⓙ Mortality
- 80% Within 4 Years of Onset of Progressive Symptoms[19]

AORTIC VALVE DISEASE

Ⓚ AORTIC VALVE REPLACEMENT

Ⓛ Morbidity
- REOPERATION   1% Within 5 Years
- Occasional Paravalvular Leak
- Embolus
- Infection
- Hemolysis
- Mechanical Problems

Ⓜ Mortality
- Operative 2–10%[22–24]
- Late
  5 Yr. 20–30%[25]
  6 Yr. 33%[26]

Ⓝ Aortic Insufficiency

Ⓞ Nonoperative Treatment
- Asymptomatic ± 10 Years[21]
- Survival ± 20 Years[18]
- Complications
  - Sudden Death (Rare)[18]
  - Left Ventricular Failure
  - Effort Dyspnea
  - Arrhythmia

ANGINA PECTORIS BY ALAN D. HILGENBERG, M.D.

Comments

A. The extent of coronary artery disease and the functional status of the left ventricle are the key factors that influence each patient's prognosis. This information is obtained via an invasive procedure that carries a small but definite incidence of complications, including death.[1]

B. The goal of the coronary bypass operation is to increase the flow of blood to the ventricular myocardium supplied by obstructed coronary arteries. This is usually achieved by placing a bypass graft of saphenous vein between the ascending aorta and the coronary arteries distal to their obstructions. Some surgeons use the left internal mammary artery to bypass the left anterior descending coronary artery in young subjects. Operative mortality should be 1 to 3 per cent, perioperative myocardial infarction 5 per cent, and long-term graft patency 80 to 85 per cent.[2]

C. Medical treatment includes propranolol, nitrates, and control of hypertension and congestive heart failure.

D. There is a debate concerning the contribution of coronary artery surgery to longevity. It is clear that surgical treatment prolongs the lives of patients with obstruction of the left main coronary artery.[3, 4] It also appears that life expectancy is increased by coronary artery bypass in patients with three-vessel disease and both normal and abnormal ventricular function.[3, 5] Survival rates of patients who have double- and single-vessel coronary disease are quite similar with medical and surgical treatment at this time. However, the lives of certain patients who have isolated left anterior descending disease should be prolonged if large left ventricular infarcts can be prevented by appropriate bypass surgery.[6] Surgery will have the greatest influence on survival in cases in which the operative mortality is low and the long-term graft patency high.[7]

E. There are many patients whose angina cannot be satisfactorily controlled with medications, and this constitutes the principal indication for surgery. About 60 per cent of operated patients are completely free of angina and another 30 per cent experience less angina, resulting in a total of 90 per cent improvement with surgical treatment.[7]

References

1. Conti, C. R.: Coronary arteriography. Circulation, 55:227–237, 1977.
2. Mundth, E. D., and Austen, W. G.: Surgical measures for coronary heart disease. N. Engl. J. Med., 293:13–130, 1975.
3. Read, R. C., et al.: Survival of men treated for chronic stable angina pectoris. J. Thorac. Cardiovasc. Surg., 75:1–13, 1978.
4. Takaro, T., et al.: The VA cooperative randomized study of surgery for coronary arterial occlusive disease. II. Subgroup with significant left main lesions. Circulation, 54:(Supp.3): 107–116, 1976.
5. Manley, J. C., et al.: The "bad" left ventricle. Results of coronary surgery and effect on late survival. J. Thorac. Cardiovasc. Surg., 72:841–848, 1976.
6. Abedin, Z., and Dack, S.: Isolated left anterior descending coronary artery disease: Choice of therapy. Am. J. Cardiol., 40:654–657, 1977.
7. Hurst, J. W., et al.: Value of coronary bypass surgery. Am. J. Cardiol., 42:308–329, 1978.

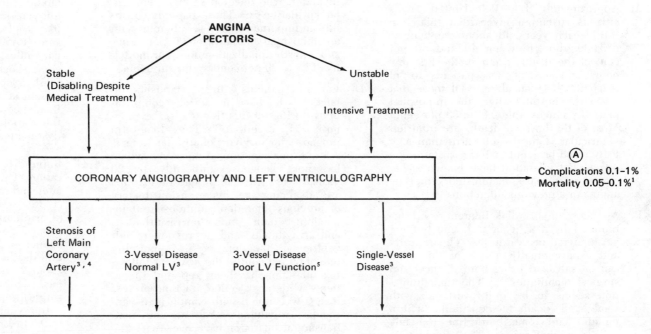

ANGINA PECTORIS

Stable
(Disabling Despite
Medical Treatment)

Unstable

Intensive Treatment

CORONARY ANGIOGRAPHY AND LEFT VENTRICULOGRAPHY

Ⓐ
Complications 0.1–1%
Mortality 0.05–0.1%[1]

Stenosis of
Left Main
Coronary
Artery[3,4]

3-Vessel Disease
Normal LV[3]

3-Vessel Disease
Poor LV Function[5]

Single-Vessel
Disease[3]

	FOUR-YEAR SURVIVAL RATE Ⓓ (%)				RELIEF OF ANGINA[7] Ⓔ (%)
Ⓑ CORONARY ARTERY BYPASS	93	89	67	98	90
Mortality 1–3%[2]					
Ⓒ Medical Treatment	63	76	40	98	65

LV = Left Ventricle

ACUTE MYOCARDIAL INFARCTION BY DONALD ELLIOT, M.D.

Comments

A. Approximately 1,300,000 United States citizens sustain a myocardial infarction (MIT) each year and about one-half, or 675,000, die.[1] Between 40 and 60 per cent of the deaths occur in the first few hours, and most of these patients do not reach the hospital alive.[1-5] Of those that reach the hospital alive, the in-hospital mortality ranges from 9.6[6] to 33 per cent.[7] Most of the hospital deaths are from left ventricular failure and arrhythmias.[8-10] Fifty to 65 per cent of those sustaining a myocardial infarction have known ischemic heart disease, manifested either by angina or a previous infarction.[1, 11-13]

B. An acute myocardial infarction is surrounded by a zone of ischemic but not yet infarcted myocardium.[14] Theoretically and experimentally, much of this zone can be salvaged using both medical and surgical techniques.[15-17] The time limitation seems to be quite variable, with some cell death demonstrable within minutes and some borderline ischemic cells surviving for days.[14] Patients who sustain a myocardial infarction in the catheterization laboratory and those who sustain an infarction while in the hospital awaiting coronary artery surgery are ideally suited for immediate revascularization.[9, 15, 18-24]

Immediate revascularization for the patient arriving at the hospital moments after sustaining a myocardial infarction is an intriguing but not yet proven mode of therapy.[15, 20, 21] Immediate bypass should prove of greatest benefit in those patients demonstrated by metabolic or radionuclide studies to have a significant amount of ischemic, but not yet infarcted, myocardium.[9, 24]

C. Mobile Coronary Care Units are resuscitating many victims of acute myocardial infarction who develop sudden ventricular fibrillation.[25, 26] These patients constitute an important high-risk subgroup with an in-hospital mortality of 60 per cent[26] and a posthospitalization one-year mortality of 28 to 29 per cent[25, 26] for survivors.

D. For those patients with an established infarction who have no serious complications during the first few days, the prognosis is excellent.[27] The long-term prognosis for survivors of all infarctions is a 5 to 8 per cent annual mortality, which has not changed significantly in 20 years.[1, 11, 27-31] Adverse prognostic features are advancing age, hypertension, history of previous infarction, nontransmural infarction, certain conduction disturbances and arrhythmias, and depression of left ventricular function.[1, 29, 30] A mortality rate of 66 per cent in the first year following infarction has been reported in patients with an ejection fraction of less than 0.40 coupled with complicated ventricular arrhythmias.[32] Patients with nontransmural infarction have over twice the incidence of postinfarction sudden death as those with transmural infarction.[11] A recent report of the Anturane Reinfarction Trial Research Group demonstrates a nearly 50 per cent reduction in postinfarction sudden deaths with Anturane therapy.[3]

E. Approximately one half to two thirds of patients hospitalized with an acute myocardial infarction will demonstrate a serious complication.[1, 27, 29] The most common complication is an arrhythmia. The table on page 200 (top), adapted from Chatterjee,[1] shows the hospital mortality rate for the various atrial and ventricular arrhythmias.

F. Approximately 55 per cent of patients hospitalized with an acute myocardial infarction demonstrate signs of significant left ventricular dysfunction, evidenced by increased pulmonary artery wedge pressure (PAWP), third heart sound, pulmonary rales, pulmonary edema, or cardiogenic shock.[29] The table on page 200 (bottom), adapted from Yu[29] and using the classification of Killip,[33] gives the relative incidence and hospital mortality rates for the various degrees of left ventricular dysfunction.

G. Rupture of the heart muscle as a complication of infarction occurs days to weeks later and may be observed in three sites: (1) free wall, (2) ventricular septum, and (3) papillary muscle. Rupture complicates about 3 per cent of all infarctions but accounts for 5 to 16 per cent of all infarction deaths.[29] Free wall rupture occurs in about 2 per cent of all infarctions and is fatal, with only a few reported successful surgical repairs.[34-37]

Interventricular septum rupture occurs in 0.5 to 1.0 per cent of myocardial infarctions and accounts for 2 per cent of the deaths.[29, 38] The acute onset of a large left-to-right shunt in an already compromised heart frequently causes cardiogenic shock. Intra-aortic balloon pump (IABP) support enables stabilization during diagnostic studies and surgery. Mortality in medically treated patients is 65 to 87 per cent at two weeks.[1, 21, 30] Mortality with early surgery for interventricular septal defect (IVSD) and cardiogenic shock is 30 to 50 per cent.[38, 40-43] Mortality for delayed surgery is 7 to 36 per cent.[1, 21, 40]

Papillary muscle rupture occurs in less than 1 per cent of all cases of infarction and accounts for about 1 per cent of the deaths.[38] The mortality is 70 per cent in

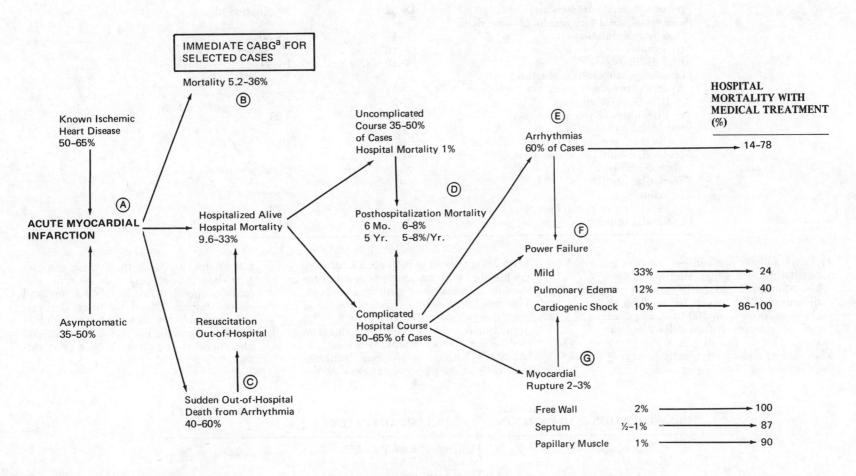

IMMEDIATE CABG[a] FOR SELECTED CASES

Mortality 5.2–36%

Ⓑ

Known Ischemic
Heart Disease
50–65%

Ⓐ

ACUTE MYOCARDIAL INFARCTION

Asymptomatic
35–50%

Hospitalized Alive
Hospital Mortality
9.6–33%

Resuscitation
Out-of-Hospital

Ⓒ

Sudden Out-of-Hospital
Death from Arrhythmia
40–60%

Uncomplicated
Course 35–50%
of Cases
Hospital Mortality 1%

Ⓓ

Posthospitalization Mortality
6 Mo.   6–8%
5 Yr.   5–8%/Yr.

Complicated
Hospital Course
50–65% of Cases

Ⓔ

Arrhythmias
60% of Cases

Ⓕ

Power Failure

Ⓖ

Myocardial
Rupture 2–3%

HOSPITAL MORTALITY WITH MEDICAL TREATMENT (%)

14–78

Mild	33%	24
Pulmonary Edema	12%	40
Cardiogenic Shock	10%	86–100

Free Wall	2%	100
Septum	½–1%	87
Papillary Muscle	1%	90

[a]CABG = Coronary artery bypass graft

199

TYPE	INCIDENCE (%)	MORTALITY (%)
Premature atrial contractions	13–52	Not increased
Paroxysmal atrial tachycardia of more than 1 minute's duration	5–18	30–50
Atrial flutter	2–10	Unknown
Atrial fibrillation	7–20	14–47
Potentially dangerous premature ventricular beats		
R on T > 6/min.	7–9	38
Bigeminy: salvos of 2 or more	32–42	23
Ventricular tachycardia (>6 consecutive PVCs, rate > 120/min.)	10	40–50
Accelerated idioventricular rhythm (rate 60–90 beats/min.)	8–36	Usually benign
Ventricular fibrillation	10	
Primary		20
Secondary to pump failure		78
Ventricular standstill	1–4	90–100

24 hours and 90 per cent in two weeks, necessitating emergency surgery in most cases. Mortality with IABP support and early surgery for cases in cardiogenic shock is reduced from 100 to 60 per cent. For those patients with papillary muscle rupture who do not manifest shock and who undergo delayed elective surgery, the mortality is 11 to 17 per cent.[1, 38]

H. Ten to 20 per cent of patients admitted to the hospital with an acute myocardial infarction will manifest cardiogenic shock. The mortality with standard medical treatment is 86 to 100 per cent.[29, 33, 44-46] Approximately 75 per cent of patients in cardiogenic shock will respond to IABP.[18, 38] Failure to respond indicates the death of 50 per cent or more of the left ventricle.[18, 38] Of those who respond to IABP, 20 per cent will become balloon-independent in 24 to 48 hours and should be considered for interval revascularization.[38] Of those who respond to IABP but remain balloon-dependent and are operated on, 40 to 55 per cent survive.[38, 47]

CLASSIFICATION	% OF TOTAL MI PATIENTS	CLINICAL FEATURES	HOSPITAL MORTALITY (%)
Class I	45	Transient ↑ PAWP in 25%	5
Class II	33	Persistent ↑ PAWP over 2 × normal	24
		Third heart sound	
		Pulmonary rales, ↑ HR, ↑ BP	
Class III	12	Pulmonary edema	40
		PAWP over 3 × normal	
		↑ HR, BP normal	
Class IV	10	↓ BP, severe ↓ CO, moderate ↑ PAWP	86–100

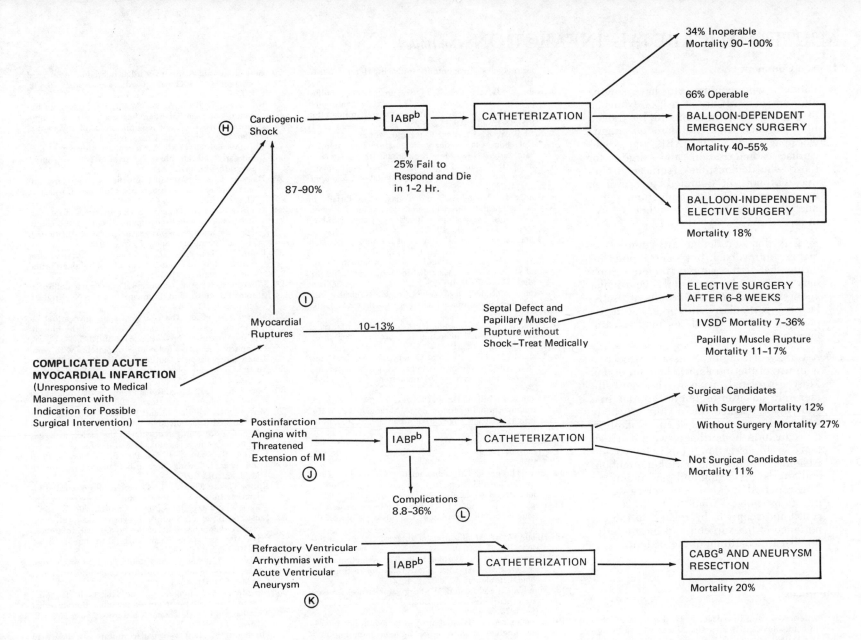

34% Inoperable
Mortality 90–100%

66% Operable

BALLOON-DEPENDENT
EMERGENCY SURGERY

Mortality 40–55%

BALLOON-INDEPENDENT
ELECTIVE SURGERY

Mortality 18%

(H) Cardiogenic
Shock

IABP[b]

CATHETERIZATION

25% Fail to
Respond and Die
in 1–2 Hr.

87–90%

(I)

Myocardial
Ruptures

10–13%

Septal Defect and
Papillary Muscle
Rupture without
Shock—Treat Medically

ELECTIVE SURGERY
AFTER 6–8 WEEKS

IVSD[c] Mortality 7–36%

Papillary Muscle Rupture
Mortality 11–17%

**COMPLICATED ACUTE
MYOCARDIAL INFARCTION**
(Unresponsive to Medical
Management with
Indication for Possible
Surgical Intervention)

Postinfarction
Angina with
Threatened
Extension of MI

(J)

IABP[b]

CATHETERIZATION

Surgical Candidates

With Surgery Mortality 12%

Without Surgery Mortality 27%

Not Surgical Candidates
Mortality 11%

Complications
8.8–36%   (L)

Refractory Ventricular
Arrhythmias with
Acute Ventricular
Aneurysm

(K)

IABP[b]

CATHETERIZATION

CABG[a] AND ANEURYSM
RESECTION

Mortality 20%

[b]IABP = Intra-aortic balloon pump
[c]IVSD = Interventricular septal defect

201

I. See Comment G.

J. Patients who continue to have angina after an acute MI are at risk of extension of the infarction and should be treated like patients with preinfarction angina (see page 196), with IABP, immediate cardiac catheterization, and surgery for those who demonstrate significant ischemic, but not yet infarcted, myocardium by myocardial lactate production, radionuclide imaging, or other technique.[9, 19, 24]

K. Surgery for ventricular arrhythmias remains controversial, but some reports indicate that if the surgery includes coronary artery bypass and ventricular aneurysm resection, the results are satisfactory, particularly if surgery can be postponed for a month or more postinfarction.[48]

L. A variety of complications are associated with use of the intra-aortic balloon pump. Most are related to passing a large catheter into an arteriosclerotic arterial tree and the presence of a foreign body within the vascular system. Complications include hemorrhage, wound hematoma, groin dissection, limb ischemia, gut ischemia, cerebral and peripheral emboli, and arterial dissection and perforation.[49-55] The reported incidence of serious complications ranges from 8.8[55] to 36 per cent[54] and seems to be related to the experience of the surgeon and the underlying disease condition of the patient.

References

1. Chatterjee, K., and Brundage, B. H.: Prognostic factors in acute myocardial infarction. Practical Cardiology, p. 23, 1978.
2. Armstrong, A., et al.: Natural history of acute coronary heart attacks: A community study. Br. Heart J., 34:67, 1972.
3. Anturane Reinfarction Trial Research Group: Sulfinpyrazone in the prevention of cardiac death after myocardial infarction: The Anturane reinfarction trial. N. Engl. J. Med., 298:289, 1978.
4. Kannel, W. B., Dawber, T. R., and McNamara, P. M.: Detection of the coronary prone adult: The Framingham study. J. Iowa Med. Soc., 56:26, 1966.
5. Prineas, R. J., and Blackburn, H.: Sudden coronary death outside the hospital. Circulation, 52(suppl. 3):1, 1975.
6. Gordis, L., Naggan, L., and Tonascia, J.: Pitfalls in evaluating the impact of coronary care units on mortality from myocardial infarctions. Johns Hopkins Med. J., 141:287–95, 1977.
7. O'Rourke, M. F., et al.: Impact of the new generation coronary care unit. Br. Med. J. 2:837–39, 1976.
8. Christensen, D., et al.: Sudden death in the late hospital phase of acute myocardial infarction. Arch. Intern. Med., 137:1675–9, 1977.
9. Wiener, L.: Selection of patients treated surgically with evolving myocardial infarction. Cardiovasc. Clin., 8:223, 1977.
10. Hunt, D., et al.: Changing patterns and mortality of acute myocardial infarction in a coronary care unit. Br. Med. J., 1:795, 1977.
11. Cannom, D., Levy, W., and Cohen, L.: The short- and long-term prognosis of patients with transmural and nontransmural myocardial infarction. Am. J. Med., 61:452, 1976.
12. Fulton, M., Julian, D., and Oliver, M.: Sudden death and myocardial infarction. AHA Monograph #27, Research in acute myocardial infarction. Circulation, 40:(suppl. 4):182, 1969.
13. Kuller, L.: Epidemiology of cardiovascular diseases: Current perspectives. Am. J. Epidemiol., 104:425, 1976.
14. Cox, J. L., et al.: The ischemic zone surrounding acute myocardial infarction: Its morphology as detected by dehydrogenase staining. Am. Heart J., 76:650, 1968.
15. Engler, R., and Ross, J.: Is there a role for surgery in acute myocardial infarction? Cardiovasc. Clin. 8:213, 1977.
16. Hood, W. B.: Modification of infarction size. Cardiovasc. Clin., 7:259, 1975.
17. Braunwald, E., and Maroko, P. L.: The reduction of infarction size — An idea whose time (for testing) has come. Circulation, 50:206, 1974.
18. Mundth, E., and Austen, W.: Surgical measures for coronary heart disease. N. Engl. J. Med., 293:13, 75, 124; 1975.
19. Bardet, J., et al.: Treatment of post–myocardial infarction angina by intra-aortic balloon pumping and emergency revascularization. J. Thorac. Cardiovasc. Surg., 74:299, 1977.
20. Berg, R., et al.: Acute myocardial infarction: A surgical emergency. J. Thorac. Cardiovasc. Surg., 70:432, 1975.
21. Brockman, S., Brest, A., and Majid, N.: Surgery for impending myocardial infarction, acute evolving myocardial infarction, and complications of myocardial infarction. Cardiovasc. Clin., 7:291, 1975.
22. Cheanvechai, C., et al.: Aortocoronary artery graft during early and late phases of acute MI. Ann. Thorac. Surg., 16:249, 1973.
23. Dawson, J., et al.: Mortality in patients undergoing coronary artery bypass surgery after MI. Am. J. Cardiol., 33:483, 1974.
24. Wiener, L., et al.: Therapeutic implications of myocardial lactate metabolism in patients considered candidates for emergency myocardial revascularization. J. Thorac. Cardiovasc. Surg., 75:612, 1978.
25. Baum, R., Alvarez, H., III, and Cobb, L.: Survival after resuscitation from out-of-hospital ventricular fibrillation. Circulation, 50:1231, 1974.
26. Liberthson, R., et al.: Prehospital ventricular defibrillation: Prognosis and followup course. N. Engl. J. Med., 291:317, 1974.
27. McNeer, F., et al.: The course of acute myocardial infarction: Feasibility of early discharge of the uncomplicated patient. Circulation, 51:410, 1975.
28. Humphries, J.: Expected course of patients with coronary artery disease. Cardiovasc. Clin., 8:41, 1977.
29. Yu, P.: The acute phase of myocardial infarction. Cardiovasc. Clin., 7:45, 1975.
30. Norris, R., et al.: Prognosis after myocardial infarction: Six-year followup. Br. Heart J., 36:786, 1974.
31. Moss, A., DeCamilla, J., and Davis, H.: Cardiac death in the first 6 months after myocardial infarction: Potential for mortality reduction in the early posthospital period. Am. J. Cardiol., 39:816, 1977.
32. Schulze, R., Strauss, H., and Pitt, B.: Sudden death in the year following myocardial infarction. Am. J. Med., 62:192, 1977.
33. Killip, T., and Kimball, J.: Treatment of myocardial infarction in a coronary care unit: A two-year experience with 250 patients. Am. J. Cardiol., 20:457, 1967.
34. Lofstrom, B., et al.: Studies of myocardial rupture with cardiac tamponade in acute myocardial infarction. III. Attempts at emergency surgical treatment. Chest, 61:10, 1972.
35. Cobbs, B., Hatcher, C., and Robinson, P.: Cardiac rupture: Three operations with two long-term survivors. JAMA, 223:532, 1973.
36. Fitzgibbon, G., Hooper, G., and Heggtveit, H.: Successful surgical treatment of postinfarction external cardiac rupture. J. Thorac. Cardiovasc. Surg., 63:622, 1972.
37. Montegut, F.: Left ventricular rupture secondary to myocardial infarction. Report of survival with surgical repair. Ann. Thorac. Surg., 14:75, 1972.

38. Mundth, E.: Surgical treatment of cardiogenic shock and of acute mechanical complications following myocardial infarction. Cardiovasc. Clin., 8:241, 1977.

39. Sanders, R., Kern, W., and Blount, S.: Perforation of the interventricular septum complicating myocardial infarction. Am. Heart J., *51*, 736, 1956.

40. Daggett, W., et al.: Surgery for post–myocardial infarction ventricular septal defect. Ann. Surg., *186*:260, 1977.

41. Hill, J., et al.: Acquired ventricular septal defects. J. Thorac. Cardiovasc. Surg., 70:440, 1975.

42. Kitamura, S., Mendoz, A., and Kay, J.: Ventricular septal defect following myocardial infarction: Repair through a left ventriculotomy and review of literature. J. Thorac. Cardiovasc. Surg., *61*:186, 1971.

43. Mundth, E., et al.: Surgery for complications of acute myocardial infarction. Circulation, *45*:1279, 1972.

44. Cohen, L.: Early and late prognosis of myocardial infarction. Cardiovasc. Clin., 7:57, 1975.

45. Rackley, C., et al.: Cardiogenic shock: Recognition and management. Cardiovasc. Clin., 7:251, 1975.

46. Scheidt, S., Ascheim, R., and Killip, T.: Shock after myocardial infarction: A clinical and hemodynamic profile. Am. J. Cardiol., *26*:556, 1970.

47. Resnekov, L.: Circulatory support and early cardiac surgery in the management of cardiogenic shock complicating acute MI. Ann. Clin. Res., 9:134, 1977.

48. Ricks, W., et al.: Surgical management of life-threatening ventricular arrhythmias in patients with coronary artery disease. Circulation, 56:38, 1977.

49. Austen, W., et al.: Intra-aortic balloon counterpulsation: Current applications. Cardiovasc. Clin., 7:285, 1975.

50. Curtis, J., et al.: Intra-aortic balloon assist: Initial Mayo Clinic experience and current concepts. Mayo Clin. Proc., 52:723, 1977.

51. Bolooki, H.: Complications of Intra-Aortic Balloon Pump and Their Treatment. Clinical Application of Intra-Aortic Balloon Pump. Mount Kisco, N. Y., Futura Publishing Co., 1977.

52. Pace, P., et al.: Peripheral arterial complications of balloon counterpulsation. Surgery, 82:685, 1977.

53. Beckman, C., et al.: Results and complications of intra-aortic balloon counterpulsation. Ann. Thorac. Surg., 24:550, 1977.

54. Alpert, S., et al.: Vascular complications of intra-aortic balloon pumping. Arch. Surg., *111*:1190, 1976.

55. McEnany, M. T., et al.: Clinical experience with intra-aortic balloon pump support in 728 patients. Circulation, *58* (supp. 1), 1978.

CARDIAC CATHETERIZATION BY P. S. WOLF, M.D., D. SHANDER, M.D., AND R. S. BAUM, M.D.

Comments

A. Hospitalization is for 24 to 48 hours. Time of procedure is 0.3 to 2 hours. Sedation consists of diazepam, meperidine, diphenhydramine hydrochloride, and secobarbital (singly or in combination). Heparin, 3000 to 5000 units, is advisable for both the brachial and femoral approaches.

B. Mortality risk is increased 5- to 10-fold with left main coronary artery stenosis greater than or equal to 50 per cent.[7] Recent studies suggest that the mortality rates from the brachial and femoral approaches are about equal.[1, 4, 7]

C. The brachial approach is preferable in patients with severe atherosclerosis in the lower extremities or aorta. Its detriments are the smaller caliber of vessel and the increased frequency of arterial injury requiring arterial repair.[3]

D. The femoral approach usually requires less time (20 to 60 minutes). No incision is necessary, and there is less discomfort.[9]

E. Of 19,295 retrograde brachial catheterizations performed at the Cleveland Clinic Foundation, 0.33 per cent of the patients required surgical correction. Thrombectomy and primary repair were required in most instances, and early exploration of the artery was recommended if signs of ischemia were present.[2]

F. Complications encountered less frequently are shown in the following table.[1, 3, 4, 6, 9]

COMPLICATION	BRACHIAL	FEMORAL
Subintimal dissection of aorta	0.9%	0.1%
Dissection of coronary artery	0.07%	0.06%
Hemorrhage at entry site	0.07%	0.16%

The following complications are seen very infrequently. Although specific figures for incidence are not available, the estimated frequency is less than 0.1 per cent.

Median or femoral nerve injury
Catheter entrapment
Infective endocarditis
Amputation of limb
Air emboli
Renal failure
Cardiac or vascular perforation
Anaphylaxis from contrast agent

G. Temporary heart block (most common with right heart catheterization in left bundle branch block) is a complication of this procedure.

H. Hemothorax may occur when the subclavian artery is punctured. This complication, although rare, may be rapidly fatal. Thoracotomy may be required if the hemothorax accumulates rapidly.[11] Pneumothorax may occur from puncture of the pleura.

References

1. Adams, D. F., Fraser, D. B., and Abrams, H. L.: The complications of coronary arteriography. Circulation, 48:609–618, 1973.
2. Beven, E. G.: Surgical treatment of angiographic complications. In Meaney, T. F., Lalli, A. F., and Alfidi, R. J., Complications and Legal Implications of Radiologic Special Procedures. St. Louis, C. V. Mosby Co., 1973, p. 69.
3. Bolasny, B. L., and Killen, D. A.: Surgical management of arterial injuries secondary to angiography. Ann. Surg., 174:962–964, 1971.
4. Bourassa, M. G., and Noble, J.: Complication rate of coronary arteriography. A review of 5250 cases studied by a percutaneous femoral technique. Circulation, 53:106–114, 1976.
5. Braunwald, E., and Swan, H. J. C., (eds.): Cooperative Study on Cardiac Catheterization. American Heart Association Monograph No. 20. New York, American Heart Association, 1968.
6. Chahine, R. A., Herman, M. V., and Gorlin, R.: Complications of coronary angiography: A comparison of the brachial to the femoral approach. Ann. Intern. Med., 76:882, 1972.
7. Davis, K., et al.: Complications of coronary arteriography from the collaborative study of coronary artery surgery (CASS). Circulation, 59:1105, 1979.
8. Gensini, G. G.: Coronary Arteriography. Mount Kisco, N.Y., Futura Publishing Co., 1975, pp. 157–163.
9. Page, H. L., Jr., and Campbell, W. B.: Percutaneous transfemoral coronary arteriography: Prevention of morbid complications. Chest, 67:221–225, 1975.
10. Ryan, J. A., Jr., et al.: Catheter complications in total parenteral nutrition. A prospective study of 200 consecutive patients. N. Engl. J. Med., 290:757–760, 1974.
11. Wennevold, A., Christiansen, I., and Lindeneg, O.: Complications in 4413 catheterizations of the right side of the heart. Am. Heart J., 68:173–180, 1965.

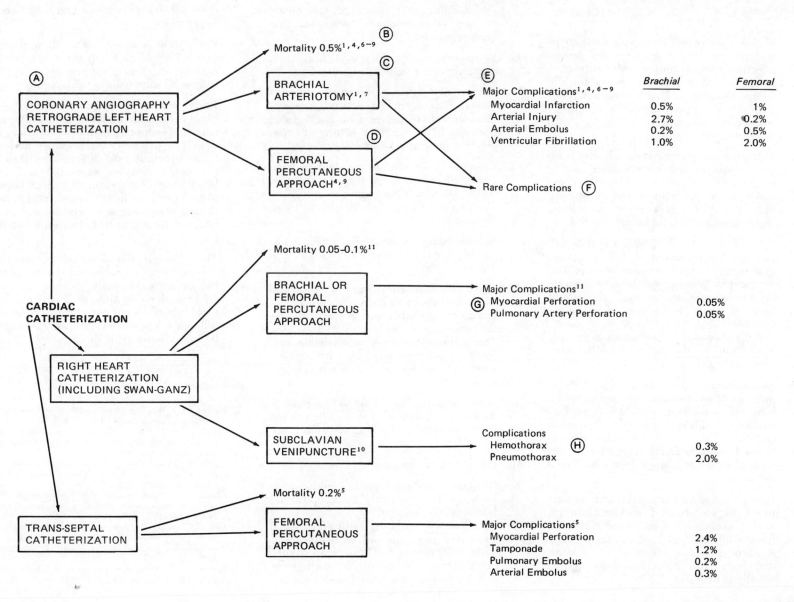

Ⓐ CORONARY ANGIOGRAPHY RETROGRADE LEFT HEART CATHETERIZATION

Ⓑ Mortality 0.5%[1,4,6-9]

Ⓒ BRACHIAL ARTERIOTOMY[1,7]

Ⓓ FEMORAL PERCUTANEOUS APPROACH[4,9]

Ⓔ Major Complications[1,4,6-9]

	Brachial	Femoral
Myocardial Infarction	0.5%	1%
Arterial Injury	2.7%	0.2%
Arterial Embolus	0.2%	0.5%
Ventricular Fibrillation	1.0%	2.0%

Ⓕ Rare Complications

CARDIAC CATHETERIZATION

RIGHT HEART CATHETERIZATION (INCLUDING SWAN-GANZ)

Mortality 0.05-0.1%[11]

BRACHIAL OR FEMORAL PERCUTANEOUS APPROACH

Major Complications[11]

Ⓖ
Myocardial Perforation	0.05%
Pulmonary Artery Perforation	0.05%

SUBCLAVIAN VENIPUNCTURE[10]

Complications
Ⓗ
Hemothorax	0.3%
Pneumothorax	2.0%

TRANS-SEPTAL CATHETERIZATION

Mortality 0.2%[5]

FEMORAL PERCUTANEOUS APPROACH

Major Complications[5]

Myocardial Perforation	2.4%
Tamponade	1.2%
Pulmonary Embolus	0.2%
Arterial Embolus	0.3%

CARDIAC PACEMAKERS BY BARRY L. MOLK, M.D.

Comments

A. This is a temporary technique until an alternative method is available and proved effective. Obesity and chronic obstructive airway disease increase probability of failure to capture. Heavy sedation is required if use is prolonged. Use of a transcutaneous pacemaker interferes with electronic monitoring.[1, 24]

B. Transthoracic pacemakers are used for brief emergencies when other access routes are unavailable. Electrodes are easily dislodged with closed chest massage. Pneumothorax, coronary laceration, and tamponade should be anticipated.[25]

C. Epicardial pacemakers offer a specific advantage for management following cardiac surgery where they can be employed for several weeks. Advantages include (1) atrioventricular pacing, (2) patient mobility, and (3) absence of thrombophlebitis.
    A disadvantage is the hazard of causing fibrillation of the heart via electronic monitoring devices.[1, 22, 23]

D. Disadvantages of access include[1, 3, 10] dislodgment from the arm and thrombophlebitis. When the femoral vein is used, pulmonary embolus is a possible complication; when the subclavian vein is used, pneumothorax occurs in 0.7 per cent of cases and arterial puncture in 3 per cent.

E. Infection may be from metastatic implantation to an abraded endocardium or, more commonly, from local infection from a foreign body (generator or lead). Antibiotics and replacement of endocardial lead with epicardial lead system usually is necessary.[4, 8, 11, 12]

F. Perforation usually is benign; tamponade is rare. Pericardotomy syndrome has been reported.

G. Ventricular tachycardia and fibrillation primarily occur only during insertion.[3, 16]

H. Failure of temporary transvenous pacemakers may occur for several reasons:[3] dislodgment (18 per cent of cases), loose connection or incorrect setting (21 per cent), or generator failure (4 per cent).

I. Currently used lithium pacemakers have projected battery lives of up to 15 years, while atomic (plutonium-powered) devices have a theoretical lifespan of up to 35 years.

J. Ectopic beat after each paced beat is frequently seen but usually subsides in 2 to 3 days.[16]

K. Endocardial abrasions and long wound exposure time with transvenous lead implantation probably are responsible for the increased incidence of infection. Thus, administration of prophylactic antibiotics is recommended for wire replacement but not for generator replacement alone.[11, 12]

L. Serous effusions are effectively aspirated. Repeated aspiration of pouch hematoma leads to infection. Early evacuation is advised.[13, 21]

M. Local revision frequently is successful.[13]

N. Hospital morbidity with endocardial leads is 19 per cent; with epicardial leads it is 35 per cent.
    Pulmonary morbidity with endocardial leads is 2 per cent and with epicardial leads is 20 per cent. There is no significant difference between the transthoracic (left anterior thoracotomy) and transmediastinal (left parasternal and subxiphoid) approaches.

O. Perforation generally occurs during insertion with stiff stylet in place. Failure to capture is the most common consequence. Tamponade is infrequent.

P. Early and late system failure rate is higher in transvenous systems (38 per cent in 24 months) than in epicardial systems (14 per cent in the same period). Causes include lead dislocation (10 to 20 per cent), elevated threshold and exit block (5 to 13 per cent), generator failure (0 to 5 per cent in two years), perforation during placement of electrode, and insulation defects and technical errors at implantation.[19, 27]

Q. There is no significant difference between the operative mortality rates of the two systems. Mortality probably is related to underlying disease. Five-year survival rate of 65 per cent levels off for the following 5 years — significant early attrition from underlying disease.[6, 7, 21]

References

1. Escher, D. J. W.: Types of pacemakers and their complications. Circulation, 47:119, 1973.
2. Grogler, F. M., et al.: Complications of permanent transvenous cardiac pacing. J. Thorac. Cardiovasc. Surg., 69:895–904, 1975.
3. Lumia, F. J., and Rios, J. C.: Temporary transvenous pacemaker therapy: An analysis of complications. Chest, 64:604–608, 1975.
4. Corman, L. C., and Levison, M. E.: Sustained bacteremia and transvenous cardiac pacemakers. JAMA, 233:264, 1975.
5. Kaye, D., Frankl, W., and Arditi, L. I.: Probable postcardiotomy syndrome following implantation of transvenous pacemaker. Am. Heart J., 90:627–63, 1975.
6. Parsonnet, V.: Permanent pacing of the heart 1952–1976. Am. J. Cardiol., 39:250–6, 1977.

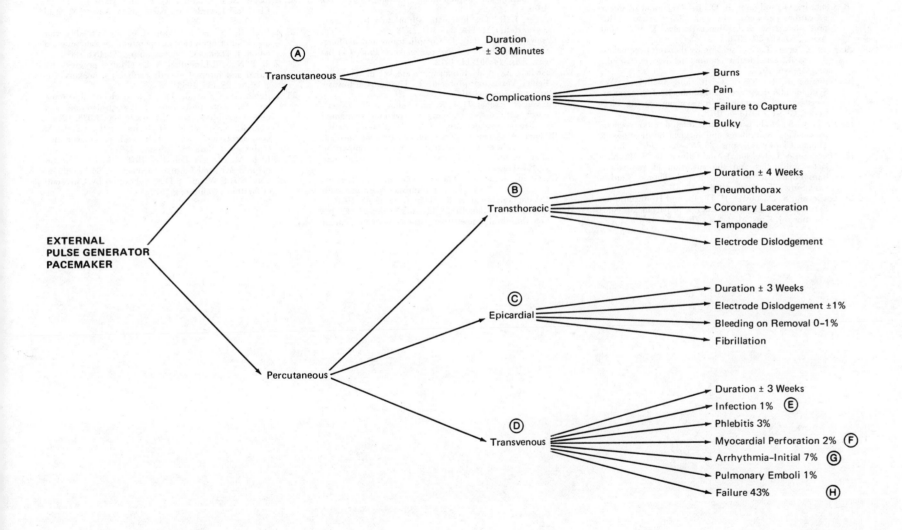

EXTERNAL
PULSE GENERATOR
PACEMAKER

(A) Transcutaneous
- Duration ± 30 Minutes
- Complications
  - Burns
  - Pain
  - Failure to Capture
  - Bulky

Percutaneous

(B) Transthoracic
- Duration ± 4 Weeks
- Pneumothorax
- Coronary Laceration
- Tamponade
- Electrode Dislodgement

(C) Epicardial
- Duration ± 3 Weeks
- Electrode Dislodgement ±1%
- Bleeding on Removal 0-1%
- Fibrillation

(D) Transvenous
- Duration ± 3 Weeks
- Infection 1% (E)
- Phlebitis 3%
- Myocardial Perforation 2% (F)
- Arrhythmia-Initial 7% (G)
- Pulmonary Emboli 1%
- Failure 43% (H)

7. Rubin, J. W., et al.: Permanent cardiac pacemakers: Twelve-year experience with 287 patients. Ann. Thorac. Surg., 22:74–9, 1976.

8. Contariri, O., and Goff, R. O., Jr.: Treatment of infected cardiac pacemaker site with closed irrigation. Report of a case and subject review. J. Fla. Med. Assoc., 63:349–50, 1976.

9. Vera, Z., et al.: Lack of sensing by demand pacemakers due to intraventricular conduction defects. Circulation, 51:815, 1975.

10. Williams, E. H., Tyers, G. R., and Shaffer, C. W.: Symptomatic deep venous thrombosis of the arm associated with permanent transvenous pacing electrodes. Chest, 73:613–5, 1978.

11. Bryan, C. S., et al.: Endocarditis related to transvenous pacemakers. Syndromes and surgical implications. J. Thorac. Cardiovasc. Surg., 75:758–62, 1978.

12. Hartstein, A. I., Jackson, J., and Gilbert, D. N.: Prophylactic antibiotics and the insertion of permanent transvenous cardiac pacemakers. J. Thorac. Cardiovasc. Surg., 75:219–23, 1978.

13. Dickerson, S. D., Lewis, H. D., Jr., and Heilbrunn, A.: Permanent pacemaker: Incidence of pacemaker complications. J. Kans. Med. Soc., 79:49–54, 1978.

14. Chamorro, H., and Rad, G., and Wholey, M. H.: Superior vena cava syndrome: A complication of transvenous pacemaker implantation. Radiology, 126:108, 1978.

15. Hedges, J. R.: Diaphragmatic stimulation by a pacemaker (letter). JAMA, 239:108, 1978.

16. Kosowsky, B. D., Barr, I.: Complications and malfunctions of electrical cardiac pacemakers. Prog. Cardiovasc. Dis., 14:501–14, 1972.

17. Nasrallah, A., et al.: Runaway pacemaker in seven patients: Persisting problem. J. Thorac. Cardiovasc. Surg., 69:365–368, 1975.

18. Furman, S., Escher, D. J. W., and Solomon, N.: Experiences with myocardial and transvenous implanted cardiac pacemakers. Am. J. Cardiol., 23:66–72, 1969.

19. Brenner, A. S., et al.: Transvenous, transmediastinal, and transthoracic ventricular pacing: A comparison after complete two-year followup. Circulation, 49:407–414, 1974.

20. Goldstein, S., et al.: Transthoracic and transvenous pacemakers. A comparative clinical experience with 131 implantable units. Br. Heart J., 32:35–45, 1970.

21. Conklin, E. F., Gianelli, S., Jr., and Nealon, T. F., Jr.: Four hundred consecutive patients with permanent transvenous pacemakers. J. Thorac. Cardiovasc. Surg., 69:1–7, 1975.

22. Whalen, R. E., Starmer, C. F., and McIntosh, H. D.: Electrical hazards with pacemakers. Ann. N.Y. Acad. Sci., 3:922–31, 1964.

23. Litwak, R. S., et al.: Support of myocardial performance after open cardiac operations by rate augmentation. J. Thorac. Cardiovasc. Surg., 56:484, 1968.

24. Zoll, P. N., and Linenthal, A. L.: Clinical progress. External and internal electric cardiac pacemakers. Circulation, 28:455, 1963.

25. Lillehei, W. C., et al.: Direct wire electrical stimulation for acute postsurgical and postinfarction complete heart block. Ann. N.Y. Acad. Sci., 3:938, 1964.

26. Crook, B. R. M., et al.: Occlusion of the subclavian vein associated with cephalic vein pacemaker electrodes. Br. J. Surg., 64:329–331, 1977.

27. Bilitch, M. (Project Director, 1976): Registry for Implanted Artificial Cardiac Pacemakers. 24-Month Report to H.E.W. and F.D.A. Submitted by University of Southern California, 1976.

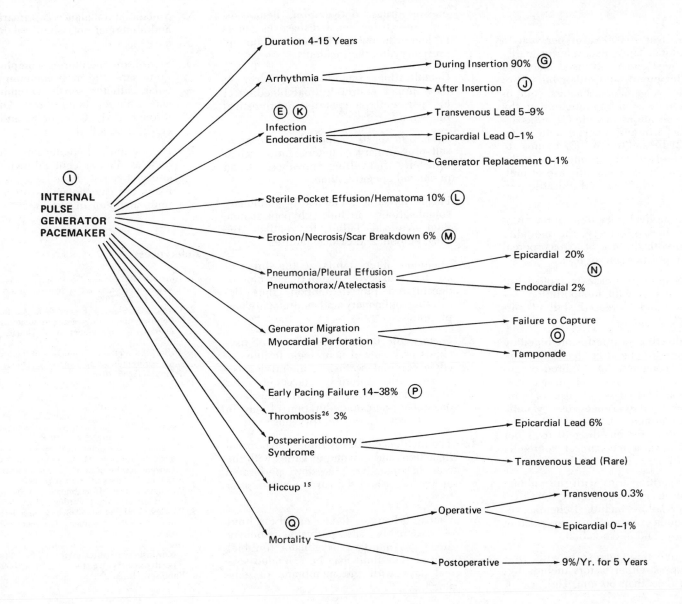

CARDIOPULMONARY BYPASS BY E. LANCE WALKER, M.D., AND BEN EISEMAN, M.D.

Comments

A. There are over 70,000 cases per year in the U.S. alone. These data refer primarily to the 2 most commonly used machines using roller pumps and either bubble or membrane oxygenators. Factors complicating their use and production of the listed complications include (1) anticoagulation (heparin and reversal with protamine), (2) hemodilution, (3) trauma to blood and platelet by pump, (4) inadequacy of organ perfusion, (5) use of multiple drugs, and (6) lack of pulsatile perfusion.

B. Based on survival data from aortocoronary artery bypass surgery, the mortality associated with the use of extracorporeal circulation is 1 per cent or less.[1]

C. Zero to 8 units per case is typical but tends to be less with hemodilution, sequestration, and increased skill of surgery.[5, 39, 40]

D. Factors affecting postperfusion bleeding in addition to operative technique include[41] (1) congenital or acquired coagulation defects, (2) type of oxygenator, (3) duration of bypass, (4) use of anticoagulation, (5) presence of cyanotic heart disease, and (6) type of operation. At reoperation for bleeding (0 to 3 per cent of cases), a mechanical source is found in 75 per cent.[4]

E. Risk of hepatitis varies with the volume of blood used. Factors affecting liver dysfunction or failure include ischemia, venous cannula obstruction, pre-existing liver disease, and microemboli.

F. Renal dysfunction increases with prolonged bypass. Other factors include hypotension (less than 80 mm. Hg), use of pressor drugs, dehydration, hemolysis, and pre-existing renal disease (accounts for higher mortality). Diuretics do not appreciably alter the incidence.

G. Complications include stress ulcer or other upper gastrointestinal bleeding (1 to 3 per cent), pancreatitis, and intestinal infarction.[17, 18]

H. Sources of sepsis include the machine itself plus urinary catheters, intravascular catheters, indwelling prostheses, and prolonged operative time.

I. Factors affecting incidence of pulmonary complications include hypoperfusion, fluid overload, failure to ventilate the lung, emboli, and cardiac failure.

J. Micropore filters minimize the threat of air, fat, leukocyte, platelet, and clot or denatured protein emboli, thus decreasing pulmonary and neurologic complications.

K. Factors affecting the incidence of psychosis or localized neurologic lesions include cerebral perfusion, underlying cerebral atherosclerosis (accounts for higher mortality rate), emboli, underlying emotional state, and duration of stay in the Intensive Care Unit (psychosis).

L. The incidence of arrhythmias, myocardial infarction, and low output varies with the type of operative procedure performed on the heart and the cardiac status prior to surgery.

M. Four to 6 hours is the accepted top limit of reasonably safe perfusion when a direct gas interface oxygenator (bubble) is used. The limit may be extended several days with the membrane oxygenator.[36]

N. Metabolic imbalance is primarily acidosis and abnormal potassium, calcium, or glucose values.

O. Significant monitoring complications are quite rare, the most common being vascular catheter sepsis, thrombophlebitis, and catheter embolism.[42] Air embolus through LAP, CVP, or Swan-Ganz catheter can be lethal.

P. Postpumping hypertension may be as high as 48 per cent following coronary artery bypass. Pathologic factors most likely are catecholamine release and the renin-angiotensin system.[37, 38]

References

1. Hurst, J. W., et al.: Controversies in cardiology. I. Value of coronary artery bypass surgery. Am. J. Cardiol., 42:308, 1978.
2. Carey, J. S., Skow, J. R., and Scott, C.: Retrograde aortic dissection during cardiopulmonary bypass: "Nonoperative" management. Ann. Thorac. Surg., 24:44, 1977.
3. Taylor, P. C., et al.: Cannulation of the ascending aorta for cardiopulmonary bypass. J. Thorac. Cardiovasc. Surg., 71:255, 1976.
4. Gomes, M. M. R., and McGoon, D. C.: Bleeding patterns after open heart surgery. J. Thorac. Cardiovasc. Surg., 60:87, 1970.
5. Yeh, T., Jr., Shelton, L., and Yeh, T.: Blood loss and bank blood requirement in coronary bypass surgery. Ann. Thorac. Surg., 26:11, 1978.
6. Freeman, R.: Microbiological aspects of open-heart surgery. In Ionescu, M. I., and Wooler, G. H. (eds.): Current Techniques in Extracorporeal Circulation. London, Butterworths, 1976, p. 333.
7. Wisch, N., et al.: Hematologic complications of open heart surgery. Am. J. Cardiol., 31:282, 1973.
8. Proskey, V. J., et al.: Anicteric and icteric hepatitis after open heart surgery. Gastroenterology, 58:203, 1970.
9. Grady, G. F., and Bennett, A. J.: Risk of posttransfusion hepatitis in the United States. A prospective cooperative study. JAMA, 220:692, 1972.
10. Rubinson, R. M., et al.: Serum hepatitis after open

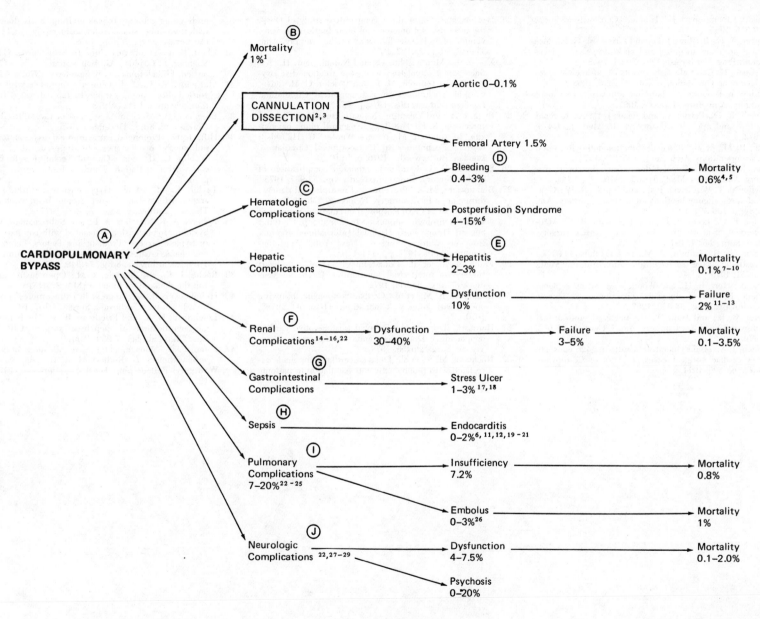

(B) Mortality
1%[1]

CANNULATION
DISSECTION[2,3]

Aortic 0–0.1%

Femoral Artery 1.5%

(C) Hematologic
Complications

Bleeding (D)
0.4–3%

Mortality
0.6%[4,5]

Postperfusion Syndrome
4–15%[6]

Hepatic
Complications

Hepatitis (E)
2–3%

Mortality
0.1%[7–10]

Dysfunction
10%

Failure
2%[11–13]

Renal (F)
Complications[14–16,22]

Dysfunction
30–40%

Failure
3–5%

Mortality
0.1–3.5%

(G) Gastrointestinal
Complications

Stress Ulcer
1–3%[17,18]

(H) Sepsis

Endocarditis
0–2%[6,11,12,19–21]

Pulmonary (I)
Complications
7–20%[22–25]

Insufficiency
7.2%

Mortality
0.8%

Embolus
0–3%[26]

Mortality
1%

Neurologic (J)
Complications[22,27–29]

Dysfunction
4–7.5%

Mortality
0.1–2.0%

Psychosis
0–20%

heart operations. J. Thorac. Cardiovasc. Surg., 50:575, 1965.

11. Kloster, F. E., Bristow, J. D., and Griswold, H. E.: Medical problems in mitral and multiple valve replacement. Prog. Cardiovasc. Dis., 7:504, 1965.

12. Duvoisin, G. E., et al.: Late results of cardiac valve replacement. Circulation, 37(suppl. 2):75, 1968.

13. Sanderson, R. G., et al.: Jaundice following open heart surgery. Ann. Surg., 165:217, 1967.

14. Yeboah, E. D., Petrie, A., and Pead, J. L.: Acute renal failure and open heart surgery. Br. Med. J., 1:415, 1972.

15. Abel, R. M., et al.: Renal dysfunction following open heart operations. Arch. Surg., 108:175, 1974.

16. Bhat, J. G., et al.: Renal failure after open heart surgery. Ann. Intern. Med., 84:677, 1976.

17. Lawhorne, T. W., Davis, J. L., and Smith, G. W.: General surgical complications after cardiac surgery. Am. J. Surg., 136:254, 1978.

18. Taylor, P. C., Loop, F. D., and Hermann, R. E.: Management of acute stress ulcer after cardiac surgery. Ann. Surg., 178:1, 1973.

19. Wilson, W. R., Jaumin, P. M., and Danielson, G. K.: Prosthetic valve endocarditis. Ann. Intern. Med., 82:751, 1975.

20. Starr, A., Herr, R. H., and Wood, J. A.: Mitral replacement. Review of six years' experience. J. Thorac. Cardiovasc. Surg., 54:333, 1967.

21. Shafer, R. B., and Hall, W. H.: Bacterial endocarditis following open heart surgery. Am. J. Cardiol., 25:603, 1970.

22. Crouch, J. A., et al.: Operative results in 1426 consecutive cardiac surgical cases. J. Thorac. Cardiovasc. Surg., 68:606, 1974.

23. Iverson, L. I. G., et al.: A comparative study of IPPB, the incentive spirometer, and blow bottles: The prevention of atelectasis following cardiac surgery. Ann. Thorac. Surg., 25:197, 1978.

24. Kay, E. B., Mendelsohn, D., and Naraghipour, H.: Extracorporeal circulation using the rotating disc oxygenator. *In* Ionescu, M. I., and Wooler, G. H. (eds.): Current Techniques in Extracorporeal Circulation. London, Butterworths, 1976, p. 45.

25. Rygg, I. H., and Valantine, N., with Henriksen, B., and Jorgensen, S. P.: The Rygg-Kyvsgaard pump oxygenator. *In* Ionescu, M. I., and Wooler, G. H. (eds.): Current Techniques in Extracorporeal Circulation. London, Butterworths, 1976, p. 139.

26. Barnhorst, D. A.: Extracardiac thoracic complications of cardiac surgery. Surg. Clin. North Am., 53:937, 1973.

27. Branthwaite, M. A.: Prevention of neurological damage during open heart surgery. Thorax, 30:258, 1975.

28. Hill, J. D., et al.: Extracorporeal circulation: Sources of subtle neurologic sequelae. *In* Davila, J. C. (ed.): Second Henry Ford Hospital International Symposium on Cardiac Surgery. New York, Appleton-Century-Crofts, 1977, pp. 111–119.

29. Frank, K. A., et al.: Long-term effects of open-heart surgery on intellectual functioning. J. Thorac. Cardiovasc. Surg., 64:811, 1972.

30. Engelman, R. M., et al.: Cardiac tamponade following open heart surgery. Circulation, 41(suppl. 2):165, 1970.

31. Hardesty, R. L., et al.: Delayed postoperative cardiac tamponade: Diagnosis and management. Ann. Thorac. Surg., 26:155, 1978.

32. Hochberg, M. S., et al.: Delayed cardiac tamponade associated with prophylactic anticoagulation in patients undergoing coronary bypass grafting: Early diagnosis with two-dimensional echocardiography. J. Thorac. Cardiovasc. Surg., 75:777, 1978.

33. Ebert, P. A.: The pericardium. *In* Sabiston, D. C., and Spencer, F. C. (eds.): Gibbon's Surgery of the Chest, 3rd ed. Philadelphia, W. B. Saunders, 1976, p. 978.

34. McEnany, M. T., et al.: Clinical experience with intra-aortic balloon pump support in 728 patients. Circulation, 58(suppl. 1):124, 1978.

35. Bregman, D.: Mechanical support of the failing heart. Curr. Probl. Surg., December 1975.

36. Hill, J. D.: Prolonged extracorporeal oxygenation for pulmonary insufficiency. *In* Ionescu, M. I., and Wooler, G. H. (eds.): Current Techniques in Extracorporeal Circulation. London, Butterworths, 1976, p. 517.

37. Taylor, K. M., et al.: Hypertension and the renin-angiotensin system following open heart surgery. J. Thorac. Cardiovasc. Surg., 74:840, 1977.

38. Roberts, A. J., Niarchos, A. P., and Subramanian, V. A.: Systemic hypertension associated with coronary artery bypass surgery: Predisposing factors, hemodynamic characteristics, humoral profile, and treatment. J. Thorac. Cardiovasc. Surg., 74:846, 1977.

39. Roche, J. K., and Stengle, J. M.: Open heart surgery and the demand for blood. JAMA, 225:1516, 1973.

40. Heimbecker, R. O.: Progress in extracorporeal circulation. J. Thorac. Cardiovasc. Surg., 74:157, 1977.

41. Leichtman, D. A., and Friedman, B. A.: The hemorrhagic complications of open heart surgery. CRC Crit. Rev. Clin. Lab. Sci., 7:239, 1977.

42. Paton, B. C.: Management and complications of central vein catheters. *In* Rutherford, R. B. (ed.): Vascular Surgery. Philadelphia, W. B. Saunders Co., 1977, p. 1225.

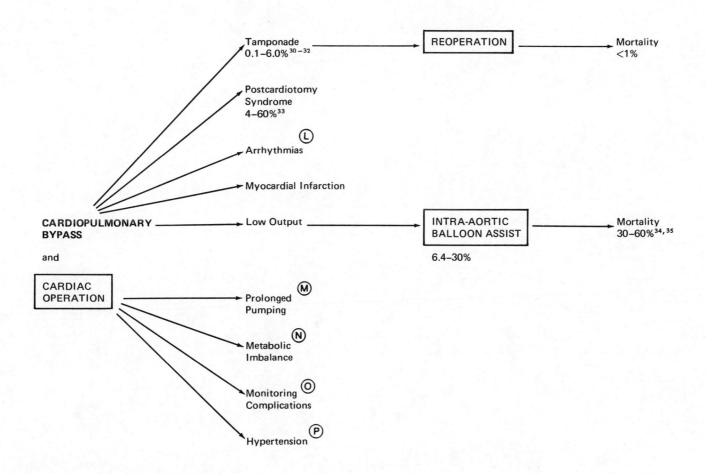

Tamponade
0.1–6.0%[30–32]

REOPERATION

Mortality
<1%

Postcardiotomy
Syndrome
4–60%[33]

(L)

Arrhythmias

Myocardial Infarction

Low Output

INTRA-AORTIC
BALLOON ASSIST

Mortality
30–60%[34, 35]

6.4–30%

**CARDIOPULMONARY
BYPASS**

and

**CARDIAC
OPERATION**

(M)
Prolonged
Pumping

(N)
Metabolic
Imbalance

(O)
Monitoring
Complications

(P)
Hypertension

Section **F**

Abdominal

HIATUS HERNIA BY E. LANCE WALKER, M.D.

Comments

A. The rate of occurrence of abnormal protrusion of the stomach through the esophageal hiatus is quoted as 5 per 100 cases, but 8 to 10 per cent of contrast x-ray studies and 33 per cent of special studies show such an abnormality. Obviously, most are not of clinical importance.

B. The stomach herniates up into the chest alongside the esophagus. The gastroesophageal junction remains in its normal position. The high probability of ulceration, bleeding, incarceration, obstruction, perforation, and gangrene makes elective surgery indicated.[3, 25]

C. Simply replacing the stomach in the abdominal cavity and closing the hiatus is all that is required, in contrast to the treatment needed for sliding hernias.

D. Sliding hernia is defined as cephalad displacement of the gastroesophageal junction and a portion of the stomach through the hiatus. It is significant when reflux exists.

E. Peptic esophagitis caused by gastroesophageal reflux with or without hiatus hernia causes symptoms and is the indication for treatment. Complications are intractability (80 to 92 per cent of cases), severe esophagitis (45 per cent), respiratory problems (35 per cent), bleeding (5 to 6 per cent), stricture (6 to 7 per cent), and ulceration (2 to 3 per cent).[7, 10, 21, 32]

F. Nonoperative therapy consists of weight reduction, postural avoidance of increased intra-abdominal pressure after meals, small meals, elevation of head of bed at night, and the use of antacids and drugs to decrease lower esophageal pressure.[8]

G. Hill repair is posterior gastropexy anchoring the cardioesophageal junction (and the gossamer phrenoesophageal membrane) to the tough median arcuate ligament.[10]

H. The transthoracic Belsey Mark IV procedure imbricates the esophagus into the gastric fundus and forms a 270-degree wrap to assist the stopcock action, thus minimizing reflux.[11]

I. Nissen fundoplication is a transabdominal 360-degree wrapping of the fundus around the esophagus and replacing it below the diaphragm.[12]

J. Historically, the initial enthusiasm for simple hernia repair, vagotomy and pyloroplasty, and gastric emptying procedures has yielded to pessimism because of high rates of recurrence of symptomatic reflux.[19]

K. Reoperation for recurrence (10 to 30 per cent of cases) in many carefully followed series is fraught with a much higher morbidity than is reflected in the reported literature. It is difficult to wrap the scarred postoperative stomach around the esophagus. Inadvertent splenectomy decreases fundic blood supply, and fistula and disaster are more common than reported.[22]

L. If vomiting, growth retardation, refractory esophagitis, stricture, or aspiration persist longer than 6 to 8 weeks of upright posture, an antireflux operation is indicated.

M. Primary reflux occurs in the presence of a hypotensive lower esophageal sphincter and no evidence of hiatus hernia or disease of stomach or esophagus. Incidence is 5 to 20 per cent.[6, 31]

N. The Boerema procedure (transabdominal anterior gastropexy) anchors the stomach to the anterior abdominal wall.[23] Nissen fundoplication is now preferred by others.[26]

References

1. Mobley, J. E., and Christensen, N. A.: Esophageal hiatal hernia: Prevalence, diagnosis and treatment in an American city of 30,000. Gastroenterology, 30:1, 1956.
2. Dyer, N. H., and Pridie, R. B.: Incidence of hiatus hernia in asymptomatic subjects. Gut, 9:696, 1968.
3. Hill, L. D., and Tobias, J. A.: Paraesophageal hernia. Arch. Surg., 96:535, 1968.
4. Pridie, R. B.: Incidence and coincidence of hiatus hernia. Gut, 7:188, 1966.
5. Crozier, R. E., and Jonasson, H.: Symptomatic esophageal hiatus hernias: Study of 105 patients. Arch. Intern. Med., 113:737, 1964.
6. Herrington, J. L., et al.: Conservative surgical treatment of reflux esophagitis and esophageal stricture. Ann. Surg., 181:552, 1975.
7. Iverson, L. I., May, I. A., and Samson, P. C.: Pulmonary complications in benign esophageal disease. Am. J. Surg., 126:223, 1973.
8. Bennett, J. R.: Medical management of gastroesophageal reflux. Clin. Gastroenterol., 5:175, 1976.
9. Raphael, H. A., et al.: Surgical repair of sliding esophageal hiatus hernia: Long-term results. Arch. Surg., 91:228, 1965.
10. Hill, L. D.: An effective operation for hiatus hernia: An eight-year appraisal. Ann. Surg., 166:681, 1967.
11. Baue, A. E., and Belsey, R. H.: The treatment of sliding hiatus hernia and reflux esophagitis by the Mark IV technique. Surgery, 62:396, 1967.
12. Nissen, R.: Gastropexy and "fundoplication" in surgical treatment of hiatus hernia. Am. J. Dig. Dis., 6:954, 1961.
13. Thomas, A. N., Hall, A. D., and Haddad, J. K.: Posterior gastropexy: Selection and management of patients with symptomatic hiatus hernia. Am. J. Surg., 126:148, 1973.
14. Hill, L. D.: Techniques of surgical management and

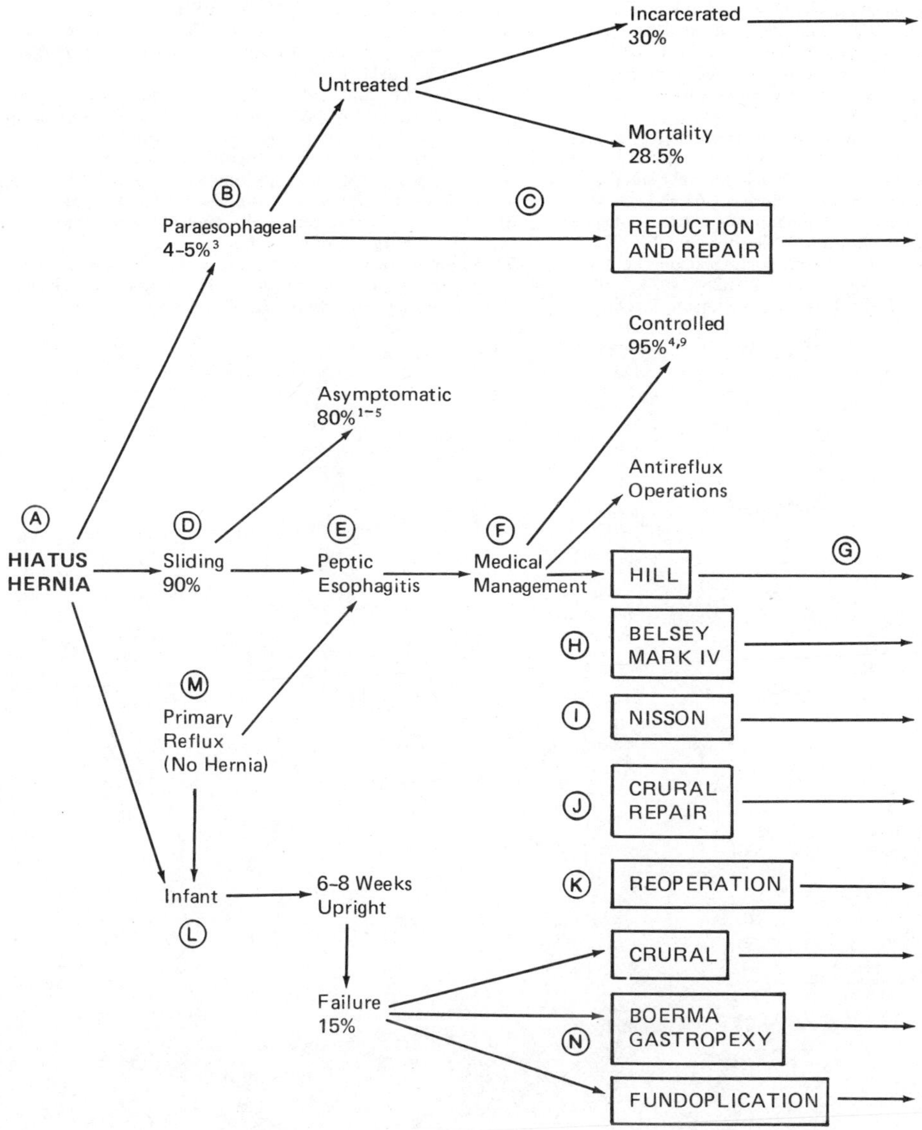

	GOOD/EXCELLENT RESULTS (%)	MORTALITY (%)	COMPLICATIONS (%)	REFERENCES
Incarcerated 30%	50–80	20–50	20–40	25, 29, 30
Mortality 28.5%				
REDUCTION AND REPAIR	90–95	1		14
Controlled 95%[4,9]				
Antireflux Operations				
HILL	66–97	0.4	20–30	10, 13, 14
BELSEY MARK IV	80–85	0–1	15–50	11, 15–18
NISSON	90–100	0–1	15–55	12, 16, 19–21
CRURAL REPAIR	45–60	0–0.3	30–40	27, 19
REOPERATION	75–80	2.9–3.3	15–50	14, 17, 18, 22
CRURAL	66	0	22	26
BOERMA GASTROPEXY	78–98	0–1	20–36	14, 28
FUNDOPLICATION	85–91	0	10–20	26

Flowchart labels:

A — HIATUS HERNIA
B — Paraesophageal 4–5%[3] → Untreated → Incarcerated 30% / Mortality 28.5%
C — REDUCTION AND REPAIR
D — Sliding 90%
E — Peptic Esophagitis → Asymptomatic 80%[1-5]
F — Medical Management → Controlled 95%[4,9] / Antireflux Operations
G — HILL
H — BELSEY MARK IV
I — NISSON
J — CRURAL REPAIR
K — REOPERATION
L — Infant → 6–8 Weeks Upright → Failure 15%
M — Primary Reflux (No Hernia)
N — BOERMA GASTROPEXY

217

results:Technique of Hill. *In* Sabiston, D. C., and Spencer, F. C. (eds.): Gibbon's Surgery of the Chest, 3rd ed. Philadelphia, W. B. Saunders Co., 1976, p. 747.

15. Belsey, R.: Technique of Belsey. *In* Sabiston, D. C., and Spencer, F. C. (eds.): Gibbon's Surgery of the Chest, 3rd ed. Philadelphia, W. B. Saunders Co., 1976, p. 764.

16. Demeester, T. R., Johnson, L. F., and Kent, A. H.: Evaluation of current operations for the prevention of gastroesophageal reflux. Ann. Surg., 180:511, 1974.

17. Orringer, M. B., Skinner, D. B., and Belsey, H. R.: Long-term results of the Mark IV operation for hiatal hernia and analyses of recurrences and their treatment. J. Thorac. Cardiovasc. Surg., 63:25, 1972.

18. Skinner, D. B., and Demeester, T. R.: Gastroesophageal reflux. Curr. Probl. Surg., 13:1, January 1976.

19. Woodward, E. R., Thomas, H. F., and McAlhany, J. C.: Comparison of crural repair and Nissen fundoplication in the treatment of esophageal hiatus hernia with peptic esophagitis. Ann. Surg., 173:782, 1971.

20. Anderson, H. A., and Payne, W. S.: Esophageal hiatus hernia, gastroesophageal reflux, and their complications. *In* Payne, S. W., and Olsen, A. M.: The Esophagus. Philadelphia, Lea & Febiger, 1974, p. 107.

21. Polk, H. C., Jr.: Fundoplication for reflux esophagitis: Misadventures with the operation of choice. Ann. Surg., 183:645, 1976.

22. Hill, L. D.: Management of recurrent hiatal hernia. Arch. Surg., 102:296, 1971.

23. Boerema, I.: Hiatus hernia: Repair by right-sided subhepatic anterior gastropexy. Surgery, 65:884, 1969.

24. Johnson, D. G., et al.: Evaluation of gastroesophageal reflux surgery in children. Pediatrics, 59:62, 1977.

25. Hill, L. D.: Incarcerated paraesophageal hernia, a surgical emergency. Am. J. Surg., 126:286, 1973.

26. Randolph, J. G., Lilly, J. R., and Anderson, K. D.: Surgical treatment of gastroesophageal reflux in infants. Ann. Surg., 180:479, 1974.

27. Allison, P. R.: Hiatus hernia: A 20-year retrospective survey. Ann. Surg., 178:273, 1973.

28. Kamal, I., and Guinery, E. J.: The treatment of hiatus hernia in children by anterior gastropexy. J. Pediatr. Surg., 7:641, 1972.

29. Bettex, M., and Kuffer, F.: Long-term results of fundoplication in hiatus hernia and cardioesophageal chalasia in infants and children. Report of 112 consecutive cases. J. Pediatr. Surg., 4:526, 1969.

30. Beardsley, J. M., and Thompson, W. R.: Acutely obstructed hiatal hernia. Ann. Surg., 159:49, 1964.

31. Gastroesophageal reflux. A panel by correspondence. Arch. Surg., 108:16, 1974.

32. Safgie-Shirazi, S., and Hardy, B. M.: Treatment of reflux esophagitis resulting in massive esophageal bleeding. Arch. Surg., 1:365, 1976.

GASTRIC ULCER

GASTRIC ULCER BY ROBERT RICHARDSON, M.D.

Comments

A. Gastric ulcer (GU) occurs in 0.4 per cent of the population and is one-fourth as common as duodenal ulcer. It occurs 2 to 5 times more often in lower than upper economic levels. Its etiology is related to bile reflux, antral stasis, and damage to the mucosal barrier. Various factors such as diet, alcohol, anti-inflammatory drugs, salicylates, corticosteroids, and smoking are causally related. Gastric ulcers are located within 2 cm. of the junction between antral and parietal mucosa in 96.4 per cent of cases.[1]

B. Although the incidence of gastric cancer is decreasing in the U.S., up to 10 per cent of all GUs show malignant changes. The risk is four times greater with histamine-fast achlorhydria and three times greater in ulcers larger than 3 cm. in diameter. In the presence of concomitant duodenal ulcers, the risk is only one-fourth that with GU alone. There is no relationship to age, sex, or location.[2,3]

C. Diagnostic accuracy of upper G.I. series is 96 per cent, with 80 per cent benign and 70 per cent malignant.[2-4] Accuracy of endoscopic biopsy is 95 per cent and of cytology, 70 per cent.[2-4]

D. Medical therapy consists of antacids or cimetidine, anticholinergics, sedation, and avoidance of nicotine, alcohol, and caffeine. Hospitalization is usually reserved for patients with maximum symptoms. There is no statistical difference in GU healing between treatment with cimetidine and with antacids. There is poor correlation between healing and symptomatic relief.[5-7]

E. Satisfactory healing is defined as a 50 per cent decrease in size at three weeks, a 90 per cent decrease at six weeks, and a 100 per cent decrease at 12 weeks. Symptomatic results are assessed by the Visik scale.[2,3]

F. A bleeding ulcer at the gastroesophageal junction (Dufoil's ulcer) is 100 per cent benign. Proper emergency treatment is conservative biopsy, oversewing of the bleeding point, vagotomy, and pyloroplasty.

G. The best reason for resecting a persistent GU is the high rate (40 to 90 per cent) of recurrence.[1,3,8]

H. Complications include hemorrhage, obstruction, and perforation developing during the treatment period and up to two years thereafter.[2,3]

I. Ulcers larger than 4 cm. in diameter are usually malignant (75 per cent of cases). Medical therapy of benign giant ulcers is usually ineffective.[2,3]

J. Eighteen to 42 per cent of GU patients have concomitant obstructing duodenal ulcers. Surgical treatment of the duodenal ulcer will cure the GU.[3,10,11]

K. One complication of antrectomy with or without vagotomy is early dumping syndrome (30 per cent of cases).[2,3,11-14]

L. Followup has not extended beyond 4.5 years, and it is too early to determine the long-term success of highly selective vagotomy.[14,15]

M. Despite the physiologic irrationality, vagotomy and pyloroplasty are curative in 60 to 93 per cent of patients with benign GU.[2,3,11]

N. Wedge excision alone has deceptively high morbidity and recurrence rates and is seldom indicated.[11]

References

1. Rudick, J.: Gastric ulcer. In Nyhus, L. M., and Wastell, C. (eds.): Surgery of the Stomach and Duodenum, 3rd ed. Boston, Little, Brown & Co., 1977, p. 191.
2. Kukral, J. C.: Gastric ulcer: An appraisal. Surgery, 63:1024, 1968.
3. Wenger, J. W., et al.: Cancer. I. Clinical aspects. The Veterans Administration cooperative study on gastric ulcer. Gastroenterology, 61:598, 1971.
4. Nelson, R. S., et al.: Evaluation of gastric ulcerations. Am. J. Dig. Dis., 21:389, 1976.
5. Frost, F.: Cimetidine in patients with gastric ulcer: A multicentre controlled trial. Br. Med. J., 2:795, 1977.
6. Dyck, W. P., et al.: Cimetidine and placebo in the treatment of benign gastric ulcer. Gastroenterology, 74:410, 1978.
7. Englert, E., Jr., et al.: Cimetidine, antacid, and hospitalization in the treatment of benign gastric ulcer. Gastroenterology, 74:416, 1978.
8. Halse, S. A., et al.: Prognosis of medically treated gastric ulcer. A prospective endoscopic study. Scand. J. Gastroenterol., 12:489, 1977.
9. Doll, R.: Perforated carcinoma of the stomach simulating perforated gastric ulcer. Br. Med. J., 1:215, 1950.
10. Athanassiades, S., and Charalambdopoulou, J.: Coexistent gastric and duodenal ulcer. Am. J. Surg., 120:381, 1970.
11. Davis, Z., et al.: The surgically treated chronic gastric ulcer: An extended followup. Ann. Surg., 185:205, 1977.
12. Zahn, R. L., et al.: Delayed recurrence of gastric ulcer following vagotomy and drainage procedures. Am. Surg., 34:757, 1968.
13. Duthie, H. L., and Kwong, N. K.: Vagotomy or gastrectomy for gastric ulcer. Br. Med. J., 4:79, 1973.
14. Hedenstedt, S., and Moberg, S.: Gastric ulcer treated with selective proximal vagotomy. Acta Chir. Scand., 140:309, 1974.
15. Johnston, D.: Current status of parietal cell vagotomy. Ann. Surg., 184:659, 1976.
16. Desmond, A. M., et al.: Further surgical management of gastric ulcer with unsuspected malignant change. Ann. R. Coll. Surg. Engl., 57:101, 1975.

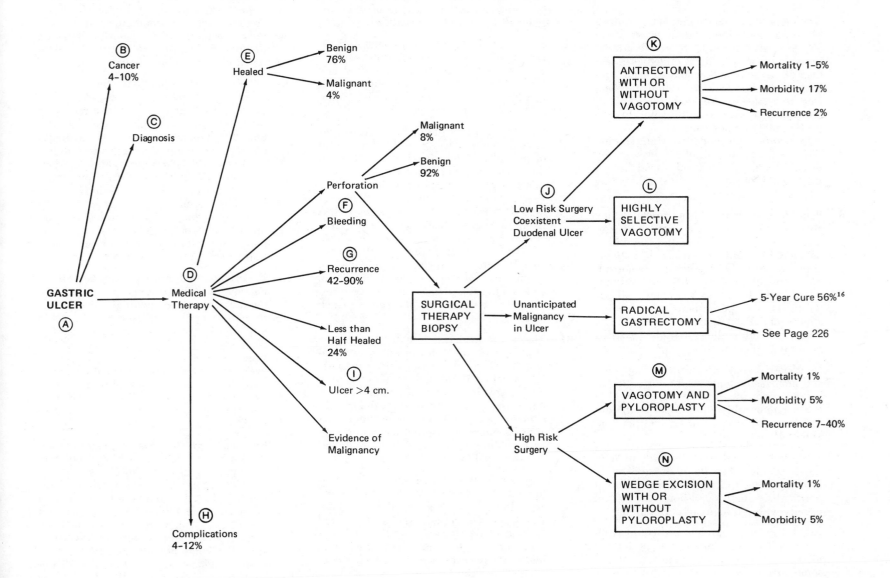

(A) **GASTRIC ULCER**

(B) Cancer 4–10%

(C) Diagnosis

(D) Medical Therapy

(E) Healed
→ Benign 76%
→ Malignant 4%

(F) Perforation
→ Malignant 8%
→ Benign 92%

Bleeding

(G) Recurrence 42–90%

Less than Half Healed 24%

(I) Ulcer >4 cm.

Evidence of Malignancy

(H) Complications 4–12%

SURGICAL THERAPY BIOPSY

(J) Low Risk Surgery Coexistent Duodenal Ulcer

Unanticipated Malignancy in Ulcer

High Risk Surgery

(K) **ANTRECTOMY WITH OR WITHOUT VAGOTOMY**
→ Mortality 1–5%
→ Morbidity 17%
→ Recurrence 2%

(L) **HIGHLY SELECTIVE VAGOTOMY**

RADICAL GASTRECTOMY
→ 5-Year Cure 56%[16]
→ See Page 226

(M) **VAGOTOMY AND PYLOROPLASTY**
→ Mortality 1%
→ Morbidity 5%
→ Recurrence 7–40%

(N) **WEDGE EXCISION WITH OR WITHOUT PYLOROPLASTY**
→ Mortality 1%
→ Morbidity 5%

DUODENAL ULCER BY LAWRENCE W. NORTON, M.D.

Comments

A. Nonoperative management controls bleeding from duodenal ulcer in about 85 per cent of patients. Selective arterial infusion of vasopressin is effective in less than 50 per cent and is seldom used. Preliminary results in a controlled, randomized trial suggest that cimetidine, an H_2 receptor blocker, is of little value in controlling ulcer hemorrhage.[1]

Indications for operative intervention include (1) 2500 ml. blood loss in the first 24 hours, (2) 1500 ml. blood loss in the second 24 hours, and (3) rebleeding after 24 hours' cessation.

B. Patients are considered poor risks if they are over age 65 or have another disease that could increase operative morbidity or mortality. Survival of such patients after operation for bleeding is comparable to that of good-risk patients if a limited procedure such as vagotomy and pyloroplasty is performed.[2] Rebleeding after V and P is about 10 per cent. The source of rebleeding may be gastritis rather than ulcer.[2]

C. In good-risk patients, truncal vagotomy and hemigastrectomy are preferred to vagotomy and pyloroplasty because of a lower rate of rebleeding (5 per cent)[2] and less frequent ulcer recurrence (4 per cent versus 10 per cent).[3-5]

D. Definitive operation after perforation of duodenal ulcer can be performed safely in the presence of minimal, nonpurulent peritonitis. Such conditions are found usually within 6 hours of perforation.[6, 7]

E. In a prospective, randomized comparison of definitive operations for perforated ulcer, vagotomy and drainage offered some advantage over hemigastrectomy in terms of mortality (0 per cent versus 1.6 per cent) but not in terms of ulcer recurrence (6.1 per cent versus 1.8 per cent).[8]

F. In a limited experience, parietal cell vagotomy after closure of a perforated ulcer was followed by no mortality and no late ulcer recurrence.[9] The procedure is still considered experimental in such circumstances.

G. Simple closure of perforated ulcer is curative for approximately 35 to 50 per cent of patients.[10-12] Duodenal ulcer recurs in the remainder, and about one-half of this group require an ulcer operation within 5 years. A patient with no evidence of ulcer disease prior to perforation is less likely to have recurrence after simple closure.[6] Since closure is used in all patients with severe peritonitis, it is associated with a higher incidence of subphrenic abscess, wound infection, and septicemia than other procedures. Mortality averages 13 per cent in such patients.[12]

H. The saline load test assesses the degree of pyloric obstruction caused by duodenal ulcer. Through a nasogastric tube, 700 ml. of saline is infused. If after 30 minutes a gastric volume of more than 350 ml. is aspirated (positive test), pyloric obstruction is significant. A positive test after 72 hours of nasogastric suction suggests failure of nonoperative treatment and the need for operation.

I. Vagotomy and hemigastrectomy performed for obstructing duodenal ulcer are followed by recurrent ulcer in about 2 to 3 per cent of patients. Vagotomy and drainage have lower mortality (1.7 per cent versus 2 to 3 per cent) but much higher recurrence rates (10 to 12 per cent versus 3 per cent).[13, 14]

J. Recurrence of ulceration is similar after either vagotomy and pyloroplasty or vagotomy and gastroenterostomy.[15] The only consideration in choosing between the two procedures for obstructing duodenal ulcer is technical ease.

K. Of all elective operations for duodenal ulcer, vagotomy and hemigastrectomy give the best protection against recurrent ulceration (1.5 to 2.5 per cent recurrence rate).[16-18] Operative mortality averages about 1 per cent.[16] Significant gastrointestinal morbidity (dumping syndrome, diarrhea, or alkaline reflux gastritis) occurs in 5 to 10 per cent of cases. Serious weight loss and anemia only rarely complicate hemigastrectomy. Wound infection and other septic complications are no greater than after other gastrointestinal operations such as cholecystectomy.

L. Experience with elective parietal cell vagotomy in 5000 patients shows that the operation has an exceedingly low mortality rate (0.3 per cent)[19] and an acceptable rate of ulcer recurrence (4 per cent).[20] Necrosis of the lesser curvature of the stomach occurs in approximately one of every 500 operations. Diarrhea occurs in only 5 per cent of patients and mild dumping in an equal number. Bilious vomiting is significant in only 2 per cent.[19]

M. Subtotal gastrectomy is no longer recommended as an elective, primary operation for duodenal ulcer because of its higher mortality (2 per cent) and significant morbidity.[16] The dumping syndrome is both more common (10 to 25 per cent) and more severe after subtotal gastrectomy than after operations without resection. Iron deficiency anemia and, rarely, vitamin B_{12} deficiency may follow a 75 per cent gastric resection. Weight loss is

DUODENAL ULCER

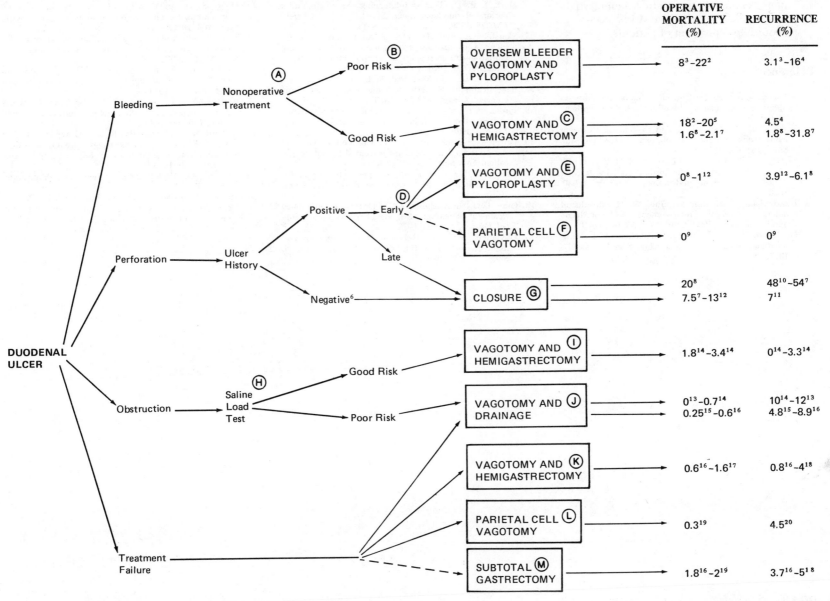

DUODENAL ULCER *Continued*

more common than after hemigastrectomy. Alkaline reflux gastritis occurs in about 2 to 3 per cent of patients.

1. Eden, K., and Kern, F.: Current status of cimetidine in upper gastrointestinal bleeding. Gastroenterology, 74:466, 1978.
2. Yajko, R. D., Norton, L. W., and Eiseman, B.: Current management of upper gastrointestinal bleeding. Ann. Surg., 181:474, 1975.
3. McGregor, D. B., Savage, L. E., and McVay, C. B.: Massive gastrointestinal hemorrhage: A 25-year experience with vagotomy and drainage. Surgery, 80:530, 1976.
4. Buckingham, J. M., and Remine, W. H.: Results of emergency surgical management of hemorrhagic duodenal cancer. Mayo Clin. Proc., 50:223, 1975.
5. Heideman, M., et al.: Surgical management of gastroduodenal hemorrhage. Acta Chir. Scand., 143:307, 1977.
6. Mark, J. B. D.: Factors influencing the treatment of perforated duodenal ulcer. Surg. Gynecol. Obstet., 129:325, 1969.
7. Skarstein, A., and Høisgeter, P. A.: Perforated peptic ulcer: A comparison of long-term results following partial gastric resection or simple closure. Br. J. Surg., 63:700, 1976.
8. Jordon, P. H., and Korompai, F. L.: Evolvement of a new treatment of perforated duodenal ulcer. Surg. Gynecol. Obstet., 142:391, 1976.
9. Jordon, P. H., et al.: Vagotomy of the fundic gland area of the stomach without drainage. Am. J. Surg., 131:523, 1976.
10. Griffin, G. E., and Organ, C. H.: The natural history of the perforated duodenal ulcer treated by suture plication. Ann. Surg., 183:382, 1976.
11. Skovgaard, S.: Late results of perforated duodenal ulcer treated by simple suture. World J. Surg., 1:521, 1977.
12. Gray, J. G., and Roberts, A. K.: Definitive emergency treatment of perforated duodenal ulcer. Surg. Gynecol. Obstet., 143:890, 1976.
13. DeMatteis, R. A., and Hermann, R. E.: Vagotomy and drainage for obstructing duodenal ulcers. Am. J. Surg., 127:237, 1974.
14. Hoerr, S. O., and Ward, J. T.: Late results of three operations for chronic duodenal ulcer. Ann. Surg., 176:403, 1972.
15. Kennedy, F., et al.: Truncal vagotomy and drainage for chronic duodenal ulcer disease: A controlled trial. Br. Med. J., 2:71, 1973.
16. Postlethwait, R. W.: Five-year followup results of operations for duodenal ulcer. Surg. Gynecol. Obstet., 137:387, 1973.
17. Herrington, J. L., Sawyers, J. L., and Scott, H. W.: A 25-year experience with vagotomy-antrectomy. Arch. Surg., 106:469, 1973.
18. Howard, R. J., Murphy, W. R., and Humphrey, E. W.: A prospective study of the elective treatment of duodenal ulcer: Two to ten-year followup study. Surgery, 73:256, 1973.
19. Johnston, D.: Highly selective vagotomy. Prog. Surg., 14:1, 1975.
20. Amdrup, E., Andersen, D., and Jensen, H. E.: Parietal cell (highly selective or proximal gastric) vagotomy for peptic ulcer disease. World J. Surg., 1:19, 1977.

POSTGASTRECTOMY AND VAGOTOMY SYNDROMES

Comments

A. Early dumping syndrome (0 to 4 hours after eating) occurs in 0 to 50 per cent of cases. Nonoperative management can be used in 99 per cent of cases and includes small meals, a low-carbohydrate diet, and no fluids with meals. Patients who have dumping and diarrhea treated by multiple small feedings need to receive supplemental iron, vitamin B_{12}, and pancreatic enzymes.[1, 14, 21]

Operation is necessary for early dumping in 1 per cent or less of the patients. Alteration of gastroenteric anastomosis produces 20 to 50 per cent good-excellent results. A jejunal loop interposition procedure produces 20 to 94 per cent good-excellent results, whereas a short reversal of an isoperistaltic piece of jejunum produces 94 per cent good-excellent results.

B. Late dumping syndrome (more than 4 hours after eating) occurs in 5 per cent of cases.

C. Diarrhea occurs in 10 to 70 per cent of cases. Medical treatment gives an 80 to 95 per cent cure rate. Of surgical treatments, jejunal reversal gives a 90 to 100 per cent cure and procedures utilizing the ligament of Treitz give a 90 per cent cure.

Operation is not indicated unless the diarrhea is so severe that there is excessive weight loss, anemia, and malnutrition.

D. Chronic afferent limb obstruction occurs in less than 5 per cent of patients. The cause is a long afferent loop. Treatment is by Roux-en-Y anastomosis in 90 per cent of cases.

Acute obstruction of the afferent loop may require early operation. When operation becomes necessary, the entire stroma should be revised because lysis of adhesions alone is inadequate.

E. Alkaline reflux gastritis has an overall cure rate of approximately 5 to 35 per cent. Nonoperative treatment is by diet. Operative treatment is Roux-en-Y biliary diversion, which has approximately a 60 to 90 per cent cure rate with vagotomy. Medical therapy for alkaline reflux has been tried intensively but is notably unsuccessful. Patients with alkaline reflux esophagitis require an antireflux procedure as well as a biliary diversion.[1, 25]

F. Recurrent ulceration of all ulcers occurs in 3 per cent of cases. Of these, duodenal ulcers have a 95 per cent recurrence rate; for gastric ulcers the rate is 2 to 4 per cent.[1, 5, 7, 13]

Causes include incomplete vagotomy (78 per cent of cases), retained antrum (40 per cent), insufficient gastric resection (10 per cent), long afferent limb of jejunum (2 per cent), and Zollinger-Ellison syndrome (less than 2 per cent).[1, 5, 7, 13, 15]

Nonsurgical treatment has a 15 per cent mortality rate and a 42 per cent failure rate. Vagotomy and gastrectomy have a possible 93 per cent cure rate. Vagotomy alone has a 40 to 80 per cent cure rate.

G. Gastric cancer is twice as common in the postgastrectomy stomach as in the unoperated stomach.[2, 14]

References

1. Bushkin, F. L., and Woodward, E. R.: Postgastrectomy Syndromes. Philadelphia, W. B. Saunders Co., 1976.
2. Herrington, J. L., Jr.: Remedial operations for postgastrectomy syndromes. Curr. Probl. Surg., 1:63, April 1970.
3. Way, L.: Surgical treatment of late postgastrectomy syndromes. Am. J. Surg., 129:71, 1975.
4. Thompson, B.: Secondary operations for duodenal ulcer. Am. J. Surg., 134:758, 1977.
5. Anchos, G., et al.: Anastomotic ulcer. Am. Surg., 165:955, 1967.
6. Cody, J. H., et al.: Gastrocolic and gastrojejunocolic fistulae: Report of twelve cases and review of the literature. Ann. Surg., 187:376, 1975.
7. White, T. T., and Harrison, R. C.: Late complications of gastric surgery, diagnosis and treatment. Surg. Annu. 8:197, 1976.
8. Boiselle, C. J., and Montalier, de H.: Recurrent peptic ulcers after ulcer or biliary bypass operations: 50 patients. Ann. Chir., 31:685, 1977. (Abstract in 560 July 1978.)
9. Duncomb, V. M., Bohn, T. D., and Davis, A. E.: Double-blind trial of cholestyramine in postvagotomy diarrhea. Gut, 18:531, 1977.
10. Bushkin, F. L., Woodward, E. R., and O'Leary, J. L.: Experience with the jejunal loop imposition in the treatment of post-gastrectomy disorders. Am. Surg., 43:101, 1977.
11. Herrington, J. L., Jr., Sangers, J. L., and Whitehen, W. A.: Surgical management of reflux gastritis. Ann. Surg., 180:526, 1974.
12. Tanner, N. C.: Results of operations for post-

	Ⓐ DUMPING (%)	Ⓑ	Ⓒ (%)	Ⓓ OBSTRUCTION (%)		Ⓔ ALKALINE REFLUX (%)		Ⓕ Recurrence		
OPERATION FOR PEPTIC ULCER	**Early**	**Late**	**Diarrhea**	**Afferent**	**Efferent**	**Gastritis**	**Esophagitis**	**(%)**		**CURE (%)**
VAGOTOMY AND EMPTYING PROCEDURE	12[21]	15[1,14]	64[21]	0–3[23]	0	5–50[24]	30[25]	2–27[26] →	HEMIGAS-TRECTOMY PLUS REVAGOTOMY	→ 90%[26]
Ⓖ VAGOTOMY AND HEMIGAS-TRECTOMY	14–25[9,21]	27[1,22]	25[21]	1–3[23]	1[23]	5–50[24]	10–50[25]	0–4[26] →	RE-RESECTION	→ 80–90[26]
HIGH GASTRIC RESECTION	11–31[22,21]	25[1,22]	7–20[21]	1–3[23]	1[23]	5–50[24]	10–50[25]	1–5[26] →	RE-RESECTION PLUS VAGOTOMY	→ 92[26]
HIGHLY SELECTIVE VAGOTOMY	0–6[27]	0–6[27]	2–3[22]	0	0	0	0	0–9[27] →	ANTRECTOMY	→ 90[27]

gastrectomy symptoms. Gastroenterology, 92:146, 1959.

13. Woodward, E. R.: Postgastrectomy Syndromes. Springfield, Ill., Charles C Thomas, 1963.

14. Nyhus, L. M., and Wastell, C.: Surgery of the Stomach and Duodenum, 3rd ed. Boston, Little, Brown & Co., 1977.

15. Ahmad, W., and Harbrecht, P. J.: Recurrent duodenal ulcer. Arch. Surg., 108:428, 1974.

16. Beahis, O. H.: Surgical management of peptic ulcer disease recurring post-operatively. Surg. Clin. North Am., 51:879, 1971.

17. Jaffee, B. M.: Surgical management of recurrent peptic ulcer. Am. J. Surg., 117:214, 1969.

18. Neustein, C. L.: Reoperation for post-surgery ulceration. Ann. Surg., 185:169, 1977.

19. Sawyers, J. L., Herrington, J. L., Jr., and Scott, H. W., Jr.: Vagotomy and antrectomy for duodenal ulcer. *In* Najarian, J., and Delaney, J. (eds.): Surgery of the Gastrointestinal Tract. Miami, Symposia Specialists; New York, Intercontinental Book Corp., 1973, pp. 225–239.

20. Tanner, N. C.: Gastrectomy for chronic duodenal ulcer. Westminster Hospital Symposium on Chronic Duodenal Ulcer. London, Butterworths, 1974.

21. Gallagher, J. C., Pulnetaft, C. N., and DeDoubal, F. T.: Five to 8-year results of Leeds/York controlled trial of elective surgery for duodenal ulcer. Br. Med. J., 2:781, 1968.

22. Burge, H., Hutchison, J. S. F., and Langland, C. J.: Selective nerve section in the prevention of post-vagotomy diarrhea. Lancet, 1:577, 1964.

23. Mitty, W. F., Grossi, C., and Nealon, T. F.: Chronic afferent loop syndrome. Ann. Surg., 172:996, 1970.

24. Drapanas, T., and Bethea, M.: Reflux gastritis following gastric surgery. Ann. Surg., 179:618, 1974.

25. Windsor, C. W. O.: Gastroesophageal reflux after partial gastrectomy. Br. Med. J., 2:1233, 1964.

26. Stabile, B. E., and Passara, E., Jr.: Recurrent peptic ulcer. Gastroenterology, 70:124, 1976.

27. Jordan, P. H., Jr.: Current status of parietal cell vagotomy. Ann. Surg., 184:659, December 1976.

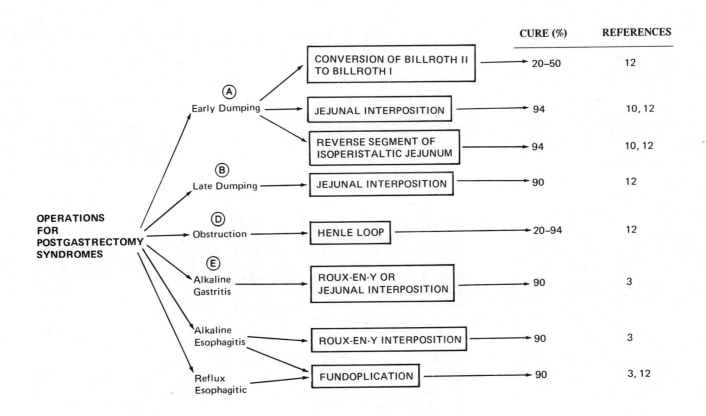

	CURE (%)	REFERENCES
CONVERSION OF BILLROTH II TO BILLROTH I	20–50	12
Early Dumping (A) — JEJUNAL INTERPOSITION	94	10, 12
REVERSE SEGMENT OF ISOPERISTALTIC JEJUNUM	94	10, 12
Late Dumping (B) — JEJUNAL INTERPOSITION	90	12
Obstruction (D) — HENLE LOOP	20–94	12
Alkaline Gastritis (E) — ROUX-EN-Y OR JEJUNAL INTERPOSITION	90	3
Alkaline Esophagitis — ROUX-EN-Y INTERPOSITION	90	3
Reflux Esophagitic — FUNDOPLICATION	90	3, 12

OPERATIONS FOR POSTGASTRECTOMY SYNDROMES

SURGERY FOR OBESITY BY ERNEST E. MOORE, M.D.

Comments

A. Indications for operation are twice ideal weight, duration exceeding 5 years, failure of dietary and psychiatric measures, no endocrinopathies, emotional stability, and less than 50 years of age.[1]

B. Gastric bypass (GB) consists of anastomosis of a 60 cc. gastric fundic pouch to the proximal jejunum. The remaining gastric remnant is left intact with the duodenum. In the morbidly obese this is not a simple technical procedure. Consequently, there has been renewed interest in a gastroplasty procedure. The stomach is stapled, as in the gastric bypass, except that 3 staples are removed, leaving an 8 mm. opening from a 50 cc. pouch. Preliminary experience is encouraging.[2]

C. There is equal weight loss with GB and jejunoileal bypass (JIB) and commensurate amelioration of hypertension, glucose intolerance, and restrictive pulmonary disease. Hyperlipidemia is reversed to a greater degree by JIB because of the malabsorptive effect of this procedure.[3, 4]

D. Transient postprandial vomiting occurs in most patients until they learn to adjust their eating habits to the small gastric reservoir. Otherwise, there are no known metabolic derangements. Surgical complications, however, are significant and reflect the technical difficulty of GB. All obese patients are liable to postoperative respiratory, thromboembolic, and wound complications.

E. The occasional revision is to narrow the gastrojejunostomy stoma or the size of the gastric pouch to improve weight reduction

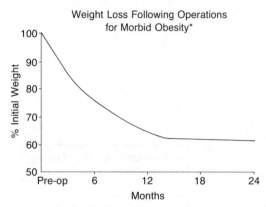

Weight Loss Following Operations for Morbid Obesity*

y-axis: % Initial Weight (50–100); x-axis: Pre-op, 6, 12, 18, 24 Months

*Weight loss is approximately the same following jejunoileal bypass and gastric bypass.

FIGURE 1

F. The Payne JIB operation involves excluding most of the small bowel by anastomosis of the jejunum transected 14 inches from the ligament of Treitz to the side of the ileum 4 inches from the ileocecal valve.[5] The Scott procedure is an end-to-end anastomosis of the jejunum 12 inches from the ligament of Treitz to the end of the ileum 6 inches from the ileocecal valve.[6]

G. The most fearsome complications include liver failure, severe diarrhea, and electrolyte imbalance and may necessitate JIB takedown. JIB revision is occasionally required to enhance weight loss.[7, 8]

H. Diarrhea is an expected consequence of JIB. Although annoying in the first several postoperative months, this usually becomes tolerable. The majority of patients have 3 to 5 soft bowel movements per day. Deficits in potassium, magnesium, and calcium are also frequent in the early postoperative period but usually are managed successfully with dietary supplements. Additional complications attributed to JIB include cholelithiasis, enteritis, colonic pseudo-obstruction, intussusception, volvulus, alopecia, vitamin deficiencies (A, B$_{12}$, C, and D), iron deficiency anemia, hyperchloremic acidosis, ataxia, and gastric hypersecretion.

I. Progressive hepatic dysfunction is a major problem following JIB. Although amino acid administration and antibiotics may partially reverse liver changes, intestinal restoration should be considered before irreversible hepatic necrosis occurs. These patients must be followed closely.

References

1. Mason, E. E., et al.: Optimizing results of gastric bypass. Ann. Surg., 182:405, 1975.
2. Pace, W. G., et al.: Gastric partitioning for morbid obesity. Ann. Surg., 190:392, 1979.
3. Alden, J. R.: Gastric and jejunoileal bypass. Arch. Surg., 112:799, 1977.
4. Griffen, W. O., Young, V L., and Stevenson, C. G.: A prospective comparison of gastric and jejunoileal bypass procedures for morbid obesity. Surg. Gynecol. Obstet., 145:661, 1977.
5. DeWind, L. T., and Payne, J. H.: Intestinal bypass for morbid obesity. JAMA, 236:2298, 1976.
6. Scott, H. W., et al.: Results of jejunoileal bypass in 200 patients with morbid obesity. Surg. Gynecol. Obstet. 145:661, 1976.
7. Halverson, J. D., et al.: Reanastomosis after jejunoileal bypass. Surgery, 84:241, 1978.
8. Hitchcock, C. T., et al.: Management of the morbidly obese patient after small bowel bypass failure. Surgery, 82:356, 1977.

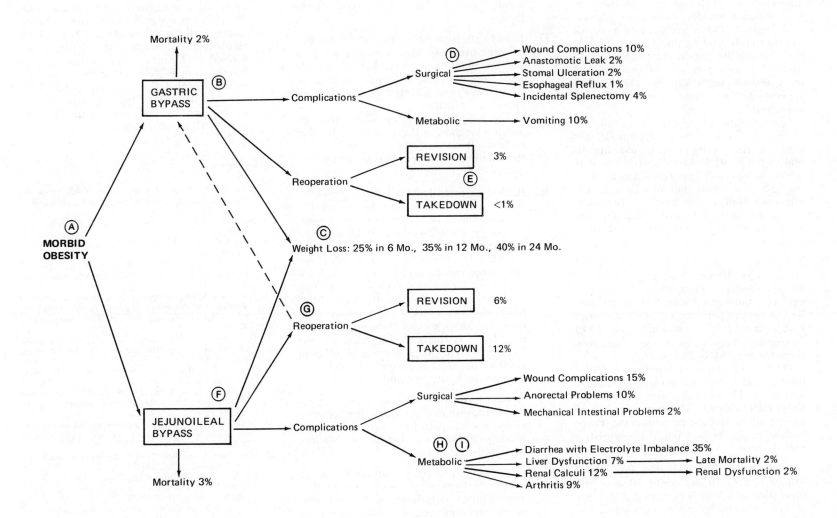

GASTRIC CANCER BY GEORGE E. MOORE, M.D.

Comments

A. Incidence of 23,000 per year in the U.S. is decreasing rapidly, as it is in Europe and Japan.[18] This means caution is required in interpreting published operability, resectability, and survival statistics.[20, 23] About 5 per cent of patients having gastric operation for benign disease develop cancers, but an etiologic relationship is unproved.[6]

Classification of cancers is as follows: ulcerative (75 per cent), polypoid (10 per cent), scirrhous (10 per cent), and superficial (5 per cent). Predominant cell type is adenocarcinoma (90 per cent). The remaining 10 per cent includes lymphoma, adenoacanthoma, carcinoid, leiomyosarcoma, and metastatic gastric wall deposits from breast, melanoma, lung, and other sites.

B. Ninety per cent of gastric ulcers (GUs) are benign, 10 per cent are cancerous; 28 per cent are prepyloric. Fifteen per cent of recurrent GUs are cancerous, and 58 per cent of patients with GUs undergo resection, which has a mortality rate of 4 to 8 per cent.[19] Flexible gastroscopy improves the accuracy of GU diagnosis.

Polyps, adenoma, and pernicious anemia are all associated with achlorhydria and a 2 to 15 per cent probability of multiple malignancies. Thirteen per cent of gastric adenomas are premalignant. Probability of cancer in a polyp is correlated with its size.

C. Overall 5-year survival rate for gastric cancer is 5 to 10 per cent;[1] 10-year survival rate is 2.5 to 5 per cent. Five-year survival rate for gastric resection is 10 to 25 per cent, for localized disease 25 to 50 per cent, and for regional disease 10 to 20 per cent. Equivalent figures from Japan[17] and Finland[12] are significantly better.

D. Direct extension into adjacent organs has a better prognosis than lymph node metastases, even though over half of patients will have occult peritoneal seeding of tumor cells, and direct invasion of blood vessels is common.[13]

The lymphatic drainage of the stomach and the location of the tumor require that individualized decisions be made about the amount of stomach that should be removed.[15, 17, 25]

E. Radical or extended total gastrectomy[10, 12] does not appreciably alter the probability of cure, which is 50 per cent for 1 year, 35 per cent for 2 years, and 15 per cent for 5 years.[16, 23]

Characteristic operative mortalities (with wide variations) for gastric cancer are 4 per cent for subtotal gastrectomy and up to 33 per cent for total gastrectomy. Morbidity following total gastrectomy is a quantum jump greater than when a gastric pouch is retained. Included are extensive weight loss, decreased vitamin absorption, and selective anorexia for milk products, sweets, and meat.

F. Neither palliative resection nor bypass gastroenterostomy prolongs life or provides useful pain-free survival except when performed for obstruction. Median survival is 2 to 3 months.

G. The relatively good prognosis of gastric lymphoma treated by resection and radiation requires debulking of unresectable tumors and outlining of residual neoplasm with silver clips at laparotomy.

H. Neither single-agent nor combinations chemotherapy given therapeutically or as an adjuvant provides significant benefit. There is a significant reduction in the tumor bulk in 10 to 20 per cent of patients, but only an occasional life is prolonged. Drugs used include 5-fluorouracil, BCNU, mitomycin, and alkylating agents.[8, 16, 20] I prefer oral 5-FU because of lack of toxicity, convenience to the patient, and equivalent effectiveness to IV administration.

References

1. Berg, J. W.: Histological aspects of the relation between gastric adenomatous polyps and gastric cancer. Cancer, *11*:1149, 1958.
2. Bush, R. S.: Primary lymphoma of the gastrointestinal tract. JAMA, *228*:1283, 1974.
3. Cain, J. C., et al.: Medically treated small gastric ulcer. JAMA, *150*:781, 1952.
4. Coller, K., and MacIntyre, R. S.: Regional lymphatic metastases of carcinoma of the stomach. Arch. Surg., *43*:748, 1941.
5. Desmond, A. M., Nicholls, J., and Brown, C.: Further surgical management of gastric ulcer with unsuspected malignant change. Ann. R. Coll. Surg. Engl., *57*:101, 1975.
6. Domellof, L., and Tanunger, K. G.: The risk for gastric carcinoma after partial gastrectomy. Am. J. Surg., *134*:581, 1977.
7. Dupont, J. B., Jr., et al.: Adenocarcinoma of the stomach: Review of 1497 cases. Cancer, *41*:941, 1978.
8. Falkson, G. S., and Falkson, H. C.: Fluorouracil and radiotherapy in gastrointestinal cancer. Lancet, *2*:1252, 1969.
9. Fujimaki, M., et al.: Total gastrectomy for gastric cancer: Clinical considerations on 431 cases. Cancer, *30*:60, 1972.
10. Gilbertsen, V. A.: Results of treatment of stomach cancer. Cancer, *23*:1305, 1969.
11. Hawley, P. R., Westerholdm, P., and Morson, B. C.: Pathology and prognosis of carcinoma of the stomach. Br. J. Surg., *57*:61, 1970.
12. Inberg, M. V., et al.: Surgical treatment of gastric carcinoma. Arch. Surg., *110*:703, 1975.
13. Iwanaga, T., et al.: Mechanisms of late recurrence after

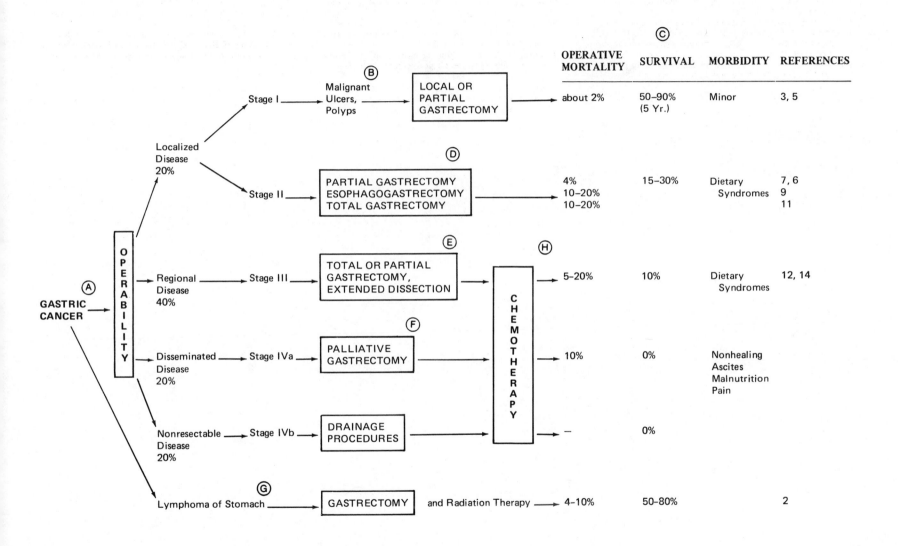

	OPERATIVE MORTALITY	SURVIVAL	MORBIDITY	REFERENCES
(B) Stage I → Malignant Ulcers, Polyps → LOCAL OR PARTIAL GASTRECTOMY	about 2%	50–90% (5 Yr.)	Minor	3, 5
(D) Stage II → PARTIAL GASTRECTOMY ESOPHAGOGASTRECTOMY TOTAL GASTRECTOMY	4% 10–20% 10–20%	15–30%	Dietary Syndromes	7, 6 9 11
(E) Stage III → TOTAL OR PARTIAL GASTRECTOMY, EXTENDED DISSECTION	5–20%	10%	Dietary Syndromes	12, 14
(F) Stage IVa → PALLIATIVE GASTRECTOMY	10%	0%	Nonhealing Ascites Malnutrition Pain	
Stage IVb → DRAINAGE PROCEDURES	—	0%		
(G) Lymphoma of Stomach → GASTRECTOMY and Radiation Therapy	4–10%	50–80%		2

Localized Disease 20%

Regional Disease 40%

Disseminated Disease 20%

Nonresectable Disease 20%

(A) GASTRIC CANCER → OPERABILITY

(C)

(H) CHEMOTHERAPY

GASTRIC CANCER *Continued*

radical surgery for gastric carcinoma. Am. J. Surg., *135*:637, 1978.

14. Moore, G. E.: Surgical therapy for gastric cancer. N. Y. J. Med., *55*:2972, 1955.

15. Moertel, C. G.: Chemotherapy. JAMA, *228*:1290, 1974.

16. Nadler, S. H., Phelan, J. T., and Moore, G. E.: Radical gastrectomy for cancer. Surg. Gynecol. Obstet., *127*:119, 1968.

17. Nakajima, T., et al.: Long-term followup study of gastric cancer patients treated with surgery and adjuvant chemotherapy with mitomycin C. Int. J. Clin. Pharmacol., *16*:209, 1978.

18. Silverberg, E., and Holleb, A. I.: Cancer statistics. Cancer, *24*:2, 1974.

19. Smith, F. H., Boles, R. S., Jr., and Jordan, S. M.: Problem of the gastric ulcer reviewed: Study of 1000 cases. JAMA, *153*:2505, 1953.

20. Tedesco, F. J., et al.: Role of gastroscopy in gastric ulcer patients: Planning a prospective study. Gastroenterology, *73*:170, 1977.

21. Wangensteen, O. H.: Cancer of the stomach. *In* Cancer of the Esophagus and the Stomach. New York, American Cancer Society, 1951, p.42.

22. Welch, C. E.: Late effects of gastrectomy. JAMA, *228*:1287, 1974.

23. White, R. R., Mackie, J. A., and Fitts, W. T., Jr.: An analysis of 20 years' experience with operations for carcinoma of the stomach. Ann. Surg., *181*:611, 975.

UPPER GASTROINTESTINAL
BLEEDING

UPPER GASTROINTESTINAL BLEEDING BY WILLIAM PEARCE, M.D., AND BEN EISEMAN, M.D.

Comments

A. Classic nonoperative therapy has now been supplemented by the use of H_2 receptor blockers. The initial enthusiasm for their use in acid peptic disease of the stomach and duodenum is waning.[29] For the acute bleeder — perhaps other than for those with stress ulcer — they may not be greatly superior to classic antacids and are much more expensive.[30]

B. Routine endoscopy for upper gastrointestinal bleeding has resulted in much more frequent diagnosis of Mallory-Weiss mucosal tears at the gastroesophageal junction than formerly, when the lesion was considered a rarity. Simple oversewing of the tear usually is curative.[12, 23]

C. Only 50 per cent of those operated upon for bleeding are resected for cure.[3, 28]

D. A wide variety of emergency operations have been advocated, most of which stop bleeding. However, the patient usually dies of liver failure in the postoperative period.

E. Massive bleeding of both gastric and duodenal ulcers has a poor long-term prognosis if not treated operatively.

WITH MEDICAL TREATMENT:

	Rebleeding Occurs	Symptoms Require Ultimate Operation
Gastric Ulcer	46%	45%
Duodenal Ulcer	53%	60–70%

F. Frequency of gastritis depends upon the nature of the hospital population. Prognosis for bleeding gastritis depends essentially on the cause of the gastritis. Although bleeding stops with operations for alcohol-induced gastritis, liver failure is frequent. The operation with the lowest mortality (vagotomy and pyloroplasty) is therefore indicated in the alcoholic patient, even though the incidence of rebleeding is higher than with resection.[9, 28]

G. The incidence of stress ulcer bleeding has fallen dramatically in the past 10 years. This probably is associated with better respiratory care. Stress ulcer in the late postinjury or postoperative period is usually (± 60 per cent of cases) associated with remote sepsis, and prognosis depends upon draining the pus.

References

1. Bryant, C. R., and Griffin, W. O.: Vagotomy and pyloroplasty: An inadequate operation for stress ulcers? Arch. Surg., 93:161, 1966.
2. Connecticut Society of American Board of Surgeons: Immediate results of emergency operations for massive upper gastrointestinal hemorrhage. Am. J. Surg., 122:387, 1971.
3. Cassell, P., and Robinson, J. O.: Cancer of the stomach. A review of 854 patients. Br. J. Surg., 63:603–607, 1976.
4. Donaldsen, R. M., et al.: Five-year followup study of patients with bleeding duodenal ulcer with and without surgery. N. Engl. J. Med., 259:201, 1958.
5. Drapanas, T., et al.: Experiences with surgical management of acute gastric mucosal hemorrhage. Ann. Surg., 173:628, 1971.
6. Dwyer, J.: Laser-induced hemostasis in canine stomach. JAMA, 231:486–489, 1975.
7. Esselstyn, C. B.: Surgical management of actively bleeding duodenal ulcer. Surg. Clin. North Am., 56:1387–1393, 1976.
8. Gaisford, W. D.: A new prototype 2-channel upper gastrointestinal operating fiberscope. Gastrointest. Endosc., 22:148, 1976.
9. Jensen, S. L., et al.: Acute hemorrhagic gastritis: Diagnosis and treatment. Acta Chir. Scand., 142:246, 1976.
10. Johnston, G. W., and Rodgers, A. W.: A review of 15 years experience in the use of sclerotherapy in the control of acute hemorrhage. Br. J. Surg., 60:797, 1973.
11. Keller, B.: Treatment of hemorrhagic gastritis by endoscopic application of acrylic polymer. Gastroint. Endosc., 21:75, 1974.
12. Knauer, C. M.: Mallory-Weiss syndrome: Characterization of 75 M-W lacerations in 528 patients with upper G.I. bleeds. Gastroenterology, 71:5–15, 1976.
13. McGregor, D. B., Savage, L. E., and McVay, C. B.: Massive gastrointestinal hemorrhage: A 25-year experience with vagotomy and drainage. Surgery, 80:530, 1976.
14. Mann, W.: Bile-induced acute erosive gastritis — Its prevention by antacids, prostaglandins E_2 and cholestyramine. Am. J. Dig. Dis., 21:89, 1976.
15. Menguy, R., Gadacz, I., and Zajtchuk, J.: The surgical management of acute gastric mucosal bleeding. Arch. Surg., 99:198, 1969.
16. Nyhus, L. M., and Wastell, C.: Surgery of the Stomach and Duodenum, 3rd ed. Boston, Little, Brown & Co., 1977.
17. Papp, J. C.: Endoscopic electrocoagulation of upper gastrointestinal hemorrhage. JAMA, 236:2076, 1976.
18. Pugh, R. N., et al.: Transection of the esophagus for bleeding esophageal varices. Br. J. Surg., 60:646–649, 1973.
19. Orloff, M. J., et al.: Portacaval shunt as emergency procedure in selected patients with alcoholic cirrhosis. Surg. Gynecol. Obstet., 141:59–68, 1975.
20. Raschke, E., and Paquet, K. T.: Management of hemorrhage from esophageal varices using the esophagoscopic sclerosing method. Ann. Surg., 177:99–102, 1973.
21. Richardson, J. D., and Bradley, J.: Gastric devascularization. Ann. Surg., 185:649–655, 1977.
22. Sandlow, L. J., et al.: Prospective randomized study of the treatment of UGI bleeding. Am. J. Gastroenterol., 61:282, 1974.
23. Saylor, J. L., and Tedesco, F. J.: Mallory-Weiss syndrome in perspective. Am. J. Dig. Dis., 20:1311, 1975.
24. Silverstein, F. E., et al.: High power argon laser treatment via standard endoscope. Gastroenterol., 71:558, 1976.
25. Smith, N. S., and Farris, J. M.: Rationale of vagotomy and pyloroplasty in the management of bleeding duodenal ulcer. JAMA, 166:878, 1958.
26. Sugiura, M., and Futagawa, S.: Further evaluation of the Sugiura procedure in the treatment of esophageal varices. Arch. Surg., 112:1317–1321, 1977.
27. Wenckert, A., Borg, I., and Lindblom, P.: Review of medically treated bleeding gastric or duodenal ulcers. Acta Chir. Scand., 120:66, 1960.
28. Yajko, R. A., Norton, L. W., and Eiseman, B.: Current management of upper gastrointestinal bleeding. Ann. Surg., 181:474, 1975.
29. Symposium on clinical results with cimetidine in peptic disease. Gastroenterol., 74:338–488, 1978.
30. Fordtran, J.: Placebo, cimetidine and antacids in peptic ulcer disease. N. Engl. J. Med., 298:1081, 1978.

UPPER GASTROINTESTINAL BLEEDING

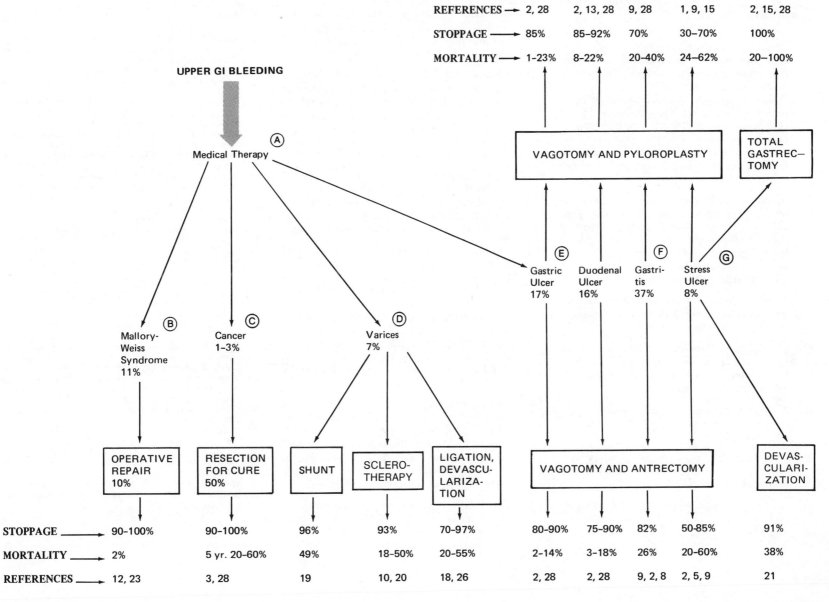

REFERENCES → 2, 28	2, 13, 28	9, 28	1, 9, 15	2, 15, 28
STOPPAGE → 85%	85–92%	70%	30–70%	100%
MORTALITY → 1–23%	8–22%	20–40%	24–62%	20–100%

UPPER GI BLEEDING

Medical Therapy   Ⓐ

VAGOTOMY AND PYLOROPLASTY

TOTAL GASTREC—TOMY

Ⓔ Ⓕ Ⓖ

Gastric Ulcer 17%   Duodenal Ulcer 16%   Gastri-tis 37%   Stress Ulcer 8%

Mallory-Weiss Syndrome 11%   Ⓑ

Cancer 1–3%   Ⓒ

Varices 7%   Ⓓ

OPERATIVE REPAIR 10%

RESECTION FOR CURE 50%

SHUNT

SCLERO-THERAPY

LIGATION, DEVASCU-LARIZA-TION

VAGOTOMY AND ANTRECTOMY

DEVAS-CULARI-ZATION

STOPPAGE →	90–100%	90–100%	96%	93%	70–97%	80–90%	75–90%	82%	50–85%	91%
MORTALITY →	2%	5 yr. 20–60%	49%	18–50%	20–55%	2–14%	3–18%	26%	20–60%	38%
REFERENCES →	12, 23	3, 28	19	10, 20	18, 26	2, 28	2, 28	9, 2, 8	2, 5, 9	21

ACUTE PANCREATITIS BY T. FARIS, M.D.

Comments

A. Prognosis in gallstone-related pancreatitis is as follows:[1] 76 per cent of cases subside spontaneously; nonoperative treatment fails in 24 per cent.

Early exploration and removal of common duct stone has a morbidity of 15 per cent and a mortality of 2 per cent. Delayed operation (cholecystectomy and common duct exploration) has a morbidity of 22 per cent and a mortality of 16 per cent.

B. Alcohol-related pancreatitis is characterized by recurrent acute attacks that subside on nonoperative treatment. Most of these do not require hospitalization. Less than 1 per cent have pancreatic ascites[12] or hemorrhage,[7] but when these occur the mortality is 35 per cent.[6]

C. Recurrence rate correlates with continued alcohol abuse and number and frequency of previous attacks.

D. Variation in the definition of hemorrhagic, necrotizing, or "malignant" pancreatitis accounts for some of the variability in reported prognoses.

E. Neither glucagon nor Trasylol (antitryptic enzyme) appreciably alters the course of pancreatitis.[17]

F. This includes gastrostomy, jejunostomy, cholecystostomy, and drainage of entire pancreatic bed.

G. All-but-total pancreatectomy (Child's procedure) leaves only a thin rim of pancreatic head containing the pancreatic- duodenal vessels and the common bile duct. Patients who undergo this operation already have a destroyed pancreas and diabetes.

H. Edema of the pancreas occurs in 100 per cent of cases, but a clinically palpable mass or phlegmon appears in about 40 per cent depending on obesity and ability to palpate the retroperitoneal area. Ultrasonography can detect a pseudocyst greater than 2 cm. in diameter.[3]

I. With routine use of sonography it can be shown that acute cysts have a 25 per cent probability of absorption and a 50 per cent chance of progressing to the chronic thick-walled stage without complication.[3]

J. Internal drainage may be accomplished by two procedures: (1) Cystogastrostomy, for which the mortality rate is 2.8 per cent, the reoperation rate 4.7 per cent, the recurrence rate 2.8 per cent, and rate of bleeding 0.9 per cent; (2) Cystoenterostomy (Roux-en-Y anastomosis), for which mortality is 2.2 per cent, reoperation rate is 4.3 per cent, recurrence rate is 2.2 per cent, and rate of bleeding is 2.2 per cent.[13]

K. The quoted mortality of 29 per cent is higher than current experience shows, when good respiratory care is available.[5, 9, 16] Most patients with acute pancreatitis have pulmonary infiltrates on chest radiographs and 8 per cent have some degree of pulmonary edema.

L. Renal failure contributes to mortality in 20 per cent of those dying of acute pancreatitis.[6]

References

1. Acosta, J. M., et al.: Early surgery for acute gallstone pancreatitis: Evaluation of a systematic approach. Surgery, 83:367, 1978.
2. Blackburn, G. I., et al.: New approaches to the management of severe acute pancreatitis. Am. J. Surg., 131:114, 1976.
3. Bradley, E. L., III, Gonzales, A. C., and Clements, J. L., Jr.: Acute pancreatic pseudocysts. Ann. Surg., 184:734, 1976.
4. Camer, S. J., et al.: Pancreatic abscess: A critical analysis of 113 cases. Am. J. Surg., 129:426, 1975.
5. Feller, J. H., et al.: Changing methods in the treatment of severe pancreatitis. Am. J. Surg., 127:196, 1974.
6. Gleidman, M. L., Bolooki, H., and Rosen, R. G.: Acute pancreatitis. Curr. Probl. Surg., August 1970.
7. Karmody, A. M., and Galloway, J. M. D.: Hemorrhagic shock in early acute pancreatitis: A rare but significant event. Br. J. Surg., 58:519, 1971.
8. Norton, L., and Eiseman, B.: Near-total pancreatectomy for hemorrhagic pancreatitis. Am. J. Surg., 127:191, 1974.
9. Ranson, J. H. C., et al.: Respiratory complications in acute pancreatitis. Ann. Surg., 179:557, 1974.
10. Rosato, E. F., Mullis, W. F., and Rosato, F. E.: Peritoneal lavage therapy in hemorrhagic pancreatitis. Surgery, 74:106, 1973.
11. Sankaran, S., and Walt, J. A.: The natural and unnatural history of pancreatic pseudocysts. Br. J. Surg., 62:37, 1975.
12. Smith, R. B., III, et al.: Pancreatic ascites: Diagnosis and management with particular reference to surgical technics. Ann. Surg., 177:538, 1973.
13. Warren, W. D., Marsh, W. H., and Sandusky, W. R.: An appraisal of surgical procedures for pancreatic pseudocyst. Ann. Surg., 147:903, 1958.
14. Warshaw, A. L.: Pancreatic abscesses. N. Engl. J. Med., 287:1234, 1972.
15. Warshaw, A. L., et al.: Surgical intervention in acute necrotizing pancreatitis. Am. J. Surg., 127:484, 1974.
16. Warshaw, A. L., et al.: The pathogenesis of pulmonary edema in acute pancreatitis. Ann. Surg., 182:505, 1975.
17. Welbourn, R B., et al.: Death from acute pancreatitis. M.R.C. multicentre trial of glucagon and aprotinin. Lancet, 2:632, 1977.

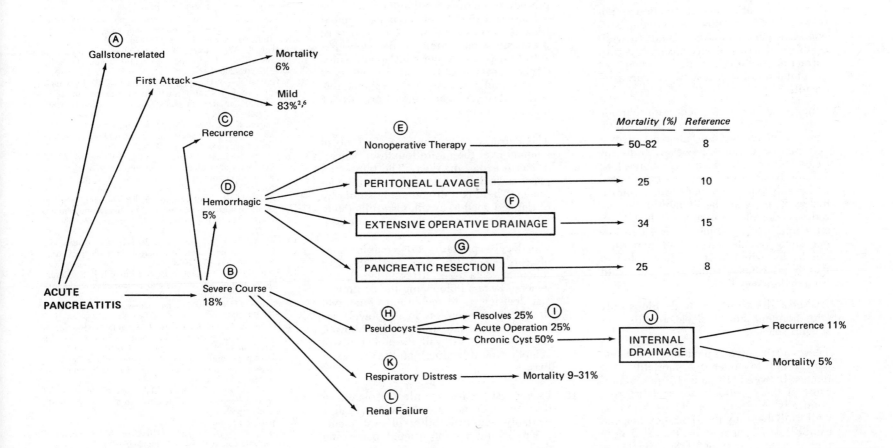

CHRONIC PANCREATITIS BY S. ENGEL, M.D., M.S. (SURG.)

Comments

A. In the U.S. 60 to 70 per cent of cases are alcohol-related.[3] The male:female ratio is 7:1[10] or 8:1.[1]

B. If the pancreatic duct obstruction is not removed and free flow guaranteed, post-operative pancreatitis is certain. In well-established cases of chronic pancreatitis, correction of biliary pathology may not give total relief as it does with acute pancreatitis.

C. Other diseases associated with chronic pancreatitis include (1) hyperparathyroidism, for which excision adenoma gives a 100 per cent cure;[1] however, transient exacerbations can occur; (2) hereditary chronic pancreatitis, which is transmitted as an autosomal dominant trait (approximately 22 cases in the literature),[11] or hereditary ductal narrowing or ductal obstruction, for which the Puestow operation provides a cure;[11] (3) hyperlipidemia, for which diet provides relief of pain;[13] (4) cancer, which leads to death from malignancy.[17]

D. Diabetes characteristically develops only after frequent attacks of pancreatitis over several years.

E. These extirpative operations exchange pain relief for operative mortality that ranges between 10 and 13 per cent.[10] Most of these patients are socially, economically, and emotionally bankrupt as well as diabetic by the time they become candidates for operation. There is only one report, consisting of 8 patients, of total pancreatectomy done for chronic pancreatitis.[6] In general, mortality for total pancreatectomy is 15 to 20 per cent and morbidity is 20 to 40 per cent.[1] Tran-

section of the pancreas with retrograde drainage into the jejunum is the DuVal operation.[8] Child's operation[5] retains a thin rim of pancreatic head, preserving duodenal blood supply. The Whipple procedure removes the duodenum.

Pancreatic duct ligation has had limited trial. It destroys the secretory pancreas, preserving what is left of the islets. Results to date are 90 per cent good results, 0 per cent mortality, and 10 per cent serious complications.[14, 15] Sphincterotomy and celiac ganglionectomy are of historical interest only.

F. The Puestow operation places a limb of jejunum over the entire length of pancreas cut to expose its duct.[7] The transected pancreas is drained retrograde into the jejunum. There is a discouraging similarity of claimed good-to-excellent results (50 to 80 per cent) among all these operations.

G. Pseudocysts primarily are complications of acute pancreatitis (see page 238). The following data refer to pseudocysts. In general, factors influencing the controversial decision as to technique of internal drainage (stomach or small bowel) include (1) adjacency to stomach or bowel, (2) maturity of cyst wall, (3) probability of complication (bleeding), and (4) personal bias.

H. Pseudocyst excision, unless isolated to the pancreatic tail, results in too high a mortality and probability of cyst recurrence behind the obstructed pancreatic duct.

I. There are occasional cases of non–alcohol-related pancreatic insufficiency secondary to pancreatitis.[16]

References

1. Howard, J. M., and Jordan, G. L.: Surgical Diseases of the Pancreas. Philadelphia, J. B. Lippincott Co., 1960, p. 607.
2. Gross, J. B., and Comfort, M. W.: Chronic pancreatitis. Am. J. Med., 21:596–617, 1956.
3. Perrier, C. V.: Symposium on the etiology and pathological anatomy of chronic pancreatitis: Marseilles, 1963. Am. J. Dig. Dis., 9:371–376, 1964.
4. Way, L. W., Gadacz, T., and Goldman, L.: Surgical treatment of chronic pancreatitis. Am. J. Surg., 127:202–209, 1974.
5. Child, C. G., III, Frey, C. F., and Fry, W. J.: A reappraisal of removal of ninety-five per cent of the distal portion of the pancreas. Surg. Gynecol. Obstet., 129:49–56, 1969.
6. Warren, K. W., Poulantzas, J. K., and Kune, G. A.: Life after total pancreatectomy for chronic pancreatitis. Ann. Surg., 164:830–834, 1966.
7. Jordan, G. L., Jr., Strug, B. S., and Crowder, W. E.: Current status of pancreatojejunostomy in the management of chronic pancreatitis. Am. J. Surg., 133:46–51, 1977.
8. DuVal, M., Jr., and Enquist, I. F.: The surgical treatment of chronic pancreatitis by pancreaticojejunostomy: An 8-year reappraisal. Surgery, 50:965–969, 1961.
9. Gilman, P. K., et al.: Unusual diagnostic aspects and current management of pancreatic pseudocysts. Ann. Surg., 40:326–334, 1974.
10. Mercadier, M. P., Clot, J. P., and Russell, T. R.: Chronic recurrent pancreatitis and pancreatic pseudocysts. Curr. Probl. Surg., July 1973.
11. Gerber, B. C.: Hereditary pancreatitis. Arch. Surg., 87:70, 1963.
12. White, T. T., and Kavlie, H.: Congenital obstruction of the pancreatic duct at the duodenum: A report of 2 cases in adulthood. Ann. Surg., 178:194–196, 1973.
13. Klatskin, G., and Gordon, M.: Relationship between relapsing pancreatitis and eventual hyperlipemia. Am. J. Med., 12:3, 1952.
14. Engel, S., et al.: Experimental study of the effect of ductal ligation in pancreatitis. Arch. Surg., 85:1031–1035, 1962.
15. Engel, S.: Unpublished data.
16. Goulston, S. J. M., and Gallagher, N. D.: Painless chronic pancreatitis. Gut, 3:252–254, 1962.
17. Gambill, E. E.: Pancreatitis associated with pancreatic carcinoma: Study of 26 cases. Mayo Clin. Proc., 46:174–177, 1971.

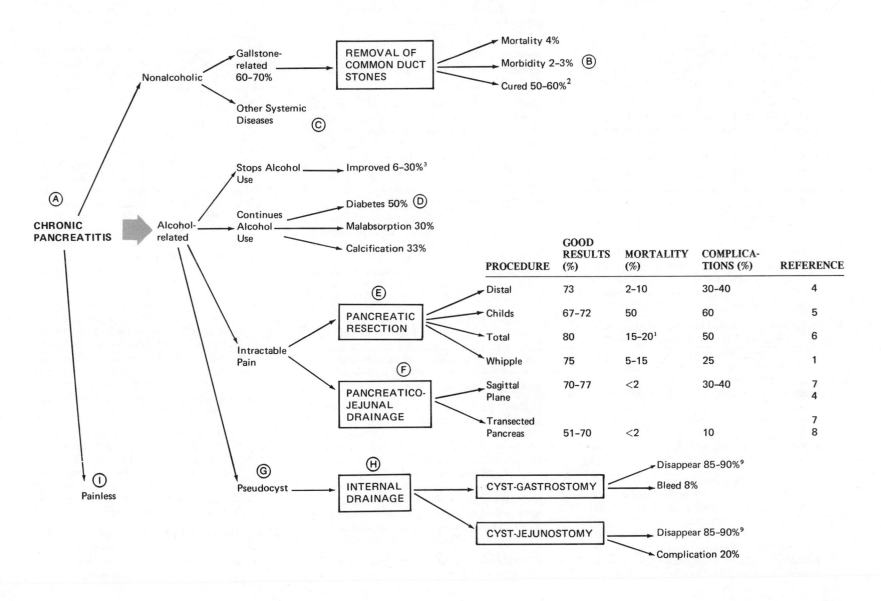

PROCEDURE	GOOD RESULTS (%)	MORTALITY (%)	COMPLICA- TIONS (%)	REFERENCE
Distal	73	2–10	30–40	4
Childs	67–72	50	60	5
Total	80	15–20[1]	50	6
Whipple	75	5–15	25	1
Sagittal Plane	70–77	<2	30–40	7 4
Transected Pancreas	51–70	<2	10	7 8

CARCINOMA OF THE PANCREAS AND RELATED CANCERS BY I. PENN, M.D.

Comments

A. This is the fourth commonest cause of death in the U.S. (behind cancer of the lung, colorectum, and breast), with nearly all of the 20,000 new cases per year dying of the disease.[6]

B. Distribution of pancreatic cancer is as follows: head (55 per cent); body and tail (20 per cent); ampulla of Vater, duodenum, and distal common bile duct (25 per cent).

C. Advanced disease with associated ascites and hepatic, pulmonary, or other widespread metastases is not treated surgically.[9]

D. Most are nonresectable because of hepatic or lymph node metastases, peritoneal spread, or involvement of the superior mesenteric vessels, portal vein, hepatic artery, or inferior vena cava.[16, 17, 22]

E. Although in several series, ranging from 31 to 56 cases, patients have had resection without any deaths,[2, 13, 24] the quoted mortality is characteristic.[20] Causes of death are pancreatitis or occlusion of mesenteric vessels, or both (9 per cent), hemorrhage (29 per cent), anastomotic leakage and sepsis (34 per cent), hepatic failure (8 per cent), acute renal failure (2 per cent), and cardiopulmonary complications (18 per cent).[12]

F. Early morbidity includes pancreatic fistulas (9 to 18 per cent), biliary fistulas (6 to 7 per cent), GI hemorrhage (8 per cent), intraperitoneal infection (5 to 9 per cent), wound infection (6 to 9 per cent), and cardiorespiratory problems (9 per cent).[2, 16, 23] Late complications include pancreatic exocrine insufficiency (22 per cent), diabetes mellitus (15 per cent), and jejunal ulcer (7.5 per cent).[20, 23]

G. Mean survival with laparotomy only is 5 months, with biliary tract bypass, 7 months, and with pancreatoduodenectomy, 15 months.[8, 12, 23]

H. Radical en bloc pancreatectomy with adjacent soft tissue, regional lymph nodes, portal vein, and other pertinent vascular structures in 18 patients resulted in 3 operative deaths. Six lived more than a year and 53 per cent are alive at 4 to 17 months.[7]

I. Quality of life can be satisfactory despite the inevitable diabetes and difficulty with adequate nutrition. Insulin should be given to prevent ketosis, rather than trying to achieve normoglycemia. Pancreatic supplements and a reduced fat intake are necessary for maintenance of body weight.[3, 14, 19]

J. Average survival time is 15 months for operative survivors.[3] Five-year survival figures usually involve small numbers of patients.[14, 19] Evidence of significantly increased longevity resulting from pancreatectomy is lacking.

K. Biliary bypass even for resectable lesions provides good palliation and minimal mortality, morbidity, and hospitalization. Survival is 10.6 months for resected patients versus 8.1 months for bypassed patients.[20] In another study, 50 per cent survival was 6 months following bypass and 21 months following resection,[12] despite attempts not to bias choice of treatment. Most surgeons use bypass solely when resection for cure is impossible.

L. Biliary bypass alone is performed in 70 per cent of patients coming to operation for cancer of the pancreatic head. This prolongs life by about 2 months over laparotomy alone[8, 23] and ensures relief of obstructive jaundice and the associated pruritus in 62 per cent of patients. Almost two thirds of patients are relieved of pain, and some even have a return of appetite and temporary weight gain.[8]

M. Gastrojejunostomy does not prolong patient survival but relieves existing obstruction or prevents imminent obstruction caused by tumor.[12, 23] If there is no actual or imminent duodenal obstruction at laparotomy, most patients die of their malignancies before becoming obstructed or hemorrhaging.

Neither pancreatojejunostomy nor pancreatogastrostomy over a T-tube prolongs survival but may diminish pain by decompressing the obstructed pancreatic duct.[23]

N. Conventional radiotherapy may afford some degree of palliation in 20 to 40 per cent of cases but has no effect on survival.[5] In contrast, 18 patients treated with high-dose, small-volume irradiation (and chemotherapy in 7 cases) have a median survival of 11.8 months, with relief of pain, increased appetite, and weight gain in approximately 70 per cent.[5]

O. Fifteen to 21 per cent of patients have an objective but short response (median duration 3 months) to 5-fluorouracil.[21, 23] Radiotherapy plus chemotherapy produces objective evidence of temporary improvement in 56 per cent of patients and a mean survival of 9½ months.[23]

P. Injection of 50 per cent alcohol into the celiac plexus may provide substantial relief of pain in occasional patients.

CARCINOMA OF THE PANCREAS AND RELATED CANCERS

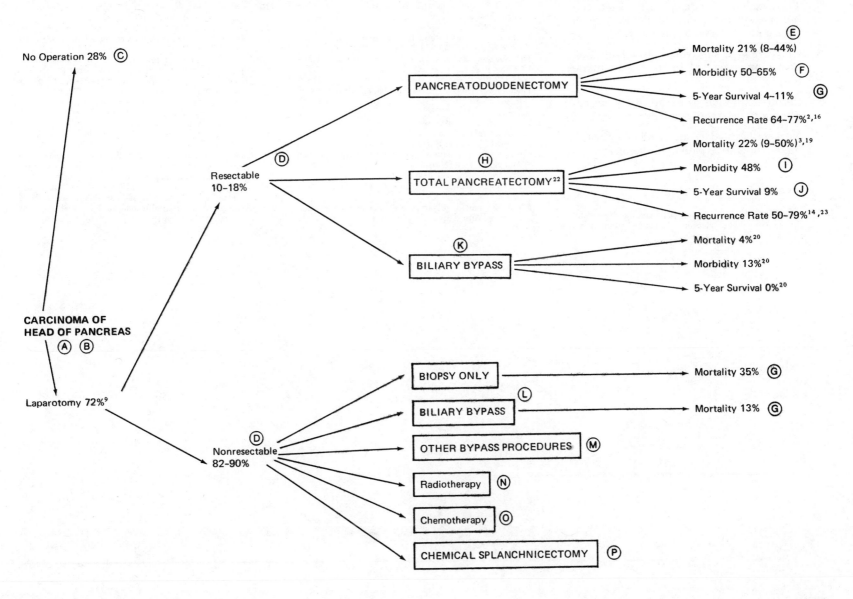

No Operation 28% Ⓒ

PANCREATODUODENECTOMY
- Mortality 21% (8–44%) Ⓔ
- Morbidity 50–65% Ⓕ
- 5-Year Survival 4–11% Ⓖ
- Recurrence Rate 64–77%[2],[16]

Resectable 10–18% Ⓓ

TOTAL PANCREATECTOMY[22] Ⓗ
- Mortality 22% (9–50%)[3],[19]
- Morbidity 48% Ⓘ
- 5-Year Survival 9% Ⓙ
- Recurrence Rate 50–79%[14],[23]

BILIARY BYPASS Ⓚ
- Mortality 4%[20]
- Morbidity 13%[20]
- 5-Year Survival 0%[20]

CARCINOMA OF HEAD OF PANCREAS Ⓐ Ⓑ

Laparotomy 72%[9]

Nonresectable 82–90% Ⓓ
- BIOPSY ONLY → Mortality 35% Ⓖ
- BILIARY BYPASS Ⓛ → Mortality 13% Ⓖ
- OTHER BYPASS PROCEDURES Ⓜ
- Radiotherapy Ⓝ
- Chemotherapy Ⓞ
- CHEMICAL SPLANCHNICECTOMY Ⓟ

CARCINOMA OF THE PANCREAS AND RELATED CANCERS *Continued*

Q. This excludes patients with islet cell tumors and cystadenocarcinomas, which have a more favorable prognosis.[4, 12, 17]

R. Only 2 5-year survivors with adenocarcinomas are recorded in the world literature.[4, 10]

S. Results with total pancreatectomy are too limited to be significant.[14]

T. No significant data are available regarding nonoperative palliative therapy.

References

1. Akwari, O. E., et al.: Radical pancreatoduodenectomy for cancer of the papilla of Vater. Arch. Surg., *112*:451, 1977.
2. Aston, S. J., and Longmire, W. P., Jr.: Pancreaticoduodenal resection. Twenty years' experience. Arch. Surg., *106*:813, 1973.
3. Diamond, D., and Fisher, B.: Pancreatic cancer. Surg. Clin. North Am., *55*:363, 1975.
4. Die Goyanes, A., Pack, G. T., and Bowden, L.: Cancer of the body and tail of the pancreas. Rev. Surg., *28*:153, 1971.
5. Dobelbower, R. R., Jr., et al.: Pancreatic carcinoma treated with high-dose, small-volume irradiation. Cancer, *41*:1087, 1978.
6. Fitzgerald, P. J.: Pancreatic cancer: The dismal disease. Arch. Path. Lab. Med., *100*:513, 1976.
7. Fortner, J. G., et al.: Regional pancreatectomy: En bloc pancreatic, portal vein, and lymph node resection. Ann. Surg., *186*:42, 1977.
8. Gallitano, A., Fransen, H., and Martin, R. G.: Carcinoma of the pancreas: Results of treatment. Cancer, *22*:939, 1968.
9. Glenn, F., and Thorbjarnarson, B.: Carcinoma of the pancreas. Ann. Surg., *159*:945, 1964.
10. Gordon-Taylor, G.: Radical surgery of cancer of the pancreas. Ann. Surg., *100*:206, 1934.
11. Hines, L. H., and Burns, R. P.: Ten years' experience treating pancreatic and peri-ampullary cancer. Am. Surg., *42*:441, 1976.
12. Howard, J. M., and Jordan, G. L., Jr.: Cancer of the pancreas. *In* Hickey, R. C. (ed.): Current Problems in Cancer, vol. 2. Chicago, Year Book Medical Publishers, 1977, p. 5.
13. Howard, J. M.: Pancreaticoduodenectomy: 41 consecutive Whipple resections without an operative mortality. Ann. Surg., *168*:629, 1968.
14. Ihse, I., et al.: Total pancreatectomy for cancer: An appraisal of 65 cases. Ann. Surg., *186*:675, 1977.
15. Kibler, C. E., and Bernatz, P. E.: Operative experience with carcinoma of the body and tail of the pancreas. Proc. Staff Meet. Mayo Clin., *33*:247, 1958.
16. Monge, J. J., Judd, E. S., and Gage, R. P.: Radical pancreatoduodenectomy: A 22-year experience with the complications, mortality rate, and survival rate. Ann. Surg., *160*:711, 1964.

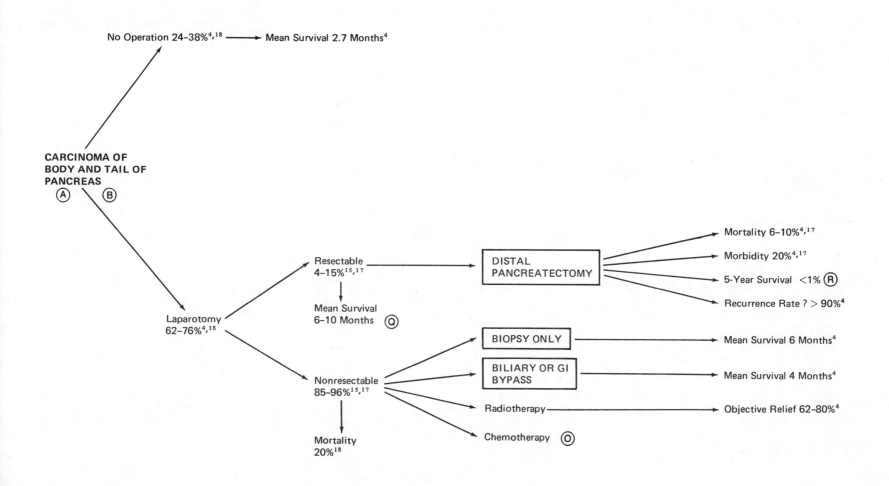

No Operation 24–38%[4],[18] ⟶ Mean Survival 2.7 Months[4]

**CARCINOMA OF
BODY AND TAIL OF
PANCREAS**
Ⓐ   Ⓑ

Laparotomy
62–76%[4],[18]

Resectable
4–15%[15],[17]

Mean Survival
6–10 Months Ⓠ

Nonresectable
85–96%[15],[17]

Mortality
20%[18]

DISTAL
PANCREATECTOMY

Mortality 6–10%[4],[17]

Morbidity 20%[4],[17]

5-Year Survival <1% Ⓡ

Recurrence Rate ? > 90%[4]

BIOPSY ONLY ⟶ Mean Survival 6 Months[4]

BILIARY OR GI
BYPASS ⟶ Mean Survival 4 Months[4]

Radiotherapy ⟶ Objective Relief 62–80%[4]

Chemotherapy Ⓞ

17. Nakase, A., et al.: Surgical treatment of cancer of the pancreas and the periampullary region. Cumulative results in 57 institutions in Japan. Ann. Surg., *185*:52, 1977.
18. Pope, N. A., and Fish, J. C.: Palliative surgery for carcinoma of the pancreas. Am. J. Surg., *121*:271, 1971.
19. Remine, W. H., et al.: Total pancreatectomy. Ann. Surg., *172*:595, 1970.
20. Shapiro, T. S.: Adenocarcinoma of the pancreas: A statistical analysis of biliary bypass vs. Whipple resection in good-risk patients. Ann. Surg., *182*:715, 1975.

21. Stolinsky, D. C., Pugh, R. P., and Bateman, J. R.: 5-Fluorouracil (NSC-19893) therapy for pancreatic carcinoma: Comparison of oral and intravenous routes. Cancer Chemother. Rep., *59*:1031, 1975.
22. Warren, K. W.: Tumors of the pancreas: Surgical aspects of exocrine tumors. *In* Bockus, H. L. (ed.): Gastroenterology, 3rd ed. Vol. 3, Philadelphia, W. B. Saunders Co., 1976, p. 1122.

23. Warren, K. W., and Jefferson, M. F.: Carcinoma of the exocrine pancreas. *In* Carey, L. C., (ed.): The Pancreas. St. Louis, C. V. Mosby Company, 1973, pp. 243–294.
24. Warren, K. W., in discussion of Howard, J. M.: Pancreaticoduodenectomy: 41 consecutive Whipple resections without an operative mortality. Ann. Surg., *168*:629, 1968.

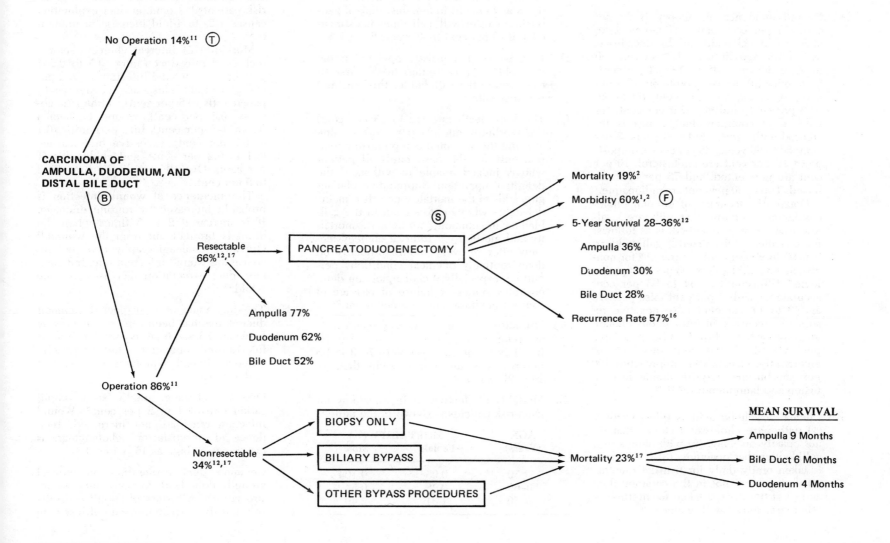

No Operation 14%[11] Ⓣ

**CARCINOMA OF
AMPULLA, DUODENUM, AND
DISTAL BILE DUCT**
Ⓑ

Resectable
66%[12,17]

Ⓢ

PANCREATODUODENECTOMY

Ampulla 77%

Duodenum 62%

Bile Duct 52%

Mortality 19%[2]

Morbidity 60%[1,2] Ⓕ

5-Year Survival 28–36%[12]

Ampulla 36%

Duodenum 30%

Bile Duct 28%

Recurrence Rate 57%[16]

Operation 86%[11]

Nonresectable
34%[12,17]

BIOPSY ONLY

BILIARY BYPASS

OTHER BYPASS PROCEDURES

Mortality 23%[17]

MEAN SURVIVAL

Ampulla 9 Months

Bile Duct 6 Months

Duodenum 4 Months

GALLSTONES BY J. HANSBROUGH, M.D., AND B. EISEMAN, M.D.

Comments

A. Overall incidence at autopsy is 20 per cent (13 per cent male, 27 per cent female).[1] Clinical incidence by decades is as follows: age 20 to 29, 1.7 per cent; 30 to 39, 2 per cent; 40 to 49, 5.4 per cent; 50 to 59, 11.9 per cent; 60 to 69, 17.3 per cent; 70 to 79, 25.6 per cent; 80 to 89, 31.3 per cent; and 90, 32.9 per cent. Incidence of common duct stones is increased with age:[2,3] 20 to 40 years, 3 per cent; 60 to 80 years, 25 per cent. Composition:[4] 10 per cent are cholesterol, 10 per cent are pigmented, and 75 per cent are mixed. Ten to 30 per cent are radiopaque.[4]

Diagnostic accuracy of an oral cholecystogram, assuming that pills are swallowed and dye is absorbed, is as follows: for opacified ("visualized") gallbladders, it is 97 to 99 per cent accurate;[5,6] for nonvisualized gallbladders, 95 per cent pathologic.[7] Ultrasound is 64 to 93 per cent accurate,[8-11] with 3 per cent false positive and 3 to 14 per cent false negative results.[8,11] Accuracy of intravenous cholangiography when bilirubin is below 3.0 mg. per 100 ml.: When done electively or emergently, visualization approaches 100 per cent but may require double-dose infusion and laminograms.[12,13,22]

B. Chenodeoxycholic acid is effective only (1) with pure cholesterol stones that do not opacify on x-ray, (2) with stones in a gallbladder that opacifies, (3) if the drug is taken orally daily for 6 to 24 months, (4) if stones are not in the common duct and (5) if the drug is taken for lifetime — otherwise, stones will reappear.[14]

C. Gallstones coexist with 85 to 90 per cent of all gallbladder cancers. Both are 3 times as frequent in females. Risk of gallbladder cancer with gallstones is estimated at 0.43 per cent in 20 years.[15]

D. Free perforation usually appears in the very old (or very young) in the first attack, before the gallbladder thickens and is walled off.

E. The high death rate (12 to 25 per cent) and morbidity rate (24 per cent) are due to using this accepted compromise operation only for the desperately ill patient who is judged unable to withstand the definitive operation. Suppurative cholangitis adds to the mortality rate. It remains debatable whether stones left in the gallbladder or common duct increase mortality and morbidity.[27] Interval cholecystectomy after recovery should probably be done routinely, medical conditions permitting, especially if cholangiogram demonstrates stones or failure of passage of contrast medium into the duodenum.[26]

F. Mortality for urgent cholecystectomy is age-related. In patients younger than 60 it is 1 per cent; in those 60 to 70 it is 1.5 to 6 per cent; and in those older than 70, 18 to 20 per cent.

G. Mortality of elective cholecystectomy for good-risk patients is shown in the table.[16]

AGE (Years)	MORTALITY (%)	
	Female	Male
<50	0.054	0.104
50–69	0.28	0.54
>70	1.31	2.49

Poor-risk patients have case fatality rates 10 to 20 times higher than those of good-risk patients.[16] Common duct exploration causes a 2- to 4-fold increase in mortality.[16]

Morbidity of interval cholecystectomy includes[25] bile duct injury (0.5 to 0.254 per cent),[23,24] wound infection (1 to 2 per cent), wound dehiscence (1 per cent), pancreatitis (0.5 per cent), subhepatic abscess (0.5 per cent), wound hematoma (0.1 to 0.2 per cent), bile peritonitis (0.1 to 0.2 per cent), excessive bile leakage (0.1 to 0.2 per cent), and cholangitis (1 per cent). Overall complication rate is 3 to 5 per cent.

The incidence of wound infection is probably increased by routine drainage. It is increased 2 to 3 times when the drain is brought out from the wound.[11] Operative cholangiography does not increase the wound infection rate, but common duct exploration increases the rate 4-fold.[28]

H. The incidence of unsuspected common duct stones has been reported as varying between 0.3 and 6 per cent.[34-36] The need for routine operative cholangiography without clinical symptoms of stones is under debate.

I. Operative cholangiography has a complication rate of 1 to 2 per cent.[29] Wound infection rates are not increased. Incidence of unsatisfactory cholangiograms may range as high as 15 per cent.

J. Common duct exploration on clinical grounds alone leads to many unnecessary procedures. A history of jaundice results in a positive exploration rate of less than

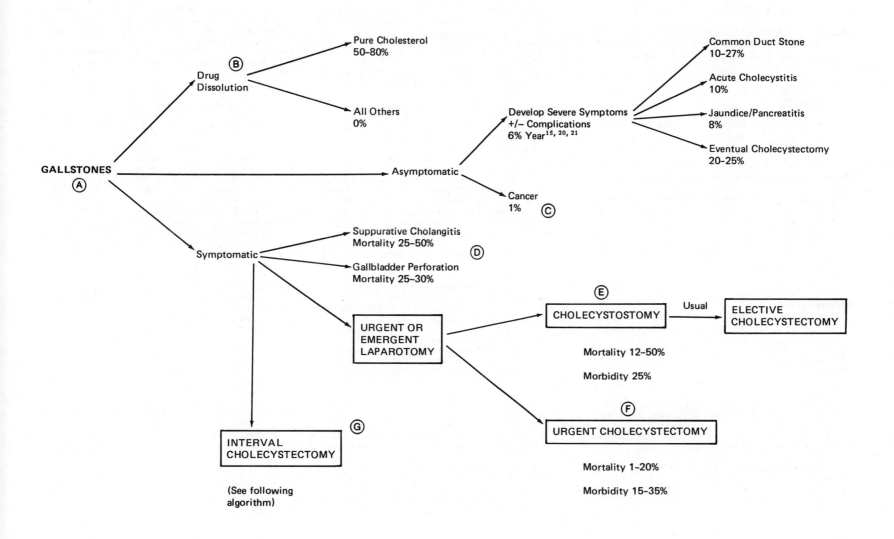

50 per cent[30, 40] and a history of pancreatitis[30] and small stones[30, 36] in a positive exploration rate of only 10 per cent.

K. Stones may pass spontaneously,[31, 32] and the rate of passage is higher when stones are small and near the T-tube site.

L. Stones up to 10 × 5 mm. in size have reportedly been removed by saline flush alone.[37]

M. Removal by forceps or Dormia basket through the T-tube tract approaches a 90 per cent success rate.[38] A T-tube of caliber no less than no. 14 French should be used routinely to facilitate such removal.

N. Re-exploration should be delayed at least 6 weeks for inflammation to subside. If nonoperative methods fail, 30 per cent of patients may require early re-exploration, and over 95 per cent may eventually require re-exploration.[39]

References

1. Torvik, A., and Hoivik, B.: Gallstones in an autopsy series. Acta Chir. Scand., *120*:168, 1960.
2. Ibach, J. R., Hume, A., and Erb, W.: Cholecystectomy in the aged. Surg. Gynecol. Obstet., *127*:523, 1968.
3. Edholm, P., and Joneson, G.: Bile duct stones related to age and duct width. Acta Chir. Scand., *124*:75, 1962.
4. Lahana, D. A., and Schoenfield, L. J.: Progress in medical therapy of gallstones. Surg. Clin. North Am., *53*:1053, 1973.
5. Berk, R. N.: Radiology of the gallbladder and the bile ducts. Surg. Clin. North Am., *53*:973, 1973.
6. Ochsner, S. F.: Performance and reliability of cholecystography. South Med. J., *63*:1268, 1970.
7. Muhajed, Z., Evans, J. P., and Whalen, J. P.: The nonopacified gallbladder on oral cholecystography. Radiology, *112*:1, 1974.
8. Leopold, G. R., et al.: Gray-scale ultrasonic cholecystography. A comparison with conventional radiographic techniques. Radiology, *121*:445, 1976.
9. Arnon, S., and Rosenquist, C. J.: Gray-scale cholecystosonography: An evaluation of accuracy. Am. J. Roentgenol., *127*:817, 1976.
10. Dompsey, P. J., et al.: Cholecystosonography for the diagnosis of cholecystolithiasis. Ann. Surg., *187*:465, 1978.
11. Bartrum, R. J., Crow, H. C., and Foote, R. T.: Ultrasonic and radiographic cholecystography. N. Engl. J. Med., *296*:538, 1977.
12. Howland, W. J., et al.: Drip-infusion cholangiography: A second look. Radiology, *107*:71, 1973.
13. Thorpe, C. D., et al.: Emergency intravenous cholangiography in patients with acute abdominal pain. Am. J. Surg., *125*:46, 1973.
14. Thistle, J. L., et al.: Chemotherapy for gallstone dissolution. JAMA, *239*:1041, 1978.
15. Fitzpatrick, G., Neutra, R., and Gilbert, J. P.: Cost-effectiveness of cholecystectomy for silent gallstones. *In* Bunker, J. P., Barnes, B. A., and Mostelles, F. (eds.): Costs, Risks, and Benefits of Surgery. New York, Oxford University Press, 1977.
16. Bishop, Y. M. M., and Mostelles, F.: Smoothed contingency table analysis. *In* Bunker, J. P., et al. (eds.): The National Halothane Study. Bethesda, Md., National Institutes of Health, National Institute of General Medical Sciences, 1969, pp. 259–266.
17. Todd, G. J., and Reemtsma, K.: Cholecystectomy with drainage. Am. J. Surg., *135*:622, 1978.
18. Thorbjarnarson, B., and Glenn, F.: Carcinoma of the gallbladder. Cancer, *12*:1009, 1959.
19. Gerst, P. H.: Primary carcinoma of the gallbladder: A 30-year summary. Ann. Surg., *153*:369, 1961.
20. Wenckert, A., and Robertson, B. The natural course of gallstone disease: 11-year review of 781 nonoperated cases. Gastroenterology, *50*:376, 1966.
21. Lund, J.: Surgical indications in cholelithiasis: Prophylactic cholecystectomy elucidated on the basis of long-term followup in 526 nonoperated cases. Ann. Surg., *151*:153, 1960.
22. Bornhurst, R. A., Heitzmann, E. R., and McAfie, J. G.: Double-dose drip-infusion cholangiography: An analysis of 107 consecutive cases. JAMA, *206*:1489, 1968.
23. Glenn, F.: Iatrogenic injuries to the biliary ductal system. Surg. Gynecol. Obstet., *146*:430, 1978.
24. Maingot, R.: Postoperative strictures of the bile ducts. *In* Maingot, R. (ed.): Abdominal Operations, 5th ed. New York, Appleton-Century-Crofts, 1969, p. 1124.
25. Hohn, J. C., Edmunds, L. H., and Baker, J. W.: Life-threatening complications after operations upon the biliary tract. Surg. Gynecol. Obstet., *127*:241, 1968.
26. Welch, J. P., and Malt, R. A.: Outcome of cholecystostomy. Surg. Gynecol. Obstet., *135*:717, 1972.
27. Moore, E. E., et al.: Reassessment of simple cholecystostomy. Arch. Surg., *114*:515, 1979.
28. Cruse, P. J. E.: Incidence of wound infection on the surgical services. Surg. Clin. North Am., *55*:1269, 1975.
29. McCormick, J. et al.: The operative cholangiogram: its interpretation, accuracy and value in association with cholecystectomy. Ann. Surg., *180*:902, 1974.
30. Mullen, J. T., et al.: One thousand cholecystectomies, extraducted palpation, and operative cholangiography. Am. J. Surg., *131*:672, 1978.
31. Bartlett, M. K.: Retained and recurrent common duct stones. Am. J. Surg., *38*:63, 1972.
32. Hampson, L. G., and Petrie, E. A.: The problem of stones in the common bile duct with particular reference to retained stones. Can. J. Surg., *7*:361, 1964.
33. Agbunag, A., Farringen, J. L., and Pickens, D. R. Operative cholangiograms. Am. Surg., *37*:746, 1971.
34. Edmunds, M. C., Emmett, J. M., and Clark, W. D.: Ten-year experience with operative cholangiography. Am. Surg., *26*:613, 1960.
35. Hight, D., Lingley, J. R., and Hurtubise, F.: An evaluation of operative cholangiograms as a guide to common duct exploration. Am. Surg., *150*:1086, 1959.
36. Jolly, P. C., et al.: Operative cholangiography: A case for its routine use. Ann. Surg., *168*:551, 1968.
37. Catt, P. B., et al.: Retained biliary calculi: Removal by a simple nonoperative technique. Ann. Surg., *180*:247, 1974.
38. Burhenne, H. J.: Complication of nonoperative extraction of retained common duct stones. Am. J. Surg., *131*:260, 1976.
39. Hicken, N. F., and McAllister, A. J.: Operative cholangiography as an aid in reducing the incidence of "overlooked" common duct stones: A study of 1293 choledocholithotomies. Surgery, *55*:753, 1964.
40. Marshall, J. F., and Bland, R. W.: Operations upon the common bile duct for stones. Ann. Surg., *149*:793, 1959.

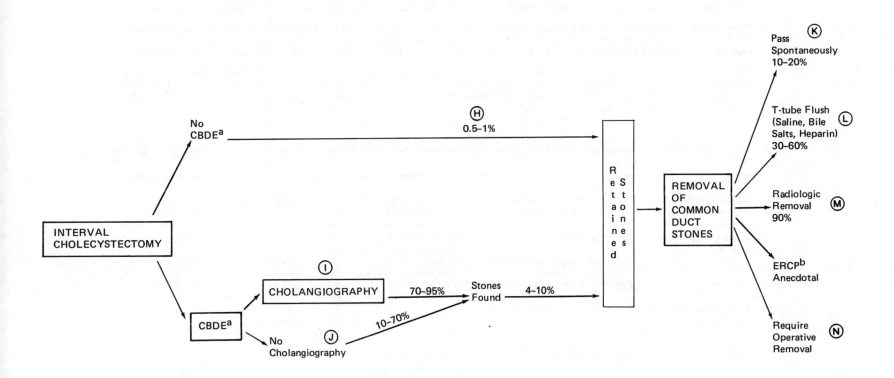

ADULT OBSTRUCTIVE JAUNDICE BY JOHN TERBLANCHE, CH.M.

Comments

A. Removal of retained stones via T-tube tract is an established procedure with a high success rate in experienced hands.[4]

B. Endoscopic sphincterotomy (papillotomy) for retained stones is still under evaluation. Proponents claim up to 90 per cent success in selected cases.[5] However, mortality is greater than 1 per cent, and complications, often severe, occur in 7 to 10 per cent of cases.

C. Direct infusion of sodium cholate via T-tube into the bile duct has had variable success.[1,2,6] Concurrently removed stones should be tested for dissolution in vitro. Mortality is 0 per cent and morbidity is minimal if technique is carefully followed. Diarrhea and occasional cholangitis are possible complications.[1,2,6] Mono-octanoin, a new solvent, is more effective in vitro and was successful in early trials.[7]

D. The most effective method of removal of residual stones is re-exploration of the bile duct. Mortality is quoted as 2 to 10 per cent but can be 0 per cent in experienced hands.[8] Associated cholangitis raises the mortality rate significantly. Lowest overall mortality and morbidity rates probably are achieved by combined use of established techniques, using simpler techniques first. That is, wait 4 to 6 weeks to determine if the stone will pass spontaneously, then have an expert extract the stone via T-tube tract or attempt to dissolve it, or both. If these fail, re-explore, unless the patient presents a prohibitive risk; in that case, endoscopic papillotomy is indicated.

E. In carcinoma of the bile ducts prognosis varies with site. The extrahepatic bile duct is divided into 5 regions, which are shown in the table.[9]

LOCATION OF CARCINOMA[9]	OPERATION OR TREATMENT	OPERATIVE MORTALITY (%)	5-YEAR SURVIVAL (%)	MEAN SURVIVAL
Main hepatic duct junction[9,10]	U-tube and radiotherapy	0–30 (mortality confined to elderly, poor-risk patients)	>20	>3 yr.
	Resection (usually not possible, except in 1 report)[11]	High (especially in inexperienced hands)	None reported	?
	Other	Variable	Very rare	3–18 mo.
Common hepatic duct and supraduodenal bile duct[9]	Resection (if possible)—rare	?	>50? (If resected)	?
Intrapancreatic bile duct and ampulla[12]	Pancreaticoduodenectomy	>15	20–30	1–3 yr.
	Palliative bypass	0–30 (esp. in elderly, poor-risk patients)	0	3–18 mo.
Diffuse carcinoma of bile ducts[9]	None	—	0	1–3 mo.
Gallbladder[13]	Right hepatic lobectomy or wide local resection	High	2–5	6–12 mo.
	None	—	0	1–3 mo.

F. Diagnosis and management of sclerosing cholangitis are controversial. There are two types, one associated with ulcerative colitis and the other truly primary. Recommended treatment is drainage via T-tube and administration of steroids with or without choleretic drugs. Prognosis is usually for an unremitting course. Survival may be a few months to 20 years. Mean survival is approximately 2 to 5 years. Complete remission has been reported.[14]

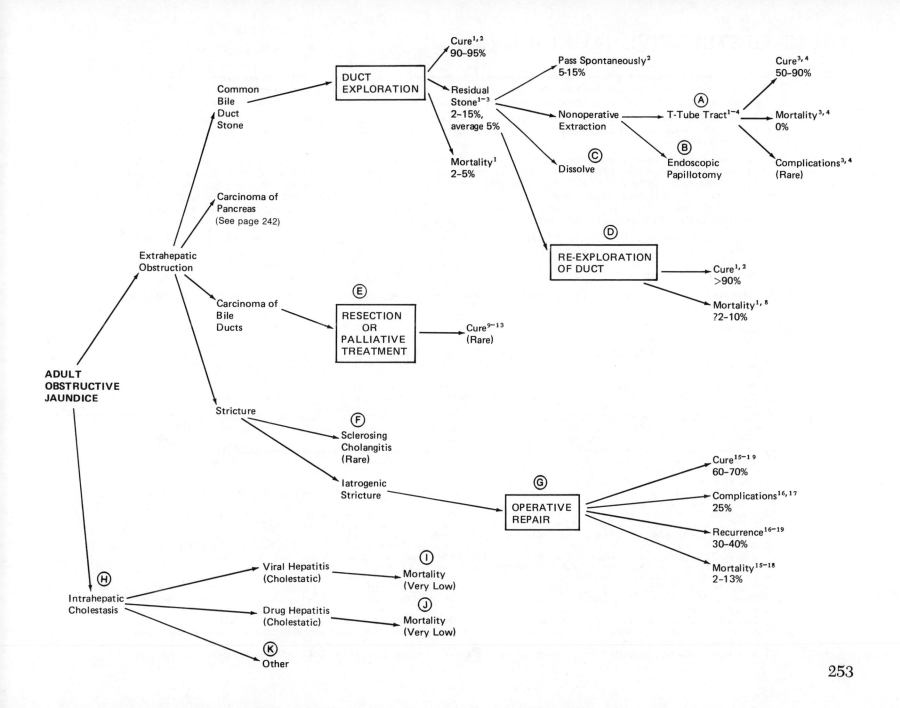

ADULT
OBSTRUCTIVE
JAUNDICE

Extrahepatic Obstruction

Common Bile Duct Stone

DUCT EXPLORATION

Cure[1,2] 90–95%

Residual Stone[1-3] 2–15%, average 5%

Mortality[1] 2–5%

Pass Spontaneously[2] 5-15%

Nonoperative Extraction

(C) Dissolve

(A) T-Tube Tract[1-4]

(B) Endoscopic Papillotomy

Cure[3,4] 50–90%

Mortality[3,4] 0%

Complications[3,4] (Rare)

Carcinoma of Pancreas (See page 242)

Carcinoma of Bile Ducts

(E) RESECTION OR PALLIATIVE TREATMENT

Cure[9-13] (Rare)

(D) RE-EXPLORATION OF DUCT

Cure[1,2] >90%

Mortality[1,8] ?2-10%

Stricture

(F) Sclerosing Cholangitis (Rare)

Iatrogenic Stricture

(G) OPERATIVE REPAIR

Cure[15-19] 60–70%

Complications[16,17] 25%

Recurrence[16-19] 30–40%

Mortality[15-18] 2-13%

(H) Intrahepatic Cholestasis

Viral Hepatitis (Cholestatic)

(I) Mortality (Very Low)

Drug Hepatitis (Cholestatic)

(J) Mortality (Very Low)

(K) Other

253

G. Quoted figures for iatrogenic strictures are from large series from major institutions. Isolated bad results are not reported in literature. To avoid prohibitive morbidity and mortality rates, this difficult surgery should only be undertaken by experts. The favored operation is hepaticojejunostomy,[15-19] preferably with mucosa-to-mucosa anastomosis. If that is not possible, a mucosal graft technique is advocated.[20,21]

H. Intrahepatic cholestasis[8,24,25] has a clinical and biochemical picture similar to that of extrahepatic obstruction. Newer diagnostic techniques (percutaneous transhepatic cholangiogram and ERCP) have improved prognosis while reducing the number of unnecessary operations being performed.[8]

I. All types of viral hepatitis can present in a cholestatic phase with obstructive jaundice. Hepatitis A (previously called infectious or short-incubation hepatitis) has a mortality less than 0.5 per cent and recovery is invariably complete,[22] although mortality from both fulminant hepatic failure and chronic liver disease has been reported recently.[23] Hepatitis B (previously called serum or long-incubation hepatitis) has mortality of 1 to 10 per cent (with the majority of deaths in the over-40 age group), and some of these patients develop chronic liver disease.[22] Hepatitis that is neither type A nor B (a recently recognized disease) has mortality and morbidity rates that are not yet defined, but perhaps more than 30 per cent of these patients develop chronic liver disease.

J. Drug hepatitis (cholestatic or hepatitic) is a hypersensitivity reaction (as opposed to a direct hepatotoxic reaction). An ever-increasing number of drugs are implicated as causing cholestatic hepatitis (see Table 1 of reference 24), with phenothiazines the most frequent offenders. Upon stopping administration of the drug, mortality becomes 0 per cent. Usually there is no residual liver disease. (Compare with the hepatitic type, which has a 20 to 50 per cent mortality and a tendency to develop chronic disease.)

K. Other causes include the familial congenital hyperbilirubinemias (Dubin-Johnson and Rotor types), primary biliary cirrhosis, and acute alcoholic hepatitis.[25]

References

1. Way, L. W., Admirand, W. H., and Dunphy, J. E.: Management of choledocholithiasis. Ann. Surg., *176*:347, 1972.
2. Way, L. W.: The retained common duct stone: Dissolution of retained common duct stones. Paper presented to the Society for Surgery of the Alimentary Tract, May 1978.
3. Patterson, H. C., Grice, O. D., and Bream, C. A.: Overlooked gallstones and their retrieval. Am. J. Surg., *125*:257, 1973.
4. Mazzariello, R.: Review of 220 cases of residual biliary tract calculi treated without reoperation: An eight-year study. Surgery, *73*:299, 1973.
5. Classen, M., and Safrany, L.: Endoscopic papillotomy and removal of gallstones. Br. Med. J., *4*:371, 1975.
6. Lansford, C., Mehta, S., and Kern, F.: The treatment of retained stones in the common bile duct with sodium cholate infusion. Gut, *15*:48, 1974.
7. Thistle, J. L., et al.: Effective dissolution of biliary tract stones by intraductal infusion of mono-octanoin. Gastroenterology, *74*:1103, 1978.
8. Blumgart, L. H.: Biliary tract obstruction: New approaches to old problems. Am. J. Surg., *135*:19, 1978.
9. Terblanche, J.: Carcinoma of the proximal extrahepatic biliary tree—Definitive and palliative treatment. Surg. Ann., *11*:249, 1978.
10. Terblanche, J.: Carcinoma of the main hepatic duct junction. *In* Way. L. W., and Dunphy, J. E., (eds.): Surgery of the Gall Bladder and Bile Ducts. Philadelphia, W. B. Saunders Co., 1979.
11. Iwasaki, Y., et al.: Treatment of carcinoma of the biliary system. Surg. Gynecol. Obstet., *144*:219, 1977.
12. Warren, K. W.: The evolution and current surgical management of periampullary carcinoma. Paper presented to the Society for Surgery of the Alimentary Tract, May 1978.
13. Kune, G. A.: Biliary tumors. *In* Kune, G. A. (ed.): Current Practice of Biliary Surgery. Boston, Little, Brown & Co., 1972, p. 249.
14. Fee, H. J., et al.: Sclerosing cholangitis and primary biliary cirrhosis—A disease spectrum. Ann. Surg., *186*:589, 1977.
15. Way, L. W., and Dunphy, J. E.: Biliary stricture. Am. J. Surg., *124*:287, 1972.
16. Warren, K. W., and Jefferson, M. F.: Prevention and repair of strictures of the extrahepatic bile ducts. Surg. Clin. North Am., *53*:1169, 1973.
17. Braasch, J. W., Warren, K. W., and Blevins, P. K.: Progress in biliary stricture repair. Am. J. Surg., *129*:34, 1975.
18. Lane, C. E., et al.: Long-term results of Roux-en-Y hepatocholangiojejunostomy. Ann. Surg., *177*:714, 1973.
19. Glenn, F.: Iatrogenic injuries to the biliary ductal system. Surg. Gynecol. Obstet., *146*:430, 1978.
20. Wexler, M. J., and Smith, R.: Jejunal mucosal graft: A sutureless technique for repair of high bile duct strictures. Am. J. Surg., *129*:204, 1975.
21. Daugherty, M., et al.: Proximal hepatic duct reconstruction. Repair using sutureless mucosal graft hepaticojejunostomy. Arch. Surg., *113*:490, 1978.
22. Aach, R. D.: Viral hepatitis—A to e. Med. Clin. North Am., *62*:59, 1978.
23. Rakela, J., et al.: Hepatitis A virus infection in fulminant hepatitis and chronic active hepatitis. Gastroenterology, *74*:879, 1978.
24. Klatskin, G.: Drug-induced hepatic injury. *In* Schaffner, F., Sherlock, S., and Leevy, C. M. (eds.): The Liver and Its Diseases. New York. Intercontinental Medical Book Corp., 1974, p. 163.
25. Sherlock, S.: Cholestasis. *In* Sherlock, S. (ed.): Diseases of the Liver and Biliary System, 5th ed. Oxford, Blackwell Scientific Publications, 1975, p. 260.

LIVER TUMORS

LIVER TUMORS BY ARTHUR F. JONES, M.D., AND JOHN TERBLANCHE, CH.M.

Comments

A. Resection is not advised because mortality is prohibitive. No other forms of treatment are of proven value. Untreated patients survive 1 to 5 months.[1] There are no 5-year cures.[2]

B. Occasional patients survive a year or more.

C. Other than infusion chemotherapy directly into the hepatic artery, which may prolong survival by months,[3] there are no forms of treatment of any value. These include systemic chemotherapy,[4] hepatic artery ligation,[5] radiotherapy,[4] and transplantation.[6]

D. In the U.S.A., about 30 per cent of cases are unassociated with cirrhosis.[7] There is marked geographic variation.

E. These are unresectable if multicentric or if both lobes are involved. They are not to be resected if distant metastases are present. (Diagnosis requires full tumor-seeking survey, especially of bones and lungs.)

F. Late mortality is due to undetected distant metastases or involvement of residual liver.

G. Few figures are available. Prognosis and treatment are similar to those for hepatocellular carcinoma.

H. Prolonged survival without treatment is fairly frequent. These tumors remain localized to the liver until late in the course of disease. Death is from biliary obstruction and liver failure.[12]

I. Radiotherapy in addition to dilatation and U-tube therapy may even hold out hope for cure.[12]

J. Although such tumors are usually unresectable and the results of resection are disappointing,[12] Iwasaki and associates[13] performed 9 "curative resections" on 23 patients, and 6 were alive and well at between 5 and 23 months.

K. After dilatation with or without stenting, survival is 6 months to 2 years, but repeated operations often are necessary.[12] Five-year survival is rare. Palliative bypass with intrahepatic duct–to–bowel anastomosis is disappointing,[12] except in one report.[14] Hepatic transplantation is not justified at present.[15]

L. Prognosis and treatment are the same as for adults.

M. Survival with untreated hepatoblastoma is 1 to 2 months.[16] Such tumors should be resected if possible.[17, 18] Resectability rate is 30 to 40 per cent,[17] and 5-year survival is 45 to 50 per cent.[18] Operative mortality is ±20 per cent.[18] Other treatment is not of proven value.

N. Unlike metastases elsewhere, liver metastases of colorectal cancer have proved to be quite resistant to systemic chemotherapy.[24] Other treatment is also of no benefit. (See Comment C.)

O. Resection other than local excision of an area of direct infiltration is not justified in most patients, because 5-year survival is almost nil[22, 23, 26] and there is no other treatment of proven value. (See Comment C.)

P. Survival with untreated tumor may be prolonged. Even palliative resection is worthwhile to reduce unpleasant symptoms.[27]

Q. More than 85 per cent are small inciden-

tal lesions that are treated by observation.[28] (See Comment W.)

R. Rupture of lesions larger than 4 cm. in diameter is fatal in 75 per cent of cases.[29] The incidence of rupture is unknown. Operative mortality is unacceptable in benign lesions, so resection must be undertaken by an expert surgeon.[10, 11] Radiation therapy has been used in cases in which resection is impossible.[30]

S. Oral contraceptives should be discontinued in all such patients, and another contraceptive method should be used or sterilization performed.[31, 32]

T. Because the lesion has only recently been recognized, valid figures are difficult to obtain. Mortality of resection is low in major centers. Patients presenting with intraperitoneal rupture and bleeding have a high mortality rate.[31] Hepatic artery interruption (ligation or embolization) is a safe alternative treatment.[31]

U. Figures are difficult to obtain. Intraperitoneal rupture and bleeding are less common than with hepatic adenoma;[32] thus, after discontinuing the contraceptive pill, more conservative treatment such as observation is justified.[31] If the lesion becomes symptomatic or does not decrease in size, hepatic artery interuption or hepatic lobectomy is indicated.[31]

V. Treatment is still controversial. Local resection, if the tumor is small and superficial, or biopsy is required in all cases; otherwise, treatment is as in Comment U.[31]

W. The only important concern with other small lesions (bile duct adenoma, cholangioadenoma) is to avoid erroneous diagnosis of hepatic metastasis when found at

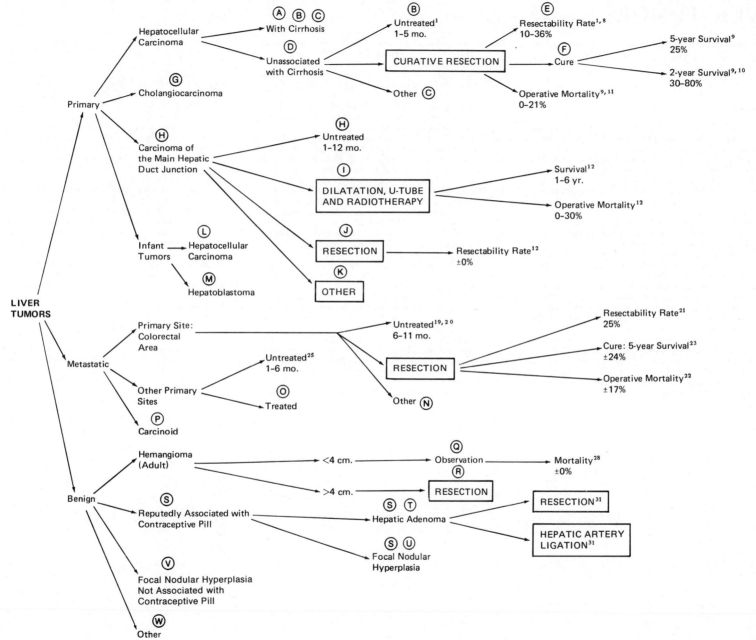

LIVER TUMORS

Primary

Hepatocellular Carcinoma
Ⓐ Ⓑ Ⓒ With Cirrhosis
Ⓓ Unassociated with Cirrhosis

Untreated[1]
1–5 mo.

CURATIVE RESECTION

Other Ⓒ

Resectability Rate[1, 8]
10–36%

Ⓔ

Ⓕ Cure

Operative Mortality[9, 11]
0–21%

5-year Survival[9]
25%

2-year Survival[9, 10]
30–80%

Ⓖ Cholangiocarcinoma

Ⓗ Carcinoma of the Main Hepatic Duct Junction

Ⓗ Untreated
1–12 mo.

Ⓘ DILATATION, U-TUBE AND RADIOTHERAPY

Survival[12]
1–6 yr.

Operative Mortality[12]
0–30%

Ⓙ RESECTION

Resectability Rate[12]
±0%

Ⓚ OTHER

Infant Tumors
Ⓛ Hepatocellular Carcinoma
Ⓜ Hepatoblastoma

Metastatic

Primary Site: Colorectal Area

Untreated[19, 20]
6–11 mo.

RESECTION

Other Ⓝ

Resectability Rate[21]
25%

Cure: 5-year Survival[23]
±24%

Operative Mortality[22]
±17%

Other Primary Sites
Untreated[25]
1–6 mo.
Ⓞ Treated

Ⓟ Carcinoid

Benign

Hemangioma (Adult)
<4 cm. ⟶ Ⓠ Observation ⟶ Mortality[28] ±0%
>4 cm. ⟶ Ⓡ RESECTION

Ⓢ Reputedly Associated with Contraceptive Pill

Ⓢ Ⓣ Hepatic Adenoma
RESECTION[31]
HEPATIC ARTERY LIGATION[31]

Ⓢ Ⓤ Focal Nodular Hyperplasia

Ⓥ Focal Nodular Hyperplasia Not Associated with Contraceptive Pill

Ⓦ Other

257

LIVER TUMORS *Continued*

laparotomy for abdominal malignancy. Biopsy and frozen section will give the diagnosis.

References

1. Bengmark, S., Börjesson, B., and Hafström, L.: The natural history of primary carcinoma of the liver. Scand. J. Gastroenterol., 6:351, 1971.
2. Lin, T-Y.: Result in 107 hepatic lobectomies with a preliminary report on the use of a clamp to reduce blood loss. Ann. Surg., 177:413, 1973.
3. Cady, B., and Oberfield, R. A.: Arterial infusion chemotherapy of hepatoma. Surg. Gynecol. Obstet., 138:381, 1974.
4. Cochrane, A. M. G., et al.: Quadruple chemotherapy versus radiotherapy in treatment of primary hepatocellular carcinoma. Cancer, 40:609, 1977.
5. Almersjö, O., et al.: Evaluation of hepatic dearterialization in primary and secondary cancer of the liver. Am. J. Surg., 124:5, 1972.
6. Starzl, T. E., et al.: Orthotopic liver transplantation in 93 patients. Surg. Gynecol. Obstet., 142:487, 1976.
7. Ihde, D. C., et al.: Clinical manifestations of hepatoma: A review of 6 years' experience at a cancer hospital. Am. J. Med., 56:83, 1974.
8. Flatmark, A., et al.: Surgical treatment of primary liver carcinoma. Scand. J. Gastroenterol., 12:571, 1977.
9. Foster, J. H., and Berman, M. M.: Primary epithelial cancer in adults. *In* Foster, J. H., and Berman, M. M. (eds.): Solid Liver Tumors. Philadelphia, W. B. Saunders, 1977, p. 62.
10. Fortner, J. G., et al.: Major hepatic resection for neoplasia: Personal experience in 108 patients. Ann. Surg., 188:363, 1978.
11. Starzl, T. E., et al.: Hepatic trisegmentectomy and other liver resections. Surg. Gynecol. Obstet., 141:429, 1975.
12. Terblanche, J.: Carcinoma of the proximal extrahepatic biliary tree: Definitive and palliative treatment. Surg. Annu., 11, 1979. (In press.)
13. Iwasaki, Y., et al.: Treatment of carcinoma of the biliary system. Surg. Gynecol. Obstet., 144:219, 1977.
14. Bismuth, H., and Corlette, M. B.: Intrahepatic cholangioenteric anastomosis in carcinoma of the hilus of the liver. Surg. Gynecol. Obstet., 140:170, 1975.
15. Terblanche, J.: Is carcinoma of the main hepatic duct junction an indication for liver transplantation or palliative surgery? A plea for the U-tube palliative procedure. Surgery, 79:127, 1976.
16. Ishak, K. G., and Glunz, R. P.: Hepatoblastoma and hepatocarcinoma in infancy and childhood: Report of 47 cases. Cancer, 20:396, 1967.
17. Clatworthy, H. W., Schiller, M., and Grosfeld, J. L.: Primary liver tumors in infancy and childhood. Arch. Surg., 109:143, 1974.
18. Foster, J. H., and Berman, M. M.: Pediatric epithelial tumors. *In* Foster, J. H., and Berman, M. M. (eds.): Solid Liver Tumors. Philadelphia, W. B. Saunders, 1977, p. 105.
19. Bengmark, S., and Hafström, L.: Natural history of primary and secondary malignant tumors of the liver. I. Prognosis for patients with hepatic metastases from colonic and rectal carcinoma by laparotomy. Cancer, 23:198, 1969.
20. Morris, M. J., et al.: Hepatic metastases from colorectal carcinoma: An analysis of survival rate and histopathology. Aust. N.Z. J. Surg., 47:365, 1977.
21. Raven, R. W.: Hepatectomy. Proc. Int. Soc. Surg., 16:1099, 1955.
22. Foster, J. H., and Berman, M. M.: Resection of metastatic tumors. *In* Foster, J. H., and Berman, M. M. (eds.): Solid Liver Tumors. Philadelphia, W. B. Saunders, 1977, p. 209.
23. Flanagan, L., and Foster, J. H.: Hepatic resection for metastatic cancer. Am. J. Surg., 113:551, 1967.
24. Rapaport, A. H., and Burleson, R. C.: Survival of patients treated with systemic fluorouracil for hepatic metastases. Surg. Gynecol. Obstet., 130:773, 1970.
25. Jaffe, B. M., et al.: Factors influencing survival in patients with untreated hepatic metastasis. Surg. Gynecol. Obstet., 127:1, 1968.
26. Almersjö, O., Bengmark, S., and Hafström, L.: Liver resection for cancer. Acta Chir. Scand, 142:139, 1976.
27. Shiu, M. H., and Fortner, J. G.: Current management of hepatic tumors. Surg. Gynecol. Obstet., 140:781, 1975.
28. Adam, Y. G., Huvos, A. G., and Fortner, J. G.: Giant hemangiomas of the liver. Ann. Surg., 172:239, 1970.
29. Sewell, J. H., and Weiss, K.: Spontaneous rupture of hemangioma of the liver. Arch. Surg., 83:729, 1961.
30. Park, W. C., and Phillips, R.: The role of radiation therapy in the management of hemangiomas of the liver. JAMA, 212:1496, 1970.
31. Terblanche, J.: Liver tumors associated with the use of contraceptive pills. S. Afr. Med. J., 53:439, 1978.
32. Klatskin, G.: Hepatic tumors: Possible relationship to use of oral contraceptives. Gastroenterology, 73:386, 1977.

LIVER TRANSPLANTATION

LIVER TRANSPLANTATION BY LAWRENCE J. KOEP, M.D., AND THOMAS E. STARZL, M.D.

Comments

A. There are only two groups of liver transplants that are large enough for statistical analysis — our own and that of Calne in England. This chapter pertains only to our own experience.[1,2]

B. The prognosis for acute hepatitis is so difficult to project that a terminal condition is recognized too late to provide adequate time for locating a suitable donor.

C. Portal vein patency is imperative in order to provide the hepatic homograft with necessary hepatotrophic factors. Portosystemic shunts are taken down at the time of surgery. We prefer to do distal splenorenal shunts in potential recipients, though an end-to-side portacaval shunt can readily be taken down also. Hepatic artery occlusion is not a contraindication, since the donor hepatic artery can be anastomosed to the aorta, but this entails considerably more dissection.

D. The Denver experience has been poor in malignant disease, and recipients with malignancies are now generally avoided. Our longest survivor, however, had a small incidental hepatoma. Calne has had a more favorable experience with malignancies.[3]

E. Metabolic diseases treated by hepatic transplants are Wilson's disease, alpha$_1$-antitrypsin deficiency, and tyrosinemia.

F. Miscellaneous causes for adult hepatic transplantation are secondary biliary cirrhosis, sclerosing cholangitis, massive hepatic necrosis, Budd-Chiari syndrome, and congenital biliary hypoplasia.

G. A number of changes were made in August 1976 that resulted in improved survival. This latest group is presented separately as an indication of the survival currently enjoyed. Survival rates beyond one year include small numbers from all disease categories. The longest survivor is in good health 9 years after transplantation.

References

1. Starzl, T. E., and Koep, L. J.: Transplantation of the liver in human subjects. *In* Maingot, R. (ed.): Abdominal Operations, 7th Ed. New York, Appleton-Century-Crofts (in press).
2. Starzl, T. E., and Putnam, C. W.: Experience in Hepatic Transplantation. Philadelphia, W. B. Saunders Co., 1969.
3. Calne, R. Y., and Williams, R.: Orthotopic liver transplantation: The first 60 patients. Br. Med. J., *1*:471, 1977.

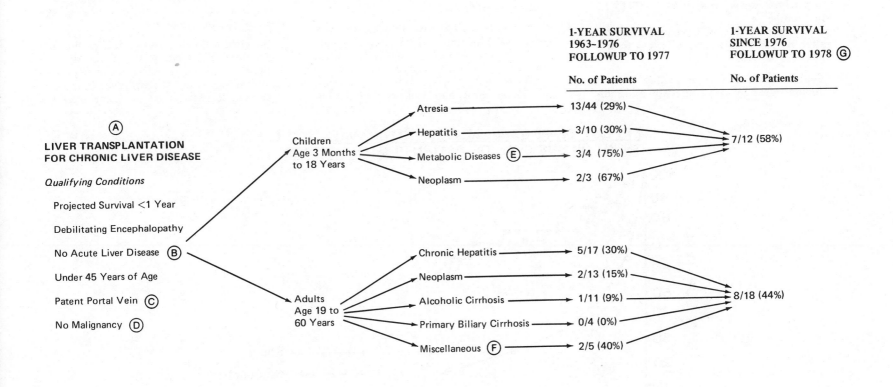

Ⓐ

**LIVER TRANSPLANTATION
FOR CHRONIC LIVER DISEASE**

Qualifying Conditions

Projected Survival <1 Year

Debilitating Encephalopathy

No Acute Liver Disease Ⓑ

Under 45 Years of Age

Patent Portal Vein Ⓒ

No Malignancy Ⓓ

Children
Age 3 Months
to 18 Years

Adults
Age 19 to
60 Years

Atresia

Hepatitis

Metabolic Diseases Ⓔ

Neoplasm

Chronic Hepatitis

Neoplasm

Alcoholic Cirrhosis

Primary Biliary Cirrhosis

Miscellaneous Ⓕ

**1-YEAR SURVIVAL
1963–1976
FOLLOWUP TO 1977**

No. of Patients

13/44 (29%)

3/10 (30%)

3/4 (75%)

2/3 (67%)

5/17 (30%)

2/13 (15%)

1/11 (9%)

0/4 (0%)

2/5 (40%)

**1-YEAR SURVIVAL
SINCE 1976
FOLLOWUP TO 1978** Ⓖ

No. of Patients

7/12 (58%)

8/18 (44%)

PORTAL HYPERTENSION BY MELVIN M. NEWMAN, M.D.

Comments

A. The etiology of cirrhosis differs geographically. In the U.S., esophageal varices are most commonly due to alcoholic cirrhosis (50 to 60 per cent of cases), postviral hepatitis (20 per cent), and other causes (drug-induced, biliary, hemochromatosis, and others) (15 to 20 per cent).[1]

   The probability of developing varices after type B viral hepatitis is less than 3 per cent.[2]

B. The incidence of nonbleeding varices demonstrated by esophagoscopy and radiography in patients with known liver disease has some influence on prognosis, but no extensive clinical reports are available. Dilated esophageal veins may occur during normal pregnancy without liver disease and disappear following delivery.[3] Prophylactic shunting of varices that have not bled in the cirrhotic patient does not prolong life.[4]

C. In the series of 476 patients with massive upper GI bleeding from Harlem Hospital in New York, endoscopy showed gastritis in 45 per cent of cases, gastric or duodenal ulcer in 27 per cent, bleeding varices in 26 per cent, and Mallory-Weiss tears and other miscellaneous causes in 1.4 per cent.[5a] Even in the 116 patients with identified liver disease, 57 per cent bled from gastritis and 27 per cent from varices. In the series from Paris reported by Franco and associates,[5b] bleeding in cirrhotic patients was caused by varices 52 per cent of the time, by acute mucosal ulceration in 41 per cent, and by chronic peptic ulcers in 7 per cent.

D. Survival following recovery from the first incident of bleeding varies greatly, depending on whether the portal hypertension is secondary to liver disease or to extrahepatic obstruction. As Clatworthy has

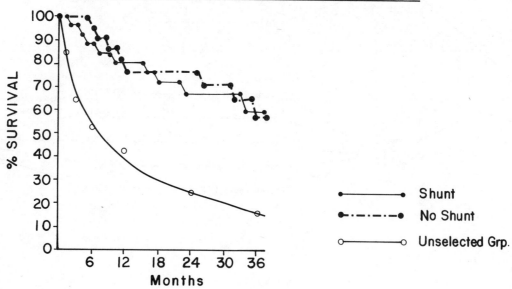

EFFECT OF PROPHYLACTIC PORTOCAVAL
SHUNT ON SURVIVAL OF PATIENTS WITH VARICES

● —— ● Shunt

● -·-·- ● No Shunt

○ —— ○ Unselected Grp.

FIGURE 1

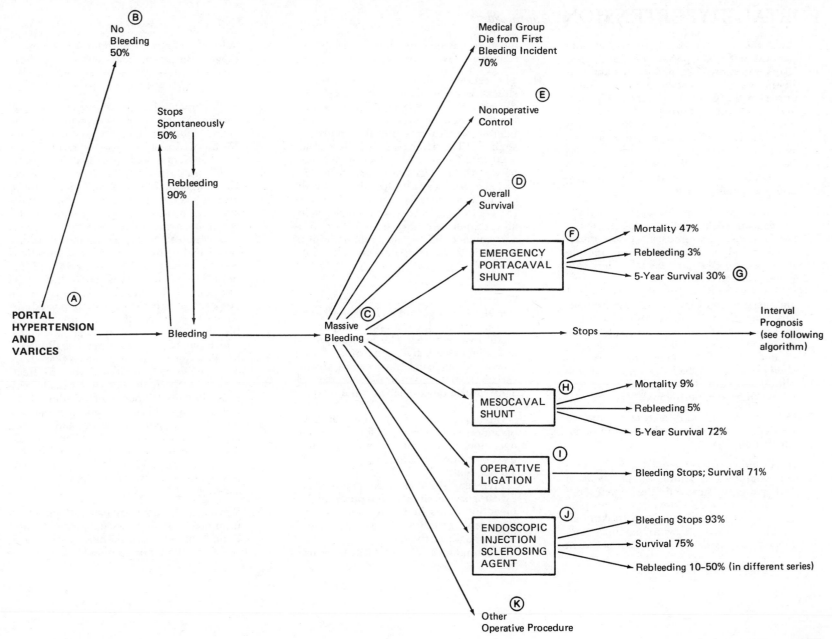

No
Bleeding
50% Ⓑ

Stops
Spontaneously
50%

Rebleeding
90%

PORTAL
HYPERTENSION
AND Ⓐ
VARICES

Bleeding

Massive
Bleeding Ⓒ

Medical Group
Die from First
Bleeding Incident
70%

Nonoperative Ⓔ
Control

Overall Ⓓ
Survival

EMERGENCY
PORTACAVAL Ⓕ
SHUNT

Mortality 47%

Rebleeding 3%

5-Year Survival 30% Ⓖ

Stops ——— Interval
Prognosis
(see following
algorithm)

MESOCAVAL Ⓗ
SHUNT

Mortality 9%

Rebleeding 5%

5-Year Survival 72%

OPERATIVE Ⓘ
LIGATION

Bleeding Stops; Survival 71%

ENDOSCOPIC Ⓙ
INJECTION
SCLEROSING
AGENT

Bleeding Stops 93%

Survival 75%

Rebleeding 10–50% (in different series)

Other Ⓚ
Operative Procedure

said,[6] there is a vast difference between patients with bad portal veins and good livers and those with good veins and bad livers. As can be seen from the lower curve on the graph in Figure 1 (Garceau and coworkers[4a]), 60 per cent of patients with cirrhosis and nonbleeding varices have died by 12 months, and nearly 65 per cent have died by 24 months. Even if he does not bleed, the cirrhotic patient is at high risk of dying from liver failure and encephalopathy.[7]

E. Nonoperative means of control include Sengstaken-Blakemore tube (84 per cent)[8] and Pitressin (vasopressin) given either intravenously or into the superior mesenteric artery (95 per cent).[9] They are equally effective.

  Selective embolization of the esophageal and gastric coronary veins gave temporary control in 15 of 21 patients treated by Lunderquist and associates at the University of Lund, Sweden. However, reexamination of 16 long-term survivors showed that 13 had recannulized the obliterated vein. The procedure must still be considered experimental.[10b]

F. Orloff has found no difference in survival between end-to-side or side-to-side portacaval shunt.[11]

G. In Orloff's patients undergoing emergency portacaval shunt, 53 per cent of 146 patients survived the operation.[12] Twenty-six per cent developed encephalopathy, 59 per cent stopped drinking alcohol, 57 per cent were gainfully employed, 3 per cent rebled, 99 per cent

retained patency of shunt, and 37 per cent were alive at 10 years.

H. The patient with extrahepatic portal obstruction, often a child or young adult, can sometimes be treated by anastomosing the superior mesenteric vein to the inferior vena cava, called the "mesocaval shunt."[13] The Drapanas H-graft employs a 20 to 22 mm. wide Dacron prosthesis between the superior mesenteric vein and the vena cava.[14] Operative mortality of this procedure is 9 per cent. Eleven per cent of patients develop encephalopathy, 22 per cent have liver failure, 5 per cent rebleed, 95 per cent retain shunt patency, and 72 per cent are alive at 5 years.

I. With ligation of varices under direct vision through a gastrotomy, 95 per cent of patients stop bleeding but 30 per cent die of liver failure.[15] The Sugiura procedure is more extensive, consisting of transthoracic esophageal transection and devascularization and transabdominal esophageal-gastric devascularization and splenectomy.[16]

  Operative mortality for the emergency operation is 12 per cent; for the elective operation in patients who have had at least one previous bleeding incident, it is 1.8 per cent.

  Five-year survival is 83 per cent and 7-year survival is also 83 per cent. Rebleeding occurs in 1.5 per cent of cases. Recurrent bleeding is usually due to hemorrhagic gastritis.

  When mesocaval or portacaval shunting

failed to control life-threatening hemorrhage, Bernstein and colleagues have used total esophagectomy or total gastrectomy as a "last ditch" measure.[17]

J. Endoscopic injection of varices has had varying degrees of acceptance for 40 years. Johnston and Rogers of Belfast, Northern Ireland,[18] use a rigid Negus esophagoscope with proximal lighting to avoid obscuring of the light by blood. Ethanolamine oleate (2 to 3 ml.) is injected into each varix, which is then tamponaded by turning the scope until the tip compresses the injection site for one to two minutes. A total of 25 ml. of sclerosant can be used per session. Injections were carried out 217 times in 117 patients. Hemorrhage was controlled in 93 per cent of the admissions; however, 18 per cent of the patients died per admission: 19 out of 35 from uncontrolled bleeding, 10 out of 35 from hepatic coma, and 6 out of 35 from unrelated illnesses. Similar figures have been reported by Terblanche of Cape Town with 51 treatments in 22 patients: Hemorrhage was controlled in 92 per cent of admissions, but mortality in the bleeding patient was 25 per cent per admission and 18 per cent per injection session. This was far lower than the 60 per cent mortality previously experienced with other emergency treatments of varices in Cape Town.[19]

K. Warren and associates have attempted to minimize hepatic encephalopathy and liver failure by maintaining perfusion of the liver with portal blood while selec-

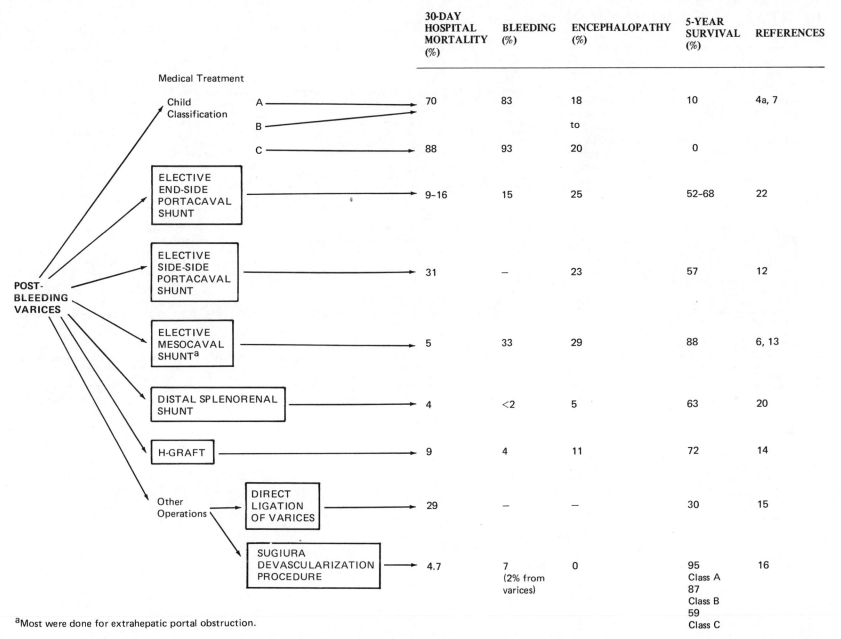

	30-DAY HOSPITAL MORTALITY (%)	BLEEDING (%)	ENCEPHALOPATHY (%)	5-YEAR SURVIVAL (%)	REFERENCES
Medical Treatment					
Child Classification A	70	83	18	10	4a, 7
B			to		
C	88	93	20	0	
ELECTIVE END-SIDE PORTACAVAL SHUNT	9–16	15	25	52–68	22
ELECTIVE SIDE-SIDE PORTACAVAL SHUNT	31	—	23	57	12
ELECTIVE MESOCAVAL SHUNT[a]	5	33	29	88	6, 13
DISTAL SPLENORENAL SHUNT	4	<2	5	63	20
H-GRAFT	9	4	11	72	14
Other Operations — DIRECT LIGATION OF VARICES	29	—	—	30	15
SUGIURA DEVASCULARIZATION PROCEDURE	4.7	7 (2% from varices)	0	95 Class A 87 Class B 59 Class C	16

POST-BLEEDING VARICES

[a]Most were done for extrahepatic portal obstruction.

265

tively decompressing esophageal varices by a distal splenorenal shunt and ligation of the gastric coronary vein.[20] However, the final answer has not yet been found. Extensive studies of pre- and postshunt pressures and flows were done by Burchell and associates in 145 patients. There was no relationship between large or small portal flows and the hospital mortality rate, incidence of encephalopathy, or long-term survival.[21]

References

1a. Mackay, I.: Chronic hepatitis. Can. Med. Assoc. J. *106*:519–524, 1972.

1b. Martini, G., and Bode, C. H.: The epidemiology of cirrhosis of the liver. *In* Engel, A., and Larssen, T. (eds.): Alcoholic Cirrhosis and Other Toxic Hepatopathies. Stockholm, Nordiska Bokhandelns Vorlag, 1970, pp. 315–335.

2a. Redeker, A. E.: Viral hepatitis: Clinical aspects. Am. J. Med. Sci., *270*:9–16, 1975.

2b. Fauerholdt, L., et al.: Significance of suspected "chronic aggressive hepatitis" in acute hepatitis. Gastroenterology, *73*:543–548, 1977.

3. Palmer, E. B.: Endoscopic contributions to the understanding of portal hypertension. Ann. N.Y. Acad. Sci., *170*:164–175, 1970.

4a. Garceau, A., et al. (Boston Inter-Hospital Group): A controlled trial of prophylactic portacaval-shunt surgery. N. Engl. J. Med., *270*:496–500, 1964.

4b. Jackson, F. C., et al. (Cooperative VAH study): A clinical investigation of the portacaval shunt. II. Survival analysis of the prophylactic operation. Am. J. Surg., *115*:22–42, 1968.

5a. Josen, A. S., et al. (Harlem Hospital): Immediate endoscopic diagnosis of upper gastrointestinal bleeding. Arch. Surg., *111*:981–986, 1976.

5b. Franco, D., et al.: Upper gastrointestinal haemorrhage in hepatic cirrhosis: Causes and relation to hepatic failure and stress. Lancet, *1*:218–220, 1977.

6. Clatworthy, H. W., Jr.: Extrahepatic portal hypertension. *In* Child, C. G., 3rd (ed.): Portal Hypertension. Philadelphia, W. B. Saunders Co., 1974, pp. 243–266.

7. Garceau, A. J., Chalmers, T. C., and the Boston Inter-Hospital Liver Group: The natural history of cirrhosis. I. Survival with esophageal varices. N. Engl. J. Med., *268*:469–473, 1963.

8. Bauer, J. J., Kreel, I., and Kark, A. E.: The use of the Sengstaken-Blakemore tube for immediate control of bleeding esophageal varices. Ann. Surg., *179*:273–277, 1974.

9. Johnson, W. C., et al.: Control of bleeding varices by vasopressin. A prospective randomized study. Ann. Surg., *186*:369–276, 1977.

10a. Rösch, J., and Dotter, C. T.: Angiography in the diagnosis and therapy of bleeding from gastroesophageal varices. Yale J. Biol. Med., *49*:361–372, 1976.

10b. Lunderquist, A., et al.: Followup of patients with portal hypertension and esophageal varices treated with percutaneous obliteration of gastric coronary vein. Radiology, *122*:59–63, 1977.

11. Orloff, M. J., et al.: Comparison of end-to-side and side-to-side portacaval shunts in dogs and human subjects with cirrhosis and portal hypertension. Am. J. Surg., *128*:195–201, 1974.

12. Orloff, M. J., et al.: Criteria for selection of patients for emergency portacaval shunt. Am. J. Surg., *134*:146–151, 1977.

13. Voorhees, A. B., and Price, J. B.: Extrahepatic portal hypertension. Arch. Surg., *108*:338–341, 1974.

14. Drapanas, T.: Interposition mesocaval shunt for treatment of portal hypertension. Ann. Surg., *176*:435–456, 1972.

15. Wirthlin, L. S., et al.: Transthoracoesophageal ligation of bleeding esophageal varices. Arch. Surg., *109*:688–692, 1974.

16. Sugiura, M., and Futagawa, S.: Further evaluation of the Sugiura procedure in the treatment of esophageal varices. Arch. Surg., *112*:1317–1321, 1977.

17. Bernstein, E. F., et al.: Treatment of bleeding esophageal varices in portal-systemic shunt failures. Arch. Surg., *99*:171–178, 1969.

18. Johnston, G. W., and Rodgers, H. W.: A review of 15 years' experience in the use of sclerotherapy in the control of acute haemorrhage from oesophageal varices. Br. J. Surg., *60*:797–800, 1973.

19. Terblanche, J.: The use of injection sclerotherapy in the management of esophageal varices. Seminar given at the University of Colorado Medical Center, Denver, 25 March 1978.

20. Galambos, J. T., et al.: Selective and total shunts in the treatment of bleeding varices. A randomized controlled trial. N. Engl. J. Med., *295*:1089–1095, 1976.

21. Burchell, A. R., et al.: Hemodynamic variables and prognosis following portacaval shunts. Surg. Gynecol. Obstet., *138*:359–369, 1974.

22. McDermott, W. V., Jr.: Surgery of the Liver and Portal Circulation. Philadelphia, Lea & Febiger, 1974, Chapter 7.

SPLENECTOMY

SPLENECTOMY BY G. E. ARAGON, M.D.

Comments

A. Course following therapeutic splenectomy for congenital hemolytic anemia (CHA), idiopathic thrombocytopenia (ITP), reticuloendothelial diseases, and malignancies is primarily that of the disease and not of the treatment (splenectomy). Much of the controversy surrounding sepsis thus arises. Overall mortality is slightly over 3 per cent,[1, 2] of which sepsis accounts for 11 per cent. Mortality for ITP is 1.1 to 1.4 per cent; for CHA, 0.25 per cent; for advanced malignancy, 7.5 per cent. Late sepsis after splenectomy for Hodgkin's disease is 11.5 per cent, with 5 per cent mortality, now believed to be strongly related to the treatment administered for the primary disease (chemotherapy) rather than to the splenectomy.[3]

B. Incidental splenectomy as a result of intraoperative damage still accounts for one quarter of all splenectomies in most hospitals.[4, 5] Mortality is 3 to 15 per cent and complications are 13 to 50 per cent.[4, 6, 7] Hospital stay is increased 70 per cent (29 vs. 19 days). Sixty per cent of cases occur in conjunction with vagus nerve or stomach surgery.[5]

C. The data base for observation (total 26 cases), suture repair (total 20 cases), and partial splenectomy (total 8 cases) is meager and highly selective.[6, 8-10, 13-17] Observation has been primarily in children.[8-10] Recent availability of microfibrillar collagen (Avitene) and other hemostatic agents has increased the feasibility of such tissue-preserving procedures.

D. The spleen is ruptured in one third of blunt abdominal injuries, necessitating laparotomy.[8, 23] Mortality (11 to 13 per cent and morbidity (45 to 55 per cent) are primarily due to associated injuries, including those to the head, kidney, pancreas, duodenum, liver, and colon. Mortality for isolated splenic injury is less than 1 per cent.[7, 18]

E. Growth of implanted splenic tissue within the peritoneal cavity is well known. There is growing evidence that developing splenic nodules produce at least partial restoration of splenic function, with significant protection against subsequent infection in children.[19] This is in contradistinction to accessory spleens, which seem to impart no such protection.

F. Overwhelming infection with pneumococcus (over 50 per cent incidence), meningococcus or *Haemophilus influenzae*, months to years following therapeutic splenectomy, occurs in an occasional child. Incidence of thalassemia is 11 per cent and of reticuloendothelial disease 10 per cent, but after removal in a normal child is 0.68 per cent compared to an expected 0.05 per cent in children 1 to 14 years old,[20] and 0.01 per cent in the general population.[25]

G. Despite little evidence of protection when given for prophylaxis, antibiotics have been used for periods of two years in some splenectomized children.[12] There may be longer intervals between splenectomy and sepsis.[2, 20] In normal adults, despite administration of antibiotics, mortality of bacteremic pneumococcal pneumonia is 17 per cent; it is 28 per cent among those over 50.[21]

H. Immunization of splenectomized patients with polyvalent pneumococcal vaccine may protect against vaccine-specific pneumococci. Over a two-year period of observation, 70 patients with sickle cell anemia, 7 with thalassemia and 19 asplenic children who were vaccinated with polyvalent pneumococcal vaccine failed to contract pneumonia. There were 8 cases of pneumonia in 106 unvaccinated, age-matched patients with sickle cell anemia who were used as controls.[22] Obviously, this approach does not protect against infection by other microorganisms.

I. Reported incidence of delayed rupture as 11 to 15 per cent, with mortality of 10 per cent, is far too high.[11, 23] Latent period before rupture is one week in 50 per cent of patients, two weeks in 25 per cent, and over one month in 10 per cent. With current use of diagnostic peritoneal lavage, arteriography, ultrasound, and isotope scans, splenic rupture should be recognized early, thus avoiding high mortality and morbidity rates.

J. Most occur following minor trauma or infectious mononucleosis, in acute or chronic leukemia, and where malaria is endemic. A few occur with no apparent cause.[24]

References

1. Eraklis, A. J., and Feller, R. M.: Splenectomy in childhood: A review of 1413 cases. J. Pediatr. Surg., 7:382–88, 1972.
2. Singer, D. B.: Postsplenectomy sepsis. *In* Rosenberg, H. S., and Bolande, R. P. (eds.): Perspectives in Pediatric Pathology, vol. I. Chicago, Year Book Medical Publishers, 1973, pp. 285–311.
3. Donaldson, S. H., Glatstein, E., and Vosti, K. L.: Bacterial infections in pediatric Hodgkin's disease. Cancer, 41:1949–1958, 1978.
4. Osen, W. R., and Beaudoin, D. E.: Surgical injury to the spleen. Surg. Gynecol. Obstet., 131:57–62, 1970.
5. Roy, M., and Geller, Y.: Increased morbidity of iatro-

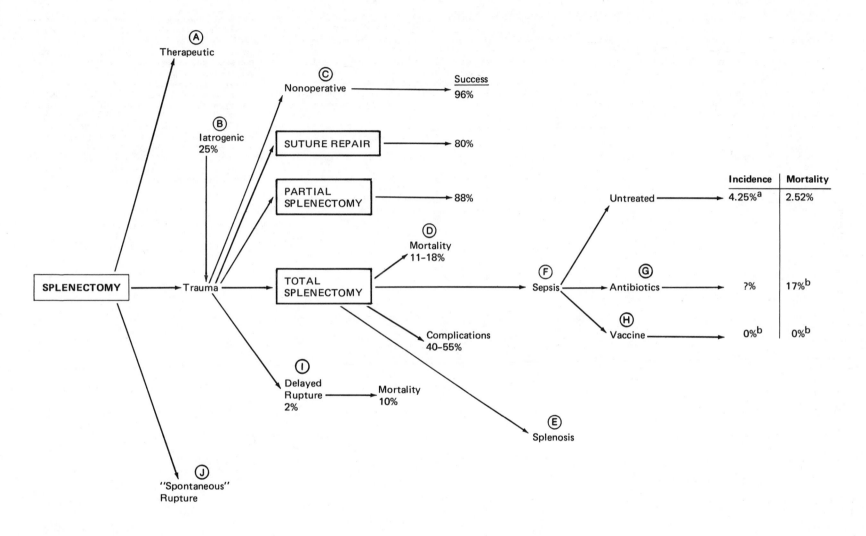

ⓐAll bacteria
ᵇPneumococcus bacteria

genic splenectomy. Surg. Gynecol. Obstet., *139*:392, 1974.

6. Morgenstern, L.: Avoidable complications of splenectomy. Surg. Gynecol. Obstet., *145*:525–528, 1977.

7. Steele, M., and Lim, R. C., Jr.: Advances in management of splenic injuries. Am. J. Surg., *130*:159–164, 1975.

8. Upadhyaya, P., and Simpson, J. S.: Splenic trauma in children. Surg. Gynecol. Obstet., *126*:781–790, 1968.

9. Douglas, G. J., and Simpson, J. S.: The conservative management of splenic trauma. J. Pediatr. Surg., *6*:565–570, 1971.

10. Shafer, R., et al.: Nonoperative treatment of splenic injury. Report of a case. J. Trauma, *15*:935–936, 1975.

11. Lorimer, W. S., Jr.: Occult rupture of the spleen. Arch. Surg., *89*:434–440, 1964.

12. Balfans, J. R., et al.: Overwhelming sepsis following splenectomy for trauma. J. Pediatr., *88*:458–460, 1976.

13. Sherman, N. J., and Asch, M. J.: Conservative surgery for splenic injuries. Pediatrics, *61*:267–271, 1978.

14. Mishalany, H.: Repair of the ruptured spleen. J. Pediatr. Surg., *9*:175–178, 1974.

15. La Mura, J., Chung-Fat, S. P., and San Filipo, J. A.: Splenorraphy for the treatment of splenic rupture in infants and children. Surgery, *81*:497–501, 1977.

16. Campos Christo, M.: Segmented resection of the spleen: Report of the first 8 cases operated on. O. Hospital Rio, *62*:187–204, 1962.

17. Burrington, J. D.: Surgical repair of a ruptured spleen in children. Arch. Surg., *112*:417–419, 1977.

18. Naylor, R., Coln, D., and Shirer, G. T.: Morbidity and mortality from injuries to the spleen. J. Trauma, *14*:773, 1974.

19. Pearson, H. A., et al.: Splenosis after splenectomy for trauma. N. Engl. J. Med., *398*:1389–1392, 1978.

20. Dickerman, J. D.: Bacterial infection and the asplenic host: A review. J. Trauma, *16*:8, 1976.

21. Austrian, R.: Pneumococcal infection and pneumococcal vaccine (Editorial). N. Eng. J. Med., *297*:938–39, 1977.

22. Amman, A. J., et al.: Polyvalent pneumococcal-polysaccharide immunization of patients with sickle-cell anemia and patients with splenectomy. N. Eng. J. Med., *297*:896–900, 1977.

23. Siser, J. S., Wayne, E. R., and Frederick, P.: Delayed rupture of the spleen: Review of the literature and report of 6 cases. Arch. Surg., *92*:362–366, 1966.

24. Orloff, M. J., and Peskin, G. W.: Collective review of spontaneous ruptures of the normal spleen: A surgical enigma. Int. Abst. Surg., *106*:1, 1958.

25. Krivit, W., Scott-Giebink, G., and Leonard, A.: Overwhelming postsplenectomy infection. Surg. Clin. North Amer., *59*:223–233, 1979.

IDIOPATHIC THROMBOCYTOPENIC PURPURA

IDIOPATHIC THROMBOCYTOPENIC PURPURA BY ELLEN MONCY, M.D.

Comments

A. Primary idiopathic thrombocytopenic purpura (ITP) results from increased platelet destruction (survival 1 to 3 days). Splenectomy diminishes antiplatelet factor and stops platelet destruction.[1, 4, 12] Incidence is 3:1 female:male, and 85 per cent of patients are younger than 8 years of age.[1]

B. Secondary ITP is a manifestation of another disease: 50 per cent of cases are the result of viral infections in children.[12] Splenectomy is rarely performed (±1 to 2 per cent of cases).[15]

C. Children are not routinely given steroids[12] unless there is serious epistaxis, gastrointestinal tract bleeding, or hematuria. One to 2 per cent will have intracranial bleeding, which has a 20 to 100 per cent mortality.[12]

D. Active ITP in pregnancy warrants steroid trial, then splenectomy with elective cesarean section. Half of the infants of these mothers will have ITP.[2, 8]

E. For the probability of postsplenectomy infection, see page 268 and references 5, 9 to 11, and 15.

Although accessory spleens are found in 14 to 30 per cent of patients, recurrent ITP caused thereby is exceedingly rare.[14]

References

1. Krupp, M. A., and Chatton, M. J. (eds.): Medical Diagnosis and Treatment 1977. Los Altos, Calif., Lange Medical Publications, 1977, pp. 314–315.
2. Homan, W. P., and Dineen, P.: The role of splenectomy in the treatment of thrombocytopenic purpura due to systemic lupus erythematosus. Ann. Surg., 187:52–56, 1978.
3. Thompson, R. L.: Idiopathic thrombocytopenic purpura. Arch. Intern. Med., 130:730–734, 1972.
4. Baldini, M. G.: Idiopathic thrombocytopenic purpura and the ITP syndrome. Med. Clin. North Am., 56:47–64, 1972.
5. Caplan, S. N., and Berkman, E. M.: Immunosuppressive therapy of idiopathic thrombocytopenic purpura. Med. Clin. North Am., 60:977, 1976.
6. Rouben, M.: Chronic idiopathic thrombocytopenic purpura. Arch. Intern. Med., 132:380–383, 1973.
7. Laros, R. K., and Sweet, R. L.: Management of idiopathic thrombocytopenic purpura during pregnancy. Am. J. Obstet. Gynecol., 122:182–191, 1975.
8. Murray, J. M., and Harris, R. E.: Management of the pregnant patient with idiopathic thrombocytopenic purpura. Am. J. Obstet. Gynecol., 126:449–451, 1976.
9. Kassum, D., and Thomas, E. J.: Morbidity and mortality of incidental splenectomy. Can. J. Surg., 20:209–214, 1977.
10. Ein, S. H., et al.: Morbidity and mortality of splenectomy in childhood. Ann. Surg., 185:307–310, 1977.
11. Joseph, T. P., Wyllie, G. G., and Savage, J. P.: Nonoperative management of splenic trauma. Aust. N.Z. J. Surg., 47:179–182, 1977.
12. McClure, P. D.: Idiopathic thrombocytopenic purpura in children: Diagnosis and management. Pediatrics, 55:68–74, 1975.
13. Sabiston, D. C., Jr. (ed.): Davis-Christopher Textbook of Surgery, 11th ed. Philadelphia, W. B. Saunders Co., 1977, pp. 1325–1326.
14. Verheyden, C. N., et al.: Accessory splenectomy in management of recurrent idiopathic thrombocytopenic purpura. Mayo Clin. Proc., 53:442–446, 1978.
15. Sandusky, W. R., Leavell, B. S., and Benjamin, B. I.: Splenectomy: Indications and results in hematologic disorders. Ann. Surg., 159:695–710, 1964.

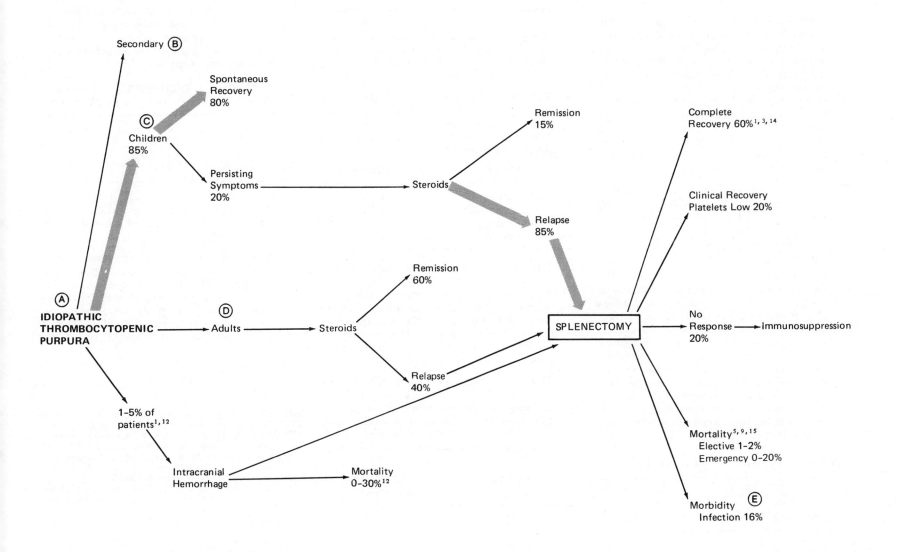

MECHANICAL SMALL BOWEL OBSTRUCTION BY JOHN B. MOORE, M.D.

Comments

A. Mechanical small bowel obstruction accounts for up to 20 per cent of acute surgical admissions.[1] In the early 1900's mortality ranged from 30 to 50 per cent, but more recently mortality is less than 10 per cent. The overall incidence of strangulation is 25 per cent with mortality doubled or tripled if resection is necessary.[2-4] In most series, adhesions, hernia, and malignancy account for more than 75 per cent of small bowel obstruction.[3, 5-8]

B. More than 90 per cent of cases of adhesive obstruction are associated with previous surgery.[9] The incidence of gangrenous bowel ranges from 6 to 12 per cent with adhesions versus 30 to 35 per cent with hernia.[4, 10]

C. Indications for a trial of nonoperative therapy include[1, 9] (1) partial small bowel obstruction, (2) cases of repeated adhesive obstruction less likely to be strangulated, (3) recent postoperative occurrence with adynamic ileus, (4) malignant carcinomatosis, and (5) obstruction secondary to inflammation that is expected to subside with therapy. Other factors affecting the decision for continued tube decompression versus laparotomy include duration of obstruction[5] (see table) and clinical evidence of strangulation.

DURATION (hours)	MORTALITY (%)
<24	0
24–48	11
>48	17

Clinical evidence to differentiate simple from strangulation obstruction is missing in 50 to 75 per cent of cases.[1, 11, 12] There is considerable overlap in signs of strangulation.[8, 9, 11, 14] According to Wangensteen,[13] "There are no absolute criteria by which simple and gangrenous bowel obstruction can be differentiated with finality short of operation."

D. The likelihood of subsequent obstruction requiring operation following original lysis of adhesions or bowel resection ranges from 8 to 16 per cent over 10-year followup periods.[1, 7]

AFTER:	LIKELIHOOD IS:
2nd operation	13%
3rd operation	17%
4th operation	30%
5th operation	43%

E. Hernia as a cause has decreased in incidence since more aggressive indications for elective herniorrhaphy are now known.[4, 13] The figure was higher than 50 per cent in the early 20th century but is 15 to 25 per cent now. Hernia still accounts for 20 per cent of deaths from small bowel obstruction.[16]

F. Due to a narrow neck and difficulty in diagnosis, femoral hernias account for a disproportionate incidence of strangulation leading to increased morbidity and mortality.[2, 10, 13, 15] The following table gives data about unreduced femoral hernias.[16]

DURATION (hours)	RESECTION RATE (%)
12	10
24	13
48	30
>48	50

G. Small bowel tumors constitute 3 per cent of all gastrointestinal malignancies.[17, 18] Their commonest presenting symptom (30 to 45 per cent of cases) is obstruction.[18, 19] At diagnosis two-thirds of these tumors have metastasized.[19, 20]

TUMOR TYPE[17-21]	INCIDENCE (%)	5-YEAR SURVIVAL[19, 21]
Adenocarcinoma	30–48	15–25
Carcinoid	21–35	40–50
Lymphoma	10–20 ⎫	20–40
Leiomyosarcoma	13–15 ⎭	

The incidence and survival data given in the table are not limited to obstructing lesions only.

H. Miscellaneous causes of acute small bowel obstruction include regional enteritis (0 to 4 per cent of cases), gallstone ileus (0 to 4 per cent), Meckel's diverticulum (0 to 2 per cent), intussusception (0 to 6 per cent), food obturation (0 to 4 per cent), and volvulus (1 to 3 per cent).[1, 3, 5-8]

References

1. Davis, S. E., and Sperling, L.: Obstruction of the small intestine. Arch. Surg., 99:424, 1969.
2. Eleason, E. L., and Welty, R. F.: A ten-year survey of intestinal obstruction. Ann. Surg., 125:57, 1947.
3. Lo, A. M., Evans, W. E., and Carey, L. C.: Review of small bowel obstruction at Milwaukee County General Hospital. Am. J. Surg., 111:884, 1966.
4. Waldron, G. W., and Hampton, J. M.: Intestinal obstruction: A half-century comparative analysis. Ann. Surg., 153:839, 1961.
5. Bollinger, J. A., and Fowler, E. F.: Results of treatment of acute small bowel obstruction: Clinical study of 205 consecutive cases. Arch. Surg., 66:888, 1953.
6. Playforth, R. H., Holloway, J. B., and Griffen, W. O.: Mechanical bowel obstruction: A plea for earlier surgical intervention. Ann. Surg., 171:783, 1970.

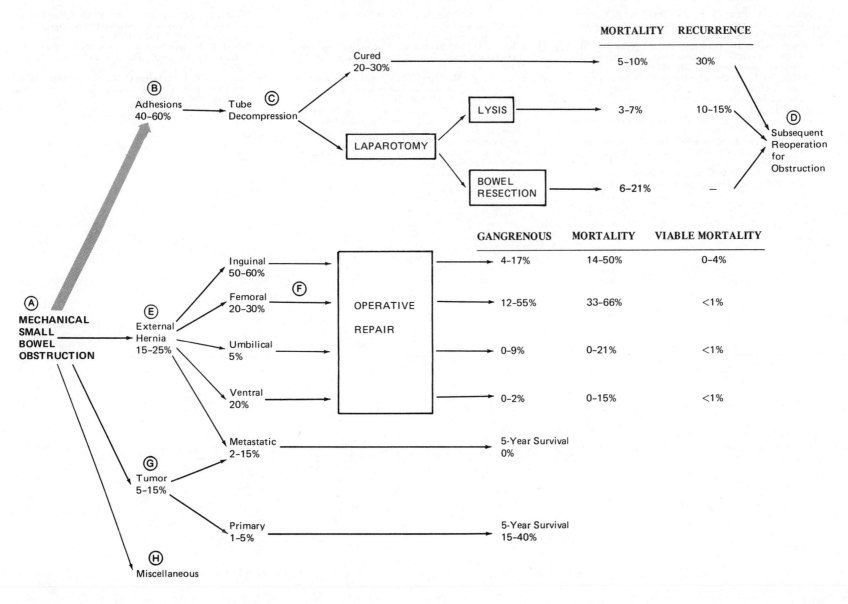

Ⓐ
MECHANICAL SMALL BOWEL OBSTRUCTION

Ⓑ
Adhesions
40–60%

Ⓒ
Tube Decompression

Cured
20–30%

LAPAROTOMY

LYSIS

BOWEL RESECTION

	MORTALITY	RECURRENCE
Cured	5–10%	30%
LYSIS	3–7%	10–15%
BOWEL RESECTION	6–21%	—

Ⓓ
Subsequent Reoperation for Obstruction

Ⓔ
External Hernia
15–25%

Ⓕ
OPERATIVE REPAIR

	GANGRENOUS	MORTALITY	VIABLE MORTALITY
Inguinal 50–60%	4–17%	14–50%	0–4%
Femoral 20–30%	12–55%	33–66%	<1%
Umbilical 5%	0–9%	0–21%	<1%
Ventral 20%	0–2%	0–15%	<1%

Ⓖ
Tumor
5–15%

Metastatic
2–15%
5-Year Survival
0%

Primary
1–5%
5-Year Survival
15–40%

Ⓗ
Miscellaneous

MECHANICAL SMALL BOWEL OBSTRUCTION *Continued*

7. Smith, G. A., Perry, J. F., and Yonehiro, E. G.: Mechanical intestinal obstructions. Surg. Gynecol. Obstet., *100*:651, 1955.
8. Stewardson, R. H., Bombeck, T., and Nyhus, L. M.: Critical operative management of small bowel obstruction. Ann. Surg., *187*:189, 1978.
9. Becker, W. F.: Acute adhesive ileus: A study of 412 cases with particular reference to the abuse of tube decompression in treatment. Surg. Gynecol. Obstet., *95*:472, 1952.
10. Coletti, L., et al.: Mechanical small bowel obstruction. Am. J. Surg., *104*:370, 1962.
11. Silen, W., Hein, M. F., and Goldman, C.: Strangulation obstruction of the small intestine. Arch. Surg., *85*:137, 1962.
12. Snyder, E. N., and McCranie, D.: Closed loop obstruction of the small bowel. Am. J. Surg., *111*:398, 1966.
13. Barnett, W. O., Petro, A. B., and Williamson, J. W.: A current appraisal of problems with gangrenous bowel. Ann. Surg., *183*:653, 1976.
14. Leffall, L. D., and Syphax, B.: Clinical aids in strangulation intestinal obstruction. Am. J. Surg., *120*:756, 1970.
15. MaGee, R. B., MacDuffee, R. C., and Isanyawongse, P.: Abdominal hernias associated with small intestinal obstruction. P. Med., *47*:1973.
16. Wangensteen, O. H.: Understanding the bowel obstruction problem. Am. J. Surg., *135*:131, 1978.
17. Croom, R. D., and Newsome, J. F.: Tumors of the small intestine. Am. Surg., *41*:160, 1975.
18. Sager, G. F.: Primary malignant tumors of the small intestine. A 22 year experience with 30 patients. Am. J. Surg., *135*:601, 1978.
19. Goel, I. P., Didolkar, M. S., and Elias, E. G.: Primary malignant tumors of the small intestine. Surg. Gynecol. Obstet., *143*:717, 1976.
20. Ratner, M. H., and Aust, J. C.: Primary malignant neoplasms of the small intestine. Rev. Surg., *32*:449, 1975.
21. Pagtalunar, R. J. G., Mayo, C. W., and Dockerty, M. B.: Primary malignant tumors of the small intestine. Am. J. Surg., *108*:13, 1964.

APPENDICITIS

APPENDICITIS BY JOHN B. GRAMLICH, M.D.

Comments

A. One of every 15 people will have acute appendicitis during his lifetime.[1] The rate stabilized at 2 to 3 per cent of all operations in the United States after the introduction of antibiotics. There were 822 deaths from appendicitis in the U.S. in 1975.[2]

Appendicitis is very rare during the first year of life. That occurring during the first month is often associated with Hirschsprung's disease.[1] Appendicitis is uncommon until about 5 years of age.[3] Thereafter it occurs with increasing frequency through young adulthood and decreases slowly by middle age, becoming less common with advancing age. Conversely, the mortality and morbidity rates are greatest at the extremes of life.[2-4] Appendicitis with gangrene, perforation, or abscess in children 16 years of age or younger increased steadily in the decade prior to 1968.[3] In patients 60 years of age and older, the morbidity and mortality rates increase progressively with advancing age.[4]

B. In the only recorded study of untreated appendicitis, Howie[5] estimated that 30 per cent of patients admitted to a hospital for suspected acute appendicitis were discharged without appendectomy. Of 35,000 patients in this category there were 6 deaths in the 12 to 29 year age group among those subjected to appendectomy at a later date, which is a mortality rate of 0.017 per cent. While the number of deaths from appendicitis has diminished annually (14,113 fatalities in 1939,[6] 5285 in 1946,[6] and 822 in 1975,[2] there is no way to estimate the number of persons who have appendicitis that resolves spontaneously and so recover without operation.

C. Howie found the gross death rate to be 0.02 to 0.8 per cent for patients undergoing appendectomy for a "normal appendix."[5] In a study of 7810 patients who had a preoperative diagnosis of acute appendicitis and were operated on between 1937 and 1959 at the Massachusetts General Hospital, Barnes[7] found a 15.2 per cent rate of error in diagnosis, with 2.4 per cent of patients undergoing negative exploration. Those in the remaining group (12.8 per cent) were found to have mesenteric lymphadenitis (4.6 per cent), ovarian pathology (2.0 per cent), pelvic inflammatory disease (1.3 per cent), gastroenteritis (0.9 per cent), small bowel pathology (0.7 per cent), and inflamed Meckel's diverticulum (0.4 per cent). The remaining diagnoses (2.9 per cent) were diverticulitis, infarction of omentum, cholecystitis, renal and ureteral pathology, nonspecific peritonitis, perforated peptic ulcer, regional enteritis, endometriosis, mesenteric thrombosis, carcinoma of the colon, pancreatitis, carcinoid, tuberculous mesenteric lymphadenitis, appendicitis epiploica, incarcerated inguinal hernia, ectopic pregnancy, infarcted leiomyoma of the uterus, carcinoma of the ovary, inguinal abscess, infected urachal cyst, mesenteric vein thrombosis, ileocolic artery embolism, seminal vesiculitis, carcinoma of the liver, and hematoma of the abdominal wall.

D. The necessity for an interval appendectomy following simple drainage of appendiceal abscess is not as compelling as once considered. About one third of Barnes' 218 patients who underwent interval appendectomy showed no evidence of inflammation of the appendix on microscopic section.[7] Bradley and Isaacs[8] followed 13 patients in the same category for 5.2 ± 1.2 years, and only one patient developed a recurrent abscess. They suggested that 10 to 20 per cent of patients undergoing drainage without appendectomy will develop recurrent appendicitis. Their complication rate for interval appendectomy was 19 per cent! Babcock[9] performed no interval appendectomies during the study period 1936 to 1955.

References

1. Condon, R. E.: Appendicitis. *In* Sabiston, D. C., Jr. (ed.): Davis-Christopher Textbook of Surgery, 11th ed. Philadelphia, W. B. Saunders Co., 1977, pp. 1062–1078.
2. Vital Statistics of the United States: Mortality. Vol. 2, part B. Hyattsville, Md. U.S. Depart. of Health, Education, and Welfare, Public Health Services, 1975, pp. 7–146, 7–147.
3. Stone, H. H., Sanders, S. L., and Martin, J. D., Jr.: Perforated appendicitis in children. Surgery, *69*:673–679, 1971.
4. Peltokallio, P., and Jauhiainen, K.: Acute appendicitis in the aged patient. Arch. Surg., *100*:140–143, 1970.
5. Howie, J. G.: Death from appendicitis and appendicectomy. Lancet, *2*:1334–1337, 1966.
6. Slattery, L. R., Yannitelli, S. A., and Hinton, J. W.: Acute appendicitis. Evaluation of factors contributing to the decrease in mortality in a municipal hospital over a 20-year period. Arch. Surg., *60*:31–41, 1950.
7. Barnes, B. A., et al.: Treatment of appendicitis at the Massachusetts General Hospital (1937–1959). JAMA, *180*:122–126, 1962.
8. Bradley, E. L., III, and Isaacs, J.: Appendiceal abscess revisited. Arch. Surg., *113*:130–132, 1978.
9. Babcock, J. R., and McKinley, W. M.: Acute appendicitis: An analysis of 1662 consecutive cases. Ann. Surg., *150*:131–141, 1959.
10. Campbell, J. A., and McPhail, D. C.: Acute appendicitis. Br. Med. J., *1*:852–855, 1958.
11. Stafford, E. S., and Scott, H. W.: Mortality of appendiceal perforation, South. Med. J., *41*:834–837, 1948.
12. Gilmour, I. E. W., and Lowdon, A. G. R.: Acute appendicitis. Edinburgh Med. J., *59*:361–373, 1952.
13. Kazarian, K. K., Roeder, W. J., and Mersheimer, W. L.: Decreasing mortality and increasing morbidity from acute appendicitis. Am. J. Surg., *119*:681–685, 1970.
14. Cantrell, J. R., and Stafford, E. S.: The diminishing mortality from appendicitis. Ann. Surg., *141*:749–758, 1955.
15. Howie, J. G.: The place of appendicectomy in the treatment of young adult patients with possible appendicitis. Lancet, *1*:1365–1367, 1968.

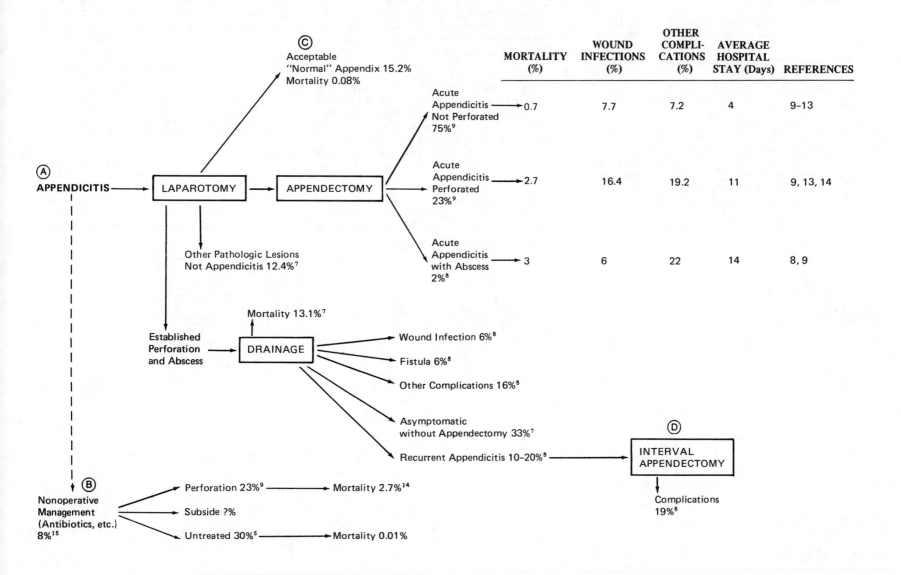

Ⓒ Acceptable
"Normal" Appendix 15.2%
Mortality 0.08%

	MORTALITY (%)	WOUND INFECTIONS (%)	OTHER COMPLI- CATIONS (%)	AVERAGE HOSPITAL STAY (Days)	REFERENCES
Acute Appendicitis Not Perforated 75%[9]	0.7	7.7	7.2	4	9–13
Acute Appendicitis Perforated 23%[9]	2.7	16.4	19.2	11	9, 13, 14
Acute Appendicitis with Abscess 2%[8]	3	6	22	14	8, 9

Ⓐ **APPENDICITIS**

LAPAROTOMY → APPENDECTOMY

Other Pathologic Lesions Not Appendicitis 12.4%[7]

Established Perforation and Abscess → DRAINAGE

Mortality 13.1%[7]

Wound Infection 6%[8]

Fistula 6%[8]

Other Complications 16%[8]

Asymptomatic without Appendectomy 33%[7]

Recurrent Appendicitis 10–20%[8] → Ⓓ INTERVAL APPENDECTOMY

Complications 19%[8]

Ⓑ Nonoperative Management (Antibiotics, etc.) 8%[15]

Perforation 23%[9] ——→ Mortality 2.7%[14]

Subside ?%

Untreated 30%[5] ——→ Mortality 0.01%

CROHN'S DISEASE BY GILBERT HERMANN, M.D.

Comments

A. Once thought primarily to affect Jews, Crohn's disease is now acknowledged to be present in all populations. Its incidence does vary markedly among subcultures. It seems to be increasing in frequency. It has been reported in all age groups, but its incidence is highest in the young adult population.[1,2]

B. Acute ileitis is diagnosed in patients with no previous history of GI symptoms who are found to have a thickened, inflamed terminal ileum at laparotomy for presumed appendicitis. Its relationship to classic regional enteritis is not clear. Appendectomy should be carried out unless the cecum is involved in the inflammatory process.

C. The word *management* rather than *treatment* is used purposely to indicate the roles of medicine and surgery in this disease of uncertain etiology and extremely variable clinical course.[4,5]

D. A low operative mortality may be an indication of operative skill and perioperative management. It may also reflect management policy. An approach that favors desperate measures in seriously ill patients will have a different mortality than one in which more conservative but possibly more numerous operations are carried out.[3,7,9]

E. Inflammatory bowel disease (IBD) of the colon involves a broad spectrum of clinical, pathologic, and radiographic changes, with Crohn's disease at one end and chronic ulcerative colitis on the other. There is a large indeterminate middle ground of colonic IBD whose exact classification remains to be delineated.[10]

F. Indolent (painless) fissures and fistulas occur in from 20 to 75 per cent of patients with Crohn's disease, the higher figure associated with the colonic pattern. Experience has shown that they should be managed conservatively if possible.

G. Recurrences in Crohn's disease vary considerably, depending on length of follow-up and the criteria one chooses to determine recurrence, i.e., clinical symptoms, radiographic findings, or need for further surgery. The literature on the subject should be considered with this in mind.

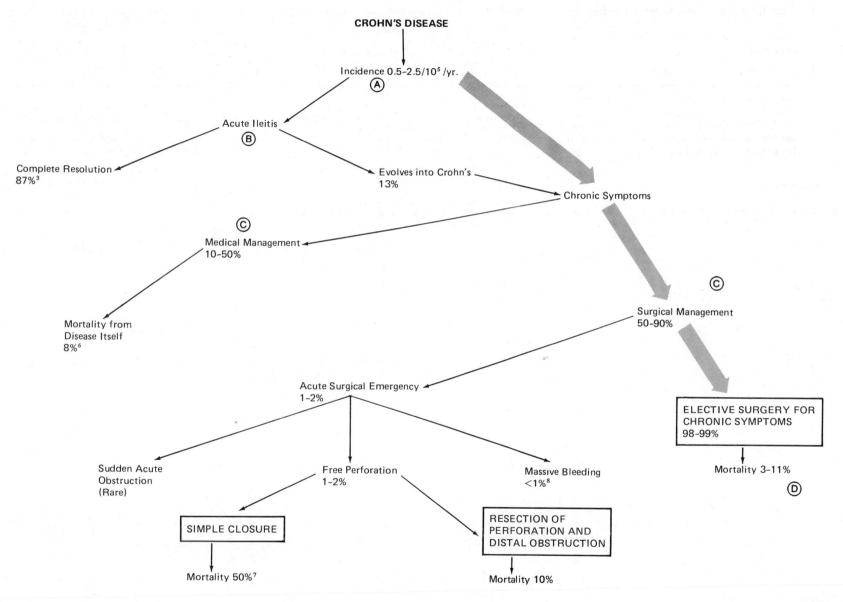

CROHN'S DISEASE

Incidence 0.5–2.5/10^5/yr.
Ⓐ

Acute Ileitis
Ⓑ

Complete Resolution
87%[3]

Evolves into Crohn's
13%

Chronic Symptoms

Ⓒ
Medical Management
10–50%

Surgical Management
50–90%
Ⓒ

Mortality from
Disease Itself
8%[6]

Acute Surgical Emergency
1–2%

ELECTIVE SURGERY FOR
CHRONIC SYMPTOMS
98–99%

Sudden Acute
Obstruction
(Rare)

Free Perforation
1–2%

Massive Bleeding
<1%[8]

Mortality 3–11%
Ⓓ

SIMPLE CLOSURE

RESECTION OF
PERFORATION AND
DISTAL OBSTRUCTION

Mortality 50%[7]

Mortality 10%

CROHN'S DISEASE *Continued*

H. This high figure was obtained using the actuarial (life-table) method rather than crude analysis. It may well be the more accurate.[11, 12]

I. Reactivation or persistence of disease, perforation, and development of carcinoma in totally bypassed segments have been reported. Fistulas do not always heal, although they may do so. Unless resection would be extremely hazardous it is strongly preferred over bypass.[13]

References

1. Gjone, E., Orning, O. M., and Myren, J.: Crohn's disease in Norway 1956–1963. Gut, 7:372, 1966.

2. Monk, M., et al.: An epidemiological study of ulcerative colitis and regional enteritis among adults in Baltimore. I. Hospital prevalence 1960–1963. Gastroenterology, 53:198, 1967.

3. Banks, B. M., Zetzel, L., and Richter, H. S.: Morbidity and mortality in regional enteritis. Am. J. Dig. Dis., 14:369, 1969.

4. de Dombal, F. T.: Results of surgery for Crohn's disease. Clin. Gastroenterol., 1:349, 1972.

5. Farmer, R. G., Hawk, W. A., and Turnbull, R. B., Jr.: Clinical patterns in Crohn's disease — A statistical study of 615 cases. Gastroenterology, 68:627, 1975.

6. Edwards, H.: Crohn's disease: An enquiry into its nature and consequences. Ann. R. Coll. Surg. Engl., 44:121, 1969.

7. Alexander-Williams, J.: Surgery and the management of Crohn's disease. Clin. Gastroenterol., 1:349, 1972.

8. Barber, K. W., et al.: Indications for and the results of the surgical treatment of regional enteritis. Ann. Surg., 156:472, 1962.

9. de Dombal, F. T., Burton, I. L., and Goligher, J. C.: The early and late results of surgical treatment of Crohn's disease. Br. J. Surg., 58:805, 1971.

10. Farmer, R. G., Hawk, W. A., and Turnbull, R. B., Jr.; Indications for surgery in Crohn's disease — Analysis of 500 cases. Gastroenterology, 71:245, 1976.

11. Lennard-Jones, J. E., and Stalder, G. A.: Prognosis after resection of chronic regional ileitis. Gut, 8:332, 1967.

12. Greenstein, A. J., Reoperation and recurrence in Crohn's colitis and ileocolitis. N. Engl. J. Med., 293:685, 1975.

13. Schofeld, P. F.: The natural history and treatment of Crohn's disease. Ann. R. Coll. Surg. Engl., 36:258, 1965.

14. Nugent, F. W., et al.: Prognosis after colonic resection for Crohn's disease of the colon. Gastroenterology, 65:398, 1973.

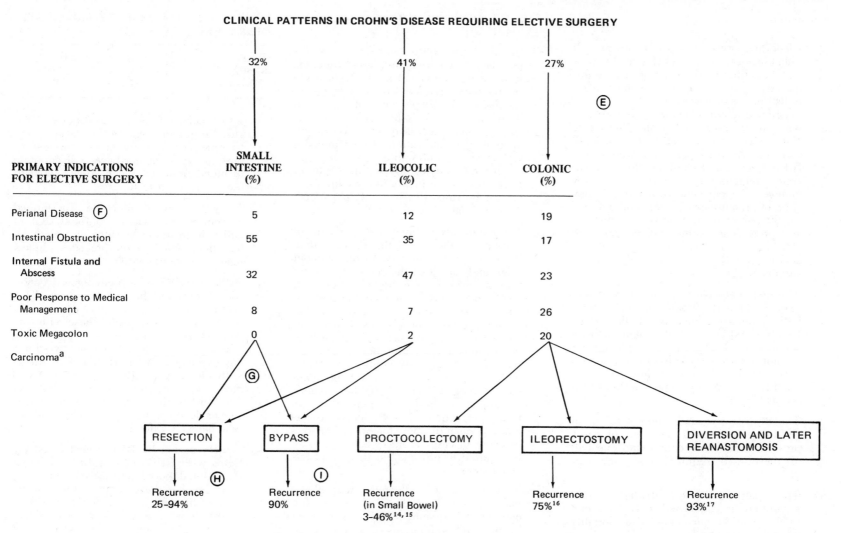

CLINICAL PATTERNS IN CROHN'S DISEASE REQUIRING ELECTIVE SURGERY

Ⓔ

PRIMARY INDICATIONS FOR ELECTIVE SURGERY	SMALL INTESTINE (%)	ILEOCOLIC (%)	COLONIC (%)
	32%	41%	27%
Perianal Disease Ⓕ	5	12	19
Intestinal Obstruction	55	35	17
Internal Fistula and Abscess	32	47	23
Poor Response to Medical Management	8	7	26
Toxic Megacolon	0	2	20
Carcinoma[a]			

Ⓖ

RESECTION	BYPASS	PROCTOCOLECTOMY	ILEORECTOSTOMY	DIVERSION AND LATER REANASTOMOSIS
Ⓗ Recurrence 25–94%	Ⓘ Recurrence 90%	Recurrence (in Small Bowel) 3–46%[14, 15]	Recurrence 75%[16]	Recurrence 93%[17]

[a]Carcinoma is reported with increasing frequency. The risk of colonic carcinoma associated with Crohn's colitis is increased up to twentyfold in age-matched groups.[18] At present there is no statistically valid increase in small bowel malignancy associated with small bowel regional enteritis, although the evidence tends that way.[19]

ULCERATIVE COLITIS BY ROBERT BEART, M.D., AND JON THOMPSON, M.D.

Comments

A. Ulcerative colitis is a partial bowel wall inflammatory disease starting at the anus and extending orad. Onset of disease frequently is associated with another infectious process or pregnancy.[1, 2]

Clinical features include pain (60 to 70 per cent of cases), rectal bleeding (90 to 100 per cent), fever (18 to 43 per cent), diarrhea (78 to 93 per cent), weight loss (18 per cent), and vomiting (14 to 27 per cent). Diagnostic accuracy of barium enema is 75 per cent; of history, 75 per cent; of proctoscopy, 75 per cent; of biopsy, 90 per cent; and of enema, history, and proctoscopy combined, 90 per cent. One third to one half of patients with ulcerative colitis will eventually require surgery.[3]

B. The first attack carries a mortality of 3 to 9 per cent and 10 per cent of patients will undergo colectomy at this time. Eighty to 90 per cent of patients will respond to medical therapy, which consists of antibiotics (Azulfidine), steroids, a milk-free diet (lactose intolerance is frequently a cause), and antidiarrheal agents.[1-3]

C. The disease is usually more virulent in children. Ten to 15 per cent of cases present with severe colitis, and one half of these will require emergency surgery.[4, 5]

D. Those patients whose colitis has a chronic continuous course will have an operative rate of 81 per cent and a mortality rate of 25 per cent.[6]

E. Those whose disease follows a relapsing-remitting course will have an operative rate of 28 per cent and a mortality rate of 14 per cent. Eighty-five per cent relapse at 10 years and 100 per cent by 17 years.[6, 7]

F. Acute, severe colitis (more than 6 stools per day, rectal bleeding, fever, anemia, tachycardia, and elevated erythrocyte sedimentation rate) will respond to medical therapy in 50 per cent of cases and have a mortality of 10 to 40 per cent. Surgery becomes necessary with the development of complications (see Comment G) or if there is no improvement from intensive medical therapy within 48 to 72 hours. Remission is less likely with a history of previous disease and in patients more than 60 years of age.[8, 9]

G. Perforation occurs in 3 to 5 per cent of cases and is the most lethal complication. It occurs most commonly in the sigmoid colon and increases the mortality rate of toxic megacolon from 13 to 42 per cent. Thirty per cent of medical failures are due to perforation.[3] Toxic megacolon occurs in 5 per cent of cases. It becomes an indication for operation with perforation or impending perforation, lack of improvement in 24 to 48 hours, clinical deterioration, and recurrence (75 per cent will require colectomy if they recur). Successful medical management occurs in 25 per cent of cases.[1] Rectal hemorrhage is an indication for operation in 3 per cent of cases. Total proctocolectomy is required to prevent bleeding from the rectal stump.[3]

H. Total or subtotal colectomy with ileostomy is the procedure of choice for emergency treatment. In suspected "sealed off" perforations of toxic megacolon, the "blowhole" ileostomy-colostomy may have a role.[10-13]

Seventy-five per cent of patients with subtotal colectomy will later require rectal excision, which has a mortality rate of

OPERATION	MORBIDITY (%)	MORTALITY (%)
Total	60	10[10]
Subtotal	80	8–10
"Blowhole"	68	10[11]

1 to 4 per cent and a 2 to 3 per cent incidence of carcinoma in the rectal stump. Five per cent of patients with procedures performed for hemorrhage will continue to bleed from the rectal stump and will require rectal resection.[10]

I. Forty per cent of colectomies performed for chronic ulcerative colitis (CUC) in children are done because of growth retardation, which often precedes clinical manifestation of colitis.[14]

J. Because CUC is a premalignant condition, endoscopic biopsy should be of the entire colon and not just the rectum, which may be spared. Of those with cancer, 88 per cent have precancer elsewhere in the colon, but only two-thirds have precancer in the rectum. Of patients with ulcerative colitis, 5.7 per cent will have precancer on rectal biopsy, but only one-third of these will have cancer. Precancer develops in 20 per cent of patients who have CUC for 10 years.[15]

K. Cancer occurs in 3.5 per cent of all patients with CUC. This is 10 to 15 times the normal population's risk. Three per cent develop the disease in the first decade of life and 20 per cent in the subsequent decade. After 35 years of CUC, 48 per cent of patients will have cancer.[16] Factors increasing the risk include[3] early onset, duration of disease (there is a 20 times greater risk after 20 years of disease compared with after only 5 years of disease), and extent of colon

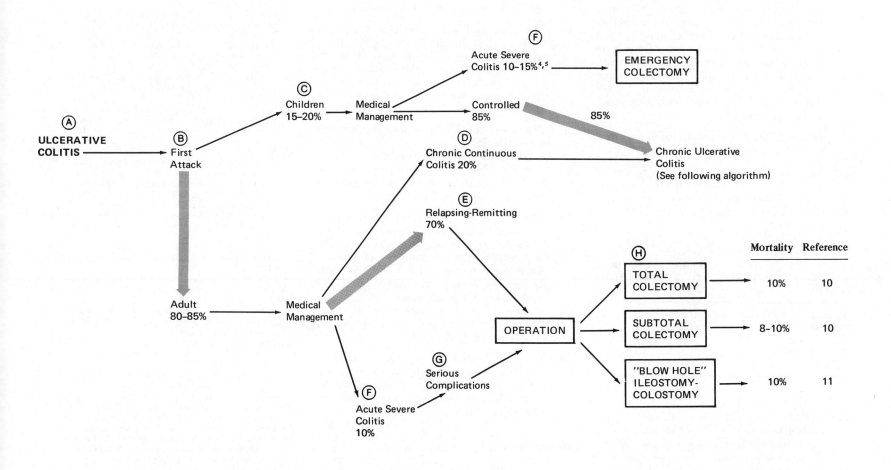

Ⓐ
ULCERATIVE COLITIS

Ⓑ First Attack

Ⓒ Children 15–20%

Medical Management

Ⓕ Acute Severe Colitis 10–15%[4,5] → EMERGENCY COLECTOMY

Controlled 85%

85%

Chronic Ulcerative Colitis (See following algorithm)

Ⓓ Chronic Continuous Colitis 20%

Ⓔ Relapsing-Remitting 70%

Adult 80–85%

Medical Management

Ⓕ Acute Severe Colitis 10%

Ⓖ Serious Complications

OPERATION

Ⓗ

TOTAL COLECTOMY

SUBTOTAL COLECTOMY

"BLOW HOLE" ILEOSTOMY-COLOSTOMY

	Mortality	Reference
TOTAL COLECTOMY	10%	10
SUBTOTAL COLECTOMY	8–10%	10
"BLOW HOLE" ILEOSTOMY-COLOSTOMY	10%	11

involved (7.2 per cent if the whole colon is involved vs. 1.3 per cent if not).[3] Factors that differentiate the CUC patient from the non-CUC patient for risk of developing colon cancer[3] include earlier age of onset (mean 37 years vs. 53 years), occurrence more common in the rectum (76 per cent) than in the sigmoid (47 per cent), and lesions more frequently multiple (20 per cent vs. 2 to 4 per cent). Survival is comparable for a given stage *but* the CUC cancers are usually poorly differentiated, resulting in only 40 per cent 5-year survival.

L. Intractability is the most common indication for resection.

M. Strictures occur in 6 to 11 per cent of cases and are usually in the rectum. Long-standing strictures may be benign. Other local complications are shown in the table.[17]

COMPLI-CATION	INCIDENCE (%)	NON-OPERA-TIVE CURE (%)	REQUIRE COLECTOMY (%)
Fissure	12.3	100	0
Abscess	6.0	85	0
Fistula-in-ano	5.4	52	0
Rectovaginal fistula	36	0	90

N. Systemic complications include[1, 2] liver dysfunction (30 to 50 per cent of cases), sclerosing cholangitis (3 per cent), cirrhosis (3 to 5 per cent), bile duct cancer (5 per cent), ankylosing spondylitis (1 to 5 per cent), uveitis (3 to 10 per cent), urethritis (5 to 15 per cent), erythema nodosum (5 to 10 per cent), clubbing (5 per cent), and urinary tract disorders (5 to 6 per cent). Most complications parallel the course of the disease and improve with colectomy. Less likely to improve are spondylitis, sclerosing cholangitis, and liver dysfunction. Colectomy has no effect on the incidence of bile duct cancer.

O. The conventional operation requires about 14 days' hospitalization. Complications include wound infection (2 to 20 per cent), persistent perineal sinus (10 to 40 per cent), ileostomy dysfunction requiring reoperation (10 per cent), and sexual impotence (5 per cent).

P. The Koch pouch[19] in experienced hands gives the following results: continence in 90 per cent of cases, mortality of 3 per cent, reoperation rate of 18 per cent, prolapse of stoma in 20 to 30 per cent of cases, and fistula in 8 per cent.

Q. The role of this procedure remains controversial.[20] Acceptable result occurs in 70 to 80 per cent of patients, conversion to ileostomy in 2 per cent; cancer develops in rectal stump in 1 per cent; morbidity rate is 35 per cent. Complications include anorectal precipitancy (40 per cent of cases), fecal incontinence (45 per cent), stricture (14 per cent), and fistula or abscess (6.9 per cent).

R. This modification of the Suave operation involves pulling the ileum through the rectum after excision of the mucosa. As yet the data are too meager to evaluate the procedure fully.[22]

References

1. Kirsner, J. B., and Shorter, R. G.: Inflammatory Bowel Disease. Philadephia, Lea & Febiger, 1975.
2. Sloan, W. P., Borgen, J. P., and Gage, R. P.: Life histories with chronic ulcerative colitis—A review of 2000 cases. Gastroenterology, *16*:35–38, 1950.
3. Bockus, H. L. (ed.): Gastroenterology, 3rd ed. Vol. 2: Small Intestine and Colon. Philadelphia, W. B. Saunders, 1976, pp. 645–750.
4. Foglia, R., et al.: Surgical management of ulcerative colitis in childhood. Am. J. Surg., *134*:58–63, 1977.
5. Werlin, S. L.: Severe colitis in children and adolescents: Diagnosis, course, and treatment. Gastroenterology, 73:828–832, 1977.
6. Jalan, K. N., Prescott, R. J., and Sirius, W.: An experience of ulcerative colitis. Gastroenterology, 59:589–609, 1970.
7. Edwards, F. C., and Truelove, S. C.: The course and prognosis of ulcerative colitis — Long-term prognosis. Gut, *4*:309, 1963.
8. Goligher, J. C.: Surgical aspects of ulcerative colitis and Crohn's disease of the large bowel. Adv. Surg., *11*:71–99, 1977.
9. Goligher, J. C., et al.: Surgical treatment of severe attacks of ulcerative colitis with special reference to the advantage of early operation. Br. Med. J. *4*:703–706, 1970.
10. Binder, S. C., et al.: Emergent and urgent operations for ulcerative colitis. Arch. Surg., *110*:284–289, 1975.
11. Fazio, W., and Turnbull, R.: Ileostomy-colostomy for the megacolon of toxic ulcerative colitis. *In* Clearfield, H. R., and Dinoso, V. P. (eds.): Gastrointestinal Emergencies. New York, Grune & Stratton, 1976.
12. Turnbull, R. B., Hawkins, A., and Weakley, F. L.: The surgical treatment of toxic megacolon. Am. J. Surg., *122*:325–331, 1971.
13. Patel, S. C., and Stone, R. M.: Toxic megacolon: Results of emergency colectomy. Can. J. Surg., *20*:36–38, 1977.
14. Frey, R., et al.: Colectomy in children with ulcerative colitis and granulomatous colitis. Arch. Surg., *104*:414–423, 1972.
15. Dobbins, W. O., et al.: Early detection and prevention of carcinoma in patients with ulcerative colitis. Cancer, *40*:2542–2548, 1977.
16. Devroede, G. J., et al.: Cancer risk and life expectancy of children with ulcerative colitis. N. Engl. J. Med., *285*:17–21, 1971.
17. de Dombal, F. T., et al.: Incidence and management of anorectal abscess, fistula and fissure in patients with ulcerative colitis. Dis. Colon Rectum, *9*:201, 1966.
18. Arlson, N. A.: Surgical treatment of ulcerative colitis. Proc. Staff Meet. Mayo Clin., *36*:484–491, 1961.
19. Kock, N.: Ileostomy. Curr. Probl. Surg., August 1977.
20. Aylett, S.: Three hundred cases of diffuse ulcerative colitis treated by total colectomy and ileorectal anastomosis. Br. Med. J., *1*:1001, 1966.
21. Watts, J. M., and Hughes, E. J.: Ulcerative colitis and Crohn's disease: Results after colectomy and ileorectal anastomosis. Br. J. Surg., *64*:72–83, 1977.
22. Martin, L., et al.: Total colectomy and mucosal proctectomy with preservation of continence in ulcerative colitis. Ann. Surg., *186*:477–480, 1977.

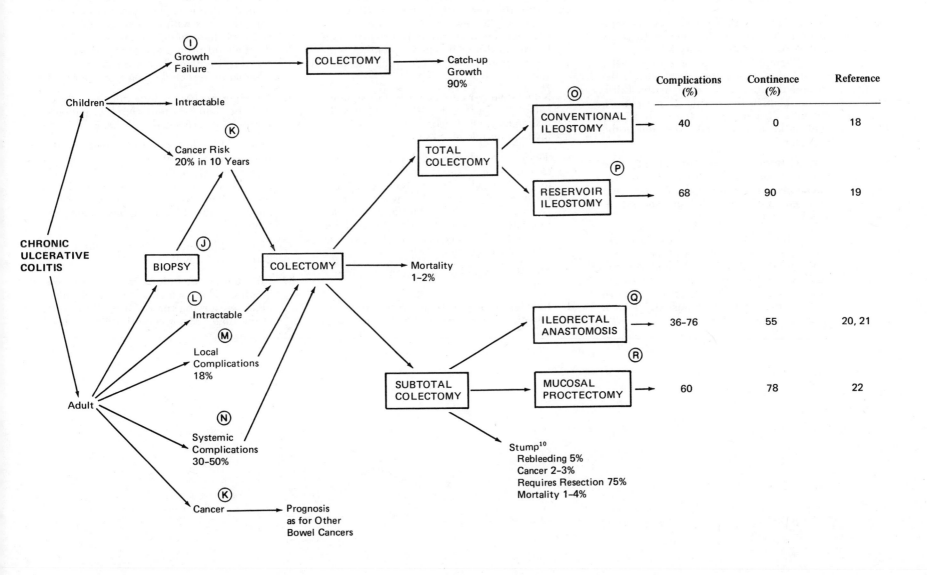

	Complications (%)	Continence (%)	Reference
CONVENTIONAL ILEOSTOMY	40	0	18
RESERVOIR ILEOSTOMY	68	90	19
ILEORECTAL ANASTOMOSIS	36–76	55	20, 21
MUCOSAL PROCTECTOMY	60	78	22

DIVERTICULAR DISEASE OF THE COLON BY DAVID HUTCHISON, M.D.

Comments

A. Ten per cent of patients become symptomatic in 5 years, 25 per cent in 10 years, and 37 per cent in 18 years.[7, 23]

   Radiographic findings of asymptomatic colonic diverticula are 1 per cent in the second decade, 6 per cent in the third, 12 per cent in the fourth, 22 per cent in the fifth, 30 per cent in the sixth, 27 per cent in the seventh, and 7 per cent in the eighth.[15-17]

B. Twenty-three per cent of patients who have had one attack will have these complications. An additional 58 per cent have complications after the second attack.[1, 6, 9, 12, 18, 22, 23]

C. Perforation includes local mesenteric abscesses (14 per cent), local perforation with abscess (25 per cent), and generalized peritonitis (5 per cent).[17] Primary anastomosis is usually avoided in the presence of free abdominal pus. Breakdown is 82 per cent.[5, 8, 9, 21]

D. Mortality for medical treatment alone is 75 to 100 per cent[9, 21] and for drainage alone is 66 per cent.[9] Colostomy plus drainage for perforation is usually done for the critically ill but is attended with greater morbidity, lengthening hospital stay as much as twice.[3, 10, 12, 17]

E. Ninety-five per cent occur in the sigmoid colon; 2.9 per cent are associated with malignancy. Obstruction often occurs following multiple attacks.[1, 15, 23]

F. Three-stage closure (delayed colostomy closure) is now rarely performed. Colostomy is usually closed with resection. Closures are done earlier when disease is excised primarily. Mortality for delayed resections is 11 per cent and for colostomy closure 4 per cent. Recurrence rate is 2.1 per cent.[3, 6, 11, 15]

G. Mortality in older age group is 50 per cent.

H. Infectious complications present as anastomotic leaks; recurrent pelvic, subphrenic, or subhepatic abscesses; and wound infections, but the frequency of complications within each operative procedure is hard to determine. Leaks in the presence of primary anastomosis and pus are very frequent. Recurrence rate for an adequately resected colon is 2.1 per cent.

I. Bleeding occurs in hypertensive, obese, diabetic, and arterosclerotic patients. Rarely is it associated with pain.[5, 13, 14, 19]

J. Sites of bleeding are 50 per cent in the right colon and 50 per cent in the left colon and sigmoid, but they are rarely away from the site of radiographically documented diverticula. Many cases of multiple sites of bleeding have been documented.[5]

K. Massive bleeding is defined as more than 2000 cc. per day.[13]

L. Colectomy includes *all* diverticula-bearing colon, which means total colectomy, preserving the rectum, 50 per cent of the time.[4] Major complications include

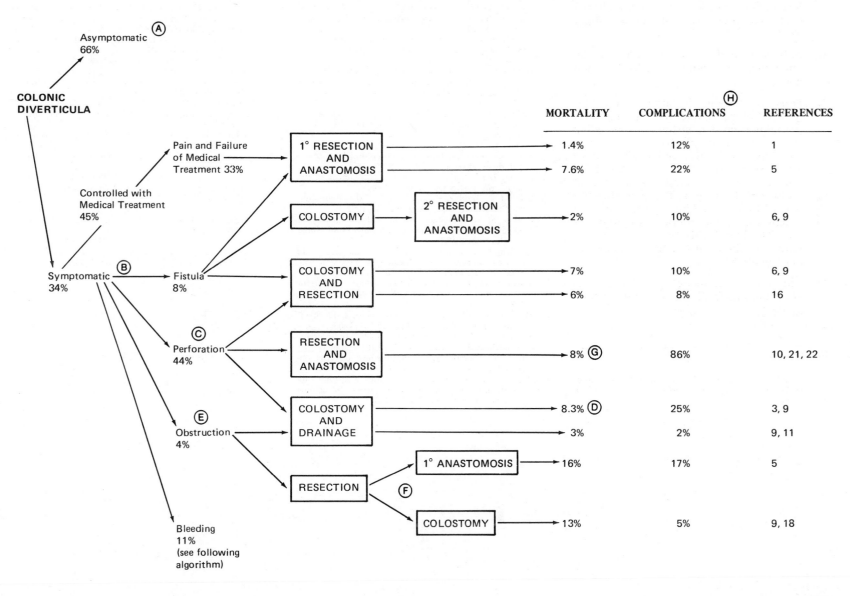

leak (3 per cent), wound infection (10 per cent) and vascular complications (10 per cent).

M. This is defined as local resection of the "bleeding site," determined by educated guess.[13]

N. Selective mesenteric arteriography requires a bleeding rate of more than 2 cc. per minute for demonstration of bleeding site and is most effective for recurrent bleeders. AV fistulas and malformations are best demonstrated with this technique, but they are rare — 2 per cent of all lower GI bleeders. The procedure remains time-consuming, particularly in demonstrating the inferior mesenteric artery. The high incidence of surgical mortality is often attributed to delay in operation.[2, 19, 20]

O. This procedure, though promising, is as yet experimental (2 cases, results of both good).[19, 20]

References

1. Boles, R. S., Jr., and Jordan, S. M.: Clinical significance of diverticulosis. Gastroenterology, *35*:579, 1958.

2. Blaisdell, F. W.: Management of acute complications of diverticular disease: Hemorrhage. Dis. Colon Rectum, *19*:287, 1976.

3. Classen, J. N., et al.: Surgical treatment of acute diverticulitis by staged procedures. Ann. Surg., *184*:582, 1976.

4. Draparias, T., et al.: Emergency subtotal colectomy: Preferred approach to management of massively bleeding diverticular disease. Ann. Surg., *177*:519, 1973.

5. Griffin, J. M., Butcher, H. R., Jr., and Ackerman, L. V.: Surgical management of colonic diverticulitis. Arch. Surg., *94*:619, 1967.

6. Hafner, C. D., Ponka, J. L., and Brush, B. E.: Genitourinary manifestations of diverticulitis of the colon: A study of 500 cases. JAMA, *179*:76, 1962.

7. Horner, J. L.: Natural history of diverticulosis of the colon. Am. J. Dig. Dis., 3:343, 1958.

8. Leigh, J. E., Judd, E. S., and Waugh, J. M.: Diverticulitis of the colon. Am. J. Surg., *103*:51, 1962.

9. Localio, S. A., and Stahl, W.: Diverticular disease of the alimentary tract. I. The colon. Curr. Probl. Surg., 4:1, December 1967.

10. Madden, J. L.: Primary resection and anastomosis in the treatment of perforated lesions of the colon. Am. Surg., *31*:781, 1965.

11. Marsh, J., et al.: One hundred consecutive operations for diverticulitis of the colon. South. Med. J., *68*:133, 1975.

12. Marshall, S. F.: Earlier resection in one stage for diverticulitis of the colon. Am. Surg., 29:337, 1963.

13. McGuire, H. H., Jr., and Haynes, B. W., Jr.: Massive hemorrhage from diverticulosis of the colon: Guidelines for therapy based on bleeding patterns observed in 50 cases. Ann. Surg., *175*:847–55, 1972.

14. Rigg, B. M., and Ewing, M. R.: Current attitudes on diverticulitis with particular reference to colonic bleeding. Arch. Surg., *92*:321, 1966.

15. Rodkey, G. U., and Welch, C. E.: Diverticulitis of the colon: Evaluation in concept and therapy. Surg. Clin. North Am., *45*:1231, 1965.

16. Rodkey, G. U., and Welch, C. E.: Surgical management of colonic diverticulitis with free perforation or abscess formation. Am. J. Surg., *117*:265, 1969.

17. Rodkey, G. U., and Welch, C. E.: Colonic diverticular disease with surgical treatment. Surg. Clin. North Am., *54*:655, 1974.

18. Smithwick, R. H.: Experiences with surgical management of diverticulitis of the sigmoid. Ann. Surg., *115*:969, 1942.

19. Taylor, F. W., and Epstein, L. I.: Treatment of massive diverticular hemorrhage. Arch. Surg., *98*:505, 1969.

20. Walter, S. F., et al.: Therapeutic angiography: Its value to surgical patients. Arch. Surg., *113*:432, 1978.

21. Watkins, C. L., and Oliver, G. A.: Surgical treatment of acute perforative sigmoid diverticulitis. Surgery, 69:215, 1971.

22. Waugh, J. M., and Walt, A. J.: Changing concepts in treatment of diverticulitis of the sigmoid. Lancet, 76:373, 1956.

23. Young, E. S., and Young, E. S., III: Diverticulitis of the colon: A review of literature and an analysis of 91 cases. N. Engl. J. Med., *230*:33, 1944.

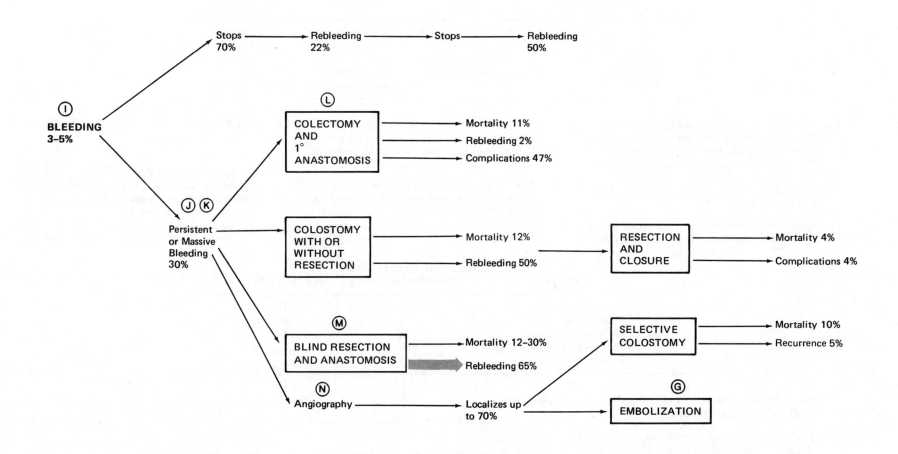

COLONIC POLYPS BY C. PRATT, M.D.

Comments

A. Infantile polyps are hamartomas without malignant potential alleged to occur in 1 per cent of children, with the peak incidence at 5 years of age. Seventy per cent occur singly. Polyps present as bleeding and rarely as intussusception.[1]

B. Inherited gastrointestinal polyposis syndromes are shown in the table below.[2]

SYNDROME	SITE	PATHOLOGY	CANCER RISK
Familial polyposis coli	Colon and rectum	Adenomatous	80–100%
Peutz-Jeghers	Small intestine	Hamartoma	2–3%
Gardner's	Colon and rectum	Adenomatous	80–100%
Juvenile	Colon and rectum	Hamartoma	± 0%
Turcot's	Colon	Adenomatous	Brain tumor

C. Average age for appearance of polyps is 24.5 years.[3] Symptoms usually appear at 33 years. Polyps are usually diagnosed by age 36, at which time two thirds of patients have cancer and 50 per cent of these have multiple cancers. Average age of death from this cancer is 42.

D. Incidence of the cancer in the rectal stump developing subsequent to subtotal colectomy is as follows:[4] within 5 years, 5 per cent; within 10 years, 13 per cent; within 15 years, 25 per cent; within 20 years, 42 per cent; and within 23 years, 59 per cent.

E. The relationship between the size of the polyps and the incidence of cancer is as follows:[5] smaller than 1 cm., 1.3 per cent; 1 to 2 cm., 9.5 per cent; larger than 2 cm., 46 per cent.

F. Locations of polyps in the colon are shown in the table below.[6]

G. Pseudopolyps of chronic ulcerative colitis are inflammatory and of questionable premalignancy.[8] Locations and frequency of pseudopolyps are as follows: cecum (44 per cent), ascending colon (76 per cent), transverse colon (84 per cent), descending colon (92 per cent), sigmoid colon (84 per cent), and rectum (40 per cent).

LOCATION	BARIUM ENEMA AND SIGMOIDOSCOPE	AT AUTOPSY
Ascending colon	2%	37%
Transverse colon	2%	25%
Descending colon	3%	11%
Mid and upper sigmoid	20%	27%
Rectum and sigmoid	73%	

H. Risk of colonic cancer increases with the duration of ulcerative colitis.[9] The risk also varies with the extent of the disease. Duration of 10 years carries a 5 per cent risk; of 15 years, 12 per cent; of 20 years, 22 per cent; of 25 years, 42 per cent; and of 30 years, 56 per cent.

References

1. Gathright, J. B., and Cofer, T. W.: Familial incidence of juvenile polyposis coli. Surg. Gynecol. Obstet., 138:185–188, 1974.
2. Erbe, R. W.: Inherited gastrointestinal polyposis syndromes. N. Engl. J. Med., 294:1101, 1976.
3. Bussey, H. J. R.: Familial Polyposis Coli. Baltimore, The Johns Hopkins University Press, 1975.
4. Moertel, C. G., Hill, J. R., and Adson, M. A.: Surgical management of multiple polyposis. Arch. Surg., 100:521, 1970.
5. Morson, B.: The polyp-cancer sequence in the large bowel. Proc. R. Soc. Med., 67:451, 1974.
6. Schwartz, S. I.: Principles of Surgery, 2nd ed. New York, McGraw-Hill, 1974, p. 1128.
7. Wolff, W. I., and Shinya, H.: Colonofibroscopic management of colonic polyps. Dis. Colon Rectum, 16:87, 1973.
8. Kleinfeld, G., and Gump, F. E.: Complications of colotomy and polypectomy. Surg. Gynecol. Obstet., 111:726, 1960.
9. DeDombal, F. T., et al.: Local complications of ulcerative colitis. Br. Med. J., 1:1442, 1966.

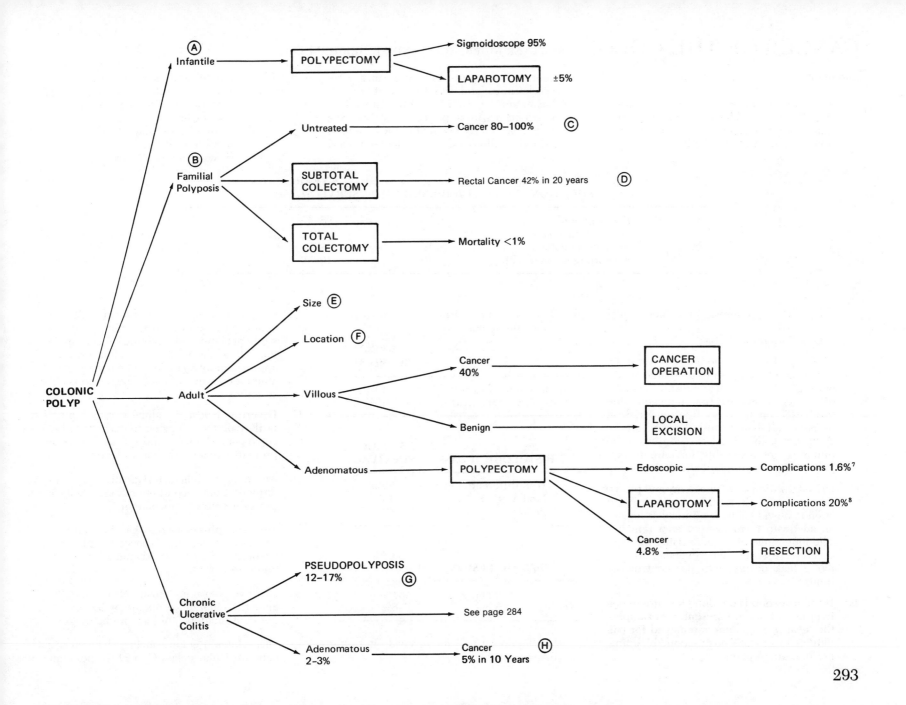

COLONIC POLYP

(A) Infantile → **POLYPECTOMY** → Sigmoidoscope 95%
→ **LAPAROTOMY** ±5%

(B) Familial Polyposis
→ Untreated → Cancer 80–100% (C)
→ **SUBTOTAL COLECTOMY** → Rectal Cancer 42% in 20 years (D)
→ **TOTAL COLECTOMY** → Mortality <1%

Adult
→ Size (E)
→ Location (F)
→ Villous
  → Cancer 40% → **CANCER OPERATION**
  → Benign → **LOCAL EXCISION**
→ Adenomatous → **POLYPECTOMY**
  → Edoscopic → Complications 1.6%[7]
  → **LAPAROTOMY** → Complications 20%[8]
  → Cancer 4.8% → **RESECTION**

Chronic Ulcerative Colitis
→ PSEUDOPOLYPOSIS 12–17% (G)
→ See page 284
→ Adenomatous 2-3% → Cancer 5% in 10 Years (H)

293

CANCER OF THE COLON BY PETER MURR, M.D., AND M. REICH, M.D.

Comments

A. This discussion excludes rectal cancer. (See page 298.) The mean age of occurrence of colon cancer is 65 years.[15] Location is shown in the table below.[15]

One to 3 per cent of colonic cancers are synchronous[3] and 3 to 4 per cent are metachronous.[1,3] An identifiable preceding polyp occurs in 50 per cent of cases. (See page 292.) Thirty per cent of these cancers arise in villous adenomas larger than 2 cm.[14]

B. Duke's classification is as follows:[24]
A = Limited to submucosa layer
B_1 = Into but not through the muscularis layer
B_2 = Through muscularis layer but confined to wall
C_1 = B_2 with nodes positive

LOCATION	INCIDENCE (%)	5-YEAR SURVIVAL (%)
Rectosigmoid	70	25–45
Descending colon	7	40
Transverse colon	12	45
Ascending colon (cecum)	10	40–50

C_2 = Through serosa with nodes positive
D = Distant metastases

C. There is a 10-month median survival if the cancer is left completely untreated (without regard to stage).[9] There is no statistical difference in survival time between wide local excision (margins free) and radical excision (all lymph node–bearing areas). Wide rather than local excision when the tumor is not resectable for cure is performed to remove lymphatic drainage.[13]

D. Hospitalization after colectomy and primary anastomosis is for 9 to 14 days. Alteration in bowel habits is minimal as long as an adequate recto-sigmoid area remains. The long-range effect of excising the ileocecal valve still is controversial. Anastomotic leak occurs in 5 per cent of patients.

E. If the resection is not done for cure (when liver metastases are present, for example), the local lesion alone is removed for palliation, to obviate obstruction, bleeding, perforation, or pain.

F. Five-year survival rates are shown in the following tables.

	5-YEAR SURVIVAL[15]
With venous invasion	19%
Without venous invasion	40%

HISTOLOGIC CLASS	5-YEAR SURVIVAL
Well differentiated	50%
Moderate	40%
Poor	20%

SIZE OF LESION	5-YEAR SURVIVAL[15]
> 5 cm.	51%
< 5 cm.	38%

See Figures 1 to 3 for survival rates after operation for cure.

G. Colonic cancer accounts for up to 22 per cent of large bowel obstruction.[1,2,4,5] Seventy per cent of obstructing cancers are to the left of the transverse colon. Overall, approximately 50 to 75 per cent are resectable for cure even though the lesion is obstructive.

H. Diverting colostomy alone is only temporarily palliative, leaving the cancer to become painful, bleed, and spread. The poor prognosis reflects this pre-selection.

I. Anastomosis characteristically is performed at the second operation; a 3-stage procedure now is uncommon.

J. Resection plus colostomy has the mortality rate of an emergency procedure plus colectomy but has the advantage of early tumor resection.

K. Elective colostomy closure 1 to 3 months after the emergency operation carries a 5 per cent incidence of leak or obstruction.

L. Of perforated colon cancers,[1,2,4,5] 90 per cent are Duke's class C or D, 75 per cent

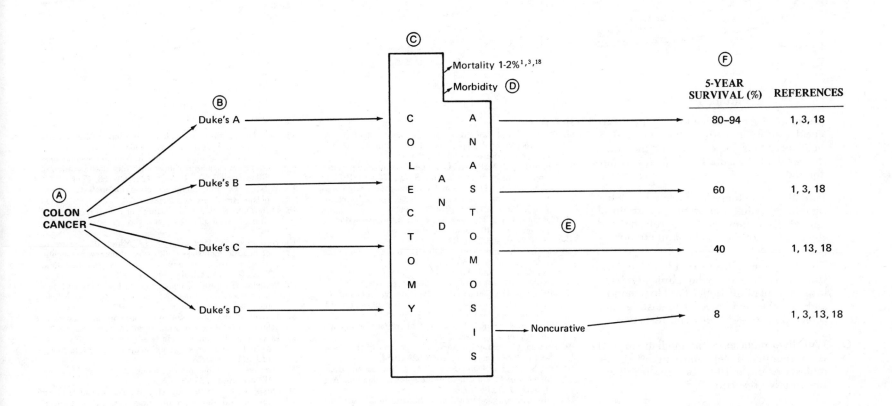

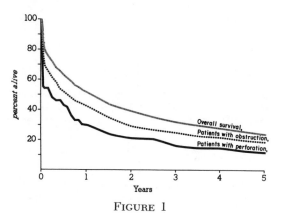

FIGURE 1

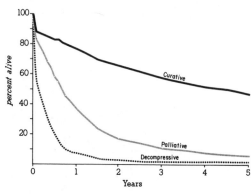

FIGURE 2

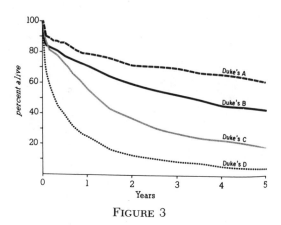

FIGURE 3

perforate at the lesion, and 20 per cent are cecal perforations (blowout). Overall 5-year survival is 28 per cent, and the rate is 40 per cent if a curative resection is performed.

M. Palliative colectomy is indicated to avoid bleeding, pain, perforation, and local spread. Resection can be merely beyond the confines of the local colonic tumor.

N. There is great self-selection in these data, since only patients who clinically have local control of the tumor for 3 to 6 months and no other evidence of metastases are selected for thoracotomy and resection.

O. With liver metastases the median survival is 5 months if left untreated.[19] Liver metastases occur 10 to 14 months following curative resection.[19]

P. Adjuvant chemotherapy does not effect 5-year survival.[21-23] Neither does local chemotherapy alter the 20 to 45 per cent incidence of local recurrence, two thirds of which appear within 2 years.[1, 3, 7]

Q. Radiation is variously said to increase the 5-year survival rate of *rectal* cancer by ± 10 per cent.[6, 25, 26]

References

1. Welch, J., and Donaldson, G.: Management of severe obstruction of the large bowel due to malignant disease. Am. J. Surg., *127*:472, 1974.
2. Glenn, F., and McSherry, C. K.: Obstruction and perforation in colorectal cancer. Ann. Surg., *173*:983, 1971.
3. Welch, J. P., and Donaldson, G. A.: Recent experience in the management of cancer of the colon and rectum. Am. J. Surg., *127*:258, 1974.
4. Goligher, J. C.: The treatment of acute obstruction or perforation with carcinoma of the colon and rectum. Br. J. Surg., *450*:270, 1957.
5. Floyd, C. E., and Cohn, I.: Obstruction in cancer of the colon. Ann. Surg., *165*:721, 1967.
6. Homsdahl, M., and Witkus, R.: Radiotherapy combined with curative surgery. Arch. Surg., *113*:446, 1978.
7. Silverman, D.: Estimated median survival times of patients with colorectal cancer based on experience with 9745 patients. Am. J. Surg., *133*:286, 1977.
8. Vidne, B. A.: Surgical treatment of solitary pulmonary metastases. Cancer, *38*:256, 1976.
9. Peatana, C.: Natural history of carcinoma of the colon and rectum. Am. J. Surg., *108*:826, 1964.
10. Welch, J. P., and Donaldson, G. A.: Detection and treatment of recurrent cancer of the colon and rectum. Am. J. Surg., *135*:505, 1978.
11. Wilson, S.: Surgical treatment of hepatic metastases from colorectal cancer. Arch. Surg., *111*:330, 1976.
12. Beahis, O.: Cancer of the colon and rectum: A review of the newer techniques, diagnosis and treatment. Adv. Surg., *9*:235, 1975.
13. Busuhil, R. W., Foglia, R., and Longmire, W., Jr.: Treatment of carcinoma of the sigmoid colon and upper rectum: A comparison of local segmental resection and left hemicolectomy. Arch. Surg., *112*:920, 1977.
14. Morson, B. C., and Bussey, H. J.: Predisposing causes of intestinal cancer. Curr. Probl. Surg., February 1970, pp. 18–20.
15. Copeland, E. M.: Anatomic distribution of carcinoma of colon. Am. J. Surg., *116*:875, 1968.
16. Mackman, S., et al.: A second look at the second look operation in colonic cancer after the administration of 5-fluorouracil. Am. J. Surg., *128*:763–766, 1974.
17. Wilkins, E.: Pulmonary resection for metastatic neoplasm. Am. J. Surg., *135*:480, 1978.
18. Falterman, K. W., et al.: Cancer of colon, rectum, and anus: Review of 2313 cases. Cancer, *34*(Suppl.):951, 1974.
19. Herlisman, H., Hassan, A., and Gardner, B.: Treatment of hepatic metastases with a combination of hepatic artery infusion, chemotherapy and external radiation. Surg. Gynecol. Obstet., *147*:13, 1978.
20. Wanebo, H.: Surgical management of patients with primary operable colorectal cancer and synchronous liver metastases. Am. J. Surg., *135*:81, 1978.
21. Lawrence, W.: Chemotherapy as an adjuvant to surgery for colorectal cancer. Ann. Surg., *181*:616–623, 1975.
22. Lawrence, W.: Chemotherapy as an adjuvant to surgery for colorectal cancer: A followup report. Arch. Surg., *113*:164–168, 1978.
23. Nystrom, J.: Adjuvant treatment of colorectal cancer. West J. Med., *126*:95–101, 1977.
24. Dukes, C. E., and Bussey, H. J. R.: The spread of rectal cancer and its effect on prognosis. Br. J. Cancer, *12*:309–320, 1958.
25. Kilgerman, M. M.: Irradiation of the primary lesion of the rectum and rectosigmoid. JAMA, *231*:1381, 1975.
26. Roswit, B., Higgins, G. A., Jr., and Keehn, R. J.: Preoperative irradiation for carcinoma of the rectum and rectosigmoid colon: Report of a national Veterans' Administration randomized study. Cancer, *35*:1597–1602, 1975.
27. Mountain, C. F., et al.: Contribution of surgery to the management of carcinomatous pulmonary metastases. Cancer, *41*:833–840, 1978.

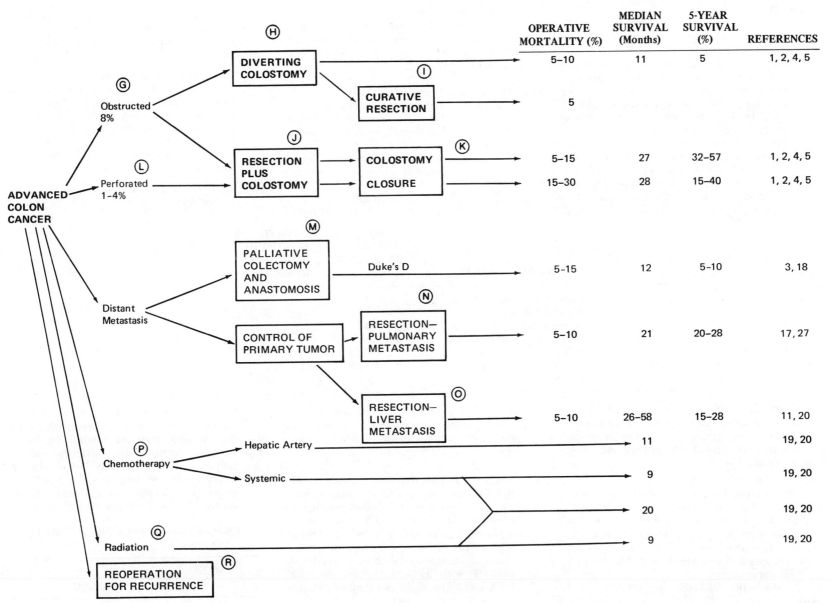

	OPERATIVE MORTALITY (%)	MEDIAN SURVIVAL (Months)	5-YEAR SURVIVAL (%)	REFERENCES
Ⓗ DIVERTING COLOSTOMY	5–10	11	5	1, 2, 4, 5
Ⓘ CURATIVE RESECTION	5			
Ⓙ RESECTION PLUS COLOSTOMY → COLOSTOMY Ⓚ	5–15	27	32–57	1, 2, 4, 5
CLOSURE	15–30	28	15–40	1, 2, 4, 5
Ⓜ PALLIATIVE COLECTOMY AND ANASTOMOSIS — Duke's D	5–15	12	5–10	3, 18
Ⓝ RESECTION— PULMONARY METASTASIS	5–10	21	20–28	17, 27
Ⓞ RESECTION— LIVER METASTASIS	5–10	26–58	15–28	11, 20
Hepatic Artery	11			19, 20
Systemic	9			19, 20
	20			19, 20
Radiation	9			19, 20

ADVANCED COLON CANCER

Ⓖ Obstructed 8%

Ⓛ Perforated 1–4%

Distant Metastasis

CONTROL OF PRIMARY TUMOR

Ⓟ Chemotherapy

Ⓠ Radiation

Ⓡ REOPERATION FOR RECURRENCE

RECTAL CANCER BY R. FARACI, M.D.

Comments

A. Mean age of onset is 60 years. Male:female predominance is 1.5:1.[14] There are a number of premalignant diseases of the rectum. At diagnosis of villous adenoma, one third of cases will be *in situ* cancer and one third will be invasive cancer.[23] With familial polyposis, overall 5-year survival is 20 per cent.[16]

   In ulcerative colitis, incidence is 20 per cent per decade,[4] with poor prognosis.[14]

   It is not clear whether adenomatous polyps are premalignant. Polypoid lesions less than 1.2 cm. in diameter rarely become malignant. Pedunculated polypoid cancer rarely metastasizes.[23] A synchronous or metachronous colonic lesion is present in 4 per cent of cases.[11] Colonic polyps accompany rectal cancer in 20 to 30 per cent of cases.

B. Duke's classification is as follows:
   Type A = Limited to bowel wall
   Type B = Involves contiguous tissue but lymph nodes are negative
   Type C = Positive lymph nodes (5-year survival decreased 50 per cent[1]
   Type D = Distant metastases
   Subclassification of type B (B_1 and B_2) as to depth of penetration and of type C (C_1 and C_2) for equivalent penetration with involved lymph nodes further refines the prognosis.

C. Recurrence at the suture line occurs in 25 to 30 per cent of cases and usually appears within 2 years of operation.[17] This usually reflects systemic spread. Re-resection (abdominoperineal), although rarely curative, results in a 21 to 34 month mean survival period. There is an incidence of 21 per cent ureteral injury.[21]

D. Complications are shown in the table below.[12, 24]

COMPLICATION	WITH ANTERIOR RESECTION (%)	WITH ABDOMINO-PERINEAL RESECTION (%)
Urinary obstruction/infection	14	35
Wound infection	12	6
Anastomotic leak	17	—
Perineal wound bleeding	—	8
Pulmonary	8.2	9
Thromboembolism	10.4	16.2
Cardiovascular	4.8	12

E. Three cm. of distal rectum should remain for continence. A temporary diverting colostomy protecting the suture line decreases the probability of leak and other complications.[10]

F. Fulguration requires an average of 4 separate 75-minute sessions over a 6 to 9 month period and is performed with the patient under general or spinal anesthesia. It is used for small lesions or in the very poor risk patient who has limited life expectancy.

   Morbidity includes bleeding (1 to 4 units) (22 per cent), perforation (5 per cent), cardiovascular complications (1.2 per cent), and rectovaginal fistula (5 per cent).

G. Positive carcinoembryonic antigen levels (CEA+) are found in 63 per cent of new cases of colon cancer.[15] Patients with preoperative CEA levels of 2.5 ng/ml. have a 5 per cent recurrence rate, whereas those with levels of 20 ng/ml. are virtually assured of recurrence. Although nearly all patients with metastases have elevated CEA levels, up to 25 per cent of patients with local recurrence have normal concentrations of CEA.[27, 30] Weak false-positive results may be caused by heavy smoking, pancreatitis, cirrhosis, colonic polyps, and inflammatory bowel disease. A postoperative drop in CEA levels followed by elevation means tumor recurrecence in 75 to 100 per cent of cases.

CEA LEVEL (ng./ml.)	RECURRENCE RATE (%)
< 2.5	5
> 20	±100

RECTAL CANCER

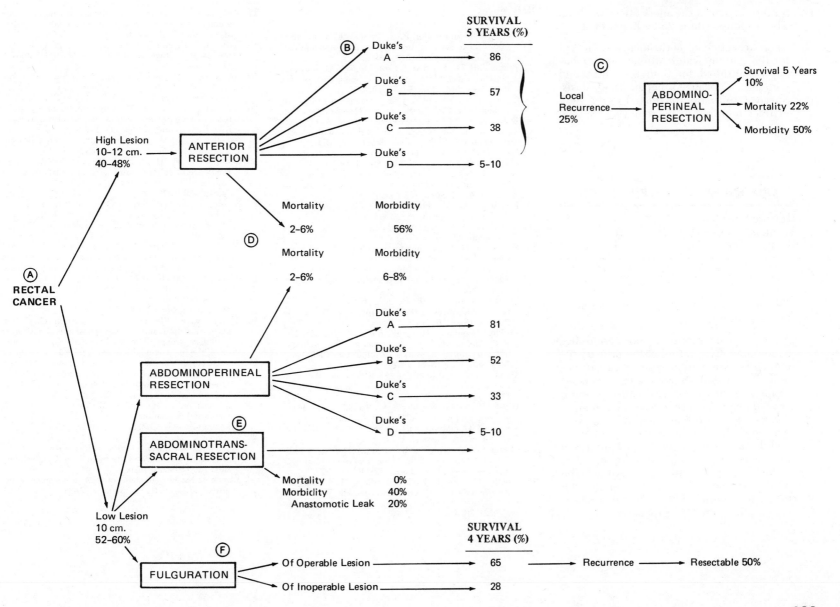

SURVIVAL 5 YEARS (%)

- Ⓑ Duke's A ——→ 86
- Duke's B ——→ 57
- Duke's C ——→ 38
- Duke's D ——→ 5-10

Ⓒ

Local Recurrence 25% ——→ ABDOMINO-PERINEAL RESECTION

Survival 5 Years 10%
Mortality 22%
Morbidity 50%

High Lesion 10-12 cm. 40-48% ——→ **ANTERIOR RESECTION**

Mortality 2-6% Morbidity 56%

Ⓓ Mortality 2-6% Morbidity 6-8%

Ⓐ **RECTAL CANCER**

ABDOMINOPERINEAL RESECTION

- Duke's A ——→ 81
- Duke's B ——→ 52
- Duke's C ——→ 33
- Duke's D ——→ 5-10

Ⓔ **ABDOMINOTRANS-SACRAL RESECTION**

Mortality 0%
Morbidity 40%
Anastomotic Leak 20%

Low Lesion 10 cm. 52-60%

SURVIVAL 4 YEARS (%)

Ⓕ **FULGURATION**

- Of Operable Lesion ——→ 65 ——→ Recurrence ——→ Resectable 50%
- Of Inoperable Lesion ——→ 28

299

RECTAL CANCER *Continued*

H. 5-Fluorouracil is the most effective drug. The response rate is 25 to 30 per cent.[19]

I. Liver resection is occasionally indicated for the patient whose primary tumor has been controlled for 3 to 6 months and who has a localized hepatic metastasis. Survival and cure are related to the bulk of liver required to be removed for total excision.[2, 5]

PROCEDURE	5-YEAR SURVIVAL (%)
Hepatic lobectomy	13
Segmental resection	21
Wedge resection	24

The metastases usually are *not* confined to a single lobe.[18]

J. An even longer observation period between operative control of the primary tumor and consideration of pulmonary resection is indicated—6 months to 2 years.[3-22] Fifteen to 20 per cent of patients dying of colorectal cancer have pulmonary metastases.[15] Most are multiple; 2 to 5 per cent develop a solitary pulmonary nodule, and half of them are benign. Of the cancerous nodules developing after abdominoperineal resection, half will be new primary tumors.[3] The longer the tumor-free period before the metastases appear, the better the prognosis.

References

1. Astler, V. B., and Coller, F. A.: Prognostic significance of direct extension of carcinoma of the colon and rectum. Ann. Surg., *139*:845–51, 1954.
2. Brasfield, R. D., Bowden, L., and McPeak, C. J.: Major hepatic resection for malignant neoplasms of the liver. Ann. Surg., *176*:171–77, 1972.
3. Cahan, W. G.: Multiple primary cancers, one of which is lung. Surg. Clin. North Am., *49*:323–35, 1969.
4. Debroede, G. J., Taylor, W. F., and Sauer, W. G.: Cancer risk and life expectancy of children with ulcerative colitis. N. Engl. J. Med., *285*:17–21, 1971.
5. Foster, J. A.: Survival after liver resection for secondary tumors. Am. J. Surg., *135*:389–94, 1978.
6. Grage, T. B., et al.: Adjuvant chemotherapy with 5-fluorouracil after surgical resection of colorectal carcinoma. Am. J. Surg., *133*:59–66, 1977.
7. Kligerman, M. M.: Preoperative radiation therapy in rectal cancer. Cancer, *36*:691–95, 1975.
8. Kligerman, M. M.: Radiation therapy for rectal carcinoma. Semin. Oncol., *3*:407–13, 1976.
9. Kligerman, M. M.: Radiotherapy and rectal carcinoma. Cancer, *39*:896–900, 1977.
10. Localio, S. A.: Abdominal transsacral resection and anastomosis for midrectal carcinoma. Surg. Gynecol. Obstet., *132*:123–27, 1971.
11. Lockhart-Mummery, H. E., and Heald, R. J.: Metachronous cancer of the large intestine. Dis. Colon Rectum, *15*:261–64, 1972.
12. Lockhart-Mummery, H. E., Ritchie, J. K., and Hawley, P. R.: The results of surgical treatment for carcinoma of the rectum at St. Mark's Hospital from 1948–1972. Br. J. Surg., *63*:673–77, 1976.
13. Madden, J. L., and Kandalaft, S.: Electrocoagulation in the treatment of cancer of the rectum. Ann. Surg., *174*:530–40, 1971.
14. Hawley, P. R., and Morson, B. C.: Tumors of the rectosigmoid, rectum, and anal canal. *In* Maingot, R. Abdominal Operations, 6th ed. New York, Appleton-Century-Crofts Medical, 1974, pp. 2029–2113.
15. Martin, E. W., et al.: The use of CEA as an early indicator for gastrointestinal tumor recurrence and second-look procedures. Cancer, *39*:440–46, 1977.
16. Moertel, C. G., Hill, J. R., and Adson, M. A.: Surgical management of multiple polyposis: The problem of cancer in the retained bowel segment. Arch. Surg., *100*:521–26, 1970.
17. Polk, H. C., and Spratt, J. S.: Recurrent colorectal carcinoma: Detection, treatment and other considerations. Surgery, *69*:9–23, 1971.
18. Raffucci, F. L., and Ramirez-Schon, G.: Management of tumors of the liver. Surg. Gynecol. Obstet., *130*:371–85, 1970.
19. Rapaport, A. H., and Burleson, R. L.: Survival of patients treated with systemic fluorouracil for hepatic metastases. Surg. Gynecol. Obstet., *130*:773–78, 1970.
20. Rider, W. D., et al.: Preoperative irradiation in operable carcinoma of the rectum: Report of the Toronto trial. Can. J. Surg., *20*:335–38, 1977.
21. Sanella, N. A.: Abdominoperineal resection following anterior resection. Cancer, *38*:378–81, 1976.
22. Schulter, M. F., Heiskell, C. A., and Shields, T. W.: Incidence of solitary pulmonary metastasis from carcinoma of the large intestine. Surg. Gynecol. Obstet., *143*:727–29, 1976.
23. Storer, E. H., Goldberg, S. M., and Nivetvongs, S.: Colon, rectum and anus. *In*: Schwartz, S. I.: Principles of Surgery. New York, McGraw Hill, 1974, pp. 1109–1165.
24. Slanetz, C. A., Herter, F. P., and Grinnell, R. S.: Anterior resection versus abdominoperineal resection for carcinoma of the rectum and rectosigmoid. Am. J. Surg., *123*:110–16, 1972.
25. Stevens, K. R., Allen, C. V., and Fletcher, W. S.: Preoperative radiotherapy for adenocarcinoma of the rectosigmoid. Cancer, *37*:2866–74, 1976.
26. Stevens, K. R., Fletcher, G. S., and Allen, C. V.: Anterior resection and primary anastomosis following high-dose preoperative irradiation for adenocarcinoma of the rectosigmoid. Cancer, *41*:2065–71, 1978.
27. Sugarbaker, P. H., Zamchek, N., and Moore, F. D.: Assessment of serial carcinoembryonic antigen (CEA) assays in postoperative detection of recurrent colorectal cancer. Cancer, *38*:2310–15, 1976.
28. Vongtama, V., et al.: End results of radiation therapy alone and in combination with 5-fluorouracil in colorectal cancers. Cancer, *36*:2020–25, 1975.
29. Watkins, E., Jr., Khazei, A. M., and Nahra, K. S.: Surgical basis for arterial infusion chemotherapy of disseminated carcinoma of the liver. Surg. Gynecol. Obstet., *130*:581–605, 1970.
30. Zamchek, N.: Present status of CEA in diagnosis, prognosis and evaluation of therapy. Cancer, *36*:2460–68, 1975.

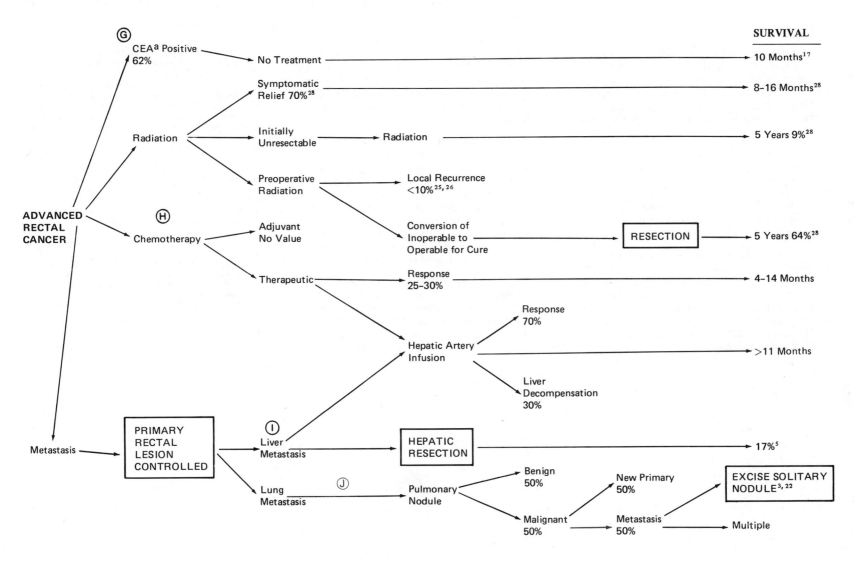

SURVIVAL

ⓖ CEA[a] Positive 62%

No Treatment —————————————→ 10 Months[17]

Radiation

Symptomatic Relief 70%[28] —————————————→ 8–16 Months[28]

Initially Unresectable —→ Radiation —————————————→ 5 Years 9%[28]

Preoperative Radiation

Local Recurrence <10%[25,26]

Conversion of Inoperable to Operable for Cure —————→ RESECTION —→ 5 Years 64%[28]

ⓗ Chemotherapy

Adjuvant No Value

Therapeutic

Response 25–30% —————————————→ 4–14 Months

Hepatic Artery Infusion

Response 70%

—————————————→ >11 Months

Liver Decompensation 30%

ADVANCED RECTAL CANCER

Metastasis —→ PRIMARY RECTAL LESION CONTROLLED

ⓘ Liver Metastasis —→ HEPATIC RESECTION —————————————→ 17%[5]

ⓙ Lung Metastasis —→ Pulmonary Nodule

Benign 50%

Malignant 50% —→ Metastasis 50%

New Primary 50% —→ EXCISE SOLITARY NODULE[3,22]

—→ Multiple

[a]Carcinoembryonic Antigen

301

PENETRATING INJURIES OF THE COLON

BY ERNEST E. MOORE, M.D., AND HENRY C. CLEVELAND, M.D.

Comments

A. Antibiotics (aminoglycosides for coliform bacteria and clindamycin for anaerobes) are only of significant value if started preoperatively.[1, 2] Missiles should be removed if possible.[3] Even with the skin left open wound infection occurs in 5 to 15 per cent of cases.

B. Contraindications to primary closure include (1) greater than 6 hours' delay in closure, (2) marked fecal contamination, (3) two or more visceral injuries, particularly of the liver and pancreas, (4) extensive colon or mesenteric injury, and (5) an unstable or debilitated patient.

C. Thirty to 50 per cent of civilian colon injuries can be closed primarily,[5, 6] but deviation from the limitations listed in Comment B results in high morbidity and mortality rates.[7] Colon injuries under military conditions are not closed primarily. Right colon injuries are treated the same as left colon trauma.[8]

D. Primary repair and exteriorization is a compromise procedure; if it breaks down it is no worse than a colostomy. The exteriorized bowel must be kept moist. Breakdowns occur before the seventh postoperative day. Complications are minimal if intraperitonealization is delayed until the tenth day.[9]

E. The morbidity rate of colostomy closure following trauma is much higher than when the stoma is created electively. This is due in part to the higher incidences of intraperitoneal abscess, adhesions, and loss of bowel that result from injuries. Morbidity and mortality rates of colostomy closure must be considered in the decision for colostomy versus primary closure or anastomosis at the initial treatment.[10]

F. The supralevator spaces do not contain infection well. The fecal stream must be diverted with a colostomy and the pelvis must be widely drained.[4, 8, 11] Fecal incontinence, impotence, and urinary tract fistula may occur with perineal wounds.

References

1. Fullen, W. D., Hunt, J., and Altemeir, W. A.: Prophylactic antibiotics in penetrating wounds of the abdomen. J. Trauma, 12:282, 1972.
2. Thadepalli, H., et al.: Abdominal trauma, anaerobes and antibiotics. Surg. Gynecol. Obstet., 137:270, 1973.
3. Flint, L. M., et al.: Missile tract infections after transcolonic gunshot wounds. Arch. Surg., 113:270, 1973.
4. Kirkpatrich, J. R.: Injuries of the colon. Surg. Clin. North Am., 57:67, 1977.
5. Mulherin, J. L., and Sawyers, J. L.: Evaluation of 3 methods for managing penetrating colon injuries. J. Trauma, 15:580, 1975.
6. Matolo, N. M., and Wolfman, E. F.: Primary repair of colonic injuries: A clinical evaluation. J. Trauma, 17:554, 1977.
7. Steele, M., and Blaisdell, F. W.: Treatment of colonic injuries. J. Trauma, 17:557, 1977.
8. Bartizal, J. F., et al.: A critical review of management of 392 colonic and rectal injuries. Dis. Colon Rectum, 17:313, 1974.
9. Kirkpatrich, J. R.: The exteriorized anastomosis: Its role in surgery of the colon. Surgery, 82:362, 1977.
10. Yajko, R. D., et al.: Morbidity of colostomy closure. Am. J. Surg., 132:304, 1976.
11. Trunkey, D., Hays, R. J., and Shires, G. T.: Management of rectal trauma. J. Trauma, 13:411, 1973.

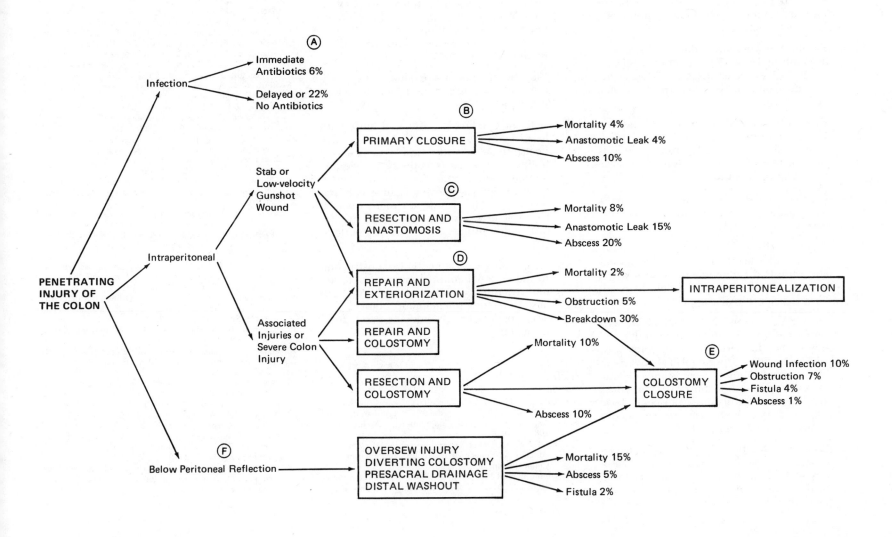

ACUTE LARGE BOWEL OBSTRUCTION BY J. B. MOORE, M.D., AND E. E. MOORE, JR., M.D.

Comments

A. Eight to 13 per cent of patients with colorectal carcinoma develop symptomatic large bowel obstruction.[2-4]

B. Partial and complete colonic obstruction account for 15 to 25 per cent of surgically treated diverticular disease.[5-10] Only one in four operations is for complete colonic obstruction.[8]

C. Complete obstruction complicating diverticulitis requires resection. Although prognosis of a resolved obstructing episode is not documented,[11] such extensive disease will require operation.

D. Comparative data on operative methods of managing obstructive diverticular disease are unavailable.[12-15]

E. There is always a lingering doubt about co-existing cancer.[16] If one can be reasonably sure that carcinoma does not exist, a waiting period of at least 3 months is advisable prior to reanastomosis.

F. Over 80 per cent of the patients in this series had penetrating colonic and rectal trauma as the indication for colostomy, while less than 5 per cent had diverticulitis. Complications of colostomy closure include wound infection (10 per cent), anastomotic obstruction (7 per cent), fecal fistula (4 per cent), and miscellaneous complications (7 per cent).[17]

G. Pseudo-obstruction of the colon is characterized by massive nonobstructive gaseous distention of the colon and is localized to the right colon and cecum in more than half of cases.[18]

H. Most patients have severe associated disease and are poor candidates for any surgical procedure. Indications for operation include failure to improve with complete bowel rest and suction over 2 to 3 days, cecal diameter greater than 12 cm., or peritoneal signs.[19, 20]

I. Flexible colonoscopy excludes the possibility of an obstructing lesion or bowel ischemia.[21]

J. Both uncomplicated cases and those with localized perforation or necrosis have been treated with tube cecostomy.[20] Splitting of teniae secondary to overdistention permits mucosal extrusion, which is an inadequate barrier against coliform organisms. This results in more than 50 per cent of cases having positive peritoneal fluid cultures even without perforation.[22]

K. Other causes of large bowel obstruction include intra-abdominal metastasis, ischemic stricture, foreign bodies, hernia, adhesive bands, inflammatory bowel disease, pancreatic pseudocyst, and fecal impaction.

References

1. Greenlee, H. B., et al.: Acute large bowel obstruction: Comparison of county, Veterans' Administration, and community hospital populations. Arch. Surg., 108:407, 1974.
2. Kronborg, O., Bacher, O., and Sprechler, M.: Acute obstruction in cancer of the colon and rectum. Dis. Colon Rectum, 18:22, 1975.
3. Glenn, F., and McSherry, C. K.: Obstruction and perforation in colorectal cancer. Am. Surg., 173:983, 1971.
4. Welch, J. P., and Donaldson, G. A.: Management of severe obstruction of the large bowel due to malignant disease. Am. J. Surg., 127:492, 1974.
5. Asch, M. J., and Markowitz, A. M.: Diverticulitis coli: A surgical appraisal. Surgery, 62:239, 1967.
6. Botsford, T. W., and Curtis, L. E.: Diverticulitis coli: Criteria of management for the physician and the surgeon. N. Engl. J. Med., 265:618, 1961.
7. Byrne, J. J., and Garich, E. I.: Surgical treatment of diverticulitis. Am. J. Surg., 121:379, 1971.
8. Petrozzi, C. A., and Lange, W. G.: Acute complications of colonic diverticulitis. Am. J. Proctol. 23:49, 1972.
9. Welch, C. E., Allen, A. W., and Donaldson, G. A.: An appraisal of resection of the colon for diverticulitis of the sigmoid. Ann. Surg., 138:332, 1953.
10. Ponka, J. L., and Shaalan, K.: Changing aspects in surgery of diverticulitis. Arch. Surg., 89:31, 1964.
11. Zollinger, R. W.: The prognosis in diverticulitis of the colon. Arch. Surg., 97:418, 1968.
12. Classen, J. N., et al.: Surgical treatment of acute diverticulitis by staged procedures. Ann. Surg., 184:582, 1976.
13. Colcock, B. P.: Surgical treatment of diverticulitis: 20 years' experience. Am. J. Surg., 115:264, 1968.
14. Hughes, L. E.: Complications of diverticular disease: Inflammation, obstruction and bleeding. Clin. Gastroenterol., 4:147, 1975.
15. Rodkey, G. U., and Welch, C. E.: Colonic diverticular disease with surgical treatment: A study of 388 cases. Surg. Clin. North Am., 54:655, 1974.
16. Morton, D. L., and Goldman, L.: Differential diagnosis of diverticulitis and carcinoma of the sigmoid colon. Am. J. Surg., 103:55, 1962.
17. Eiseman, B.: Morbidity of colostomy closure. Am. J. Surg., 132:304, 1976.
18. Ogilvie, H.: Large intestine colic due to sympathetic deprivation: A new clinical syndrome. Br. Med. J., 2:671, 1948.
19. Wojtalik, R. S., Lindenauer, S. M., and Kahn, S. S.: Perforation of the colon associated with adynamic ileus. Am. J. Surg., 125:601, 1973.
20. Adams, T. T.: Adynamic ileus of the colon: An indication for cecostomy. Arch. Surg., 109:503, 1974.
21. Kukora, J. S., and Dent, T. L.: Colonoscopic decompression of massive nonobstructive cecal dilation. Arch. Surg., 112:512, 1977.
22. Norton, L., Young, D., and Scribner, R.: Management of pseudo-obstruction of the colon. Surg. Gynecol. Obstet., 138:595, 1974.

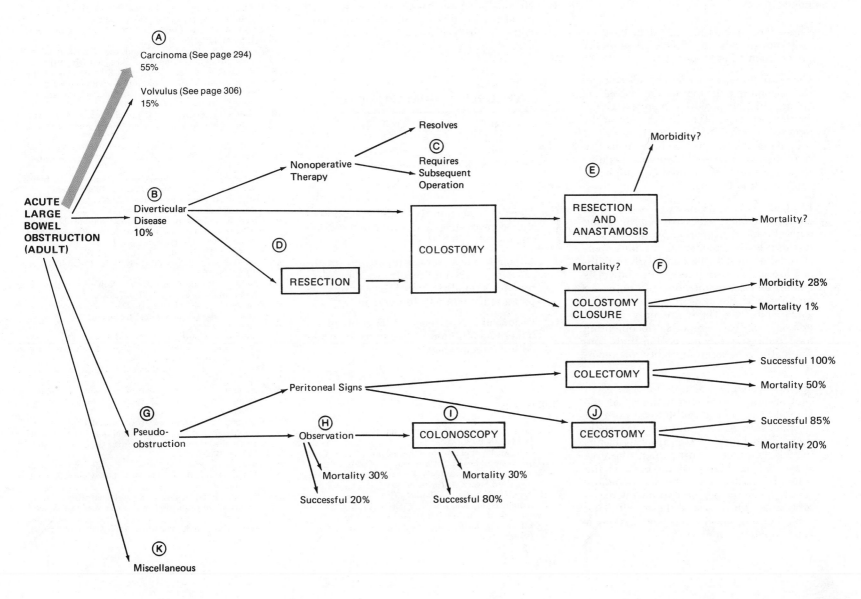

Ⓐ Carcinoma (See page 294)
55%

Volvulus (See page 306)
15%

ACUTE LARGE BOWEL OBSTRUCTION (ADULT)

Ⓑ Diverticular Disease 10%

Nonoperative Therapy

Resolves

Ⓒ Requires Subsequent Operation

Ⓓ RESECTION

COLOSTOMY

Ⓔ RESECTION AND ANASTAMOSIS

Morbidity?

Mortality?

Mortality?

Ⓕ COLOSTOMY CLOSURE

Morbidity 28%

Mortality 1%

Peritoneal Signs

COLECTOMY

Successful 100%

Mortality 50%

Ⓖ Pseudo-obstruction

Ⓗ Observation

Ⓘ COLONOSCOPY

Ⓙ CECOSTOMY

Successful 85%

Mortality 20%

Mortality 30%

Successful 20%

Mortality 30%

Successful 80%

Ⓚ Miscellaneous

VOLVULUS BY JOHN B. MOORE, M.D., AND ERNEST E. MOORE, JR., M.D.

Comments

A. Three large series are the data base for large bowel volvulus.[1-3] Overall mortality ranges from 15 to 30 per cent.

B. Cecal volvulus is associated with congenital incomplete fusion of the ascending colon with the posterior parietes. Hypofixation occurs in 10 to 15 per cent of the general population. Precipitating factors producing symptoms include constipation, increased peristalsis, a postoperative or postpartum state, overeating, a high residue diet, and trauma.[4-9]

C. Etiologic factors in this rare condition include congenital excessive length; aging with chronic constipation, weight loss, or loss of intestinal tone; and previous operative adhesions.[10] Detorsion with or without fixation is performed if the bowel is viable, and resection and colostomy are performed if the bowel is perforated or gangrenous.[11, 12] There are only a small number of case reports documenting transfixation of the mesocolon and, consequently, no solid mortality or recurrence data.

D. Sigmoid volvulus accounts for 3 to 5 per cent of large bowel obstruction[13-15] in the United States but up to 30 to 50 per cent in some East Asian countries.[15] It usually occurs in the elderly. Contributing factors include chronic constipation, laxative abuse, and a high residue diet. If the colon is viable, reduction by sigmoidoscope, colonoscope, or barium enema is preferable. Only when these fail or if compromised bowel is suspected is emergency operation indicated.[14, 16]

E. Nonoperative recurrence varies from 20 to 90 per cent,[2, 16-21] with increased mortality with successive recurrent episodes.[16, 18, 19]

EPISODE	MORTALITY (%)[19]
1st	7
2nd	17
3rd	38

Elective resection is widely supported after conservative and surgical detorsion therapy.[2, 3, 13, 15, 17, 18, 20-22]

F. Although most series report no recurrence or a very rare recurrence after elective resection,[14, 15, 17, 18, 22] two series report a range of 4.5 to 10 per cent.[13, 19]

G. Bhatnagar's experience in 35 cases of extraperitonealization of the sigmoid resulted in no recurrence.[23]

References

1. Dadoo, R. C., et al.: Volvulus of the large gut. Am. J. Proctol., 24:69, 1975.
2. Inberg, M. V., et al.: Acute intestinal volvulus. A report of 238 cases. Scand. J. Gastroenterol., 7:209, 1972.
3. Kronborg, O., and Lauritsen, K.: Volvulus of the colon. Acta Chir. Scand., 141:550, 1975.
4. Grover, N. K., et al.: Volvulus of the cecum and ascending colon. Am. J. Surg., 125:672, 1973.
5. Meyers, J. R., Heifetz, C. J., and Baue, A. E.: Cecal volvulus: A lesion requiring resection. Arch. Surg., 104:594, 1972.
6. Rahbar, A., Easley, G. W., and Mendoza, C. B.: Volvulus of the cecum. Am. Surg., 39:325, 1973.
7. Smith, W. R., and Goodwin, J. N.: Cecal volvulus. Am. J. Surg., 126:215, 1975.
8. Anderson, A., Bergdahl, L., and Van Den Linden, W.: Volvulus of the cecum. Ann. Surg., 181:876, 1975.
9. Halvorsen, J. F., and Semb, H. K.: Volvulus of the right colon: A review of 30 cases with special reference to late results of various surgical procedures. Acta. Chir. Scand., 141:804, 1975.
10. Eisenstat, T. E., Raneri, A. J., and Mason, G. R.: Volvulus of the transverse colon. Am. J. Surg., 134:396, 1977.
11. McGowan, J. M., Soriano, S., and McCausland, W.: Volvulus of the transverse colon. Am. J. Surg., 93:857, 1957.
12. Perdue, G. D., and Polesky, R.: Volvulus of the transverse colon. Am. J. Surg., 103:512, 1962.
13. Sharpton, B., and Cheek, R. C.: Volvulus of the sigmoid colon. Am. Surg., 42:436, 1976.
14. Greco, R. S., Dragon, R. E., and Kerstein, M. D.: Alternatives in management of volvulus of the sigmoid colon. Dis. Colon Rectum, 17:241, 1974.
15. Siroospour, D., and Berardi, R. S.: Volvulus of the sigmoid colon: A 10-year study. Dis. Colon Rectum, 19:535, 1976.
16. Arnold, G. J., and Nance, F. C.: Volvulus of the sigmoid colon. Ann. Surg., 177:527, 1973.
17. Drapanas, T., and Stewart, J. D.: Acute sigmoid volvulus: Concepts in surgical treatment. Am. J. Surg., 101:70, 1961.
18. Hines, J. R., Geurkink, R. E., and Bass, R. T.: Recurrence and mortality rates in sigmoid volvulus. Surg. Gynecol. Obstet., 124:567, 1967.
19. Moseson, D. L., et al.: Sigmoid volvulus. Am. Surg., 42:492, 1976.
20. Shepherd, J. J.: Treatment of volvulus of sigmoid colon: A review of 425 cases. Br. Med. J., 2:280, 1968.
21. Wuepper, K. D., Otteman, M. G., and Stahlgren, L. H.: An appraisal of the operative and nonoperative treatment of sigmoid volvulus. Surg. Gynecol. Obstet., 122:84, 1966.
22. Gama, A. H., et al.: Volvulus of the sigmoid colon in Brazil: A report of 230 cases. Dis. Colon Rectum, 19:314, 1976.
23. Bhatnagar, B. N. S., Roy, S. K., and Chakravarty, M. R.: Comparative evaluation of the commonly performed emergency procedures for the prevention of recurrence of sigmoid volvulus. Am. J. Proctol., 29:35, 1977.

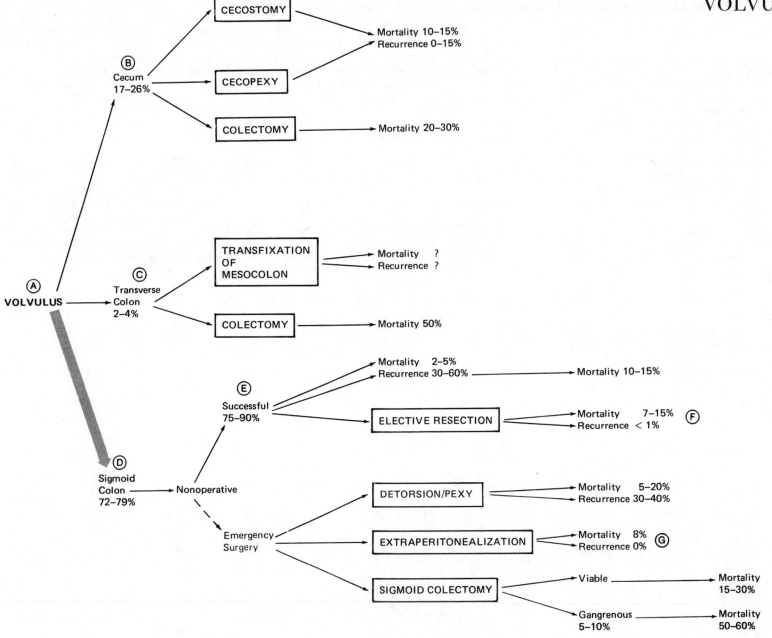

HEMORRHOIDS BY JOSEPH GREER, M.D.

Comments

A. Hemorrhoids due to increased intra-abdominal pressure may be caused by
   (1) Pregnancy. Internal and external hemorrhoids may appear in the third trimester or at delivery. Ninety-nine per cent become asymptomatic in the postpartum period.
   (2) Cirrhosis and portal hypertension. Symptomatic therapy is indicated. Injection may be helpful. Poor clotting may lead to increased bleeding after rubber-band ligation or cryosurgery.
   (3) Chronic lung disease, which characteristically produces first-degree mucosal prolapse. Localized areas may respond to office treatment but circumferential tissue is best managed with excision.

   Rectal and colon cancer mimic hemorrhoids by producing painless rectal bleeding. All such patients should have proctosigmoidoscopy. Those over 40 or who have a change in bowel habits or abdominal symptoms require x-ray examination of the colon.

B. The accepted classification of Goligher[1] is as follows:

   1st Degree: Engorgment and congestion with projection into the anal canal with defecation.

   2nd Degree: Engorged tissue prolapses into the anal canal with defecation but returns spontaneously.

   3rd Degree: Tissue prolapses through the anal canal and requires manual reduction.

   4th Degree: Prolapse persists despite attempts to reduce it.

C. Cure rates for nonexcisional methods decrease with increased severity of disease. Excisional hemorrhoidectomy is the definitive treatment of choice for third and fourth degree internal hemorrhoids. Patient request, advanced age, or poor health may dictate the use of other methods for attempted relief of symptoms.

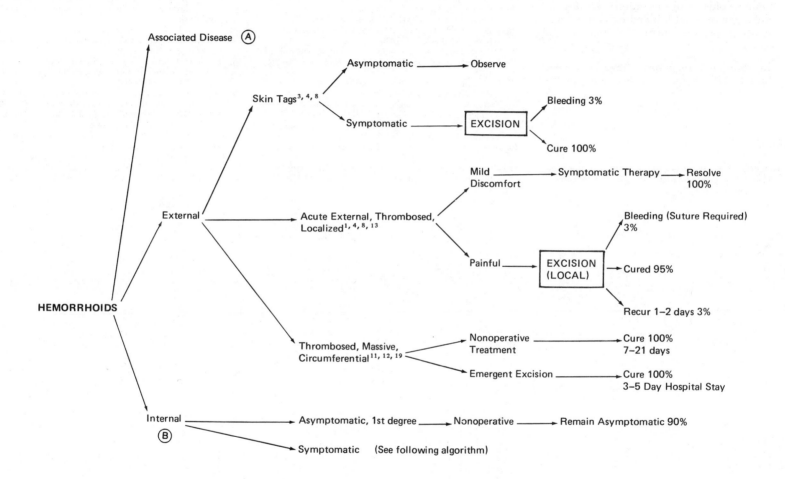

D. The Lord operation of dilatation has little following in the United States. It should not be used in third or fourth degree hemorrhoids or in the elderly. Cure is 80 to 90 per cent, with bleeding and incontinence a problem in 4 to 5 per cent of cases.

E. Ligation and cryosurgery have been combined with some improvement in results.[9, 12]

References

1. Goligher, J. C.: Surgery of the Anus, Rectum, and Colon, 2nd ed. Springfield, Ill., Charles C Thomas, 1970, pp. 111–167.
2. Goligher, J. C.: Cryosurgery for hemorrhoids. Dis. Colon Rectum, *19*:213–218, 1976.
3. Goldberg, S. M., et al.: Symposium on anal surgery. Contemp. Surg., *11*:29–55, November 1977.
4. Goldberg, S. M., et al.: Symposium on anal surgery. Contemp. Surg., *11*:34–51, December 1977.
5. Salvati, E. P.: Ligation of internal hemorrhoids. Proc. R. Soc. Med., *63*:111, 1970.
6. Oh, C.: Treatment of hemorrhoids and application of cryotechnique. Mt. Sinai J. Med., N. Y. *42*:179–204, 1975.
7. Ferguson, J. A., et al.: The closed technique of hemorrhoidectomy. Surgery, *70*:480–484, 1971.
8. Nigro, N. D.: Common guidelines for treating hemorrhoids. Consultant, February 1967, pp. 10–12.
9. Rudd, W. H.: Ligation of hemorrhoids as an office procedure. Can. Med. J., *108*:56–59, 1973.
10. Burkitt, D.: Epidemiology of large bowel disease. Recent Adv. Surg., *8*:257, 1973.
11. Mazier, W. P., et al.: Symposium: Hemorrhoidectomy — How I do it. Dis. Colon Rectum, *20*:173–208, 1977.
12. Turell, R., et al.: Symposium: Diverse methods of managing hemorrhoids. Dis. Colon Rectum, *16*:171–192, 1973.
13. Turell, R., et al.: Diseases of the Colon and Anorectum, 2nd ed. Philadelphia, W. B. Saunders, 1969, pp. 895–954.
14. Hugo, G. J., et al.: Symposium: The role of cryotherapy in the management of anorectal disease. Dis. Colon Rectum, *18*:281–303, 1975.
15. Bacon, H. E.: Anus, Rectum, Sigmoid Colon — Diagnosis and Treatment, Vol 1. Philadelphia, J. B. Lippincott, 1949, pp. 451–496.
16. Salvati, E. P.: Evaluation of ligation of hemorrhoids as an office procedure. Dis. Colon Rectum, *10*:53, 1967.
17. Wantz, G. E.: A rubberband ligation for internal hemorrhoids. Medical Times, October 1977, p. 47.
18. Lewis, M. I.: Cryosurgical hemorrhoidectomy. Dis. Colon Rectum, *15*:128–134, 1972.
19. Ganchrow, M. I.: Hemorrhoidectomy revisited: A computer analysis of 2038 cases. Dis. Colon Rectum, *14*:128–33, 1971.

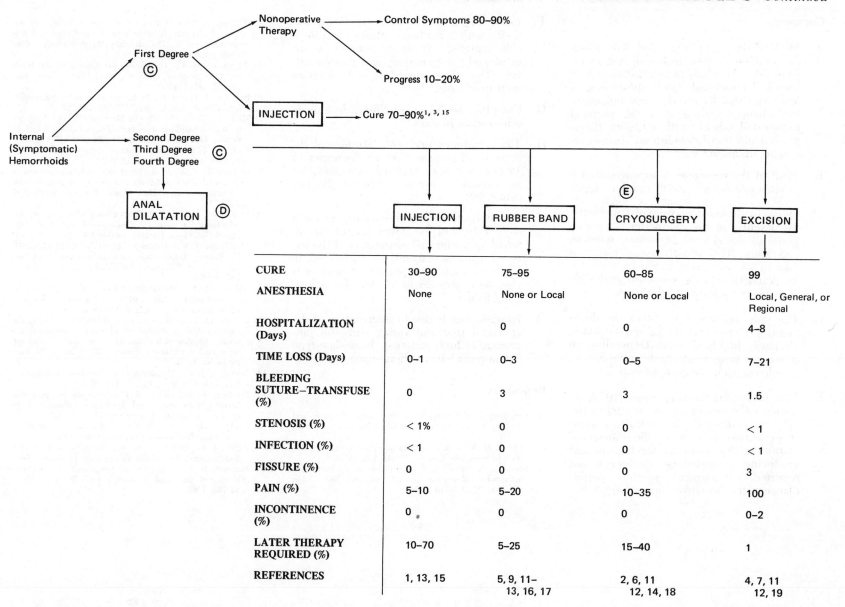

Nonoperative Therapy ────→ Control Symptoms 80–90%

First Degree ©

Progress 10–20%

INJECTION ──→ Cure 70–90%[1, 3, 15]

Internal (Symptomatic) Hemorrhoids

Second Degree
Third Degree ©
Fourth Degree

ANAL DILATATION ⓓ

Ⓔ

	INJECTION	RUBBER BAND	CRYOSURGERY	EXCISION
CURE	30–90	75–95	60–85	99
ANESTHESIA	None	None or Local	None or Local	Local, General, or Regional
HOSPITALIZATION (Days)	0	0	0	4–8
TIME LOSS (Days)	0–1	0–3	0–5	7–21
BLEEDING SUTURE–TRANSFUSE (%)	0	3	3	1.5
STENOSIS (%)	< 1%	0	0	< 1
INFECTION (%)	< 1	0	0	< 1
FISSURE (%)	0	0	0	3
PAIN (%)	5–10	5–20	10–35	100
INCONTINENCE (%)	0	0	0	0–2
LATER THERAPY REQUIRED (%)	10–70	5–25	15–40	1
REFERENCES	1, 13, 15	5, 9, 11–13, 16, 17	2, 6, 11 12, 14, 18	4, 7, 11 12, 19

ANORECTAL ABSCESS BY D. MIRELMAN, M.D.

Comments

A. Medical therapy is indicated only when concomitant disease makes operation inadvisable; these are mainly inflammatory bowel disease and blood dyscrasias. A few cases that have only early inflammatory changes (cellulitis) in the perianal region will subside with antibiotic therapy, but most will develop an abscess requiring drainage.[1, 2, 8, 9]

B. Most of the recurrences appear within 6 months following incision and drainage.[3-5]

C. Delay in drainage may involve necrotizing fasciitis of the perineum, i.e., gangrene of the skin of perineum, scrotum, and groin. This ghastly complication is fatal in 6.5 per cent of cases. Treatment is by defunctionalizing colostomy and wide incision or excision and drainage.[1, 6, 7]

D. The sole reference in literature documents a 6.5 per cent mortality rate[7] but is obviously highly skewed. Depending on degree of prior neglect, the mortality of simple excision should approach zero.[7]

E. The prolonged healing time (49 days) counters the reported cure rate (96 to 100 per cent). Although theoretically a more cost-effective procedure, the danger of disrupting the sphincter mechanism and producing incontinence (incidence not reported) discourages routine performance of the "curative" operation.[5, 10, 11]

F. Incise and drain the abscess, closing the cavity with 3 mattress sutures of absorbable material. Systemic antibiotics are employed preoperatively and postoperatively. The whole procedure is done on an outpatient basis.[1, 12, 15]

G. Complete healing with this technique is achieved in 10 days.[13-15]

H. The recurrence rate with ischiorectal abscess is 33 per cent, which decreases to 15 per cent with perianal abscesses, for an overall recurrence rate of 20 per cent.[1, 12, 13]

I. Hospitalization characteristically is for 5 days. Fibers of the lower part of the internal sphincter and sometimes of the external sphincter should be transected to achieve a cure. The process of healing is slow and takes 28 to 35 days for a low-lying fistula.[1, 16]

J. Incontinence is due to interruption of the anorectal ring and varies with the percentage of high variety or horseshoe-type fistula included in different reports.[1, 17, 18]

· References

1. Goligher, J. C.: Surgery of the Anus, Rectum and Colon, 3rd ed. Springfield, Ill., Charles C Thomas, 1975.
2. Sehdev, M. K., et al.: Perianal and anorectal complication in leukemia. Cancer, 31:149–152, 1973.
3. Scoma, J. A., Salvati, E. P., and Rubin, R. T.: Incidence of fistulas subsequent to anal abscesses. Dis. Colon Rectum, 17:357–359, 1974.
4. Hughes, E. S. R.: Inflammations and infections of the anus. In Turell, R.: Diseases of the Colon and Anorectum, vol. 2. Philadelphia, W. B. Saunders Co., 1969, pp. 955–996.
5. Waggener, H. U.: Immediate fistulotomy in the treatment of perianal abscess. Surg. Clin. North Am., 49:1227–1233, 1969.
6. Bevans, D. W., et al.: Perirectal abscess: a potentially fatal illness. Am. J. Surg., 126:765–768, 1973.
7. Mark, G., Chase, W. V., and Mervine, T.: The fatal potential of fistula-in-ano with abscess: Analysis of 11 deaths. Dis. Colon Rectum, 16:224–230, 1973.
8. Fielding, J. F.: Perianal lesions in Crohn's disease. J. R. Coll. Surg. Edinb., 17:32, 1972.
9. DeBombal, F. T., et al.: Incidence and management of anorectal abscess, fistula and fissure in patient with ulcerative colitis. Dis. Colon Rectum, 9:201–206, 1966.
10. McElwain, J. W., et al.: Experience with primary fistulectomy for anorectal abscess—A report of 1000 cases. Dis. Colon Rectum, 18:646–649, 1975.
11. McElwain, J. W., Alexander, R. M., and MacLean, M. D.: Primary fistulectomy for anorectal abscess: Clinical study of 500 cases. Dis. Colon Rectum, 9:181–185, 1966.
12. Wilson, D. H.: Late results of anorectal abscess treated by incision, curettage and primary suture under antibiotic cover. Br. J. Surg., 51:828–831, 1964.
13. Leaper, D. T., et al.: A controlled study comparing the conventional treatment of idiopathic anorectal abscess with that of incision, curettage and primary suture under antibiotic cover. Dis. Colon Rectum, 19:46–50, 1976.
14. Goligher, J. C.: Management of perianal suppuration. Dis. Colon Rectum, 19:516–517, 1976.
15. Buchan, R., and Grace, R. H.: Anorectal suppuration: Results of treatment and the factors influencing the recurrence rate. Br. J. Surg., 60:537–540, 1973.
16. Lockhart-Mummery, H. E.: Symposium on anorectal problems. Dis. Colon Rectum, 18:650–651, 1975.
17. Parks, A. G., and Stitz, R. W.: The treatment of high fistula-in-ano. Dis. Colon Rectum, 19:487–499, 1976.
18. Bennett, R. C.: A review of the results of orthodox treatment for anal fistulae. Proc. R. Soc. Med., 55:756, 1962.

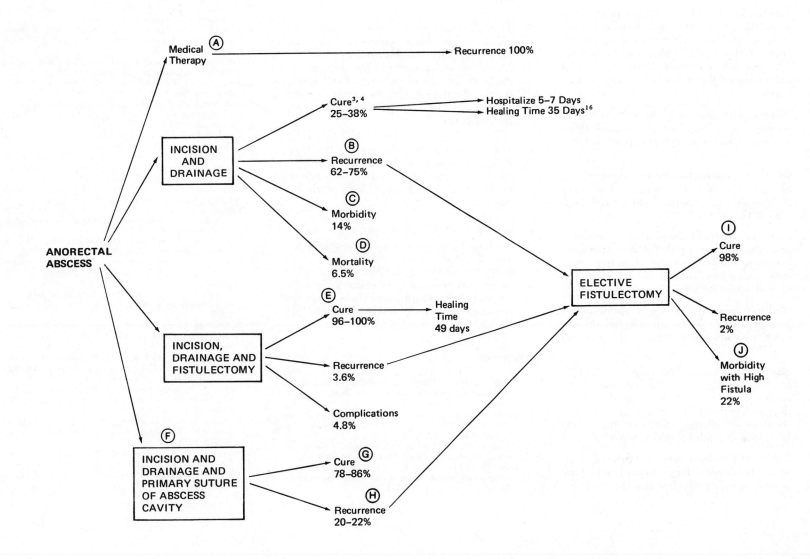

PILONIDAL SINUS BY R. COHEN, M.D.

Comments

A. Pilonidal sinus occurs in 5 per cent of the population,[13] and the male:female ratio is 3 or 4:1.[10] Free hair is found in 50 per cent of the cysts.[10] Most asymptomatic cysts are left untreated.[10] There is caudal extension of the sinus in 7 per cent of cases.

B. Abscess formation is influenced by hypertrichosis or a deep internatal cleft along with poor hygiene[5, 12, 16] and trauma.[11, 21]

C. Belief in congenital versus acquired etiology determines the surgical treatment philosophy, i.e., complete or partial excision of the cyst.[7, 10, 11]

D. I and D is usually used as a preliminary procedure prior to definitive operation but many authors advocate that the definitive procedure should be done in the face of acute abscess.[1, 18]

E. Multiple phenol injections given under general anesthesia in noninfected sinuses have a good cure rate with minimal cost.[16, 19]

F. Marsupialization to the edge of the cyst tract is similar to the laying-open technique, but if it is "marsupialized" to deeper tissue the recurrence and morbidity rates are greater. The cyst tract must be strong enough to hold sutures.[1, 10, 11]

G. This is the time-honored method of treatment. It leaves a large wound with long period of morbidity but has the least recurrence rate if judicious followup is done.[14]

H. This is a most controversial operation because of the high recurrence rate and long hospitalization (10 to 15 days).[9, 11, 18] Many series using plastic flap procedures or angulated incisions that obliterate the deep cleft and those with careful patient selection have better cure rates (90 per cent).[4, 8, 13]

I. This operation, popularized by the English and similar to marsupialization, is the least traumatic procedure with consistently good results and low morbidity rates.[10, 11, 18]

J. Recurrences depend mostly upon the existence of hair, so it must be carefully removed in the postoperative courses of all operative procedures. Other contributing factors are proximity to the anus, deep internatal cleft, complicated sinus tracts (50 per cent of cases), and incomplete followup.[1-7, 10, 18]

References

1. Abramson, D. J.: A simple marsupialization technic for treatment of pilonidal sinus. Ann. Surg., 151:261, 1960.
2. Abramson, D. J.: An open semi-primary closure operation for pilonidal sinus using local anesthesia. Dis. Colon Rectum, 13:215, 1970.
3. Abramson, D. J.: Excision and delayed closure of pilonidal sinus. Surg. Gynecol. Obstet., 144:205, 1977.
4. Aldav, F. S.: Pilonidal cyst and sinus: radical excision and primary closure. Surg. Clin. North Am., 53:559, 1973.
5. Bernhoft, W. H.: Pilonidal disease. Arch. Surg., 94:418, 1967.
6. Edwards, M. H.: Pilonidal sinus — excision and closure. Proc. R. Soc. Med., 63:8, 1970.
7. Eftaiha, M., and Abcarian, H.: The dilemma of pilonidal disease: Surgical treatment. Dis. Colon Rectum, 20:279, 1977.
8. Farringer, J. L., and Pickens, D. R.: Pilonidal cyst — an operative approach. Am. J. Surg., 135:262, 1978.
9. Foss, M. V.: Pilonidal sinus: Excision and closure. Proc. Soc. Med., 63:8, 1970.
10. Goligher, J. C.: Pilonidal sinus. In Surgery of the Anus, Rectum and Colon, 3rd ed. Springfield, Ill., Charles C Thomas, 1975, p. 256.
11. Goodall, P.: Etiology and treatment of pilonidal sinus. Br. J. Surg., 49:212, 1961.
12. Healy, M. J., and Hoffert, P. W.: Pilonidal sinus and cyst: A comparative evaluation of various surgical methods. Am. J. Surg., 87:578, 1954.
13. Karydakis, G. E.: New approach to the problem of pilonidal sinus. Lancet, 2:1414, 1973.
14. Lamke, L. O., Larsson, J., and Nylen, B.: Results of different types of operations for pilonidal sinus. Acta Chir. Scand., 140:321, 1974.
15. Lord, P. H., and Millar, D. M.: Pilonidal sinus: A simple treatment. Br. J. Surg., 52:298, 1965.
16. Maurice, B. A., and Greenwood, R. K.: A conservative treatment of pilonidal sinus. Br. J. Surg., 51:510, 1964.
17. McCaughan, J. S.: The results of the surgical treatment of pilonidal cysts. Surg. Gynecol. Obstet., 121:316, 1965.
18. Noraras, M. J.: A review of 3 popular methods of treatment of postnatal (pilonidal) sinus disease. Br. J. Surg., 57:886, 1970.
19. Stephens, F. O., and Sloane, D. R.: Conservative management of pilonidal sinus. Surg. Gynecol. Obstet., 129:786, 1969.
20. Shons, A. R., and Mountjoy, J. R.: Pilonidal disease: The case for excision with primary closure. Dis. Colon Rectum, 14:353, 1971.
21. Swinton, N. W., and Markee, R. K.: Present status of treatment of pilonidal sinus disease. Am. J. Surg., 86:562, 1953.
22. Weinstein, M. A., Rubin, R. J., and Salvati, E. P.: The dilemma of pilonidal disease — pilonidal cystectomy: Reappraisal of an old technic. Dis. Colon Rectum, 20:287, 1977.

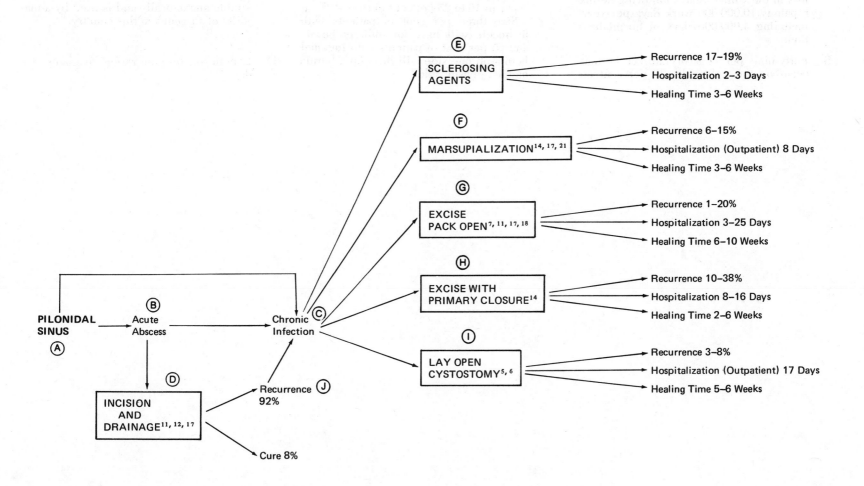

PILONIDAL SINUS (A)

Acute Abscess (B)

Chronic Infection (C)

INCISION AND DRAINAGE[11, 12, 17] (D)

Recurrence 92% (J)

Cure 8%

SCLEROSING AGENTS (E)
→ Recurrence 17–19%
→ Hospitalization 2–3 Days
→ Healing Time 3–6 Weeks

MARSUPIALIZATION[14, 17, 21] (F)
→ Recurrence 6–15%
→ Hospitalization (Outpatient) 8 Days
→ Healing Time 3–6 Weeks

EXCISE PACK OPEN[7, 11, 17, 18] (G)
→ Recurrence 1–20%
→ Hospitalization 3–25 Days
→ Healing Time 6–10 Weeks

EXCISE WITH PRIMARY CLOSURE[14] (H)
→ Recurrence 10–38%
→ Hospitalization 8–16 Days
→ Healing Time 2–6 Weeks

LAY OPEN CYSTOSTOMY[5, 6] (I)
→ Recurrence 3–8%
→ Hospitalization (Outpatient) 17 Days
→ Healing Time 5–6 Weeks

ADULT GROIN HERNIAS BY JACK GALLAGHER, M.D., AND T. K. EARLEY, M.D.

Comments

A. Incidence is 40 cases per 1000 adults, and 90 per cent occur in males.[17] Work loss in the United States following hernia repair is 10,000,000 work days per year, including 4,000,000 days of hospitalization.

B. Forty-nine per cent of indirect hernias occur on the right side, 38 per cent on the left side and 13 per cent are bilateral. Sliding hernias make up 2 to 5 per cent with the left side predominant. Direct and indirect hernias (on the same side) occur in 10 to 25 per cent of cases.[4, 15]

Sixty-three per cent of patients with hydrocele will have an indirect hernia and 25 per cent of patients with inguinal hernia on one side will develop a hernia on the opposite side.[8]

C. Although there is controversy and although reports in the literature definitely vary with individual series, a Cooper's ligament (McVay) repair seems most desirable anatomically and is used by a majority of surgeons in this country.

D. Length of hospitalization averages 4.2 days.[19]

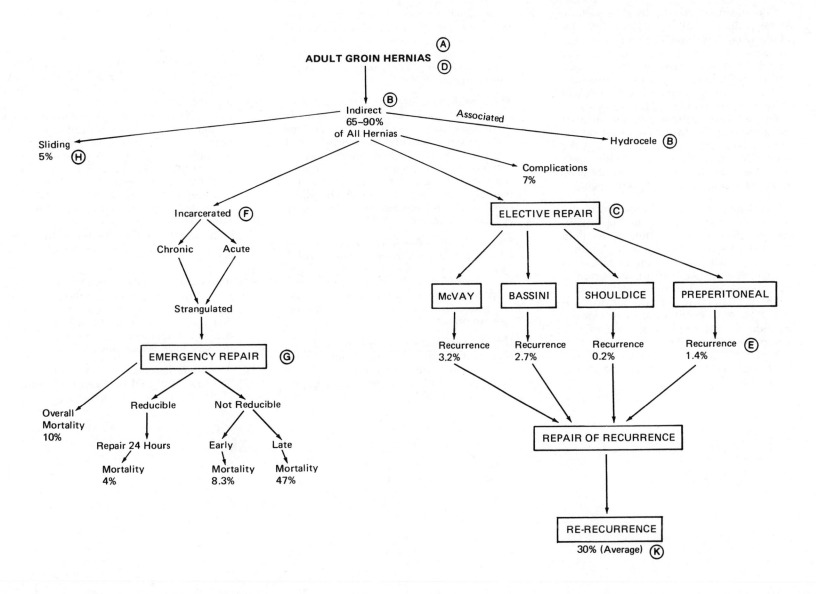

Complications may be local or systemic for patients of all ages. Local ones include major infection (1.3 per cent), hematoma (0.7 per cent), and testicular atrophy (1.8 per cent). Systemic complications include cardiovascular-pulmonary (4.1 per cent), urinary (1.5 per cent), and miscellaneous problems (1.3 per cent).

Overall complication rate for all ages is 6.9 per cent.[2, 5] In patients over 60 the complication rate is 27 per cent and the mortality rate is 2 per cent. With emergency surgery the complication rate is 52 per cent and mortality is 12.5 per cent.[9]

E. More than 50 per cent of recurrences are associated with indirect hernia repair, and 62 per cent of recurrences occur in the first 5 years.[3, 11] Causes for recurrence include a 16.3 per cent rate of failure to recognize a concomitant direct hernia at operation.[4] The recurrence rate is 2 to 5 times if bilateral repair is done originally.[2, 13] Factors contributing to recurrence include chronic respiratory problems (36 per cent), urinary distention or infection (35 per cent), anorectal disease (12 per cent), and ascites or multiple pregnancy (5 per cent).[20]

F. An associated chronic illness was found in 26 per cent of cases and an associated acute illness in 17 per cent to be contributing to incarceration. Therefore, one should look for a contributing cause for the incarceration.[10]

G. The overall mortality rate associated with emergency operations is 10 per cent. If the incarceration is reduced and the hernia repaired electively, the mortality is 4 per cent.[7] Emergency herniorrhaphy in patients more than 60 years old carries a complication rate of 56 per cent and a mortality rate of 12 per cent.[9] Therefore, early repair is mandatory if the hernia cannot be reduced.

H. Sliding hernia constitutes 5 per cent of all indirect inguinal hernias and occurs 5 times more more frequently on the left side. Over 95 per cent occur in men, and 28 per cent are bilateral.[5] These hernias are generally associated with advanced age and obesity.

I. Direct hernias make up less than 10 per cent of all inguinal hernias and can be found in association with indirect hernias in 7 per cent of cases.[15, 20] Direct hernia is unusual in women. The incidence increases with age.

J. Femoral hernias are more commonly found in women and often are associated with obesity. Average age of occurrence is 58 for women and 52 for men. They occur bilaterally in 3 to 4 per cent of cases. There is an associated inguinal hernia found in 9 per cent of female patients and 50 per cent of male patients.[6] Seventy per cent of strangulated hernias occurred in patients over 60 years of age, with an overall mortality of 13 per cent; mortality is 26 per cent if strangulation is associated with resection or gangrene. Mortality is 8.3 per cent if the operation is performed within 24 hours of occurrence and 47 per cent if done after that time.[18]

K. Reports of the rate of re-recurrence vary from 3 to 40 per cent, but the average of several authors is 30 per cent. A relaxing incision appears to be even more important in the repair of re-recurrence than in primary herniorrhaphies.[2, 12, 13]

L. Use of Marlex mesh is very rarely necessary. It should be used between the conjoined

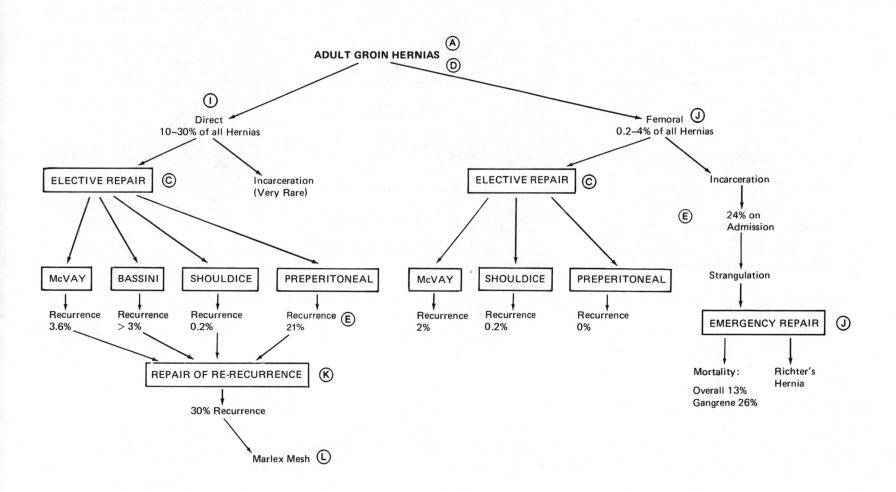

tendon and Cooper's ligament. Rerecurrence rate using this technique is reported at 3 per cent.[21]

INGUINAL HERNIA IN A 65 YEAR OLD MAN

M. All data are from Neuhauser, D.: Elective inguinal herniorrhaphy versus truss in the elderly. *In* Burker, J. P., Barnes, B. A., and Mosteller, F. (eds.): Costs, Risks, and Benefits in Surgery. New York, Oxford University Press, 1977, pp. 223–239. Adapted and used with permission of the author and publisher.

N. An inguinal hernia in a 65 year old man has a ±90 per cent probability of being a *direct* rather than an indirect hernia. The probability of incarceration, obstruction, and strangulation would be significantly greater with an indirect hernia. These data give no weight to the quality of life with an untreated hernia, with a truss, or following a successful repair.

References

1. Weinstein, M., and Roberts, M.: Recurrent inguinal hernia. Am. J. Surg., 129:564–569, 1975.
2. Halverson, K., and McVay, C. B.: Inguinal and femoral hernioplasty. A 22-year study of the authors' methods. Arch. Surg., 101:127–135, 1970.
3. McVay, C. B., and Ravitch, M. N.: Inguinal hernia. Curr. Probl. Surg., October, 1967.
4. Palumbo, L. T., and Sharpe, W. S.: Primary inguinal hernioplasty in the adult. Surg. Clin. North Am., 51:1293–1307, 1971.
5. Ryan, E. A.: An analysis of 303 consecutive cases of indirect sliding inguinal hernias. Surg. Gynecol. Obstet., 102:45–58, 1956.
6. Glassow, F.: Femoral hernia: Review of 1143 consecutive repairs. Ann. Surg., 163:227–232, 1966.
7. Kauffman, H. M., and O'Brien, D. P.: Selective reduction of incarcerated inguinal hernia. Am. J. Surg., 119:660, 1970.
8. Schwartz, S. I. (ed.): Principles of Surgery, 2nd ed. New York, McGraw-Hill, 1974.
9. Williams, J. S., and Hale, H. W.: The advisability of inguinal herniorrhaphy in the elderly. Surg. Gynecol. Obstet., 122:100, 1966.
10. Craighead, C. C., Coltar, A. M., and Moore, K.: Associated disorders with acute incarcerated groin hernia. Ann. Surg., 159:987, 1964.
11. Postlethwait, R. W.: Causes of recurrence after inguinal herniorrhaphy. Surgery, 69:772, 1971.
12. Thieme, E. T.: Recurrent inguinal hernia. Arch. Surg., 103:238, 1971.
13. Madden, J. L., Hakim, S., and Agorogiannis, A. B.: Anatomy and repair of inguinal hernias. Surg. Clin. North Am., 51:1269, 1971.
14. Sheraburn, K., and Myers, B.: Shouldice repair for inguinal hernia. Surgery, 66:450, 1969.
15. Rhoads, J., et al.: Surgery: Principles and Practice, 4th ed. Philadelphia, J. B. Lippincott, 1970.
16. Nyhus, L. M., and Harkins, H. N.: Hernia. Philadelphia, J. B. Lippincott, 1964.
17. Lichtenstein, I.: Hernia Repair Without Disability. St. Louis, C. V. Mosby Co., 1970.
18. Rogers, F. A.: Strangulated femoral hernias: A review of 170 cases. Ann. Surg., 149:9, 1959.
19. Commission on Professional and Hospital Activities: Length of stay in P.A.S. hospitals. Ann Arbor, Michigan, October 1977.
20. Martin, J. D., and Stone, H. H.: Recurrent inguinal hernia. Ann. Surg., 156:713, 1962.
21. Usher, F. C.: Repair of incisional and inguinal hernias. Surg. Gynecol. Obstet., 131:525, 1970.

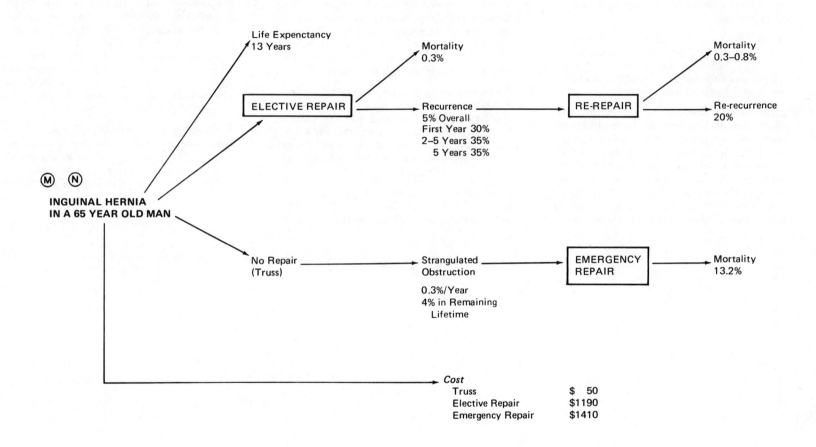

INGUINAL HERNIA
IN A 65 YEAR OLD MAN

Life Expenctancy
13 Years

ELECTIVE REPAIR

Mortality
0.3%

Recurrence
5% Overall
First Year 30%
2–5 Years 35%
 5 Years 35%

RE-REPAIR

Mortality
0.3–0.8%

Re-recurrence
20%

No Repair
(Truss)

Strangulated
Obstruction

0.3%/Year
4% in Remaining
 Lifetime

EMERGENCY
REPAIR

Mortality
13.2%

Cost

Truss	$ 50
Elective Repair	$1190
Emergency Repair	$1410

ELECTIVE LAPAROTOMY BY ERNEST DUNN, M.D., AND BEN EISEMAN, M.D.

Comments

A. Hospitalization the night before operation permits final evaluation of unsuspected disease. Factors affecting mortality and postoperative course include the type of operation and the age and health of the patient.

B. Representative examples of mortality rates include[1-4] 0.2 per cent for appendectomy, 1.0 per cent for cholecystectomy, 1.5 per cent for gastric operation, and 2.1 per cent for colonic operation.

C. *Clean* means that the operation did not enter the gastrointestinal or respiratory tract, and no inflammation was encountered. *Clean contaminated* means that the procedure entered the gastrointestinal or respiratory tract but there was no gross spillage. *Contaminated* means that there was gross spillage from a hollow viscus and acute inflammation without pus.

Dirty means there was a perforated viscus or that pus was encountered. Factors that increase the incidence of infection include obesity, diabetes, and prolonged prior hospitalization.[5, 6]

D. Wound evisceration usually occurs on the fifth to eighth postoperative day and is associated with pulmonary complications, wound sepsis, and abdominal distention. The mortality rate is improved with early recognition and immediate repair.[7-10]

E. Incidence of incisional hernia (skin and subcutaneous tissues intact) varies with the type of incision used and the underlying surgical procedures. Seventy-five per cent of incisional hernias occur within the first year. Wound infection is found in 14 per cent of cases.[11-14]

F. Ileus (absence of normal peristalsis) is normal for the first 24 hours. Prolonged ileus may be due to paralysis secondary to intra-abdominal sepsis or mechanical obstruction secondary to adhesions. Gastric and colonic surgery are the most frequent precursors of mechanical obstruction.[10, 15]

G. Pulmonary complications include hypoventilation, atelectasis, and pneumonia and are associated with obesity, oversedation, immobilization, and a history of cigarette smoking. The incidence depends on the postoperative diagnostic procedures used: physical examination, chest film, or calculation of per cent shunt.[16, 17]

H. Intraoperative aspiration of gastric contents occurs in 7 to 16 per cent of patients. The majority of these events do not produce clinical symptoms. There is an increased rate of aspiration postopera-

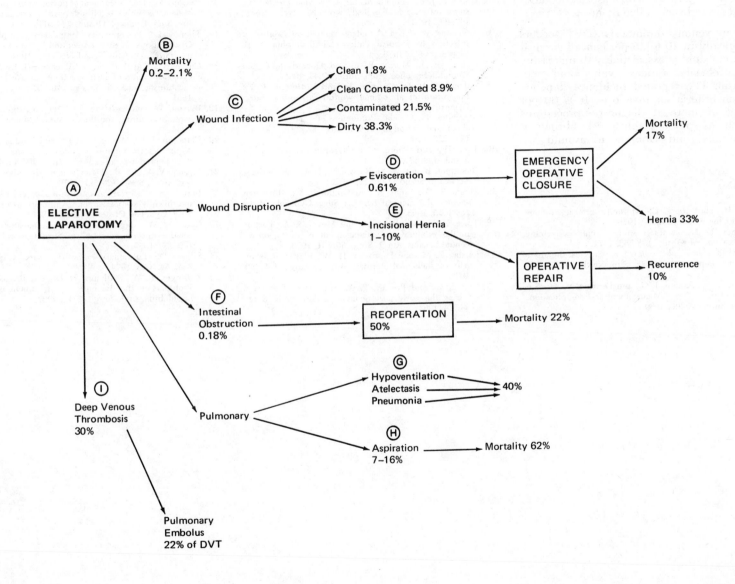

ELECTIVE LAPAROTOMY *Continued*

tively in patients with nasogastric tubes and altered states of consciousness.[18-20]

I. Deep venous thrombosis (DVT) occurs clinically in 10 to 15 per cent of surgical patients and is associated with increasing age, obesity, varicose veins, and neoplasm. The reported incidence depends upon criteria for diagnosis. It is 30 per cent or more if diagnostic procedures such as phlebography, ^{125}I fibrinogen scanning, and Doppler ultrasound are used.[21-25]

References

1. Tera, H., and Aberg, C.: Mortality after laparotomy. Acta Chir. Scand., *142*:67, 1976.
2. Bremner, D. N., et al.: A study of cholecystectomy. Surg. Gynecol. Obset., *138*:752, 1974.
3. Dodworth, J. M., and Fischer, J. E.: Surgical therapy of chronic peptic ulcer. Surg. Clin. North Am., *54*:529, 1974.
4. Beahrs, O. H., Hoehn, J. G., and Dearing, W. H.: Surgery of the colon — Management and complications. Arch. Surg., *98*:480, 1969.
5. Cruse, P. J. E., and Foord, R.: A five-year prospective study of 23,649 surgical wounds. Arch. Surg., *107*:206, 1973.
6. Altemeier, W. A., et al. (eds.): Manual on Control of Infection in Surgical Patients. Philadelphia, J. B. Lippincott Co., 1976.
7. Guiney, E. J., Morris, P. J., and Donaldson, G. A.: Wound dehiscence. Arch. Surg., *92*:47, 1966.
8. Lehman, J. A., Jr., Cross, F. S., and Partington, P. F.: Prevention of abdominal wound disruption. Surg. Gynecol. Obset., *126*:1235, 1968.
9. Alexander, H. C., and Prudden, J. F.: The causes of abdominal wound disruption. Surg. Gynecol. Obstet., *122*:1223, 1966.
10. Tera, H., and Aberg, C.: Relaparotomy. Acta Chir. Scand., *141*:637, 1975.
11. Blomstedt, B. and Welin-Burger, T.: Incisional hernias. Acta Chir. Scand., *138*:275, 1972.
12. Moore, S. W., Conn, J., and Guida, P. M.: Recurrent abdominal incisional hernias. Surg. Gynecol. Obstet., *126*:1015, 1968.
13. Trace, H. D., Kozoll, D. D., and Meyer, K. A.: Factors in the etiology and management of postoperative ventral hernias. Am. J. Surg., *80*:531, 1950.
14. Larson, G. M., and Harrower, H. W.: Plastic mesh repair of incisional hernias. Am. J. Surg., *135*:559, 1978.
15. Coletti, L., and Bossart, P. A.: Intestinal obstruction during the early postoperative period. Arch. Surg., *88*:774, 1964.
16. Becker, A., et al.: Treatment of postoperative pulmonary atelectasis with intermittent positive pressure breathing. Surg. Gynecol. Obstet., *111*:517, 1960.
17. Thoren L.: Postoperative pulmonary complications. Observations on their prevention by means of physiotherapy. Acta Chir. Scand., *107*:193, 1954.
18. Culver, G., Makel, H. P., and Beecher, H. K.: Frequency of aspiration of gastric contents by the lungs during anesthesia and surgery. Am. J. Surg., *133*:289, 1951.
19. Berson, W., and Adriane, J.: Silent regurgitation and aspiration during anesthesia. Anesthesiology, *15*:644, 1954.
20. Cameron, J. L., Mitchell, W. H., and Zuidema, G. D.: Aspiration pneumonia: Clinical outcome following documented aspiration. Arch. Surg., *106*:49, 1973.
21. Kakkar, V. V., et al.: Deep venous thrombosis of the leg. Am. J. Surg., *120*:527, 1970.
22. Barnes, R. W., et al.: Accuracy of Doppler ultrasound in clinically suspected venous thrombosis of the calf. Surg. Gynecol. Obstet., *143*:425, 1976.
23. Coon, W. W., and Coller, F. A.: Clinicopathologic correlation in thromboembolism. Surg. Gynecol. Obstet., *109*:259, 1959.
24. Silver, D.: Pulmonary embolism. Surg. Clin. North Am., *54*:1089, 1974.
25. Zollinger, R. W., Williams, R. D., and Briggs, D. O.: Problems in the diagnosis and treatment of thrombophlebitis. Arch. Surg., *85*:18, 1962.

ESOPHAGOSCOPY, GASTROSCOPY, AND DUODENOSCOPY

ESOPHAGOSCOPY, GASTROSCOPY, AND DUODENOSCOPY BY BARRY W. FRANK, M.D.

Comments

A. These procedures do not require hospitalization. They are performed using local pharyngeal spray anesthesia and light intravenous sedation with diazepam or meperidine or both. To minimize bradycardia or arrhythmia and gastric secretion, premedication with atropine is useful.

B. Factors influencing the incidence of minor complications include[1-3, 7] (1) careful determination of any history of allergies and chronic medications, (2) slow injection of sedative via a large peripheral vein, and (3) removal of patient's dental prostheses and care to avoid trauma to teeth, gums, and pharynx.

C. Several factors influence the incidence of major complications. Perforation[3-5, 7, 8] may be a result of (1) physician's lack of experience, (2) oversedation of the patient, (3) traversing strictured or inflamed areas with undue force, (4) exploration and/or biopsy of a penetrating lesion, and (5) overdistention of the stomach with air.

Bleeding may be minimized by having knowledge of bleeding disorders and any anticoagulant therapy the patient has received prior to biopsy or polyp removal. Cardiopulmonary complications[7] can be reduced by (1) awareness of the patient's other medical problems and (2) immediate availability of cardiopulmonary emergency equipment.

Infection[7] may be avoided by (1) proper cleansing of instruments and (2) avoidance of pulmonary aspiration.

D. An experienced endoscopist using a modern flexible endoscope should not encounter blind spots in the upper gastrointestinal tract unless hindered by blood, mucus, or food. To achieve significant results with esophageal and gastric cytology, the importance of meticulous technique is stressed.[12]

References

1. Adriani, J., and Campbell, D.: Fatalities following topical application of local anesthetics to mucous membranes. JAMA, *162*:1527–1530, 1956.
2. Castiglioni, L., Allen, T., and Patterson, M.: Intravenous diazepam: An improvement in pre-endoscopic medication. Gastrointest. Endosc., *19*:134–136, 1973.
3. Katz, D.: Morbidity and mortality in standard and flexible gastrointestinal endoscopy. Gastrointest. Endosc., *15*:134–141, 1969.
4. Mandelstam, P., et al.: Complications associated with esophagogastroduodenoscopy and with esophageal dilation. Gastrointest. Endosc., *23*:16–20, 1976.
5. Bombeck, T., Boyd, D., and Nyhus, L.: Esophageal trauma. Surg. Clin. North Am., *52*:219–230, 1972.
6. Papp, J. P.: Electrosurgical gastric polytectomy via the Olympus GIF endoscope. Gastrointest. Endosc., *20*:70–73, 1973.
7. Work Group XII: Human experimentation in digestive disease research. Gastroenterology, *69*:1165–1182, 1975.
8. Manier, J. W.: Fiberoptic gastrointestinal endoscopy in the aged. Gastrointest. Endosc., *23*:155–156, 1977.
9. Cameron, A. J., and Ott, B. J.: The value of gastroscopy in clinical diagnosis: A computer assisted study. Mayo Clin. Proc., *52*:806–808, 1977.
10. Belber, J. P.: Endoscopic examination of the duodenal bulb: A comparison with x-ray. Gastroenterology, *61*:55–61, 1971.
11. Yoshii, Y.: Endoscopic biopsy and cytology in esophageal and gastric carcinoma with fiberesophagoscope. Gastrointest. Endosc., *17*:150–152, 1971.
12. Waters, E. D.: Initial experience of gastric cytology in a routine cytologic service. Acta Cytol., *13*:637–644, 1969.

ESOPHAGOSCOPY, GASTROSCOPY, AND DUODENOSCOPY

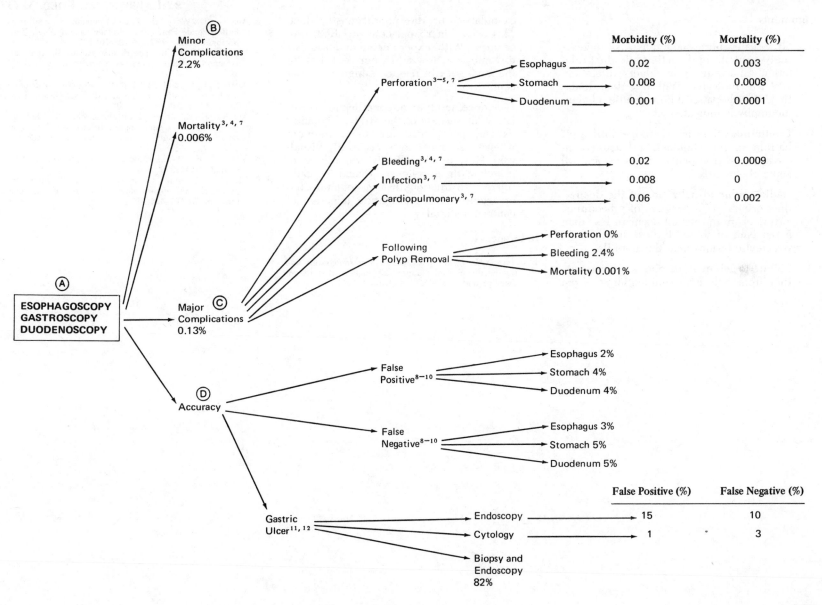

	Morbidity (%)	Mortality (%)
Esophagus	0.02	0.003
Stomach	0.008	0.0008
Duodenum	0.001	0.0001
Bleeding[3,4,7]	0.02	0.0009
Infection[3,7]	0.008	0
Cardiopulmonary[3,7]	0.06	0.002

Following Polyp Removal
- Perforation 0%
- Bleeding 2.4%
- Mortality 0.001%

(B) Minor Complications 2.2%

Mortality[3,4,7] 0.006%

(A) ESOPHAGOSCOPY GASTROSCOPY DUODENOSCOPY

Perforation[3-5,7]

(C) Major Complications 0.13%

(D) Accuracy

False Positive[8-10]
- Esophagus 2%
- Stomach 4%
- Duodenum 4%

False Negative[8-10]
- Esophagus 3%
- Stomach 5%
- Duodenum 5%

Gastric Ulcer[11,12]

	False Positive (%)	False Negative (%)
Endoscopy	15	10
Cytology	1	3

Biopsy and Endoscopy 82%

ENDOSCOPIC RETROGRADE CHOLANGIOPANCREATOGRAPHY (ERCP)

BY LAWRENCE J. KOEP, M.D.

Comments

A. Gray-scale ultrasonography is increasingly accurate in detecting bile duct dilatation. Lacking bile duct dilatation, ERCP is indicated. With bile duct dilatation, transhepatic skinny-needle cholangiography is indicated.[1, 2]

B. Contraindications are (1) inoperability, (2) barium in the abdomen, (3) acute pancreatitis, (4) true pancreatic cysts, and (5) acute cholangitis.

C. Radiographic visualization of the desired duct occurs in 70 per cent of procedures. Errors of interpretation occur in less than 5 per cent of these studies, mainly from pancreatic lesions near the ampulla.

D. Failure to achieve a diagnosis can arise either from failure of cannulation or from cannulation of the nondiagnostic duct. This occurs in 25 per cent of ERCP procedures. With experienced endoscopists this rate is as low as 15 per cent, but for the novice it can rise to as high as 62 per cent.

E. Incidence and type of complication correlate with success of the study. Cholangitis and pancreatitis are more frequent when these ducts are successfully visualized. Hospital mortality is primarily associated with unrelieved ductal (usually biliary) obstruction that is contaminated or aggravated by retrograde injection of contrast material.

References

1. Goldstein, L. I., et al.: Gray-scale ultrasonography and thin-needle cholangiography. Evaluation in the jaundiced patient. JAMA, 238:1041–1044, 1977.
2. Anacker, H., Weiss, H. D., and Kramann, B.: Endoscopic Retrograde Pancreatico cholangiography. New York, Springer-Verlag, 1977, pp. 25–26.
3. Longmire, W. P., Jr.: The diverse causes of biliary obstruction and their remedies. Curr. Probl. Surg.,14(7), 1977.
4. Arvanitakis, C., and Cooke, A. R.: Diagnostic tests of exocrine pancreatic function and disease. Gastroenterology, 74:932–948, 1978.
5. Kessler, R. E., et al.: Indications, clinical value and complications of endoscopic retrograde cholangiopancreatography. Surg. Gynecol. Obstet., 142:865–870, 1976.
6. Silvis, S. E., et al.: Endoscopic complications. JAMA 235:928–930, 1976.
7. Bilbao, M. K., et al.: Complications of endoscopic retrograde cholangiopancreatography (ERCP). Gastroenterology, 70:314–320, 1976.

ENDOSCOPIC RETROGRADE CHOLANGIOPANCREATOGRAPHY (ERCP)

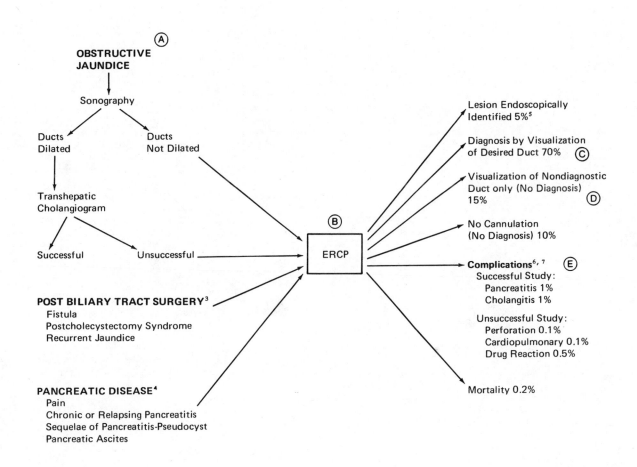

(A) **OBSTRUCTIVE JAUNDICE**

Sonography

Ducts Dilated

Ducts Not Dilated

Transhepatic Cholangiogram

Successful

Unsuccessful

POST BILIARY TRACT SURGERY[3]
Fistula
Postcholecystectomy Syndrome
Recurrent Jaundice

PANCREATIC DISEASE[4]
Pain
Chronic or Relapsing Pancreatitis
Sequelae of Pancreatitis-Pseudocyst
Pancreatic Ascites

(B) ERCP

Lesion Endoscopically Identified 5%[5]

Diagnosis by Visualization of Desired Duct 70% (C)

Visualization of Nondiagnostic Duct only (No Diagnosis) 15% (D)

No Cannulation (No Diagnosis) 10%

Complications[6,7] (E)
Successful Study:
Pancreatitis 1%
Cholangitis 1%

Unsuccessful Study:
Perforation 0.1%
Cardiopulmonary 0.1%
Drug Reaction 0.5%

Mortality 0.2%

Section **G**

Gynecologic

ABORTION BY DONALD W. APTEKAR, M.D.

Comments

A. In an uninterrupted pregnancy there are both fetal and maternal risks.

Fetal risks include spontaneous abortion (10 to 15 per cent), congenital anomaly (4 to 6 per cent), prematurity (6 to 8 per cent), and perinatal mortality (2 per cent).

Maternal risks include death (excluding that from abortion and ectopic pregnancy) at the rate of 12.4 per 100,000, operation (cesarean section) (12 to 20 per cent), and infection and hemorrhage (5 per cent).

B. Duration of pregnancy is based on the date of the last menstrual period and is confirmed by pelvic exam prior to the procedure.

More than 95 per cent of abortions of pregnancies of less than 12 weeks' gestation are done by suction curettage. Other techniques include sharp curettage or instillation when sizing has been determined inaccurately.[1]

Eighty-two per cent of abortions done in 1975 were by suction curettage in patients whose pregnancies were of less than 12 weeks' gestation.[1]

C. Total morbidity refers to a list of 100 possible complications compiled by the Joint Program for the Study of Abortion.[8]

The most common complications are[1, 7, 13] (1) perforation, (2) cervical laceration, (3) postabortion hemorrhage — usually defined as more than 250 cc., (4) septic incomplete abortion requiring a repeat curettage, and (5) endometritis or fever.

D. From the list of 100 complications, 15 were felt to be major.[6] These are (1) cardiac arrest, (2) convulsions, (3) death, (4) endotoxic shock, (5) fever lasting 3 or more days, (6) hemorrhage necessitating blood transfusion, (7) hypernatremia, (8) injury to bladder, ureter, or intestine, (9) pelvic infection, with 2 or more days of fever and a peak temperature of at least 40° C. or with hospitalization for 11 or more days, (10) pneumonia, (11) psychiatric hospitalization for 11 or more days, (12) pulmonary embolism or infarction, (13) thrombophlebitis, (14) unintended major surgery, and (15) wound disruption after hysterotomy or hysterectomy.

E. Abortion at this stage is most frequently done by dilatation and evacuation. Some are still done by instillation of various medications.

F. Mortality figures refer to crude data from all types of procedures, e.g., dilatation and evacuation and uterine instillation with saline urea, prostaglandin F_2Alpha, prostaglandin E_2 suppositories, and calcium with and without oxytocin augmentation. The data are insufficient to break down as to the safety of each individual procedure.[1, 5, 10]

G. At greater than 16 weeks' gestation the instillation techniques are still most commonly used. Much has been written recently about dilatation and evacuation of the uterus up to 20 weeks' gestation.

H. These data may be biased by the expertise of those reporting. The morbidity might be greater when the operation is performed by the casual operator.

The data are meant to be a crude summation of all types of pregnancy termination procedures.

Occasionally hysterotomy or hysterectomy may be the method of choice for pregnancy termination. In those instances, the indications for the procedure would have to be taken into account in assessing morbidity and mortality.

References

1. U.S. Center for Disease Control: Abortion Surveillance for 1975 and 1976. Washington, D.C., U.S. Department of Health, Education and Welfare. Issued in 1977 and 1978, respectively.
2. Bozorgi, N.: Termination of pregnancy in a private outpatient clinic. Am. J. Obstet. Gynecol. 127:763, 1977.
3. Wulff, G. J., Jr., and Freiman, S. M.: Elective abortion. Complications seen in a free-standing clinic. J. Obstet. Gynecol., 49:35, 1977.
4. Moberg, P.: Uterine perforation in connection with vacuum aspiration for legal abortion. Int. J. Gynecol. Obstet., 14:77, 1976.
5. Cates, W., and Tietze, C.: Standardized mortality rates associated with legal abortion: United States, 1972–1975. Fam. Plann. Perspect., 10(2), April 1978.
6. Cates, W., et al.: The effect of delay and choice of method on the risk of abortion morbidity. Fam. Plann. Perspect., 9:266–270, 1977.
7. Nemec, D., Predergast, T. J., and Trumbovli, W.: Medical abortion complications. J. Obstet. Gynecol., 51:433, 1978.
8. Joint Program for the Study of Abortion (JPSA/CDC): Forms Instruction Manual. Atlanta, Center for Disease Control. David Grimes, M.D., Personal Communication, 1978.
9. Grimes, D., et al.: Mid-trimester abortion by dilatation and evacuation. N. Engl. J. Med., 296:1141, 1977.
10. Cates, W., et al.: The risk of dying from legal abortion in the United States: 1972–1975. J. Obstet. Gynecol., 15:172, 1977.
11. Hogue, C. J.: Evaluation of studies concerning reproduction after first trimester induced abortion. Int. J. Obstet. Gynecol., 15:167, 1977.
12. Pritchard, J. A., and MacDonald, P. C.: Williams Obstetrics, 15th ed. New York, Appleton-Century-Crofts, 1976; and Hellman, L. M., and Pritchard, J. A.: Williams Obstetrics, 14th ed. 1971.
13. Stewart, G. K., and Goldstein, P.: Medical and surgical complications of therapeutic abortions. Obstet. Gynecol., 40:539–542, 1972.

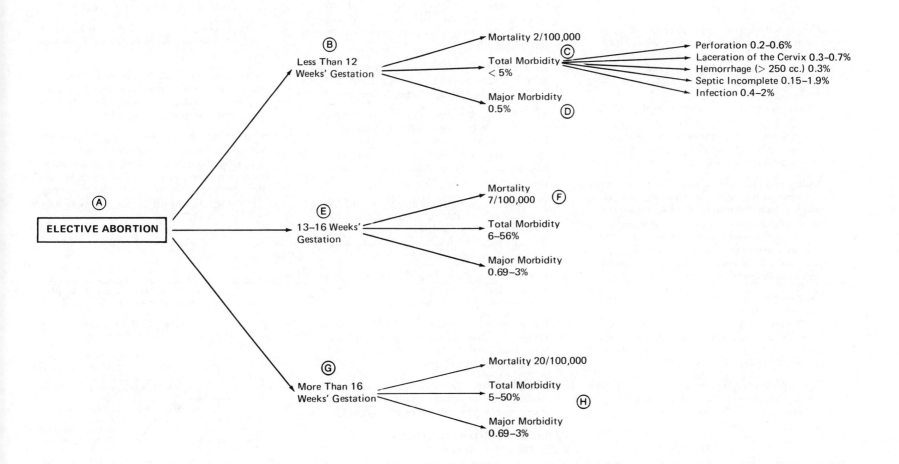

Ⓐ **ELECTIVE ABORTION**

Ⓑ Less Than 12 Weeks' Gestation
- Mortality 2/100,000
- Total Morbidity < 5% Ⓒ
- Major Morbidity 0.5% Ⓓ
  - Perforation 0.2–0.6%
  - Laceration of the Cervix 0.3–0.7%
  - Hemorrhage (> 250 cc.) 0.3%
  - Septic Incomplete 0.15–1.9%
  - Infection 0.4–2%

Ⓔ 13–16 Weeks' Gestation
- Mortality 7/100,000 Ⓕ
- Total Morbidity 6–56%
- Major Morbidity 0.69–3%

Ⓖ More Than 16 Weeks' Gestation
- Mortality 20/100,000
- Total Morbidity 5–50% Ⓗ
- Major Morbidity 0.69–3%

STERILIZATION BY T. ENGEL, M.D.

Comments

A. Omitted from this discussion is hysterectomy alone; though sometimes performed for sterilization, it is normally done for other primary reasons.

B. This is the vaginal approach. Avoiding an abdominal incision is easier when there is (1) vaginal relaxation or (2) a retroflexed uterus or (3) when performed in conjunction with other vaginal procedures such as D and C.

   Complications include[11] bowel perforation (0.3 per cent), infection requiring reoperation (1.2 per cent) and bleeding (2 per cent). Coitus is prohibited for 6 weeks postoperatively.

C. Endoscopy includes culdoscopy, carrying the same advantages and risks as colpotomy[1, 15] (see Comment B) and laparoscopy. Complications of laparoscopy include bowel perforation (1 in 3,600)[13] gas embolism (rare)[2] and cardiac arrhythmia (5 per cent). It is contraindicated following previous laparotomy or pelvic infection.[9]

D. Laparotomy for sterilization has the usual risks of elective laparotomy for other reasons (see page 322). Minilaparotomy through a small incision decreases the length of the scar but not the incidence of complication.[14]

E. One or two spring-loaded plastic clips are placed across the isthmic portion of the tubes.[6]

F. A Silastic band with "memory" is placed across a knuckle of the isthmic portion of the tube.[16]

G. Burn complications are minimized with meticulous techniques and use of low voltage and bipolar instruments. Division or division and resection increase the risk of bleeding.[3]

H. In the Uchida procedure, a segment of tube is excised and the lumen ligated. It is effective but complicated to perform.[12]

I. In the Pomeroy procedure, the midportion of the tube is formed into a loop, the base is ligated, and the knuckle is excised. Easy to perform and with no major disadvantage, it is effective except during pregnancy.[4]

J. In a fimbriectomy the ampullary and fimbriated ends of the tubes are ligated and meticulously excised. Even minute portions of residual fimbria or fimbria ovarica may allow subsequent pregnancy.[8]

K. In the Irving procedure the tube is ligated and divided and the proximal portion is buried in the myometrium.[7]

L. Experimental methods include hysteroscopic or blind transcervical use of cautery, chemicals, plastics or solid plugs. Failure and complication rates are high.[10]

M. Complications include[5] hematoma (rare), wound infection (rare), painful ejaculation (rare), sperm granuloma (rare), psychological problems (1.5 per cent). Expectancy of subsequent operative reanastomosis is 30 per cent.

N. Salpingolysis is lysis of peritubal adhesions with normal tubal architecture.[14]

O. Tubal occlusion at the distal end can be done in patients with previous fimbriectomy.[14]

P. Reimplantation can be done for cornual obstruction and in patients following cautery ligation. It works best when there is 5 cm. of tube to work with.[14]

Q. Reanastomosis can be done in patients whose ligations were performed by the clip, ring, Pomeroy, or Irving techniques. In selected cautery patients, success rate with conventional means is 50 per cent. Microsurgery improves the success rate to 70 per cent.[15]

PROCEDURE	FAILURE RATE (%)	COMPLICATION RATE (%)
Cautery alone	0.1–0.5	0.13
Cautery + division	0.1–0.5	0.12
Cautery + division and resection	0.1–0.5	0.12

References

1. Clyman, J. J.: Tubal sterilization by operative culdoscopy. In Richard, R. M., and Prager, D. J. (eds.): Human Sterilization. Springfield, Ill., Charles C Thomas, 1972.
2. Cohen, M. R.: Laparoscopy, Culdoscopy and Gynecography: Technique and Atlas. Philadelphia, W. B. Saunders, 1970.
3. Engel, T., and Harris, F. W.: The electrical dynamics of laparoscopic sterilization. J. Reprod. Med., 15:33–42, 1975.
4. Garb, A. E.: A review of tubal sterilization failures. Obstet. Gynecol. Surv., 12:291–305, 1957.
5. Hackett, R. E., and Waterhouse, K.: Vasectomy reviewed. Am. J. Obstet. Gynecol., 116:438–54, 1973.
6. Hulka, J. F., et al.: Spring clip sterilization: One-year followup of 1079 cases. Am. J. Obstet. Gynecol., 125:1039–43, 1976.
7. Irving, F. C.: A new method of insuring sterility following cesarean section. Am. J. Obstet. Gynecol., 8:335–37, 1974.
8. Kroener, W. F., Jr.: Surgical sterilization by fimbriectomy. Am. J. Obstet. Gynecol., 104:247–51, 1969.
9. Peterson, E. P., and Behrman, S. J.: Laparoscopic tubal

STERILIZATION

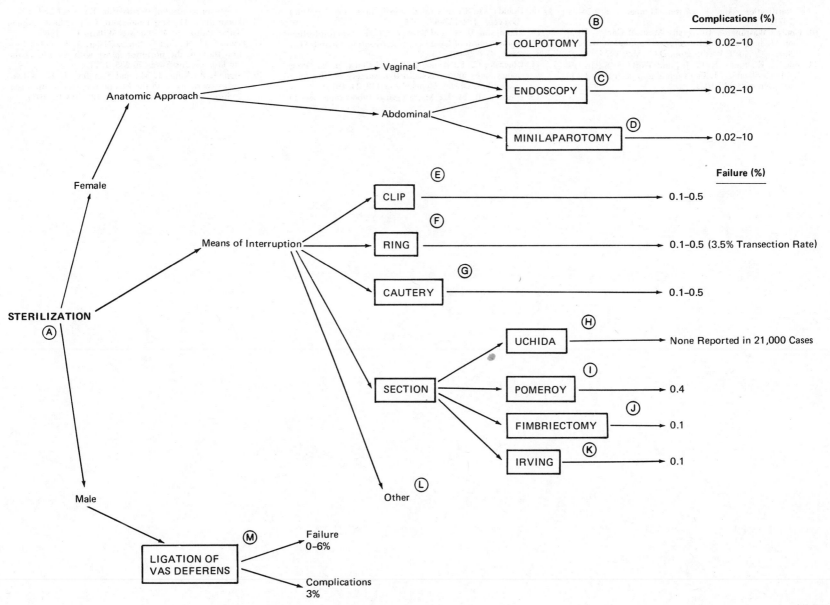

Complications (%)

COLPOTOMY (B) → 0.02–10

ENDOSCOPY (C) → 0.02–10

MINILAPAROTOMY (D) → 0.02–10

Failure (%)

CLIP (E) → 0.1–0.5

RING (F) → 0.1–0.5 (3.5% Transection Rate)

CAUTERY (G) → 0.1–0.5

UCHIDA (H) → None Reported in 21,000 Cases

POMEROY (I) → 0.4

FIMBRIECTOMY (J) → 0.1

IRVING (K) → 0.1

Other (L)

Vaginal

Abdominal

Anatomic Approach

Female

STERILIZATION (A)

Means of Interruption

SECTION

Male

LIGATION OF VAS DEFERENS (M)

Failure 0–6%

Complications 3%

STERILIZATION *Continued*

sterilization. Am. J. Obstet. Gynecol., *110*:24–31, 1971.

10. George Washington University Medical Center, Dept. of Medical and Public Affairs: Population Reports. Series C. No. 7. Washington, D.C., May 1976.

11. Roe, R. E., Laros, R. K., Jr., and Work, B. A., Jr.: Female sterilization. I. The vaginal approach. Am. J. Obstet. Gynecol., *112*:1031, 1972.

12. Uchida, H.: Uchida tubal sterilization. Am. J. Obstet. Gynecol., *121*:153–58, 1975.

13. Thompson, B. H., and Wheeless, C. P.: Gastrointestinal complication of laparoscopy sterilization. Obstet. Gynecol., *41*:669–676, 1973.

14. Umezaki, C., Katayama, P. P., and Jones, H. W.: Pregnancy rates after reconstructive surgery on the fallopian tubes. Obstet. Gynecol., *43*:418–24, 1974.

15. Winston, R. M. L.: Microsurgical tubocornual anastomosis for reversal of sterilisation. Lancet, *1*:284, 1977.

16. Woodruff, J. D., and Pauerstein, C. J.: The Fallopian Tube. Baltimore, Williams & Wilkins Co., 1969.

17. Wynter, H. H., and Gutierrez Najar, A. J.: Tubal ligation through the posterior fornix with the aid of the culdoscope. Int. Surg., *56*:235, 1971.

18. Yoon, I. B., King, T. M., and Parmley, T. H.: A two-year experience with the Falope ring sterilization procedure. Am. J. Obstet. Gynecol., *127*:109–12, 1977.

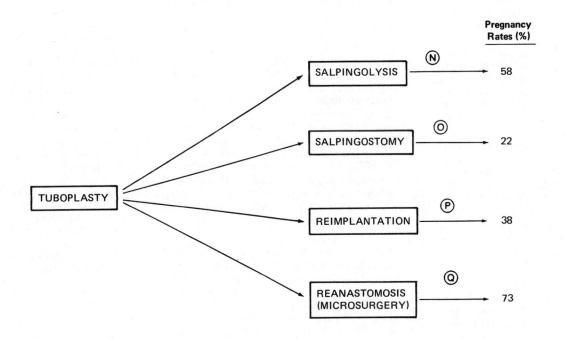

UTERINE DILATATION AND CURETTAGE BY J. McGREGOR, M.D.

Comments

A. Satisfactorily performed, formal D and C and suction curettage may have similar outcomes:
   1. Accuracy of formal D and C for diagnosis of endometrial cancer approaches 100 per cent.[15] Accuracy of suction curettage is 90 per cent.[20]
   2. Accuracy of both formal D and C and suction curettage for diagnosis of benign endometrial disorders is 90 to 98 per cent.[1, 5, 7, 10, 15, 20, 22, 26, 28]
   3. Formal D and C may miss 10 per cent of lesions found at hysterectomy.[28] Suction curettage does not allow for routine examination under anesthesia or exploration of the uterus with polyp forceps.[14, 22] Neither formal D and C nor suction curettage completely samples an endometrial cavity that is enlarged or irregular.[10]

      Vagaries of collection methods and pathological interpretation limit the accuracy of either procedure.[10, 14]
   4. Formal D and C or suction curettage appear therapeutically similar for control of bleeding at three months' followup (1/3 to 2/3 of cases).[7-10]

B. Pain occurs with all curettages done without anesthesia and syncope complicates roughly 1 per cent of suction curettage cases.[10] Curettage without anesthesia cannot be performed adequately in 10 to 25 per cent of patients because of apprehension, a stenotic cervix, a large or irregular uterus, or medical contraindication to such an outpatient procedure.[10, 14, 26] An insufficient sample of tissue is submitted in approximately 10 per cent of formal D and Cs or suction curettages.[13, 14, 22, 26]

C. The precise incidence of perforation is unknown owing to uncertain diagnosis or reluctance in reporting.[3]

   Frequency in premenopausal patients is 0.2 to 0.7 per cent,[16, 28] postmenopausal 1.5 per cent,[28] and postpartum 0.8 per cent.[28] Perforation associated with neoplasia, leiomyoma, infection, or congenital anomalies occurs in approximately 2 per cent of cases.[2, 3, 28] Perforation must be considered in every instance of illegal abortion.[19]

D. Factors making exploratory laparotomy mandatory include (1) evidence of rapid or excessive blood loss,[3, 16] such as deteriorating vital signs or a palpably expanding broad ligament hematoma, and (2) a high likelihood of visceral damage,[18, 20, 28] evidenced by visualization of abdominal contents at the cervix or in curettage material; blood found on culdocentesis, bladder catheterization, or rectal examination; or the operator's feeling of likely damage owing to the use of sharp instruments or powerful suction at the time of perforation.

E. Damage to most pelvic and lower abdominal structures has been reported. Early complications include bleeding, infection, bladder or ureteric damage, and injury to intestine or mesentery leading to abdominal soilage or bowel infarction.[3, 4, 28] Late complications include pelvic abscess, bowel obstruction from adhesions or herniation through a broad ligament rent, uterine rupture during pregnancy, intramural pregnancy, endometriosis, and gastrointestinal or genitourinary fistula.[3, 16, 20]

F. Causes of excessive bleeding include incomplete emptying of the uterus, laceration of vessels, bleeding diathesis, or inability of the uterus to contract. Cervical trauma may cause significant blood loss.[25]

G. Other late complications include (1) Endometrial damage leading to intrauterine adhesions (Asherman's syndrome) following curettage for late postpartum or post-abortion bleeding (2 to 38 per cent) and rarely after simple curettage.[6, 12] Intrauterine adhesions may cause amenorrhea, hypomenorrhea, infertility, repeated fetal wastage, and placenta accreta.[6, 11, 12] (2) Cervical incompetence from cervical dilatation leading to recurrent fetal wastage. Cervical weakness occurs after the cervix is forcibly dilated past 9 to 11 mm.[13] Other studies show no change in reproductive performance after cervical dilatation, suggesting the necessity of further investigation.[21] (3) Transient reparative changes on Pap smear,[23] and (4) Possible endometriosis.[24]

H. Incidence of infection depends on criteria and diligence used in making diagnosis. Incidence in uncomplicated formal curettage is 0.3 to 0.5 per cent[13, 15] and in uncomplicated suction curettage, 0.3 per cent.[10] Incidence of reactivation of prior pelvic infection is less than 1 per cent.[17]

References

1. Benson, R. C., and Miller, J. N.: Surgical curettage. Its value in abnormal uterine bleeding. Obstet. Gynecol., 8:523, 1956.
2. Caldwell, L. A.: Perforation of a non-pregnant uterus. Can. Med. Assoc. J., 64:533, 1951.
3. Deasy, P. P., and Anderson, G. V.: Uterine perforation as a complication of dilatation and curettage and its management. West. J. Surg., 68:294, 1960.
4. Decker, W. H., and Zaneski, B. W.: Accidental perforation of the uterus. Am. J. Obstet. Gynecol., 66:345, 1953.

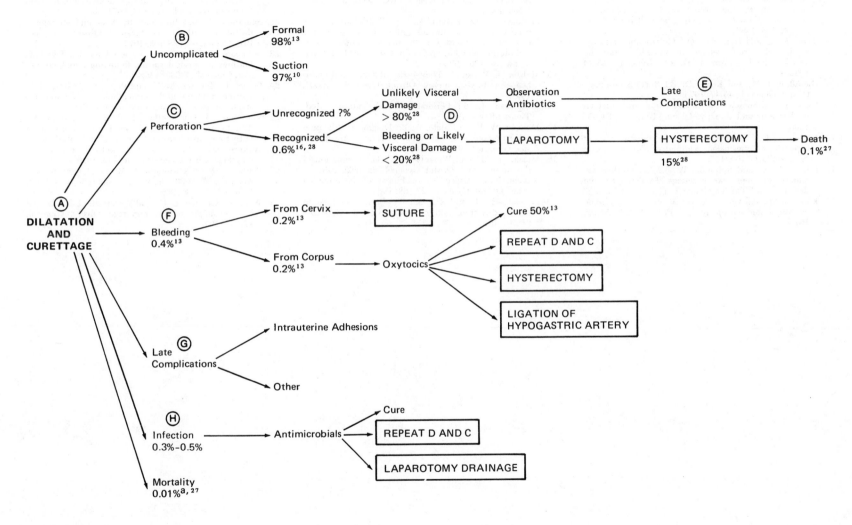

Ⓐ **DILATATION AND CURETTAGE**

Ⓑ Uncomplicated
— Formal 98%[13]
— Suction 97%[10]

Ⓒ Perforation
— Unrecognized ?%
— Recognized 0.6%[16, 28]
  — Unlikely Visceral Damage > 80%[28] → Observation Antibiotics → Ⓔ Late Complications
  — Ⓓ Bleeding or Likely Visceral Damage < 20%[28] → LAPAROTOMY → HYSTERECTOMY 15%[28] → Death 0.1%[27]

Ⓕ Bleeding 0.4%[13]
— From Cervix 0.2%[13] → SUTURE
— From Corpus 0.2%[13] → Oxytocics
  — Cure 50%[13]
  — REPEAT D AND C
  — HYSTERECTOMY
  — LIGATION OF HYPOGASTRIC ARTERY

Ⓖ Late Complications
— Intrauterine Adhesions
— Other

Ⓗ Infection 0.3%-0.5% → Antimicrobials
— Cure
— REPEAT D AND C
— LAPAROTOMY DRAINAGE

Mortality 0.01%[a, 27]

[a]Many large series with no deaths[15, 19, 25, 28]

5. Denis, R., Barnett, J. M., and Forbes, S. E.: Diagnostic suction curettage. Obstet. Gynecol., *42*:201, 1973.

6. Dmowski, W. P., and Greenblatt, R. B.: Asherman's syndrome and risk of placenta accreta. Obstet. Gynecol., *34*:288, 1965.

7. Geist, S. H., and Glassman, O.: Therapeutic and diagnostic value of curettage in so-called functional uterine bleeding. Am. J. Obstet. Gynecol., *23*:14, 1932.

8. Hamilton, J. V., and Knab, D. R.: Suction curettage. Obstet. Gynecol., *45*:47, 1975.

9. Hark, B., and Sommers, S. C.: Dilatation and curettage in diagnosis and therapy. Obstet. Gynecol., *21*:636, 1963.

10. Jensen, J. G.: Vacuum curettage — Outpatient curettage without anesthesia. A report of 350 cases. Dan. Med. Bull., *17*:199, 1970.

11. Jensen, P. A., and Stromme, W. B.: Amenorrhea secondary to puerperal curettage (Asherman's syndrome). Am. J. Obstet. Gynecol., *113*:150, 1972.

12. Klein, S. M., and Garcia, C. G.: Asherman's syndrome: A critique and current review. Fertil. Steril., *24*:722, 1973.

13. MacKenzie, I. Z., and Bibby, J. G.: Critical assessment of dilatation and curettage in 1029 women. Lancet, *2*:556, 1978.

14. Mathews, D. D., Kakani, A., and Bhattacharya, A.: A comparison of vacuum aspiration of the uterus and conventional curettage in the management of abnormal uterine bleeding. J. Obstet. Gynaecol. Brit. Commonw., *80*:176, 1973.

15. McElin, T. W., et al.: Diagnostic dilatation and curettage — A 10-year survey. Obstet. Gynecol., *33*:807, 1965.

16. McGoogan, L. S.: Perforation of the uterus. Med. Times, *98*:989, 1966.

17. Mengert, W. F., and Slate, W. B.: Diagnostic dilatation and curettage as an outpatient procedure. Am. J. Obstet. Gynecol., *79*:727, 1960.

18. Murray, P. M., and Winkelstein, L. G.: Perforation of the uterus. Am. J. Obstet. Gynecol., *62*:1262, 1951.

19. Nugent, F. B.: Office suction biopsy of the endometrium. Obstet. Gynecol., *22*:168, 1963.

20. Radman, H. M., and Korman, W.: Uterine perforation during dilatation and curettage. Obstet. Gynecol., *21*:210, 1963.

21. Roht, L. H., and Aoyama, H.: Induced abortion and its sequelae: Prematurity and spontaneous abortion. Am. J. Obstet. Gynecol., *120*:868, 1974.

22. Saunders, P., and Rowland, R.: Vacuum curettage of the uterus without anaesthesia. J. Obstet. Gynaecol. Brit. Commonw., *79*:168, 1972.

23. Soloman, C., Rosenberg, M., and Falk, H.: Cytologic findings in cervical smears following curettage. Obstet. Gynecol., *7*:630, 1956.

24. Stanca, C., Jonesco, M. V., and Popesco, C.: Role of the uterine curettage in the etiopathology of endometriosis. Gynecologie Obstetrique, *67*:377, 1968.

25. Vermeeren, J., Chamberlain, R. R., and Telinde, R. W.: Ten thousand minor gynecologic operations on an outpatient basis. Obstet. Gynecol., *9*:139, 1957.

26. Walters, D., et al.: Diagnostic outpatient aspiration curettage. Obstet. Gynecol., *46*:160, 1975.

27. Watts, W. F., and Kimbrough, R. A.: Hysterectomy — Analysis of 1000 consecutive operations. Obstet. Gynecol., *7*:483, 1956.

28. Word, B., Gravlee, L. C., and Wideman, G. L.: The fallacy of simple uterine curettage. Obstet. Gynecol., *12*:642, 1958.

ECTOPIC PREGNANCY

ECTOPIC PREGNANCY by William E. Fuller, M.D.

Comments

A. Ectopic pregnancy occurs in one of every 100 to 200 pregnancies. Location[3] may be tubal (97.7 per cent of cases), ovarian (0.15 per cent), fimbrial ovarian (1.5 per cent), cervical (0.15 per cent), or abdominal (1.4 per cent). Of tubal pregnancies, 1.2 per cent are interstitial, 12.3 per cent occur in the proximal third, 38.2 per cent occur in the middle third, and 41.3 per cent occur in the distal third; 4.7 per cent are fimbrial.

Etiologic factors include[1, 3, 7, 11] (1) pelvic inflammatory disease (44 to 53 per cent of cases), (2) use of an intrauterine device (increases risk up to 6-fold), (3) previous induced abortion (increases risk 10-fold), (4) birth control pills (may increase risk 2- to 5-fold), and (5) previous ectopic pregnancy (9 to 11.2 per cent of cases).

B. D and C is only an adjunct to other diagnostic procedures.

C. The beta subunit of human chorionic gonadotropin assay is the best pregnancy test.

D. Ultrasound may define an intrauterine gestational sac that should simply be observed. If the sac is degenerated, D and C is indicated for threatened, incomplete, or missed abortion. If an adnexal mass is present without an intrauterine gestational sac, laparoscopy is indicated.

E. Pelvic endoscopy (laparoscopy or culdoscopy) is used as a definitive diagnostic tool in 5.35 per cent[3] of cases. Mortality associated with diagnostic laparoscopy is 0.8 per 100,000.[8] Morbidity associated with laparoscopy is 5.4 per 1000.[8] Rate of bowel perforation is 1 per 3600,[13] and laceration of a mesenteric vein occurs once per 150 cases.[2]

F. Surgical management depends upon the operative findings.
1. Salpingectomy and cornual resection is the traditional operation. If the pregnancy is in the ampullar portion of the tube it may be milked out without tubal resection. Salpingostomy can be tried for patients who have had recurrent ectopic pregnancy and previous salpingectomy.[9] If the implantation site is other than the tube, resection is required.
2. A hemorrhagic corpus luteum should be weighed out without resecting the ovary.
3. Adnexal torsion should be resected.
4. A functional corpus luteum cyst resolves itself and does not require oophorectomy.

G. Mortality of ectopic pregnancy is 2 to 4 per 100,[10] or 10.6 per cent of all causes of maternal mortality. Earlier diagnosis correlates with lower mortality rate.

H. Approximately 30 per cent of women with one ectopic pregnancy will have a repeat occurrence, and 70 per cent will be unable to carry a subsequent pregnancy to viability.[11]

Complications include[3] postoperative sepsis (18.4 per cent), wound infection (5.8 per cent), pelvic infection (5.8 per cent), and upper respiratory infection (2.1 per cent), for a total morbidity rate of 26.9 per cent.

References

1. Beral, V.: An epidemiological study of recent trends in ectopic pregnancy. Br. J. Obstet. Gynaecol., 82:775, 1975.
2. Betz, G.: Personal communication.
3. Breen, J. L.: A 21-year survey of 654 ectopic pregnancies. Am. J. Obstet. Gynecol., 106:1004, 1970.
4. Hallatt, J. G.: Repeat ectopic pregnancy: A study of 123 consecutive cases. Am. J. Obstet. Gynecol., 122:520, 1975.
5. Kosasa, T. S., et al.: Use of radioimmunoassay specific for human chorionic gonadotropin in the diagnosis of early ectopic pregnancy. Obstet. Gynecol., 42:868, 1973.
6. LaIuppa, M. A., and Cavanagh, D.: The endometrium in ectopic pregnancy. Obstet. Gynecol., 21:155, 1963.
7. Panayotou, P. P., et al.: Induced abortion and ectopic pregnancy. Am. J. Obstet. Gynecol., 114:507, 1972.
8. Phillips, J. M., et al.: American Association of Gynecologic Laparoscopists' 1976 membership survey. J. Reprod. Med., 21:3, 1978.
9. Scaling, S. T., et al.: The correlation of pelvic ultrasound and laparoscopy in the diagnosis and management of gynecologic disorders. J. Reprod. Med., 21:53, 1978.
10. Schneider, J., Berger, C. T., and Cattell, C.: Maternal mortality due to ectopic pregnancy. Obstet. Gynecol., 49:557, 1977.
11. Schoen, J. A., and Nowak, P. T.: Repeat ectopic pregnancy. A 16-year clinical survey. Obstet. Gynecol., 45:542, 1975.
12. Stangel, J. J., Reyniak, J. V., and Stone, M. L.: Conservative surgical management of tubal pregnancy. Obstet. Gynecol., 48:241, 1976.
13. Thompson, B. H., and Wheeless, C. R.: Gastrointestinal complications of laparoscopy sterilization. Obstet. Gynecol., 41:669, 1973.

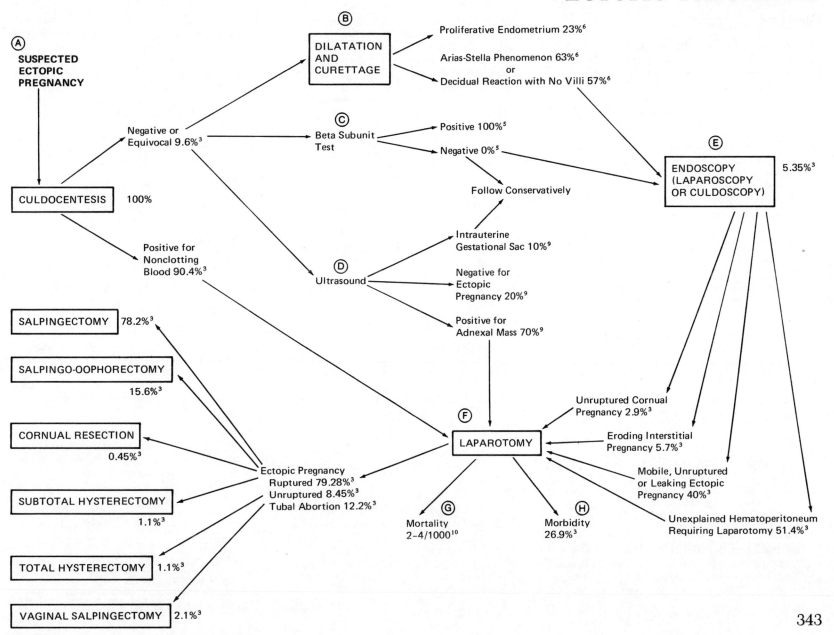

(A) **SUSPECTED ECTOPIC PREGNANCY**

CULDOCENTESIS 100%

Negative or Equivocal 9.6%[3]

Positive for Nonclotting Blood 90.4%[3]

(B) DILATATION AND CURETTAGE

Proliferative Endometrium 23%[6]

Arias-Stella Phenomenon 63%[6]
or
Decidual Reaction with No Villi 57%[6]

(C) Beta Subunit Test

Positive 100%[5]

Negative 0%[5]

Follow Conservatively

(D) Ultrasound

Intrauterine Gestational Sac 10%[9]

Negative for Ectopic Pregnancy 20%[9]

Positive for Adnexal Mass 70%[9]

(E) ENDOSCOPY (LAPAROSCOPY OR CULDOSCOPY) 5.35%[3]

SALPINGECTOMY 78.2%[3]

SALPINGO-OOPHORECTOMY 15.6%[3]

CORNUAL RESECTION 0.45%[3]

SUBTOTAL HYSTERECTOMY 1.1%[3]

TOTAL HYSTERECTOMY 1.1%[3]

VAGINAL SALPINGECTOMY 2.1%[3]

Ectopic Pregnancy
Ruptured 79.28%[3]
Unruptured 8.45%[3]
Tubal Abortion 12.2%[3]

(F) LAPAROTOMY

Unruptured Cornual Pregnancy 2.9%[3]

Eroding Interstitial Pregnancy 5.7%[3]

Mobile, Unruptured or Leaking Ectopic Pregnancy 40%[3]

Unexplained Hematoperitoneum Requiring Laparotomy 51.4%[3]

(G) Mortality 2–4/1000[10]

(H) Morbidity 26.9%[3]

343

FIBROIDS BY THEODORE COOPER, M.D.

Comments

A. Fibroids occur in 20 to 50 per cent of women[5, 17, 21] and are 3 to 9 times more common in blacks.[10] Ninety-five per cent arise in the uterine corpus, with 5 per cent from the cervical musculature.[10, 21] Most frequently they are intramural;[5] only 5 per cent are submucous.[19, 21]

B. Expectant observation is used for small, asymptomatic fibroids. *Exceptions* include (1) tumors so situated that adnexal disease could be obscured, and (2) evidence of continued growth (or lack of regression) postmenopausally.[10, 17]

C. "Symptoms" include growth to greater than 12 cm. in diameter or greater than 25 per cent of original size within 6 months. Pain, pressure, and bleeding can occur. Only bleeding necessitates the interval D and C.

D. Factors associated with poor prognosis include postmenopausal state, microscopic anaplasia, vascular invasion, submucous position of the original fibroid, and evidence of extension at operation.[5, 19, 27] Mitotic activity is important but can be misleading.[28]

E. Fractional curettage rules out coexistent cancer as a cause of bleeding.[10, 17] D and C can be curative (up to 80 per cent probability) with small, submucous fibroids.[26] Postmenopausal bleeding coexistent with fibroids is due to causes other than fibroid in more than half of patients.[17]

F. Hysterectomy rather than myomectomy is used in the majority of cases, myomectomy being reserved for those patients in whom childbearing potential is to be preserved. Ninety-seven per cent of hysterectomies for fibroids are performed via the abdominal route,[30] but this can be influenced by surgeon's experience, tumor size, and the need for colporrhaphy. Selected prolapsed, pedunculated, submucous myoma can be treated by myomectomy with or without interval hysterectomy.[2]

Adnexal management involves the patient's age and coexistent adnexal disease.[10, 25] Complete removal was performed in 12 per cent of one series of hysterectomies.[25] Carcinoma develops in 1 per cent of retained ovaries of patients over 40.[3, 28] Reoperation for adnexal disease occurs in 2 to 7 per cent of cases.[3, 17] Five to 8 per cent of patients with ovarian cancer have had previous hysterectomies.[3, 17, 29]

G. Postoperative morbidity for abdominal hysterectomy includes fever (30 to 40 per cent of cases), severe bleeding (0.7 per cent), phlebitis (0.3 to 1.4 per cent), pulmonary embolus (0.7 per cent), urinary tract infection (30 to 40 per cent), ileus or obstruction (5 per cent), vesicovaginal and rectovaginal fistulae (rare late complications), and ureteral injury (rare).[6, 11, 15, 18, 30]

Preoperative (prophylactic) antibiotics decrease infection after vaginal hysterectomy 30 per cent[12, 13] but are not required for abdominal hysterectomy because of the lower probability of infection.

H. Twenty-five to 35 per cent of patients with multiple fibroids are infertile.[8, 16, 21] This may be caused by tubal compression from a cornual tumor, interference with placentation by a submucous fibroid, interference with sperm migration by cervical myoma, or uterine irritability from a degenerating fibroid.[8, 17, 24]

I. Myomectomy is indicated only after other causes of infertility are excluded. Probability of subsequent fertility decreases with increasing age at time of myomectomy.[8] It varies from 100 per cent if the patient is younger than 25 to 29 per cent if she is between 36 and 40 years old to 0 per cent if she is over 41.[8]

J. Solitary fibroid removal resulted in 27 per cent recurrence; the rate was 59 per cent with multiple fibroids.[8]

K. There is a high rate of fetal loss (25 to 30 per cent)[16, 24] in the 30 to 50 per cent of patients who became pregnant after myomectomy.

L. Fibroids occur in 0.1 to 2.1 per cent of patients in labor.[7] Most have no effect on labor or delivery,[7, 17] although there is associated abnormal presentation in 15 per cent.[7] Rarely there is dystotic labor, tumor previa, or postpartum hemorrhage.

M. Red (carneous) degeneration is a rare complication (less than 5 per cent of cases) and is almost always treated nonoperatively. Probability of abortion after myomectomy increases if there is dissection into the uterine wall.[7, 17, 26]

N. These include the incidental epithelioid leiomyoma and plexiform tumorlet as well as intravenous leiomyomatosis, leiomyomatosis peritonealis disseminata, and benign metastasizing leiomyoma.[1, 4, 5, 20, 23, 31]

References

1. Abell, M. R., and Littler, E. R.: Benign metastasizing uterine leiomyoma — multiple lymph node metastases. Cancer, 36:2206–2213, 1975.
2. Brooks, G., and Stage, A.: Surgical management of pro-

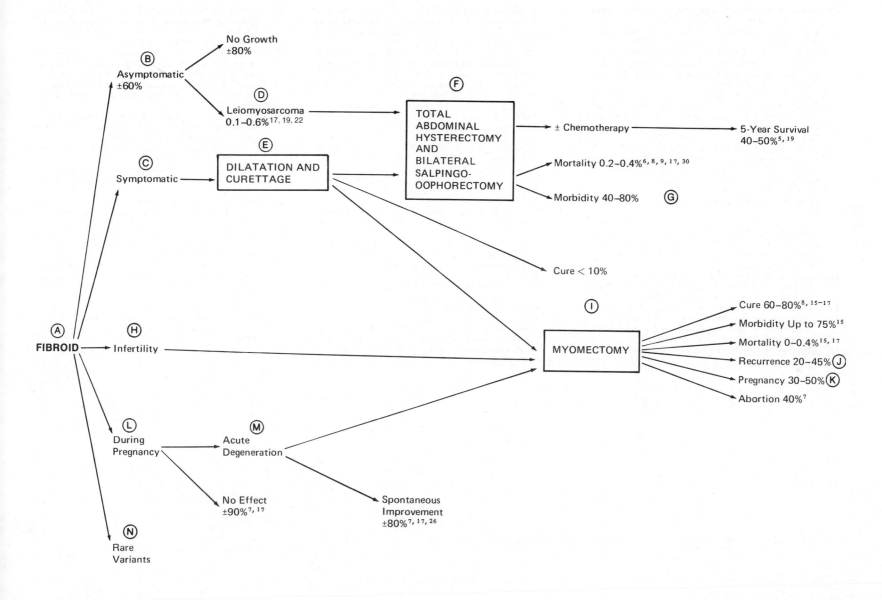

No Growth
±80%

(B)
Asymptomatic
±60%

(D)
Leiomyosarcoma
0.1–0.6%[17, 19, 22]

(F)
TOTAL ABDOMINAL HYSTERECTOMY AND BILATERAL SALPINGO-OOPHORECTOMY

± Chemotherapy

5-Year Survival
40–50%[5, 19]

Mortality 0.2–0.4%[6, 8, 9, 17, 30]

Morbidity 40–80% (G)

(E)
DILATATION AND CURETTAGE

(C)
Symptomatic

Cure < 10%

(A)
FIBROID

(H)
Infertility

(I)
MYOMECTOMY

Cure 60–80%[8, 15–17]
Morbidity Up to 75%[15]
Mortality 0–0.4%[15, 17]
Recurrence 20–45% (J)
Pregnancy 30–50% (K)
Abortion 40%[7]

(L)
During Pregnancy

(M)
Acute Degeneration

No Effect
±90%[7, 17]

Spontaneous Improvement
±80%[7, 17, 26]

(N)
Rare Variants

345

FIBROIDS *Continued*

lapsed pedunculated submucous leiomyomas. Surg. Gynecol. Obstet., *141*:397–398, 1975.

3. Christ, J. E., and Lotze, E. C.: The residual ovary syndrome. Obstet. Gynecol., *46*:551–556, 1975.

4. Goldberg, M. F., Hurt, W. C., and Frable, W. J.: Leiomyomatosis peritonealis disseminata: Report of a case and review of the literature. Obstet. Gynecol. *49*(Suppl.):46s–52s, 1977.

5. Gompel, C., and Silverberg, S.: The corpus uteri. *In* Pathology in Gynecology and Obstetrics, 2nd ed. Philadelphia, J. B. Lippincott Co., 1977, pp. 120–243.

6. Gray, L.: Open cuff method of abdominal hysterectomy. Obstet. Gynecol., *46*:42–46, 1975.

7. Hellman, L., and Pritchard, J.: Dystocia caused by abnormalities of the generative tract. *In* William's Obstetrics, 14th ed. New York, Appleton-Century-Crofts, 1971, pp. 921–931.

8. Ingersoll, F. M., and Malone, L. J.: Myomectomy: An alternative to hysterectomy. Arch. Surg., *100*:557–561, 1970.

9. Jenkins, V. R., II: Unnecessary—Elective—Indicated? Audit criteria of the American College of Obstetricians and Gynecologists to assess abdominal hysterectomy for uterine leiomyoma. Quality Review Bulletin, *3*:7–21, May 1977.

10. Kistner, R. W.: The uterine corpus. *In* Gynecology: Principles and Practice, 2nd ed. Chicago, Year Book Medical Publishers, 1971, pp. 172–280.

11. Ledger, W. J., and Child, M. A.: Hospital care of patients undergoing hysterectomy: An analysis of 12,026 patients from the professional activity study. Am. J. Obstet. Gynecol., *117*:423–433, 1973.

12. Ledger, W. J., Sweet, R. L., and Headington, J. T.: Prophylactic cephaloridine in the prevention of postoperative pelvic infections in premenopausal women undergoing vaginal hysterectomy. Am. J. Obstet. Gynecol., *115*:766–774, 1973.

13. Ledger, W. J., Gee, C., and Lewis, W. P.: Guidelines for antibiotic prophylaxis in gynecology. Am. J. Obstet. Gynecol., *121*:1038–1045, 1975.

14. Levinson, C. J.: Hysterectomy complications. Clin. Obstet. Gynecol., *15*:802–826, 1972.

15. Loeffler, F. E., and Noble, A. D.: Myomectomy at the Chelsea Hospital for Women. J. Obstet. Gynecol. Brit. Commonw., *77*:167–170, 1970.

16. Malone, L. J., and Ingersoll, F. M.: Myomectomy in infertility. *In* Behrman, S. J., and Kistner, R. W. (eds.): Progress in Infertility, 2nd ed. Boston, Little, Brown and Co., 1975, pp. 85–90.

17. Mattingly, R. F.: Myomata uteri. *In* TeLinde's Operative Gynecology, 5th ed. Philadelphia, J. B. Lippincott Co., 1977, pp. 187–222.

18. Mattingly, R. F., and Friedrich, E. G., Jr.: Difficult hysterectomy. Clin. Obstet. Gynecol., *15*:788–801, 1972.

19. Montague, A. C. W., Swartz, D. P., and Woodruff, J. D.: Sarcoma arising in a leiomyoma of the uterus. Am. J. Obstet. Gynecol., *91*:421–427, 1965.

20. Norris, H. J., and Parmley, T. L.: Mesenchymal tumors of the uterus. V. Intravenous leiomyomatosis: A clinical and pathologic study of 14 cases. Cancer, *36*:2164–2178, 1975.

21. Novak, E. R., and Woodruff, J. D.: Myoma and other benign tumors of the uterus. *In* Novak's Gynecologic and Obstetric Pathology, 7th ed. Philadelphia, W. B. Saunders Co., 1974, pp. 243–255.

22. Novak, E. R., and Woodruff, J. D.: Sarcoma and allied lesions of the uterus. *In* Novak's Gynecologic and Obstetric Pathology, 7th ed. Philadelphia, W. B. Saunders Co., 1974, pp. 272–281.

23. Parmley, T. H., et al.: Histiogenesis of leiomyomatosis peritonealis disseminata (disseminated fibrosing deciduosis). Obstet. Gynecol., *46*:511–516, 1975.

24. Pieretti, A. L.: Fibromyomas of the uterus: Cause of infertility and subfertility. Acta Eur. Fertil., *5*:235–239, 1974.

25. Randall, C. L., and Paloucek, F. P.: Frequency of oophorectomy at the time of hysterectomy. Am. J. Obstet. Gynecol., *100*:716–726, 1968.

26. Russel, K.: Fibroids — When not to operate. Postgrad. Med., *60*:245–248, 1976.

27. Silverberg, S. G.: Leiomyosarcoma of the uterus: A clinicopathologic study. Obstet. Gynecol., *38*:613–628, 1971.

28. Silverberg, S. G.: Reproducibility of the mitosis count in the histologic diagnosis of smooth muscle tumors of the uterus. Hum. Pathol., *7*:451–454, 1976.

29. Terz, J. J., Barber, H. R. K., and Brunschwig, A.: Incidence of carcinoma in the retained ovary. Am. J. Surg., *113*:511–515, 1967.

30. White, S. C., Wartel, L. J., and Wade, M. E.: Comparison of abdominal and vaginal hysterectomies: A review of 600 operations. Obstet. Gynecol., *37*:530–537, 1971.

31. Winn, K. J., Woodruff, J. D., and Parmley, T.: Electronmicroscopic studies of leiomyomatosis peritonealis disseminata. Obstet. Gynecol., *48*:225–227, 1976.

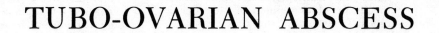

TUBO-OVARIAN ABSCESS

TUBO-OVARIAN ABSCESS BY WILLIAM B. WILSON, M.D.

Comments

A. At some time during their premenopausal period 3 to 5 per cent of U.S. women will have a tubo-ovarian abscess (TOA). Common causes are pelvic inflammatory disease, puerperal or postabortion infection, pelvic operation, malignancy, or an intrauterine contraceptive device.[1-6] Seldom is *Neisseria gonorrhoeae* involved.[1,2] Bacteroides and other anaerobes frequently are responsible. Because TOA often occurs in young women, preservation of fertility is important in many cases.

B. Accepted antibiotic regimes include penicillin, an aminoglycoside, and clindamycin or chloramphenicol (for Bacteroides).[1,4,8,10]

C. Colpotomy rather than laparotomy drainage is preferable for an abscess pointing into the rectovaginal septum in the midline.[1,2,10]

D. Seventy per cent of patients respond to antibiotics with or without colpotomy, but only 10 per cent will have a later pregnancy;[10] at least 33 per cent will have subsequent abnormal hysterosalpingograms. If there is bilateral abnormality the probability of pregnancy is zero; if abnormality is unilateral, pregnancy probability is 83 per cent.[1,10]

E. Of the 10 per cent of cases that have early failure, 4 per cent rupture and 6 per cent enlarge.[2,10,11]

F. An additional 20 per cent of patients respond at first to antibiotics (with or without colpotomy) but later the abscess reactivates (4 per cent) or they develop a persistent painful pelvic mass with menorrhagia (16 per cent). Unless these patients respond promptly to antibiotics and colpotomy, most ultimately will require operation.[10,11]

G. Hysterectomy and bilateral salpingo-oophorectomy is the classic treatment for ruptured TOA because of its lower overall mortality and subsequent reoperation rates and the infrequency of subsequent pregnancy when other techniques are used. Mortality was 0 to 15 per cent[11,13] but currently is 3 to 5 per cent with better antibiotics and operative and postoperative techniques.[1,12,14]

H. Conservation of the uterus using intraoperative and postoperative lavage is being re-evaluated. Reported mortality is 7.1 per cent. Hormonal and menstrual function is retained in 73.5 per cent of cases and potential for pregnancy in 42.5 per cent. Reoperation rate is 17.5 per cent.[17]

References

1. Mattingly, R. F.: TeLinde's Operative Gynecology. Philadelphia, J. B. Lippincott Co., 1977, pp. 259–289.
2. McNamara, M. T., and Mead, P. B.: Diagnosis and management of the pelvic abscess. J. Reprod. Med. *17*:299–304, 1976.
3. Weeks, L. R.: Ruptured tubo-ovarian abscess. J. Nat. Med. Assoc., 67:435–43, 1975.
4. Ledger, W. J., et al.: Adnexal abscess as a late complication of pelvic operation. Surg. Gynecol. Obstet., *129*:973–8, 1969.
5. Gassner, C. B., and Ballard, C. A.: Pelvic abscess: A sequela of first trimester abortion. Obstet. Gynecol. 48:716–17, 1976.
6. Taylor, E. S., et al.: The intrauterine device and tubo-ovarian abscess. Am. J. Obstet. Gynecol., *123*:338–48, 1975.
7. Eschenbach, D. A., and Holmes, K. K.: Acute pelvic inflammatory disease: Current concepts of pathogenesis, etiology and management. Clin. Obstet. Gynecol., *18*:35–56, 1975.
8. Heaton, C., and Ledger, W. J.: Postmenopausal tubo-ovarian abscess. Obstet. Gynecol., *47*:90–94, 1976.
9. Ledger, W. J., Gassner, C. A., and Gee C: Operative care of infections in obstetrics-gynecology. J. Reprod. Med. *13*:128, 1974.
10. Franklin, E. W., Hevron, J. E., and Thompson, J. D.: Management of the pelvic abscess. Clin. Obstet. Gynecol., *16*:66–79, 1973.
11. Collins, C. G., and Jansen, W. J.: Treatment of pelvic abscess infections. Clin. Obstet. Gynecol., 2:512, 1959.
12. Michal, A., Sellman, A. H., and Beebe, J. L: Ruptured tubo-ovarian abscesses. Am. J. Obstet. Gynecol., *100*:432, 1968.
13. Vermeeren, J., and Telinde, R. W.: Intra-abdominal rupture of pelvic abscesses. Am. J. Obstet. Gynecol. 68:402, 1954.
14. Pedowitz, P., Bloomfield, R.: Ruptured adnexal abscess (tubo-ovarian) with generalized peritonitis. Am. J. Obstet. Gynecol. 88:721, 1964.
15. Pedowitz, P., and Felmus, L. B.: Ruptured adnexal abscess with generalized peritonitis. Am. J. Surg., 83:507, 1952.
16. TeLinde, R. W., and Mattingly, R. F.: Operative Gynecology. Philadelphia, J. B. Lippincott Co. 1970, pp. 230–269.
17. Rivlin, M. E., and Hunt, J. A.: Ruptured tubo-ovarian abscess — is hysterectomy necessary? Obstet. Gynecol., *50*:518–22, 1977.

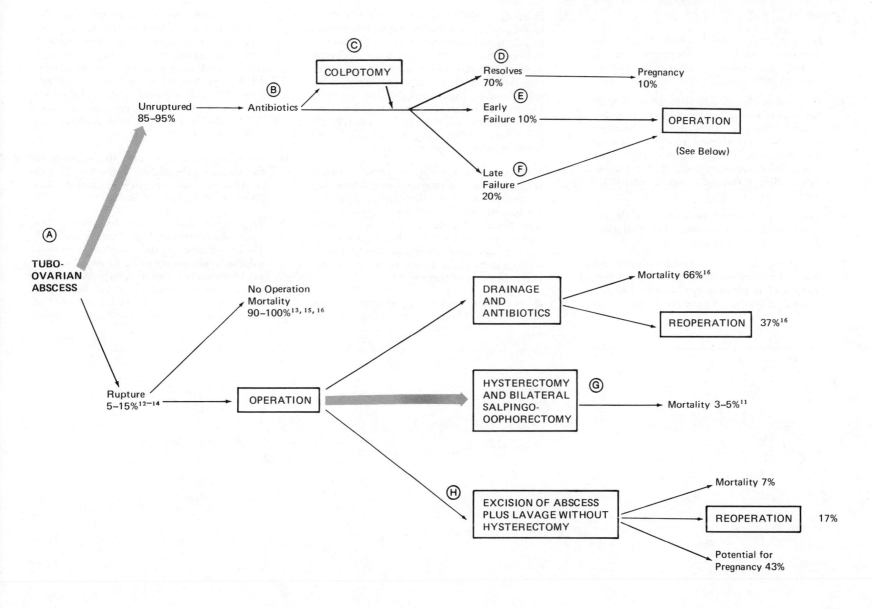

Ⓒ
COLPOTOMY

Ⓑ
Unruptured
85–95% → Antibiotics

Ⓐ
TUBO-OVARIAN ABSCESS

Ⓓ
Resolves
70% → Pregnancy 10%

Ⓔ
Early
Failure 10% → OPERATION

(See Below)

Late
Failure Ⓕ
20%

No Operation
Mortality
90–100%[13, 15, 16]

Rupture
5–15%[12–14] → OPERATION

DRAINAGE
AND
ANTIBIOTICS → Mortality 66%[16]

REOPERATION 37%[16]

HYSTERECTOMY
AND BILATERAL
SALPINGO-
OOPHORECTOMY Ⓖ → Mortality 3–5%[11]

Ⓗ
EXCISION OF ABSCESS
PLUS LAVAGE WITHOUT
HYSTERECTOMY → Mortality 7%

REOPERATION 17%

Potential for
Pregnancy 43%

ENDOMETRIOSIS BY PAUL WEXLER, M.D.

Comments

A. Incidence approximates 13 to 17 per cent of women. Definitive diagnosis depends on implants visible at laparotomy, endoscopy, or microscopic examination.[1]

B. External endometriosis is found in 15 to 20 per cent of women in the 24 to 45 year age group. Common sites are the ovaries; uterosacral, broad, and round ligaments; the peritoneum; and pelvic laparotomy scars. Other remote sites (e.g., the pleura, extremities, hernia sacs, and appendix) are rare.

C. There is poor correlation between the extent of implants and symptoms. Extensive disease may be asymptomatic.

D. If endometriosis is severe enough to cause bowel or ureteral obstruction, hysterectomy and oophorectomy should be performed at the same time to minimize sequelae.

E. Internal endometriosis (endometrial glands and stroma within the myometrium, or adenomyosis) characteristically occurs between the ages of 41 and 50 years. Eight to 40 per cent of hysterectomy specimens may demonstrate microscopic evidence of the disease. Associated lesions include leiomyomata uteri (15 per cent) and salpingitis isthmica nodosum (approximately 20 per cent). About 12 per cent have coexisting external endometriosis.[2, 3]

F. Malignant degeneration of endometriosis is infrequent. The ovary is the primary site in most cases, but other sites do occur. Microscopically the lesions are usually endometrioid. Malignant adenomatous and squamous elements may be represented. Cancer may occur in the postmenopausal woman even if she is not receiving estrogen replacement therapy.[4, 5]

G. Hysterectomy and oophorectomy is the operation of choice and the last resort when symptoms are intractable or the woman has completed childbearing. Conservation of an ovary in a young patient may be indicated. Rarely (0 to 3 per cent of cases), peritoneal implants may be activated by postoperative estrogen replacement.[5] Operative mortality for endometriosis approaches that of anesthesia alone (0.02 to 0.05 per cent) or hysterectomy (0.2 to 0.7 per cent).

H. Infertility correlates with the severity of the disease. Pregnancy rates are 75 per cent for mild, 50 per cent for moderate, and 33 per cent for severe disease.[6, 7]

I. To preserve fertility, various conservative surgical procedures have been advocated. These include partial ovarian resection, salpingolysis, electrocoagulation of peritoneal implants, uterine suspension, and uterosacral ligament plication. Remission rates may approach 20 to 35 per cent of these cases. Presacral neurectomy, once

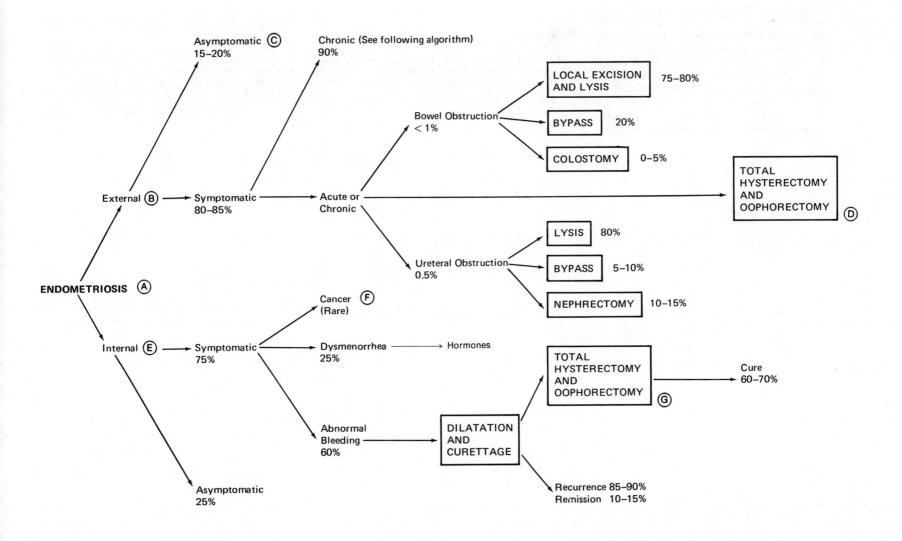

ENDOMETRIOSIS *Continued*

frequently employed for pain, is rarely required.

J. Progestins, either alone or in combination with estrogens, are effective in achieving remissions. Often surgery can be averted or pregnancy achieved with medical therapy. Danazol, a synthetic 2,3-isoxazol derivative of 17-alpha-ethinyltestosterone, produces a 50 per cent fertility rate and 85 to 90 per cent remission. (It is a weak androgen that inhibits release of gonadotropin.) It induces amenorrhea and endometrial atrophy, usually providing symptomatic relief.[8, 9]

References

1. Gold, J. J.: Gynecologic Endocrinology., 2nd ed. New York, Harper & Row, 1975, pp. 245–271.
2. Greenblatt, R. A.: Recent Advances in Endometriosis. Princeton, N.J., Excerpta Medica, 1976.
3. Mattingly, R. F.: TeLinde's Operative Gynecology, 5th ed. Philadelphia, J. B. Lippincott Co., 1977, pp. 233–252.
4. Novak, E. R.: Textbook of Gynaecology, 9th ed. Baltimore, Williams & Wilkins Co., 1975, pp. 542–565.
5. Chalmers, J. A.: Endometriosis. Woburn, Mass., Butterworths, 1975.
6. Ingersoll, F. M.: Selection of medical and surgical treatment of endometriosis. Clin. Obstet. Gynecol., 20:849–864, 1977.
7. Acosta, A. A. et al.: A proposed classification of pelvic endometriosis. Obstet. Gynecol., 42:19–25, 1973.
8. Kistner, R. W.: Management of endometriosis in the infertile patient. Fertil. Steril., 26:1151–1166, 1975.
9. Dmowski, W. P., and Cohen, M. R.: Treatment of endometriosis with an antigonadotropin, danazol: A laparoscopic and histologic evaluation. Obstet. Gynecol., 46:147–154, 1975.

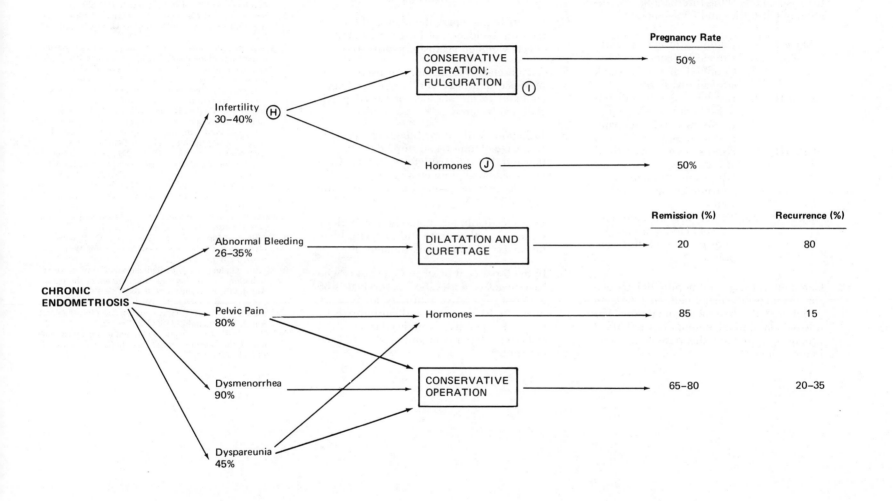

CANCER OF THE CERVIX BY FRANCIS J. MAJOR, M.D.

Comments

A. Clinical staging is accomplished according to the standards of the International Federation of Obstetrics and Gynecology.[1-5]

    Stage I: A. Confined to cervix, early stromal invasion
           B. Confined to cervix, frank stromal invasion
    Stage II: A. Involving cervix and upper two-thirds of vagina
           B. Involving cervix and parametrial tissue
    Stage III: A. Extension to lower third of vagina
           B. Extension through parametrium to lateral pelvic wall
    Stage IV: A. Tumor has invaded mucosa of bladder or bowel
           B. Spread beyond the true pelvis

B. Carcinoma *in situ* is intraepithelial neoplasia, cytologically malignant, that has not penetrated the basement membrane. Extensive gland involvement does not affect prognosis, provided the basement membrane is intact.

C. Microinvasive carcinoma is invasion to a depth of 3 mm., without confluence of tongues of invasion and no evidence of stromal vascular involvement.[6, 7]

D. Results being equal, the choice of therapy rests on avoidance of long-term radiation effects weighed against operative risk.[8-13]

E. Extrafascial hysterectomy is used in the presence of a large cervix (greater than 5 cm.) and in the absence of lateral pelvic wall involvement.[9, 11]

F. Radiation will stop bleeding, provide shrinkage of tumor, and stop bone destruction and thus will palliate symptoms. Chemotherapy will produce regression in 30 to 50 per cent of cases, but no cures are reported.[14, 18-20]

Drugs available for chemotherapy include Cytoxan, methotrexate, Adriamycin, bleomycin, *cis*-platinum, and mutamycin.

G. In the 5 per cent of stage IV patients who have negative nodes, 5-year survival is 50 per cent. Operative mortality for primary tumors is 10.2 per cent and morbidity is 67 per cent. Operative mortality for recurrent disease is 30 per cent and morbidity is 80 per cent.[15-17]

References

1. Townsend, D. E., et al.: Abnormal Papanicolaou smears: Evaluation by colposcopy, biopsies and endocervical curettage. Am. J. Obstet. Gynecol., *108*:429, 1970.
2. Eiseman, B., and Watkyns, R. S.: Surgical Decision Making. Philadelphia, W. B. Saunders Co., 1978, pp. 280–282.
3. American Joint Committee for Staging and End Results Reporting: Manual for Staging of Cancer 1977. Chicago, Am. Joint Committee, 1977, pp. 90–91.
4. Sudarsanam, A., et al.: Influence of exploratory celiotomy on the management of carcinoma of the cervix: A preliminary report. Cancer, *41*:1049–1053, 1978.
5. Delgado, G., Caglar, H., and Walker, P.: Survival and complications in cervical cancer treated by pelvic and extended field radiation after para-aortic lymphadenectomy. Am. J. Roentgenol., *130*:141–143, 1978.
6. Christopherson, W., Gray, L., and Parker, J.: Microinvasive carcinoma of the uterine cervix: Long-term followup study of 80 cases. Cancer, *38*:629–632, 1976.
7. Seski, J., Abell, M., and Morley, G.: Microinvasive squamous carcinoma of the cervix. Obstet. Gynecol., *50*:410–414, 1977.
8. Park, R., et al.: Treatment of stage I carcinoma of the cervix. Obstet. Gynecol., *41*:117–122, 1973.
9. DiSaia, P., Morrow, C., and Townsend, D.: Synopsis of Gynecologic Oncology. New York, John Wiley and Sons, 1975, pp. 40–65.
10. Morley, G., and Seski, J.: Radical pelvic surgery versus radiation therapy for stage I carcinoma of the cervix. Am. J. Obstet. Gynecol., *126*:785–789, 1976.
11. Easley, J., and Fletcher, G.: Analysis of the treatment of stage I and stage II carcinomas of the uterine cervix. Am. J. Roentgenol., *111*:243–251, 1972.
12. Villasanta, U.: Complications of radiotherapy for carcinoma of the uterine cervix. Am. J. Obstet. Gynecol., *114*:717–726, 1972.

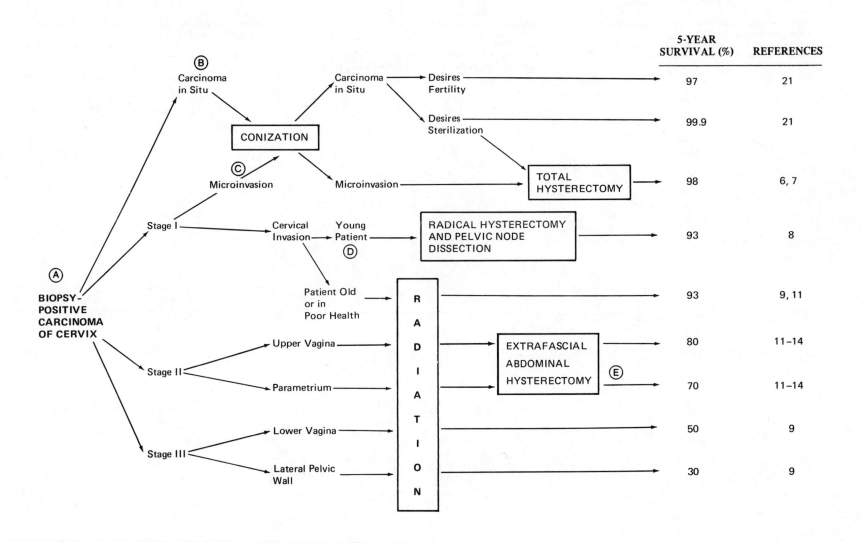

13. Abitol, M., and Davenport, J.: The irradiated vagina. Obstet. Gynecol., *44*:249–256, 1974.
14. Fletcher, G.: External radiation therapy in cancer of the uterine cervix. *In* Lewis, G. C., et al. (eds.): New Concepts in Gynecologic Oncology. Philadelphia, F. A. Davis, 1966, pp. 111–130.
15. Deckers, D., et al.: Pelvic exenteration for primary carcinoma of the uterine cervix. Obstet. Gynecol., *37*:647–659, 1971.
16. Turko, M., et al.: Pelvic exenteration 1949–1971. Gynecol. Oncol., 5:246–250, 1977.
17. Brunschwig, A.: What are the indications and results of pelvic exenteration? JAMA, *194*:204–210, 1965.
18. Malkasian, G., et al.: Chemotherapy of squamous cell carcinoma of the cervix, vagina and vulva. Clin. Obstet. Gynecol., *11*:367, 1968.
19. Omura, G.: Chemotherapy and hormone therapy in gynecologic cancer. South. Med. J., *66*:689–702, 1973.
20. Thigpen, T., and Shingleton, H.: Phase II trial of *cis*-platinum in treatment of advanced squamous cell carcinoma of the cervix. Proc. Am. Assoc. Cancer Res., *19*:332, 1978.
21. Boyes, D., Worth, A., and Fidler, H.: Results of treatment of 4389 cases of preclinical cervical squamous carcinoma. J. Obstet. Gynecol. Brit. Commonw., *77*:769–780, 1970.

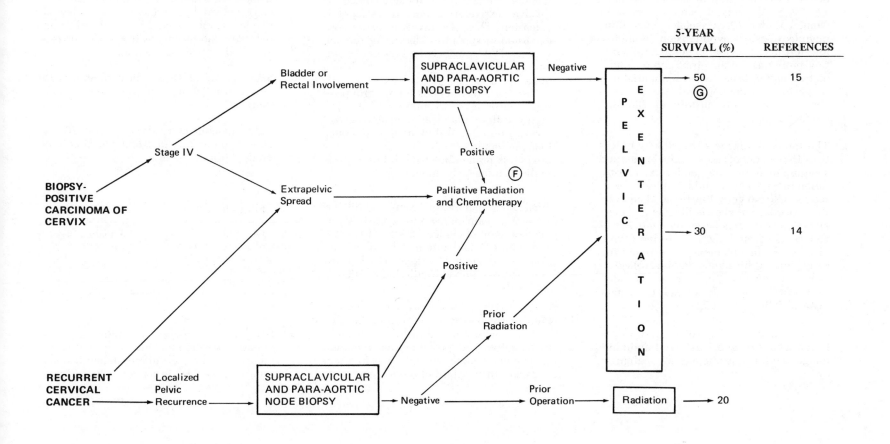

ADENOCARCINOMA OF THE ENDOMETRIUM BY STANLEY N. GOODMAN, M.D.

Comments

A. Endometrial adenocarcinoma is the commonest gynecologic cancer and constitutes 90 per cent of all endometrial neoplasms. Seventy-five per cent of cases occur after age 50, while only 4 per cent occur in women under 40. Associated conditions include obesity, hypertension, diabetes, low fertility, irregular bleeding, anovulatory problems, endometrial polyps, endometrial hyperplasia, use of sequential oral progestins, postmenopausal estrogen therapy, and a family history of the disease.[2, 3, 6, 12]

B. The source of diagnosis is cytology in less than 15 per cent of cases, vaginal pools and scraping in 40 per cent, endocervical aspiration in 65 per cent, and intrauterine aspiration in 90 per cent. Fractional D and C is the procedure of choice. Staging and classification (FIGO) is based on a number of factors: (1) 8 cm length of uterine cavity, (2) cervical involvement, (3) extrauterine extension, (4) histologic grading, (5) extrapelvic extension, (6) spread to adjacent organs, and (7) spread to distant organs.[1, 2, 12]

C. Carcinoma *in situ* (Stage 0) is a preinvasive lesion whose diagnosis is based upon histologic findings suspicious for malignancy.[1]

D. Distinctions of staging: Stage I is confined to the uterine corpus; in stage IA the uterine cavity is 8 cm. or less and in stage IB the uterine cavity is greater than 8 cm. Stage II involves the corpus and cervix without extrauterine extension. Stage III involves extrauterine but not extrapelvic extension. Stage IV involves extrapelvic extension or spread to bladder or rectum; in stage IVA spread is to adjacent organs and in stage IVB spread is to distant organs.

Histologic distinctions for subgroups of stage I lesions are as follows: Group 1 is highly differentiated adenomatous carcinoma, group 2 is differentiated adenomatous carcinoma with partly solid areas, and group 3 is predominantly solid or entirely undifferentiated carcinoma.[1, 2, 6]

E. Total abdominal hysterectomy and bilateral salpingo-oophorectomy (TAH-BSO) is the treatment of choice for stage I disease with group 1 and group 2 histologic lesions. Unexpected extension requires postoperative pelvic irradiation of 5000 to 8000 rads.[3, 8]

F. Preoperative radiation is required in stage I disease with group 3 histologic lesions. Preoperative and postoperative radiation are of equal benefit when there is invasion of greater than a third of the myometrium, occult cervical disease, or extrauterine spread.[3, 8]

G. Stage II is best managed by preoperative irradiation followed in 2 to 6 weeks by TAH-BSO. The other alternatives are primary radical hysterectomy with bilateral pelvic lymphadenectomy and followup pelvic radiation for positive nodes or primary pelvic irradiation alone.[2, 3]

H. Stages III and IV are best treated with pelvic irradiation and progestin chemotherapy.[2, 3, 5]

I. Eight per cent of grade 1 tumors, 20 per cent of grade 2 tumors, and 44 per cent of grade 3 tumors recur.

RECURRENCE	SITE	RATE (%)
After TAH-BSO	Vaginal	5–10
After adjunctive radiation	Vaginal	2–5
Without myometrial invasion		9
Superficial invasion		8.5
Deep invasion		27

J. Recurrence in pelvis or vagina requires radiation treatment. Pulmonary and bone recurrence and well-differentiated lesions require progestins to achieve a 30 to 35 per

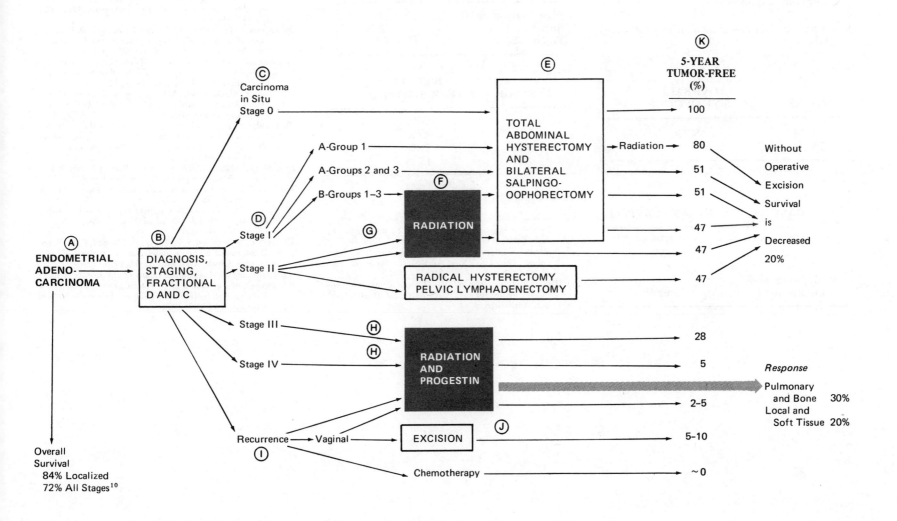

cent objective benefit. Soft tissue recurrence requires progestins to achieve a 20 per cent response.[3, 6]

K. Survival data are shown in the following tables.

AGE (yr.)	OVERALL 5-YEAR CURE
45–54	83%
75–84	47%

GRADE	5-YEAR SURVIVAL
1	82%
2	75%
3	43%
With pelvic node involvement	40%

STAGE I

DEPTH OF INVASION	5-YEAR SURVIVAL
Absent myometrial	98%
Superficial	90%
Deep	68%

STAGE	OVERALL 5-YEAR SURVIVAL
I	76%
II	47%
III	28%
IV	4.7%

References

1. American College of Obstetrics and Gynecology. Classification and Staging of Malignant Tumors in the Female Pelvis. Technical Bulletin No. 47, June 1977.
2. Rutledge, F., Boronow, R. C., and Wharton, J. T.: Gynecologic Oncology. New York, John Wiley & Sons, 1976, p. 97.
3. DiSaia, P. J., and Rich, W. M.: The management of gynecologic malignancies. J. Continuing Ed. Obstet. Gynecol., April 1978, p. 13.
4. Kistner, R. W.: Chemotherapy for carcinoma of the endometrium. OB/GYN Digest, August 1975, p. 26.
5. Hernandez, W., et al.: Stage II endometrial cancer: Two modalities of treatment. Am. J. Obstet. Gynecol., 131:171, 1978.
6. DiSaia, P. J., Morrow, C. P., and Townsend, D. E.: Synopsis of Gynecologic Oncology: Cancer of the Corpus. New York, John Wiley & Sons, 1975, p. 111.
7. Muggia, F. M., et al.: Doxorubicin-cyclophosphamide: Effective chemotherapy for advanced endometrial adenocarcinoma. J. Obstet. Gynecol., 128:314, 1977.
8. Tavares, M. A., et al.: Management and results of endometrial carcinoma treated at Instituto Portuges de Oncologia de Francisco Gentil. Cancer, 39:675, 1977.
9. Landgren, R. D., Fletcher, G. H., and Gallager, H. S.: Treatment failure sites according to irradiation technique and histology in patients with endometrial cancer. Cancer, 40:131, 1977.
10. National Cancer Institute: Cancer Patient Survival. Report No. 5, Washington, D.C., U.S. Dept. H.E.W., 1976.
11. Cancer survival among women. Surgical Rounds, March 1978, pp. 70–72.
12. Cancer in Colorado: A report of the Colorado Cancer Registry, Colorado Dept. of Health, Report No. 1, 1970–1975. May 1978.
13. Surwit, E. A., Fowler, W. C., Jr., and Rogoff, E. E.: Stage II carcinoma of the endometrium: An analysis of treatment. J. Obstet. Gynecol., 52:97, 1978.
14. Kottmeier, H. L.: Annual report of the results of treatment in carcinoma of the uterus, ovary, and vagina. Geneva, International Federation of Gynecology and Obstetrics, Vol. 15, 1973.

OVARIAN CANCER

OVARIAN CANCER BY FRANCIS MAJOR, M. D.

Comments

A. Metastases of breast and colon cancer to the ovary are more common than primary ovarian malignancies.

B. Types include serous (50 per cent of cases), mucinous (15 per cent), clear cell (5 per cent), endometrioid (15 per cent), and undifferentiated (15 per cent).[1-3]

    Stage I tumors make up 40 to 50 per cent of cases. Average age is 45 to 60 years.

C. Debulking involves removal of all possible tumor not infiltrating vital organs. This allows better response to radiation and chemotherapy.[3]

    Five-year survival without debulking is 20 per cent and with debulking is 55 per cent.

D. Staging is based on clinical, operative, and histologic evidence. It is of particular prognostic importance in epithelial tumors.

    Stage I is limited to the ovaries; stage IA has no ascites; stage IAi has no tumor on the external surface, and capsule is intact; and stage IAii has tumor present on the external surface, or capsule(s) ruptured, or both. In stage IB growth is limited to both ovaries, with no ascites; in IBi there is no tumor on the external surface, and capsule is intact; in IBii tumor is present on the external surface, or capsule(s) are ruptured, or both. Stage IC has a tumor of either stage IA or IB, but ascites is present or there are positive peritoneal washings.

    Stage II involves one or both ovaries with pelvic extension; stage IIA has extension and/or metastases to the uterus or tubes or both; stage IIB has extension to other pelvic tissues. Stage IIC has tumor of either stage IIA or IIB, but ascites is present or peritoneal washings are positive.

    Stage III is growth involving one or both ovaries with intraperitoneal metastases outside the pelvis, or positive retroperitoneal nodes, or both. Tumor is limited to the true pelvis with histologically proven malignant extension to small bowel or omentum.

    Stage IV means distant metastases, including those to liver.

E. Intraperitoneal chromic phosphate (^{32}P) is used in stage I patients in whom full surgical staging, including biopsy of the diaphragm and para-aortic nodes, confirms localized disease. Patients whose staging is incomplete receive systemic chemotherapy. Whole-abdomen radiation may compromise systemic chemotherapy in stage II and stage III.[1, 2, 3, 6]

F. This category includes dysgerminoma (2 per cent of cases), immature teratoma (2 per cent), embryonal tumors (1 per cent), choriocarcinoma (1 per cent), endodermal sinus (1 per cent), and mixed types (3 per cent).

    Except for the pure dysgerminoma, these tumors are highly malignant. Most — except dysgerminoma and immature teratoma — occur in infants and children.[1, 9]

G. This includes node biopsy for staging.

H. Dysgerminoma with an intact capsule and negative pelvic and para-aortic nodes requires no further therapy. Invasion of the capsule or a positive node biopsy necessitates adjuvant radiation.[5, 8, 9]

I. Chemotherapeutic agents include vincristine, actinomycin D, and Cytoxan, or Velban, bleomycin, and *cis*-platinum.[8, 9]

J. Incidence of granulosa cell tumors is 5 per cent. It is the most malignant of these tumors and can occur at any age. Androblastoma (0.5 per cent incidence) and gynandroblastoma (1 per cent incidence) have a low rate of malignancy in young women.

References

1. Scully, R. E.: Recent progress in ovarian cancer. Hum. Pathol. *1*:73–98, 1970.
2. DiSaia, P. J., Morrow, C. P., and Townsend, D. E.: Synopsis of Gynecologic Oncology. New York, John Wiley & Sons, 1975, pp. 152–195.
3. Aure, J. C., Hoeg, K., and Kolstad, P.: Clinical and histologic studies of ovarian carcinoma: Long-term followup of 990 cases. Obstet. Gynecol., 37:1, 1971.
4. Decker, D. G., et al.: Adjuvant therapy for advanced ovarian malignancy. Am. J. Obstet. Gynecol., 37:1, 1971.
5. Kottmeier, H. L.: Presentation of therapeutic results in carcinoma of the female pelvis: Experience of the annual report on the results of treatment in carcinoma of the uterus, vagina, and ovary. Gynecol. Oncol., 4:13, 1976.
6. Fisher, R. I., and Young, R. C.: Chemotherapy of ovarian cancer. Surg. Clin. North Am., 58:143, 1978.
7. Hreshchyshyn, M. M., and Norris, H. J.: Post operative treatment of women with resectable ovarian cancer with radiotherapy, melphalan or no further treatment. Proceedings of Am. Assoc. Cancer Res., #777, 1977.
8. Nogales, F. F., Jr., et al.: Immature teratoma of the ovary with a neural component. Hum. Pathol., 7:625–642, 1976.
9. Scully, R. E., Sturgis, S. H., and Taymor, M. L.: Ovarian tumors of germ cell origin. *In* Meigs, J. V., and Sturgis, S. H. (eds.): Progress in Gynecology, vol. 5. New York, Grune & Stratton, 1970, pp. 329–348.
10. Norris, H. J., and Taylor, H. B.: Prognosis of granulosa thecal tumors of the ovary. Cancer, 21:255, 1968.
11. O'Hern, T. M., and Neubecker, R. D.: Arrhenoblastoma. Obstet. Gynecol. 19:758, 1962.

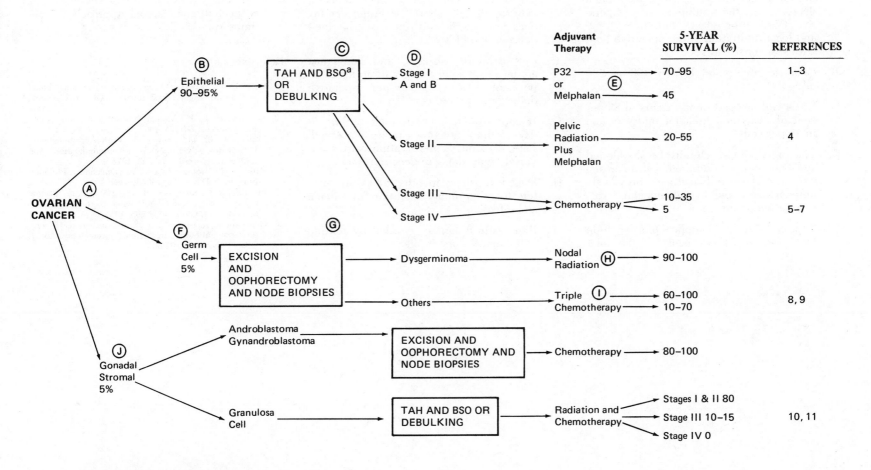

	Adjuvant Therapy	5-YEAR SURVIVAL (%)	REFERENCES

Ⓐ OVARIAN CANCER

Ⓑ Epithelial 90–95% → Ⓒ TAH AND BSO[a] OR DEBULKING → Ⓓ Stage I A and B → P32 or → 70–95 (1–3)

Ⓔ Melphalan → 45

Stage II → Pelvic Radiation Plus Melphalan → 20–55 (4)

Stage III → Chemotherapy → 10–35

Stage IV → 5 (5–7)

Ⓕ Germ Cell 5% → Ⓖ EXCISION AND OOPHORECTOMY AND NODE BIOPSIES → Dysgerminoma → Nodal Radiation Ⓗ → 90–100

Others → Triple Ⓘ Chemotherapy → 60–100 / 10–70 (8, 9)

Ⓙ Gonadal Stromal 5% → Androblastoma Gynandroblastoma → EXCISION AND OOPHORECTOMY AND NODE BIOPSIES → Chemotherapy → 80–100

Granulosa Cell → TAH AND BSO OR DEBULKING → Radiation and Chemotherapy → Stages I & II 80 / Stage III 10–15 / Stage IV 0 (10, 11)

[a]Total abdominal hysterectomy and bilateral salpingo-oophorectomy

VAGINAL HYSTERECTOMY BY WILLIAM E. FULLER, M.D., AND EDGAR L. MAKOWSKI, M.D.

Comments

A. Mortality and morbidity rates[2] have been decreased by the routine use of preoperative IVP,[16] prophylactic antibiotics,[6, 10, 12] and local infiltration of the operative field with vasoconstrictors.[7]

B. Characteristic blood loss is 190 to 290 ml.[1]

C. Unilateral ureteral injury occurs in 85 per cent of cases and bilateral injury occurs in 15 per cent.[4]

D. The vaginal approach must be abandoned and laparotomy performed instead in 0.3 per cent of cases because of previously unrecognized pelvic inflammatory disease or endometriosis.[2]

E. Reported early complications include fever (48 to 78 per cent),[6, 12] the incidence of which has been reduced by the use of prophylactic antibiotics to 0 to 8 per cent,[6, 12] and urinary tract infection (8.6 to 48 per cent).[11, 13] Adnexectomy does not significantly increase the incidence of morbidity.[11]

F. Cuff cellulitis, abscess, and hematoma are managed solely with antibiotics in 96 per cent of cases[14] and require operative drainage in 4.4 per cent.[14]

G. If nephrostomy is performed within 40 days, kidney function can be preserved. Rate of kidney preservation varies inversely with delay in decompression.

H. Staged repair 6 months following hysterectomy permits resolution of edema and infection.

I. Enterocele is largely avoided by routine uterosacral ligament plication.

J. Rate of adnexal excision at the time of vaginal hysterectomy varies from 3.8[15] to 24 per cent.[11] If ovarian neoplastic disease is suspected, the vaginal approach is contraindicated.[9]

References

1. Copenhaver, E. H.: Observations concerning blood loss during vaginal hysterectomy. Obstet. Gynecol., 24:385, 1964.
2. Copenhaver, E. H.: Vaginal hysterectomy. Am. J. Obstet. Gynecol., 84:123, 1962.
3. Coulam, C. B., and Pratt, J. H.: Vaginal hysterectomy: Is previous pelvic operation a contraindication? Am. J. Obstet. Gynecol., 116:252, 1973.
4. Falk, H. C.: Urologic Injuries in Gynecology. Philadelphia, F. A. Davis Co., 1964, p. 267.
5. Fleming, S. P., Kearns, P. R., and Lock, F. R.: Factors influencing morbidity following vaginal hysterectomy. Obstet. Gynecol., 4:295, 1954.
6. Goosenberg, J., Emich, J. P., and Schwarz, R. H.: Prophylactic antibiotics in vaginal hysterectomy. Am. J. Obstet. Gynecol., 105:503, 1969.

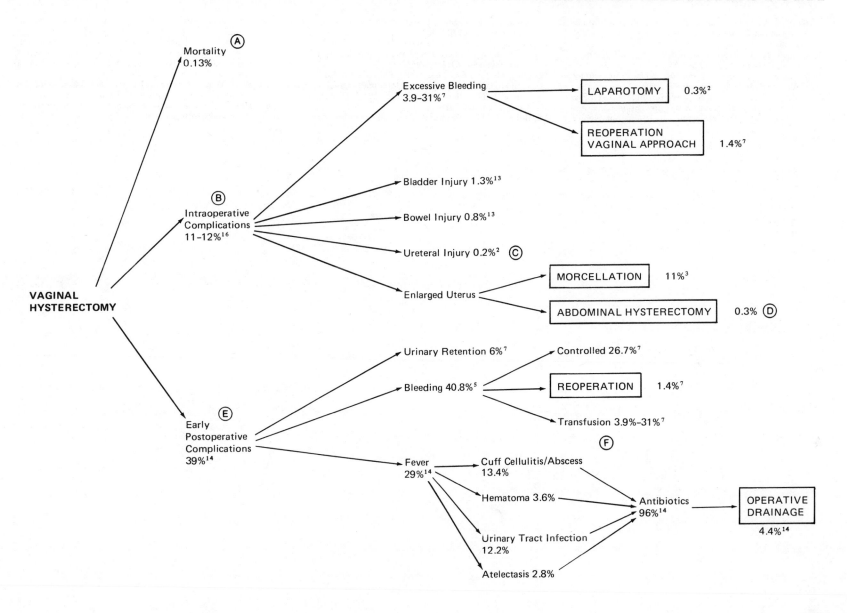

7. Gray, L. A.: Indications, techniques, and complications in vaginal hysterectomy. Obstet. Gynecol., *28*:714, 1966.

8. Grogan, R. H.: Reappraisal of residual ovaries. Am. J. Obstet. Gynecol., *97*:124, 1967.

9. Israel, S. L.: Vaginal sequelae of vaginal hysterectomy. Am. J. Obstet. Gynecol., *69*:87, 1955.

10. Ledger, W. J., Sweet, R. L., and Headington, J. T.: Prophylactic cephaloridine in the prevention of postoperative pelvic infections in premenopausal women undergoing vaginal hysterectomy. Am. J. Obstet. Gynecol., *115*:766, 1973.

11. Leventhal, M. L., and Lazarus, M. L.: Total abdominal and vaginal hysterectomy, a comparison. Am. J. Obstet. Gynecol., *61*:289, 1951.

12. Ohm, M. J., and Galask, R. P.: The effect of antibiotic prophylaxis on patients undergoing vaginal operations. I. The effect on morbidity. Am. J. Obstet. Gynecol., *123*:590, 1975.

13. Rubin, A.: Complications of vaginal operations for pelvic floor relaxation. Am. J. Obstet. Gynecol., *95*:972, 1966.

14. Sprague, A. D., and van Nagell, J. R.: The relationship of age and endometrial histology to blood loss and morbidity following vaginal hysterectomy. Am. J. Obstet. Gynecol., *118*:805, 1974.

15. Weir, W. C.: A statistical report of 1914 cases of hysterectomy. Am. J. Obstet. Gynecol., *42*:285, 1941.

16. Hard data not available. Estimates based on clinical experience ± 10 per cent.

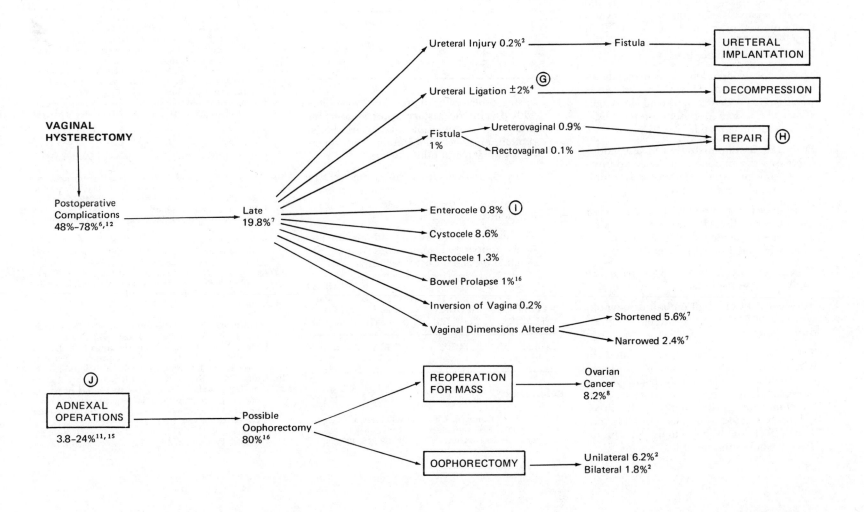

VAGINAL HYSTERECTOMY

Postoperative
Complications
48%–78%[6,12]

Late
19.8%[7]

Ureteral Injury 0.2%[2] → Fistula → URETERAL IMPLANTATION

Ureteral Ligation ±2%[4] G → DECOMPRESSION

Fistula
1%
→ Ureterovaginal 0.9%
→ Rectovaginal 0.1%
→ REPAIR H

Enterocele 0.8% I

Cystocele 8.6%

Rectocele 1.3%

Bowel Prolapse 1%[16]

Inversion of Vagina 0.2%

Vaginal Dimensions Altered
→ Shortened 5.6%[7]
→ Narrowed 2.4%[7]

J
ADNEXAL OPERATIONS
3.8–24%[11,15]

Possible
Oophorectomy
80%[16]

REOPERATION FOR MASS
→ Ovarian Cancer 8.2%[8]

OOPHORECTOMY
→ Unilateral 6.2%[2]
Bilateral 1.8%[2]

ABDOMINAL HYSTERECTOMY BY FREDRICK R. ABRAMS, M.D.

Comments

A. Reported mortality rates vary with the size of the series, e.g., 1 per cent in 300 cases[30] versus 0.085 to 0.2 per cent when the number of patients is more than 1000.[1, 11, 14] The majority of deaths are from pulmonary embolus.

B. The reported incidence of ureteral injuries varies from 1 per cent in some small series[20] to 0.2 per cent in larger series.[5, 17, 30] Many unilateral ureteral ligations go unrecognized.[7]

C. Prophylactic administration of antibiotics decreases the incidence of fever approximately 65 per cent[19] and virtually eliminates urinary tract infections.[1, 8, 14, 15, 30]

D. Differences in the techniques of incision and closure allegedly account for variations in the incidence of wound complications from 0.3 to 0.7 per cent.[2, 21, 28]

E. Risk factors as summarized on page 110 apply to these patients.

F. Fifty per cent of silent emboli discovered within ^{125}I fibrinogen scanning occurred during operation.

G. The patient's satisfaction is related to whether the hysterectomy was "desired" or "imposed,"[25] the greatest satisfaction being evidenced by those choosing hysterectomy for sterilization.[10] Erotic drive is loosely related to ovarian conservation. The effect of hysterectomy on erotic drive is shown in the table.

EROTIC DRIVE

Increased (%)	Same (%)	Decreased (%)	REFERENCE
23	45	32	18
20	62	18	18
52	44	4	10
38	56	6	25

H. Posthysterectomy depression correlates with psychiatric history, questionable indications for operation, age, marital disruption, misconceptions about the expected result, IQ, and other factors.[18, 20]

I. The reoperative rate varies from 0.89 to 3.5 per cent.[3, 4, 23] This represents removal of abnormal ovaries subsequent to hysterectomy.

J. The data refer to ovarian tumors in patients reoperated upon after either abdominal or vaginal hysterectomy.

NATURE OF TUMOR	GROGAN[9] (n = 92)	RANDALL et al.[22] (n = 345)	CHRIST and LOTZE[3] (n = 202)
Benign	14%	5.7%	23.3%
Malignant	10.8%	1.2%	3.0%

References

1. Allen, J. L., Rampone, J. F., and Wheeless, C. R.: Use of prophylactic antibiotics in elective major gynecologic operations. Obstet. Gynecol., 39:218, 1972.

2. Baggish, M. S., and Lee, W. K.: Abnormal wound disruption. Obstet. Gynecol., 46:530, 1975.

3. Christ, J. E., and Lotze, E. C.: The residual ovary syndrome. Obstet. Gynecol., 46:551, 1975.

4. DeNeef, J. C., and Hollenbeck, Z. J. R.: The fate of ovaries preserved at the time of hysterectomy. Am. J. Obstet. Gynecol., 96:1088–1097, 1967.

5. Everett, H. S., and Mattingly, R. F.: Urinary tract injuries resulting from pelvic surgery. Am. J. Obstet. Gynecol., 71:502, 1956.

6. Flanc, C., Kakkar, V. V., and Clarke, M. B.: Detection of venous thrombosis of the legs using ^{125}I-labeled fibrinogen. Br. J. Surg., 55:742, 1968.

7. Freda, V. C., and Tacchi, D.: Ureteral injury discovered after pelvic surgery. Am. J. Obstet. Gynecol., 80:406, 1962.

8. Gray, L. A.: Open cuff method of abdominal hysterectomy. Obstet. Gynecol., 46:42, 1975.

9. Grogan, R. H.: Reappraisal of residual ovaries. Am. J. Obstet. Gynecol., 97:124–129, 1967.

10. Hampton, P. T., and Tarnasky, W.: Hysterectomy and tubal ligation: A comparison of the psychological aftermath. Am. J. Obstet. Gynecol., 119:949–952, 1974.

11. Howkins, J., and Stallinorthy, J.: Bonney's Gynecological Surgery, 8th Ed. Baltimore, Williams & Wilkins, 1974, p. 808.

12. Jeffcoate, T. N. A., and Tindall, V. R.: Venous thrombosis and embolism in obstetrics and gynecology. Aust. N.Z. J. Obstet. Gynaecol., 5:119, 1965.

13. Kakkar, V. V., Corrigan, T. P., and Fossard, D. P.: Prevention of postoperative pulmonary embolism by low dose heparin. Lancet, 2:45, 1975.

14. Ledger, W. J., and Childs, M. A.: Hospital care of patients undergoing hysterectomy: An analysis of 12,026 patients from the professional activity study. Am. J. Obstet. Gynecol., 117:429, 1973.

15. Ledger, W. J., Reite, A., and Headington, J. T.: The surveillance of infection of an inpatient gynecology service. Am. J. Obstet. Gynecol., 113:662, 1971.

16. Ledger, W. J., Sweet, R. I., and Headington, J. T.: Prophylactic cephaloridine in the prevention of postoperative pelvic infections in premenopausal women undergoing vaginal hysterectomy. Am. J. Obstet. Gynecol., 115:766, 1973.

17. Mattingly, R. F.: TeLinde's Operative Gynecology, 5th Ed. Philadelphia, J. B. Lippincott Co., 1977.

ABDOMINAL HYSTERECTOMY

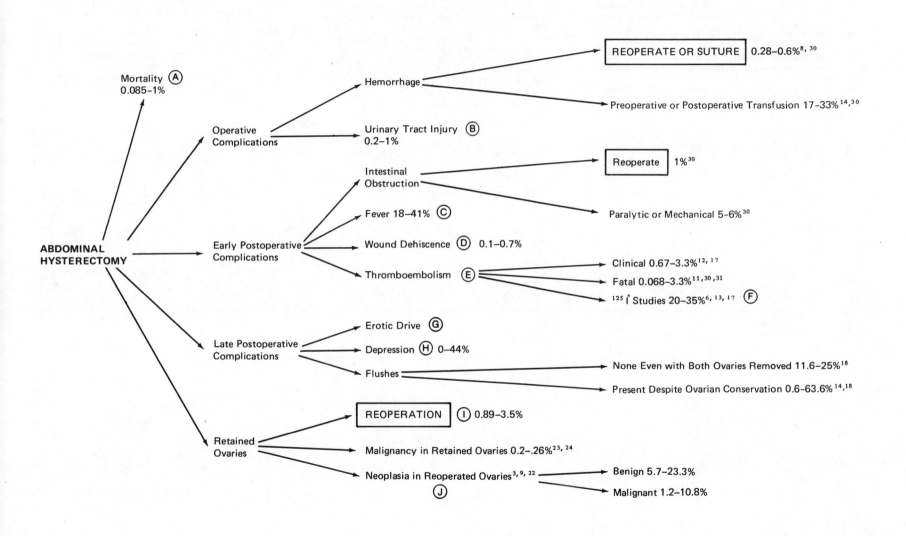

18. Newton,, N., and Baron, E.: Reactions to hysterectomy: Fact or fiction. Primary Care, 3:781, 1976.
19. Ohm, M. J. and Galask, R. P.: The effect of antibiotic prophylaxis on patients undergoing total abdominal hysterectomy. I. Effect on morbidity. Am. J. Obstet. Gynecol., 125:442, 1976.
20. Polivy, J.: Psychological reactions to hysterectomy. Am. J. Obstet. Gynecol., 118:3, 1974.
21. Pratt, J. H., and Souders, J. C.: A review of ventral hernia in gynecologic patients. Minn. Med., 45:714, 1962.
22. Randall, C. L., Hall, D. W., and Armenia, C. S.: Pathology in the preserved ovary after unilateral oophorectomy. Am. J. Obstet. Gynecol., 84:1233–1241, 1962.

23. Ranney, B.: The future function and fortune of ovarian tissue which is retained in vivo during hysterectomy. Am. J. Obstet. Gynecol., 128:6, 1977.
24. Reycraft, J. L.: Carcinoma of the ovary following hysterectomy. Am. J. Obstet. Gynecol., 69:543–544, 1955.
25. Richards, B. C.: Hysterectomy: From women to women. Am. J. Obstet. Gynecol., 131:446–452, 1978.
26. Smith, R. O., and Pratt, J. H.: Serious bleeding following vaginal or abdominal hysterectomy. Obstet. Gynecol., 26:592–595, 1965.
27. Smith, P., Roberts, M., and Slade, N.: Urinary symptoms following hysterectomy. Br. J. Urol., 42:3–9, 1970.

28. Tweedie, F. J., and Long, R. C.: Abdominal wound disruptions. Surg. Gynecol. Obstet., 99:41, 1954.
29. Turnbull, A. C.: Pulmonary embolism: Prophylactic use of anticoagulants. J. Obstet. Gynecol. Brit. Commonw., 71:482, 1964.
30. White, S. C., Wartel, L. J., and Wade, M. E.: Comparison of abdominal and vaginal hysterectomies: A review of 600 operations. Obstet. Gynecol., 37:530, 1971.
31. Young, D. D. and Wise, T. N.: Changing perspectives on elective hysterectomy. Primary Care, 3:765, 1976.

RADIOTHERAPY FOR CANCER OF THE UTERINE CORPUS

RADIOTHERAPY FOR CANCER OF THE UTERINE CORPUS BY W. MACKEY, M.D.

Comments

A. Radiation may be external (to the pelvis) (4500 to 5000 rads) or intracavitary (per vagina) (5000 mg.-hours to the uterine cavity, 4500 to 7000 rads to the vagina).[3-4]

B. Acute symptoms may start 1 to 2 weeks after the onset of therapy and subside by the twelfth week after completion of therapy. Nausea, vomiting, diarrhea, and dysuria may be controlled with antiemetics, antispasmodics, and a low residue diet.[7]

C. Tumor control and complications are closely related to dose, time, tumor volume and histology, and radiobiology.[1, 2]

D. Transient leukopenia may occur because of pelvic marrow depression. Thrombocytopenia usually is not seen. The long-bone marrow compensates.[9]

E. Complications develop after 12 weeks; most develop within 3 to 24 months after therapy.[7]

F. Previous surgery, infections, poor anatomy, and technical errors increase the risk of bowel injuries.[6]

G. Sigmoiditis may be mild, moderate, or severe. Approximately one third of cases require colostomy.[7]

H. Most bladder ulcers occur in the region of the trigone.[7, 12]

I. The majority of all fistulas (80 per cent) are caused by recurrent tumor, not by irradiation.[10]

J. Secondary malignant tumors of the bladder, bowel, bone, and other areas have been reported sporadically following pelvic irradiation, although the exact incidence is unknown and there are no studies with control populations who were treated surgically.[11]

References

1. Dritschilo, A., et al.: The complication probability factor: A method for selection of radiation treatment plans. Br. J. Radiol., 51:370–374, 1978.
2. Graham, J. B., Sotto, L. S., and Paloucek, F. P.: Carcinoma of the Cervix. Philadelphia, W. B. Saunders Co., 1962.
3. Rutledge, F., Boronow, R. C., and Wharton, J. T.: Gynecologic Oncology. New York, John Wiley & Sons, 1976.
4. Fletcher, G. H.: Textbook of Radiotherapy, 2nd Ed. Philadelphia, Lea & Febiger, 1973.
5. Fifth Annual Clinical Conference on Cancer, 1960: Carcinoma of the Uterine Cervix, Endometrium, and Ovary. Chicago, Year Book Medical Publishers, 1962.
6. Wharton, J. T., and Fletcher, G. H.: The principle of radiation therapy for malignant pelvic lesions. Surg. Clin. North Am., 58:181–199, 1978.
7. Chau, P. M., et al.: Complications in high dose whole pelvis irradiation in female pelvic cancer. Am. J. Roentgenol., 87:22, 1962.
8. Strockbine, M. F., Hancock, J. E., and Fletcher, G. H.: Complications in 831 patients with squamous cell carcinoma of the intact uterine cervix treated with 3000 rads or more whole pelvis irradiation. Amer. J. Roentgenol., 108:293, 1970.
9. Kjellgren, O., and Jonsson, L.: Bone marrow depression in the pelvis after megavoltage irradiation for ovarian cancer. A study with radioisotope scanning. Am. J. Obstet. Gynecol., 105:849, 1969.
10. Dean, R. J., and Lytton, B.: Urologic complications of pelvic irradiation. J. Urol., 119:64, 1978.
11. Seydel, H. G.: The risk of tumor induction in man following medical irradiation for malignant neoplasm. Cancer, 35:1641–1645, 1975.

RADIOTHERAPY FOR CANCER OF THE UTERINE CORPUS

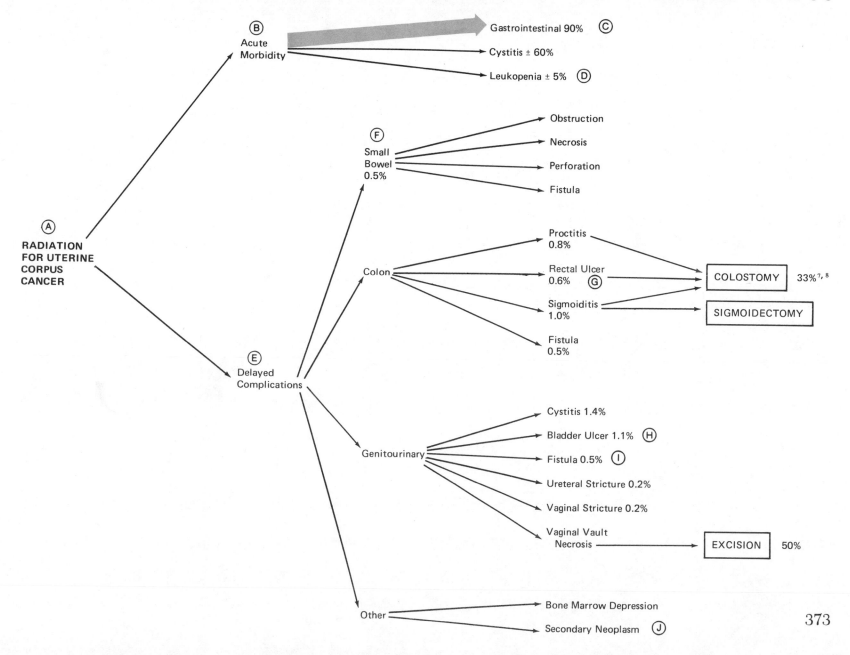

373

Section **H**

Pediatric

ESOPHAGEAL ATRESIA/TRACHEOESOPHAGEAL FISTULA BY JAMES ANDERSON, M.D.

Comments

A. There are associated congenital anomalies in 48 per cent of cases.[1] These include heart disease (19 per cent), gastrointestinal anomalies (13 per cent), genitourinary anomalies (10 per cent), imperforate anus (9 per cent), musculoskeletal anomalies (9 per cent), central nervous system anomalies (6 per cent), anomalies of the face (5 per cent), and others (9 per cent).

B. Classification is according to Gross.[2] Type differentiation requires only an x-ray localizing the nasogastric tube and confirming the presence or absence of intestinal air. Type E (TEF without EA) may require diagnostic bronchoscopy and contrast x-ray studies.

C. Delayed Primary Repair =

PROXIMAL POUCH SUCTION AND GASTROSTOMY PLUS DAILY OR TWICE DAILY DOWNWARD STRETCHING OF PROXIMAL POUCH	→	DELAYED PRIMARY REPAIR 4–10 Weeks

Delayed primary repair increasingly is used for simple atresias.[3-5] Circumferential myotomy of the proximal pouch may help relieve tension on the anastomosis.[5] Anastomotic leaks and strictures continue to be a major problem.

D. Staged repairs using colon[6] or gastric tubes[7] for esophageal replacement continue to be favored by most pediatric surgeons. All agree that this approach should be used for high-risk infants.

Staged Repair =

CERVICAL ESOPHAGOSTOMY and GASTROSTOMY	→	ESOPHAGEAL REPLACEMENT 1 Year

E. Direct drainage of secretions into the trachea in types B and D makes primary repair with division of the fistula necessary.

F. Risk factors (weight, prematurity, pulmonary status, and others) may dictate the type of repair chosen.[8, 9] Primary repair is for good-risk infants weighing more than two kg.; staged repair is for very poor-risk infants, and delayed primary repair is a compromise procedure. Fistula division requires thoracotomy;[10] diversion using gastric division laparotomy does not.[11]

G. Waterston[16] recognized that mortality is related to risk factors.[1, 9, 14-16]

In Group A (weight more than 2500 gm., no major anomalies, minimal pulmonary complications), mortality is 0 to 5 per cent.

In Group B (weight between 1800 and 2500 gm., no major anomalies), mortality is 4 to 11 per cent.

In Group C (weight less than 1800 gm. or associated major anomalies), mortality is 53 to 57 per cent.

H. Complications related to type of repair are shown in the table below.[1, 12, 13, 20, 22] Leaks tend to close spontaneously with drainage but strictures present long-term problems. Accordingly, division of the fistula plus single-layer end-to-end anastomosis is generally preferred.

I. Seventy-five per cent of strictures will respond to dilatation only, and 25 per cent will require resection.[1]

J. Recurrent bronchitis is defined as 3 episodes of respiratory disease per year. Incidence is 78 per cent in patients younger than 3 years of age and 48 per cent after age 8. Gradually the frequency of bronchitis diminishes.[17]

K. Thirty-three per cent of gastroesophageal reflux cases respond to positional therapy and 67 per cent require fundoplication.[19]

TYPE OF REPAIR	LEAK	STRICTURE	RECURRENT FISTULA
Division of fistula plus			
Haight end-to-end anastomosis	10.5%	27%	
One-layer end-to-end	21.4%	18%	6%
Two-layer end-to-end	14.6%	25%	
Ligation of fistula plus			
end-to-side anastomosis	~25%	~10%	16%

ESOPHAGEAL ATRESIA/TRACHEOESOPHAGEAL FISTULA

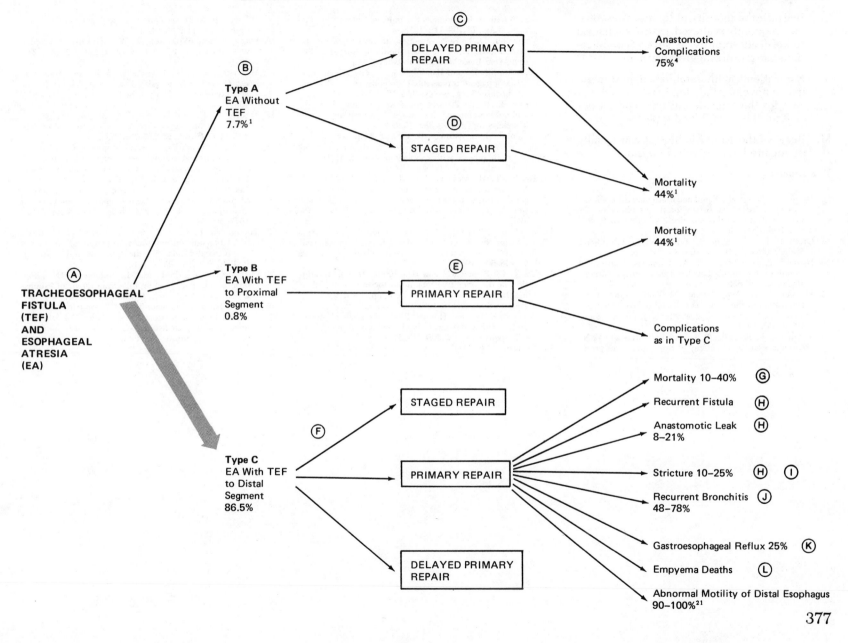

Ⓐ

TRACHEOESOPHAGEAL FISTULA (TEF) AND ESOPHAGEAL ATRESIA (EA)

Ⓑ

Type A
EA Without TEF
7.7%[1]

Ⓒ
DELAYED PRIMARY REPAIR

Anastomotic Complications 75%[4]

Ⓓ
STAGED REPAIR

Mortality 44%[1]

Type B
EA With TEF to Proximal Segment
0.8%

Ⓔ
PRIMARY REPAIR

Mortality 44%[1]

Complications as in Type C

Type C
EA With TEF to Distal Segment
86.5%

Ⓕ
STAGED REPAIR

PRIMARY REPAIR

DELAYED PRIMARY REPAIR

Mortality 10–40% Ⓖ

Recurrent Fistula Ⓗ

Anastomotic Leak 8–21% Ⓗ

Stricture 10–25% Ⓗ Ⓘ

Recurrent Bronchitis Ⓙ 48–78%

Gastroesophageal Reflux 25% Ⓚ

Empyema Deaths Ⓛ

Abnormal Motility of Distal Esophagus 90–100%[21]

377

ESOPHAGEAL ATRESIA/TRACHEOESOPHAGEAL FISTULA *Continued*

Because the motility of the distal esophagus frequently is altered, gastroesophageal reflux leads rapidly to severe complications and requires aggressive therapy.[18-20, 22]

L. For patients with established postoperative empyema, the death rate is 34 per cent for the transpleural type and 24 per cent for the extrapleural type.[1]

M. Because the fistula is high it can usually be repaired via a cervical incision.

References

1. Holder, T. M., et al.: Esophageal atresia and tracheoesophageal fistula: A survey of its members by the surgical section of the American Academy of Pediatrics. Pediatrics, *34*:542–549, 1964.
2. Gross, R. E.: The Surgery of Infancy and Childhood. Philadelphia, W. B. Saunders Co., 1953.
3. Howard, R., and Myers, N. A.: Esophageal atresia: A technique for elongating the upper pouch. Surgery, *58*:725–727, 1965.
4. Mahour, G. H., Woolley, M. M., and Gwinn, J. L.: Elongation of the upper pouch and delayed anatomic reconstruction in esophageal atresia. J. Pediatr. Surg., *9*:373–383, 1974.
5. Eraklis, A. J., Rossello, P. J., and Ballantine, T. V. N.: Circular esophagomyotomy of upper pouch in primary repair of long-segment esophageal atresia. J. Pediatr. Surg., *11*:709–712, 1976.
6. Waterston, D. J.: Reconstruction of the esophagus. *In* Mustard, W. T., et al. (eds.): Pediatric Surgery. Chicago, Year Book Medical Publishers, 1969.
7. Anderson, K. D., and Randolph, J. G.: The gastric tube for esophageal replacement in children. J. Thorac. Cardiovasc. Surg., *66*:333–342, 1973.
8. Tyson, K. R. T.: Primary repair of esophageal atresia without staging or preliminary gastrostomy. Ann. Thorac. Surg., *21*:378–381, 1976.
9. Randolph, J. G., Altman, R. P., and Anderson, K. D.: Selective surgical management based upon clinical status in infants with esophageal atresia. J. Thorac. Cardiovasc. Surg., *74*:335–342, 1977.
10. Holder, T. M., McDonald, V. G., Jr., and Woolley, M. M.: The premature or critically ill infant with esophageal atresia: Increased success with a staged approach. J. Thorac. Cardiovasc. Surg., *44*:344–358, 1962.
11. Randolph, J. G., Lilly, J. R., and Tunell, W. P.: Gastric division in the critically ill infant with esophageal atresia and tracheoesophageal fistula. Surgery, *63*:496–502, 1968.
12. Ty, T. C., Brunet, C., and Beardmore, H. E.: A variation in the operative technique for the treatment of esophageal atresia with tracheoesophageal fistula. J. Pediatr. Surg., *2*:118–126, 1967.
13. Ashcraft, K. W., and Holder, T. M.: Esophageal atresia and tracheoesophageal fistula malformations. Surg. Clin. North Am., *56*:299–315, 1976.
14. German, J. C., Mahour, G. H., and Woolley, M. M.: Esophageal atresia and associated anomalies. J. Pediatr. Surg., *11*:299–306, 1976.
15. Cozzi, F., and Wilkinson, A. W.: Mortality in esophageal atresia. J. R. Coll. Surg. Edinb., *20*:236–241, 1975.
16. Waterston, D. J., Bonham-Carter, R. E., and Aberdeen, E.: Oesophageal atresia: Tracheoesophageal fistula. A study of survival in 218 infants. Lancet, *1*:819–822, 1962.
17. Dudley, N. E., and Phelan, P. D.: Respiratory complications in long-term survivors of esophageal atresia. Arch. Dis. Child., *51*:279–282, 1976.
18. Pieretti, R., Shandling, B., and Stephens, C. A.: Resistant esophageal stenosis associated with reflux after repair of esophageal atresia: A therapeutic approach. J. Pediatr. Surg., *9*:355–357, 1974.
19. Ashcraft, K. W., et al.: Early recognition and aggressive treatment of gastroesophageal reflux following repair of esophageal atresia. J. Pediatr. Surg., *12*:317–321, 1977.
20. Tonloukian, R. J., et al.: Repair of esophageal atresia by end-to-side anastomosis and ligation of the tracheoesophageal fistula: A critical review of 18 cases. J. Pediatr. Surg., *9*:305–310, 1974.
21. Orringer, M. B., Kirsh, M. M., and Sloan, H.: Long-term esophageal function following repair of esophageal atresia. Ann. Surg., *186*:436–443, 1977.
22. Ein, S. H., and Theman, T. E.: A comparison of the results of primary repair of esophageal atresia with tracheoesophageal fistula using end-to-side and end-to-end anastomosis. J. Pediatr. Surg., *8*:641–645, 1973.

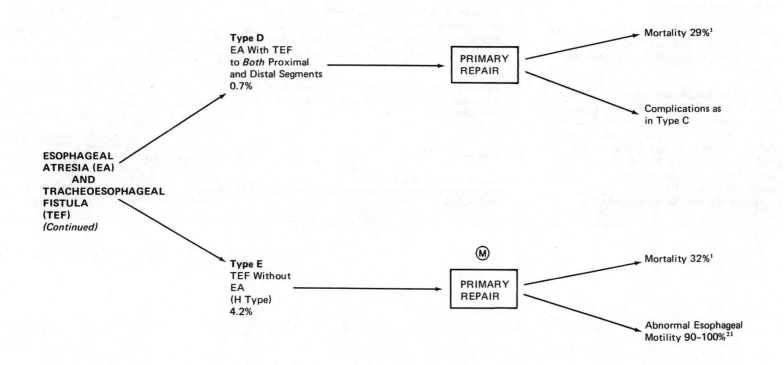

ESOPHAGEAL ATRESIA (EA) AND TRACHEOESOPHAGEAL FISTULA (TEF)
(Continued)

Type D
EA With TEF
to *Both* Proximal
and Distal Segments
0.7%

PRIMARY REPAIR

Mortality 29%[1]

Complications as in Type C

Type E
TEF Without EA
(H Type)
4.2%

Ⓜ

PRIMARY REPAIR

Mortality 32%[1]

Abnormal Esophageal Motility 90–100%[21]

UMBILICAL HERNIA BY GEORGE PETERS, M.D.

Comments

A. Umbilical hernia is common, occurring equally in both sexes and in one fourth of all black neonates.[1]

B. Seventy-five per cent of children whose birth weight is less than 1500 grams have an umbilical hernia.[1-3]

C. The diameter of the fascial defect but not the size of the protrusion at age 3 months establishes the prognosis for spontaneous closure.[4]

D. Indications for elective repair are controversial and variously include (1) persistence to age 6[4, 5] or to puberty,[7] (2) size (repair at age 2 to 4 years is advocated if the fascial defect is 1.5 cm. or larger[6]) and (3) persistence to adulthood. Some physicians advocate repair of all adult umbilical hernias.[11]

   Taping the hernia is valueless.[10]

Operation requires general anesthesia and hospitalization for 6 to 24 hours.

E. Results of emergency repair in children do not differ from those of elective repair.[5, 8, 9]

F. Ten per cent of congenital hernias will persist to adulthood.[11]

G. Increased intra-abdominal pressure may result from pregnancy, lifting, sports activities, coughing, or ascites, which allegedly precipitate the development of the hernia.[11]

H. Recurrences are infrequent, but no data are available to support this clinical observation.

References

1. Crump, E. P.: Umbilical Hernia: Occurrence of the infantile type in Negro infants and children. J. Pediatr., 40:214, 1952.
2. Woods, G. E.: Some observations on umbilical hernia in infants. Arch. Dis. Child., 8:450, 1953.
3. Vohr, B. R., Rosenfield, A. G., and Oh, W.: Umbilical hernia in the low birth weight infant (less than 1500 gm.). J. Pediatr., 90:807, 1977.
4. Walker, S. H.: The natural history of umbilical hernia. Clin. Pediatr., 6:29, 1967.
5. Lassaletta, L., et al.: Management of umbilical hernias in infancy and childhood. J. Pediatr. Surg., 10:405, 1975.
6. Morgan, W. W., et al.: Prophylactic umbilical hernia repair in childhood to prevent adult incarceration. Surg. Clin. North Am., 50:839, 1970.
7. Gellis, S. S. (ed.): Editorial comment. In Year Book of Pediatrics. Chicago, Year Book Medical Publishers, 1978, p. 396.
8. Gross, R. E.: Surgery of Infancy and Childhood. Philadelphia, W. B. Saunders Co., 1953, p. 423.
9. Benson, C. D.: In Mustard, W. T., et al. (eds.): Pediatric Surgery, 2nd ed. Chicago, Year Book Medical Publishers, 1969, p. 689.
10. Halpern, L. J.: Spontaneous healing of umbilical hernias. JAMA, 182:851, 1962.
11. Jackson, O. J., and Moglen, L. H.: Umbilical hernia: A retrospective study. Calif. Med., 113:8, 1970.
12. Baron, H. C.: Umbilical hernia secondary to cirrhosis of the liver: Complications of surgical correction. N. Engl. J. Med., 263:824, 1960.
13. Musca, A. A.: Umbilical and ventral herniorrhaphy: A review of 1000 cases. Int. Surg., 48:169, 1967.

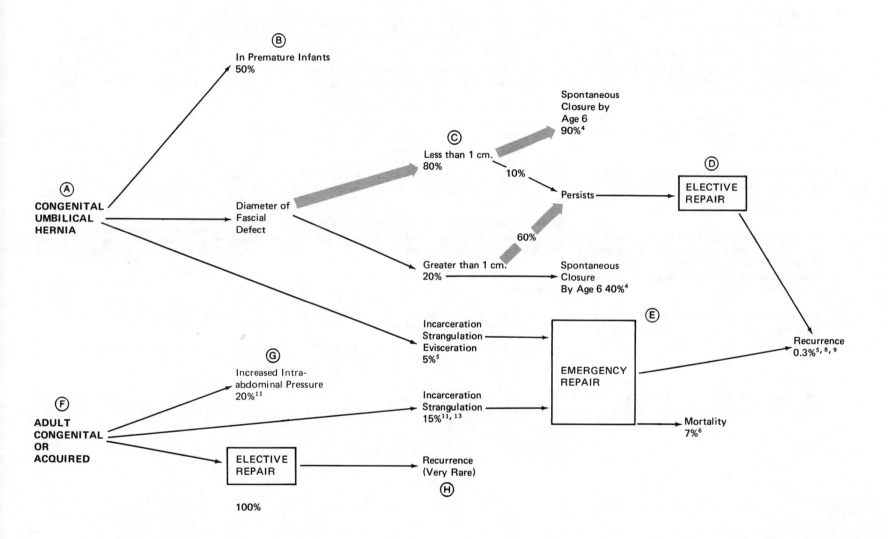

Ⓑ In Premature Infants
50%

Spontaneous
Closure by
Age 6
90%[4]

Ⓒ Less than 1 cm.
80%

10%

Ⓐ
CONGENITAL
UMBILICAL
HERNIA

Diameter of
Fascial
Defect

Persists

Ⓓ
ELECTIVE
REPAIR

60%

Greater than 1 cm.
20%

Spontaneous
Closure
By Age 6 40%[4]

Ⓔ

Incarceration
Strangulation
Evisceration
5%[5]

Ⓖ Increased Intra-
abdominal Pressure
20%[11]

EMERGENCY
REPAIR

Recurrence
0.3%[5, 8, 9]

Ⓕ
ADULT
CONGENITAL
OR
ACQUIRED

Incarceration
Strangulation
15%[11, 13]

Mortality
7%[6]

ELECTIVE
REPAIR

Recurrence
(Very Rare)

Ⓗ

100%

OMPHALOCELE AND GASTROSCHISIS BY GEORGE PETERS, M.D.

Comments

A. Although different embryologic aberrations, these conditions have similar management problems. In omphalocele the viscera lie in a friable sac derived from the amnion. In gastroschisis foreshortened, thickened cyanotic bowel extrudes through a cleft to the right of the normal umbilicus. There is no sac. The incidence of omphalocele is one per 2600 live births.[2] The ratio of omphalocele to gastroschisis is 10:1.[3]

B. Gastrointestinal defects are the most common, and cardiac anomalies occur in 8 per cent of cases.[10] Associated defects are less common in gastroschisis.

C. Primary repair of gastroschisis is indicated if abdominal wall closure will not produce respiratory insufficiency, vena cava obstruction, or pressure necrosis of the bowel.[11, 12]

D. In at least 50 per cent of cases there is prolonged ileus, requiring parenteral nutrition. There may also be sepsis and fistula.[12]

E. A nonreactive plastic bag is sutured to the edges of the fascial defect while the patient is anesthetized.[13] The viscera are gradually squeezed into the abdominal cavity over a 7 to 10 day period.[1]

F. The mobilized skin is pulled over the defect. The resulting ventral hernia repair is a formidable task.

G. Applicable only with an intact sac, this utilization of 2 per cent Mercurochrome, 70 per cent alcohol and other agents results in an eschar that contracts and pushes the intestine back into the abdominal cavity.[5] It is now used only occasionally for a very poor risk neonate. The viscera cannot be inspected for accompanying atresia; hospitalization is 8 to 14 weeks, and the resulting herniorrhaphy is difficult.[5, 15-17]

H. Small ventral hernias that are easy to repair occur in 85 per cent of cases.[8] Large defects are difficult to repair.[18-20]

References

1. Allen, R. G., and Wrenn, E. L.: Silon as a sac in the treatment of omphalocele and gastroschisis. J. Pediatr. Surg., 4:3, 1969.
2. Ravitch, M. M., and Barton, B. A.: The need for pediatric surgeons as determined by the volume of work and the mode of delivery of surgical care. Surgery, 76:754, 1974.
3. Savage, J. P., and Davey, R. B.: The treatment of gastroschisis. J. Pediatr. Surg., 6:148, 1971.
4. Wesselhoeft, C. W., and Randolph, J. G.: Treatment of omphalocele based on individual characteristics of the defect. Pediatrics, 44:101, 1969.
5. Firor, H. V.: Omphalocele — An appraisal of therapeutic approaches. Surgery, 69:208, 1971.
6. Hollabaugh, R. S., and Boles, E. T.: The management of gastroschisis. J. Pediatr. Surg., 8:263, 1973.
7. Lewis, J. E., Jr., Kraeger, R. R., and Davis, R. K.: Gastroschisis: Ten-year review. Arch. Surg., 92:218, 1973.
8. Wayne, E. R., and Burrington, J. D.: Gastroschisis. Am. J. Dis. Child, 125:218, 1973.
9. Mollitt, D. L., et al.: A critical assessment of fluid requirements in gastroschisis. J. Pediatr. Surg., 13:217, 1978.
10. Rickham, P. P., and Johnston, J. H.: Exomphalos and gastroschisis. In Neonatal Surgery. New York, Appleton-Century-Crofts, 1969, p. 254.
11. Zwiren, G. T., and Andrews, H. G.: Progress in the management of gastroschisis. Am. Surg., 40:45, 1974.
12. Mahour, G. H., Weitzman, J. J., and Rosenkrantz, J. G.: Omphalocele and gastroschisis. Ann. Surg., 177:478, 1973.
13. Aaronson, I. A., and Eckstein, H. B.: The role of the Silastic prosthesis in the management of gastroschisis. Arch. Surg., 112:297, 1977.
14. Girvan, D. P., Webster, D. M., and Shandling, B.: The treatment of omphalocele and gastroschisis. Surg. Gynecol. Obstet. 139:222, 1974.
15. Mahour, G. H.: Omphalocele. Surg. Gynecol. Obstet., 143:821, 1976.
16. Soave, F.: Conservative treatment of giant omphalocele. Arch. Dis. Child., 38:130, 1963.
17. Kim, S. H.: Omphalocele. Surg. Clin. North Am., 56:361, 1976.
18. Ravitch, M. M.: The nonoperative treatment of surgical conditions in children. Pediatrics, 57:435, 1973.
19. Boles, E. T.: Staged repair of huge ventral hernias. J. Pediatr. Surg., 6:618, 1971.
20. Talbert, J. L., Rodgers, B. M., and Moazam, F.: Surgical management of massive ventral hernias in children. J. Pediatr. Surg., 12:63, 1977.

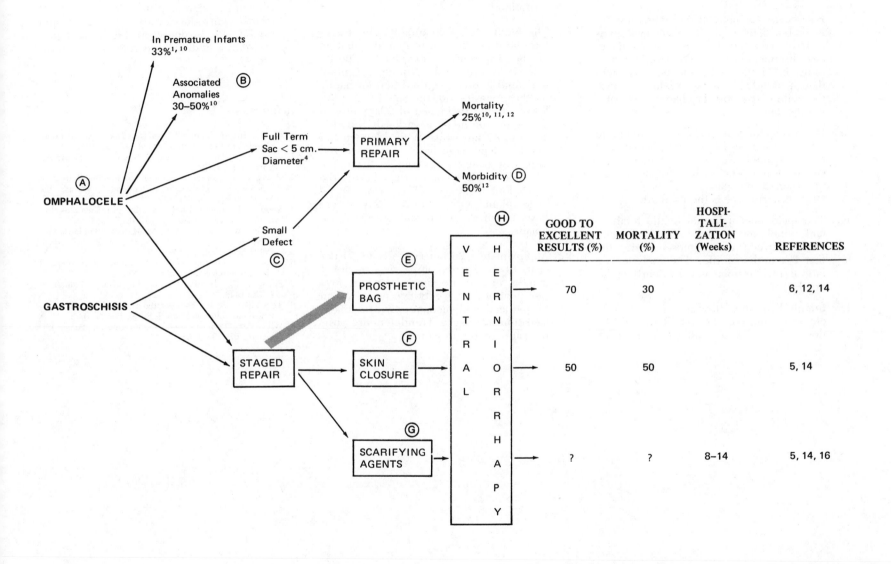

INFANT HERNIA AND HYDROCELE by Joyce A. Majure, M.D.

Comments

A. Hydrocele is common in premature infants, but data surprisingly are lacking as to frequency and likelihood of spontaneous disappearance. Groin exploration is indicated if the hydrocele persists more than 4 months, is tense, seems to cause the child discomfort, or changes size during the day.[1]

B. Hydrocelectomy is performed through an infant hernia groin incision because of the high incidence (93 per cent) of associated hernia. The hydrocele sac is simply opened and partially excised if very large. A hernia sac is then sought.

C. The incidence of hernia in the total infant population is 0.8 to 4.4 per cent. Eighty per cent are diagnosed during the first 3 months of life. The male:female ratio is 14:1 in infancy, 5:1 in early childhood.

D. Simple ligation of the sac is usually sufficient for indirect hernia. This can be done on an outpatient basis in many cases or may require a 2 or 3 day hospitalization.[1]

E. The incidence of bilaterality, and therefore the indication for routine exploration of the apparently uninvolved opposite side, is controversial. Nine per cent of unilateral hernias required herniorrhaphy on the opposite side in one 10-year followup study.[5] Incidence of bilaterality in the premature infant is variously reported as 19 to 47 per cent.[5] With a known left hernia, 74 per cent have an unsuspected hernia or patent processus on the opposite side. With a known right hernia the equivalent number is 55 per cent. In female infants with a hernia, 82 per cent have a contralateral patent processus vaginalis.

F. Approximately 26 per cent (21 to 50 per cent) of all hernias appearing before 4 months of age are incarcerated at *first* presentation.[1, 9] Seventy-five per cent can be reduced with nonoperative treatment (sedation, ice packs, Trendelenburg position, and gentle pressure).

G. Strangulation following nonoperative reduction is extremely rare (4 per cent). If the bowel reduces during anesthesia and viability is in doubt on the basis of preoperative findings, laparotomy is indicated.[5, 8]

References

1. Clatworthy, H.: Inguinal hernia, hydrocoele, and undescended testicle. Postgrad. Med., 22:122, 1957.
2. Coles, J. S.: Operative cure of inguinal hernia. Am. J. Surg., 69:366, 1945.
3. Davis, C. E.: Surgical treatment of inguinal hernia in infancy and childhood—Changing concepts. Va. Med. Monthly, 80:431, 1953.
4. Koop, C. E.: Inguinal herniorrhaphy in infants and children. Surg. Clin. North Am., 37:1675, 1957.
5. Mustard, W. T., and Ravitch, M. M. (eds.): Pediatric Surgery, 2nd ed. Vol. 1. Chicago, Year Book Medical Publishers, 1969, pp. 692–707.
6. Potts, W. J.: Treatment of inguinal hernia in infants and children. Ann. Surg., 132:566, 1950.
7. Potts, W. J.: Inguinal hernia in infancy. Pediatrics, 1:772, 1948.
8. Thorndike, A., Jr.: Incarcerated inguinal hernia in infancy and childhood. Am. J. Surg., 39:429, 1938.
9. Wiklander, O.: Incarcerated inguinal hernia. Acta Chir. Scand., 101:303, 1951.

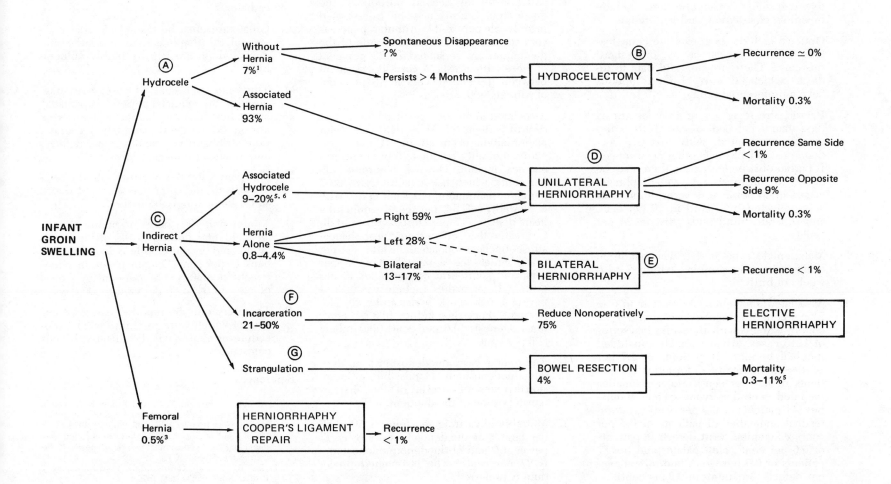

NEONATAL PYLORIC AND DUODENAL OBSTRUCTION BY WM. CARL BAILEY, M.D.

Comments

A. There being only 67 reported cases, little hard data exist on which to base objective decisions.[1,2] Complications include bleeding, obstruction, and perforation.

B. Options include cyst excision, enucleation, Billroth I gastrectomy, or cystgastrostomy.[3] There are no valid data to indicate which, if any, of these options have a preferential prognosis.

C. Pyloric atresia is a rare form of atresia (less than 1 per cent of cases).[4] It is frequently associated with maternal hydramnios and has a familial occurrence.[5] If partial obstruction exists, there may be delay in diagnosis. A web-diaphragm occurs in 66 per cent of cases, blind ends are connected by a cord in 10 per cent, and separate blind ends exist in 24 per cent.[6]

D. Male:female ratio is 4:1. The condition characteristically presents within 2 to 6 weeks of birth.

E. Associated anomalies[10,13,14] occur in 6 to 21 per cent of cases. Schärli[13] found 6 per cent of patients with anomalies in a series of 1215 cases. Minor anomalies included inguinal hernias (21 patients or 1.7 per cent) and extremity deformities (11 patients or 0.9 per cent). Major anomalies included central nervous system anomalies (11 patients or 0.9 per cent), gastrointestinal anomalies (9 patients or 0.7 per cent), congenital heart defects (8 patients or 0.6 per cent), cleft palates and lips (7 patients or 0.5 per cent), and miscellaneous defects (3 patients or 0.2 per cent).

F. Nonoperative treatment is largely of historic interest only.

G. In 79 per cent of patients the site of obstruction is the second portion of the duodenum. Emesis may be bile-stained in only 55 per cent.[18] Annular pancreas coexists in 21 per cent. The ends of the duodenum are separated in 23 per cent of those with atresia. A cord-like segment between the ends occurs in 18 per cent of patients with atresias.[15]

H. Associated anomalies occurred in 48 per cent of patients.[15-17] More than one major malformation occurred in 24 per cent, with a mortality rate of 43.5 per cent. Anomalies include Down's syndrome (30 per cent), which has a mortality of 28.7 per cent, malrotation (19.4 per cent), with a mortality of 34 per cent, congenital heart disease (17 per cent), with mortality greater than 50 per cent, esophageal atresia-tracheoesophageal fistula (7 per cent), which has a mortality of 70 per cent, and genitourinary anomalies (5 per cent). GU anomalies include cystic kidney (1.4 per cent), hydronephrosis (1.0 per cent), horseshoe kidney (0.6 per cent) renal agenesis (0.6 per cent), and others (1.6 per cent).

I. End-to-end gastroduodenostomy or duodenoduodenostomy is possible in occasional cases of atresia of the first or fourth portion of the duodenum.[15]

J. Mortality of gastrojejunostomy is 50 to 66 per cent,[19] of duodenojejunostomy is 47 per cent,[16] and of duodenoduodenostomy is 22 per cent.[16] The last-named procedure is preferred.

K. Synonyms include duodenal diaphragm, "wind-sock," or intraluminal diverticulum. Diagnosis may be difficult, requiring intraduodenal probing with a balloon catheter.[20]

L. Great care must be taken in partial excision of the diaphragm to spare the bile ducts, which are usually highly vulnerable.[16]

M. Thirty-one per cent of cases are diagnosed in the neonatal period.[21] Associated anomalies include duodenal stenosis or atresia (80 per cent), malrotation, coarctation, atrial and ventricular septal defects, and tracheoesophageal atresia.[21,22]

N. The pancreatic tissue grows into the duodenal wall and often has aberrant ducts, so it cannot simply be incised.[21,22]

O. Nonrotation (90° only) or malrotation is an incidental finding in 0.2 of the population, and cecum mobile is found in perhaps 15 per cent. Diagnosis rate in symptomatic neonates is 55 per cent by 7 days of age and 64 to 80 per cent by 30 days.

P. There are only 56 reported cases, 70 per cent of which were in children. The procedure of choice will be dictated by circumstances.

References

1. Alschibaja, T., Putnam, T. C., and Yablin, B. A.: Duplication of the stomach simulating hypertrophic pyloric stenosis. Am. J. Dis. Child., 127:120–122, 1974.
2. Anas, P., and Miller, R. C.: Pyloric duplication masquerading as hypertrophic pyloric stenosis. J. Pediatr. Surg., 6:664, 1971.
3. Parker, B. C., et al.: Gastric duplications in infancy. J. Pediatr. Surg., 7:294–298, 1972.

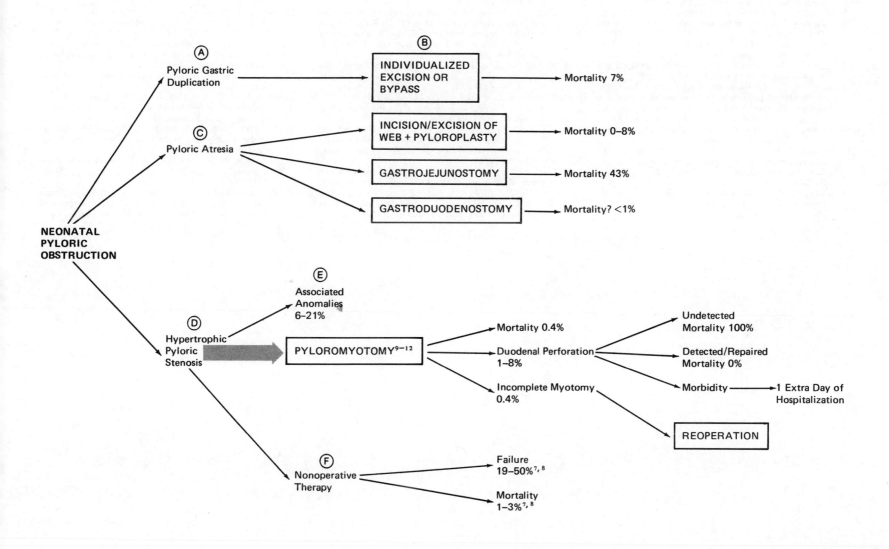

4. Bronsther, B., Nadeau, M. R., and Abrams, M. W.: Congenital pyloric atresia: A report of 3 cases and a review of the literature. Surgery, 69:130–136, 1971.
5. Olsen, L., and Grotte, G.: Congenital pyloric atresia: Report of a familial occurrence. J. Pediatr. Surg., 11:181–184, 1976.
6. Saw, E. C., Arbegast, N. R., and Comer, T. P.: Pyloric atresia: A case report. Pediatrics, 51:574–577, 1973.
7. Jacoby, N. M.: Pyloric stenosis: Selective medical and surgical treatment. Lancet, 1:119–121, 1962.
8. Berglund, G., and Rabo, E.: A long-term followup investigation of patients with hypertrophic pyloric stenosis, with special reference to heredity and later morbidity. Acta Paediatr. Scand., 62:130–132, 1973.
9. Benson, C. D., and Lloyd, J. R.: Infantile pyloric stenosis. Am. J. Surg., 107:429–433, 1964.
10. Pollock, W. F., Norris, W. J., and Gordon, H. E.: The management of hypertrophic pyloric stenosis at the Los Angeles Childrens Hospital. Am. J. Surg., 94:335–349, 1957.
11. Gibbs, M. K., Van Heerden, J. A., and Lynn, H. B.: Congenital hypertrophic pyloric stenosis. Mayo Clin. Proc., 50:312–316, 1975.

12. Bell, M. J.: Infantile pyloric stenosis: Experience with 305 cases at Louisville Children's Hospital. Surgery, 64:983–989, 1968.
13. Schärli, A., Siever, W. K., and Kiesewetter, W. B.: Hypertrophic pyloric stenosis at the Children's Hospital of Pittsburgh from 1912 to 1967: A critical review of current problems and complications. J. Pediatr. Surg., 4:108–114, 1969.
14. Ahmed, S.: Infantile pyloric stenosis associated with major anomalies of the alimentary tract. J. Pediatr. Surg., 5:660–666, 1970.
15. Fonkalsrud, E. W., deLorimier, A. A., and Hays, D. M.: Congenital atresia and stenosis of the duodenum. Pediatrics, 43:79–83, 1969.
16. Girvan, D. P., and Stephens, C. A.: Congenital intrinsic duodenal obstruction: A 20-year review of its surgical management and consequences. J. Pediatr. Surg., 9:833–839, 1974.
17. Wesley, J. R., and Mahour, G. H.: Congenital intrinsic duodenal obstruction: A 25-year review. Surgery, 82:716–719, 1977.
18. Reid, I. S.: The pattern of intrinsic duodenal obstructions. Aust. N. Z. J. Surg., 42:349–352, 1973.

19. Stauffer, U. G., and Irving, I.: Duodenal atresia and stenosis — long-term results. Prog. Pediatr. Surg., 10:49–61, 1977.
20. Rowe, M. I., Buckner, D., and Clatworthy, H., Jr.: Wind-sock web of the duodenum. Am. J. Surg., 116:444–449, 1968.
21. Merill, J. R., and Raffensperger, J. G.: Pediatric annular pancreas: 20 years' experience. J. Pediatr. Surg., 11:921–925, 1976.
22. Jackson, J. M.: Annular pancreas and duodenal obstruction in the neonate. Arch. Surg., 87:379–383, 1963.
23. Stewart, D. R., Colodny, A. L., and Daggett, W. C.: Malrotation of the bowel in infants and children: A 15-year review. Surgery, 79:716–720, 1976.
24. Brennom, W. S., and Bill, A. H.: Prophylactic fixation of the intestine for midgut nonrotation. Surg. Gynecol. Obstet. 138:181–184, 1974.
25. Imamoglu, K. H., and Walt, A. J.: Duplication of the duodenum extending into liver. Am. J. Surg., 133:628–632, 1977.
26. Parnes, I. H.: Duodenal duplication: Surgical treatment using a unique method of locating the ampulla of Vater. Am. J. Gastroenterol., 60:406–407, 1973.

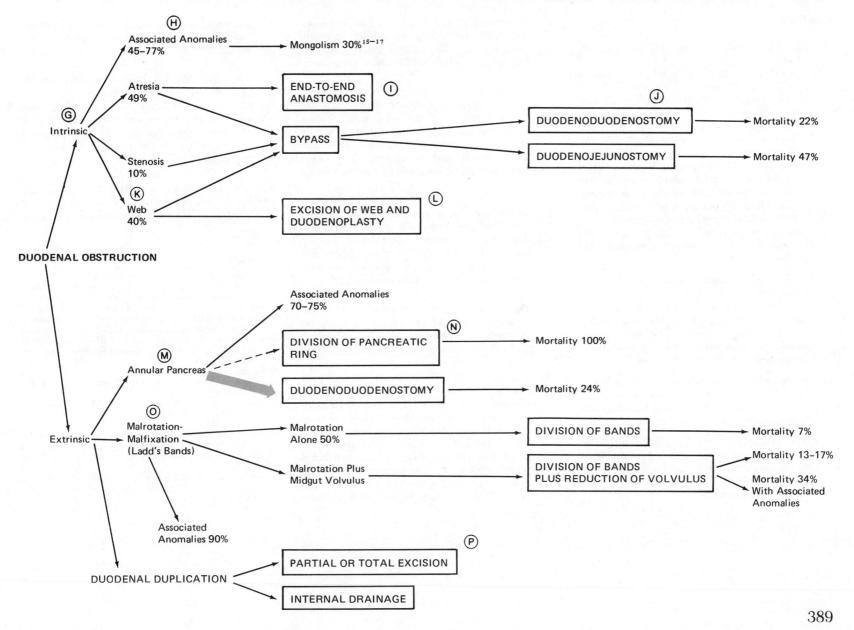

IMPERFORATE ANUS BY JACK H. T. CHANG, M.D.

Comments

A. Classification according to Ladd is as follows:

Anal stenosis: Normal rectal development with stenotic anus.

Anal membrane: Thin membrane at normal site.

Anal agenesis: Blind segment of distal bowel terminates more than 1.5 cm. (high) or less than 1.5 cm. (low) from the skin. Approximately 50 per cent of males have a fistula connecting the rectum to the urethra, bladder, or perineum. Over 80 per cent of females have fistulas to the perineum or vagina.

Anal atresia: Blind segment of rectum ends 2 to 6 cm. above a normal anal pouch.

B. Associated anomalies include those of the genitourinary tract (30 per cent of cases), vertebral column (25 per cent), and alimentary tract (10 per cent) and cardiac defects (10 per cent). The majority of deaths are accounted for by associated anomalies.

C. Blind rectal pouches less than 1.5 cm. from the skin or those with perineal fistulas can usually be treated by anoplasty anastomosing skin to anal mucosa.

D. The colostomy may be placed either in the transverse or descending colon, leaving enough length to perform the definitive procedure without having to take down the colostomy.

E. Colostomy in infants has a much higher morbidity rate than in adults. Usually prolapse may be treated conservatively, but occasionally it will require revision.[1]

F. Owing to the anterior location of the anus, several procedures have been devised to transpose the anal opening to a more normal posterior location. Usually by the teen years the perineal body will have grown and separated the vagina from the anus, producing an acceptable result.

G. There are many procedures for pulling the blind pouch through to the perineum. The key to success, however, is having the blind pouch traverse the puborectalis sling. Without the puborectalis muscle, true continence is unobtainable.

H. Dilatation is crucial for success. Most recurrent stenosis or stricture may be avoided by diligent periodic dilatation and followup for at least one year.

I. Continence is difficult to assess and may not be achieved until the teens. Many children who have had a pull-through procedure may be anatomically normal but will not develop continence until they develop a social awareness and need. On the other hand, some children who have no palpable puborectalis mechanism will lead a normal social life because of developing habits (such as daily morning enemas and avoidance of certain foods) which prevent inopportune soilage.[3-6]

J. The pull-through operation may be repeated with success if during the initial operation the puborectalis sling was missed. There now are successful reports of free transposition of the palmaris longus and sartorius muscles in place of the puborectalis.[2, 3]

K. The experience with this type of atresia is limited. Therefore the continence and mortality data may be unreliable.

References

1. Brenner, R. W., and Swenson, O.: Colostomies in infants and children. Surg. Gynecol. Obstet., 124:1239, 1976.
2. Hakelius, L., et al.: A new treatment of anal incontinence in children: Free autogenous muscle transplantation. J. Pediatr. Surg., 12:77, 1978.
3. Kiesewetter, W. B., and Chang, J. H. T.: Imperforate anus: A 5 to 30 year followup perspective. Prog. Pediatr. Surg., 10:111, 1977.
4. Nixon, H. H., and Puri, P.: The results of treatment of anorectal anomalies: A 13 to 20 year followup. J. Pediatr. Surg., 12:27, 1977.
5. Sharli, A. F., and Kiesewetter, W. B.: Defecation and continence: Some new concepts. Dis. Colon Rectum, 13:81, 1970.
6. Smith, E. I., Tunell, W. P., and Williams, G. R.: A clinical evaluation of the surgical treatment of anorectal malformations (imperforate anus). Ann. Surg., 187:583, 1978.
7. Stephens, F. D., and Smith, E. D.: Anorectal Malformations in Children. Chicago, Year Book Medical Publishers, 1971.

IMPERFORATE ANUS

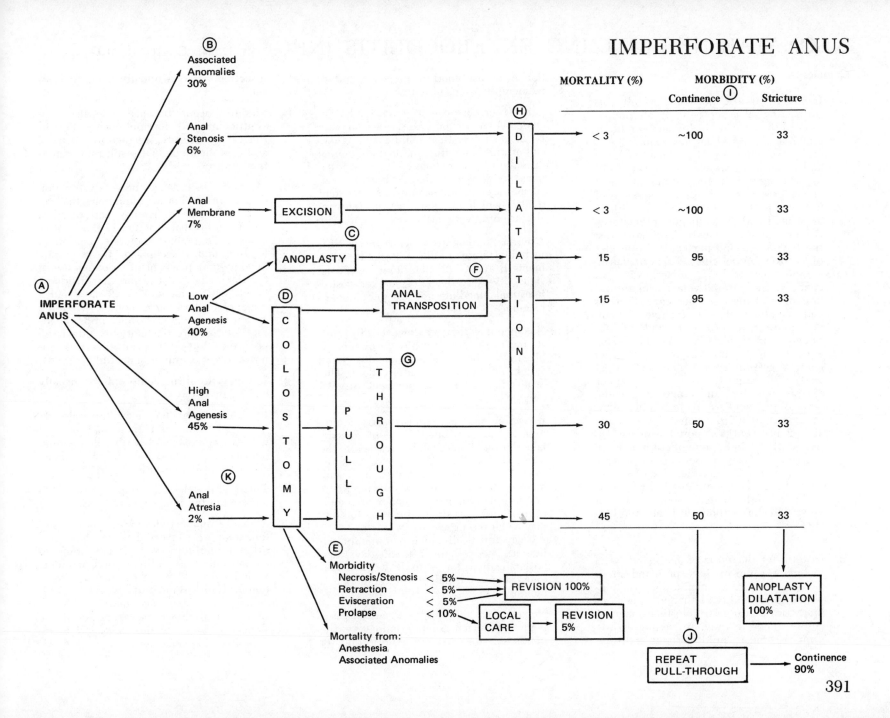

	MORTALITY (%)	MORBIDITY (%) Continence	Stricture
Anal Stenosis	< 3	~100	33
Anal Membrane	< 3	~100	33
Anoplasty	15	95	33
Anal Transposition	15	95	33
High Anal Agenesis	30	50	33
Anal Atresia	45	50	33

Ⓑ Associated Anomalies 30%
Anal Stenosis 6%
Anal Membrane 7%
EXCISION
Ⓒ ANOPLASTY
Ⓐ IMPERFORATE ANUS
Low Anal Agenesis 40%
Ⓓ COLOSTOMY
Ⓕ ANAL TRANSPOSITION
High Anal Agenesis 45%
Ⓖ PULL THROUGH
Ⓚ
Anal Atresia 2%
Ⓗ DILATATION
Ⓘ

Ⓔ Morbidity
Necrosis/Stenosis   < 5%
Retraction   < 5%
Evisceration   < 5%
Prolapse   < 10%
REVISION 100%
LOCAL CARE → REVISION 5%
Mortality from:
Anesthesia
Associated Anomalies

ANOPLASTY DILATATION 100%

Ⓙ REPEAT PULL-THROUGH → Continence 90%

391

NEONATAL NECROTIZING ENTEROCOLITIS (NEC) BY DAVID C. HITCH, M.D.

Comments

A. Incidence is 0.2 per cent of all live births[1] and 2.4 per cent of all premature births.[1, 2] The male:female ratio is equal (1.17:1).[2-5] Mean gestational age is 32 weeks (range of 24 to 40 weeks),[1, 3, 6] and mean birth weight is 1.64 kg. (0.78 to 4.11 kg.).[1-7] Average time of onset of symptoms is 5 days, with a range of 6 hours to 1 month.[1, 2, 4, 6-8] Conditions associated with NEC include prematurity (75 per cent of cases),[9] respiratory distress syndrome (58 per cent),[2-7] episodes of hypoxia (69 per cent),[1, 5, 6] perinatal infection (maternal or infant) (54 per cent),[1, 3, 5] and arterial-venous catheterization or exchange (46 per cent).[3-7] Signs and symptoms of NEC include abdominal distention (79 per cent of patients),[1, 3, 4, 8] emesis or an increasing amount of gastric aspirate (56 per cent),[3, 8] gastrointestinal bleeding (69 per cent),[1, 8] lethargy (79 per cent),[1, 8] apnea (54 per cent),[1, 4, 8] and progressive acidosis (18 per cent).[1, 2] Radiographic signs include ileus (67 per cent),[1, 3] pneumatosis (82 per cent),[1-4, 8] portal vein gas (19 per cent),[1-3, 8] and pneumoperitoneum (10 per cent).[1-3] Forty-six per cent of patients with portal vein gas die. Sixty-five per cent of all infants believed to have NEC will survive the acute episode and 47 per cent will be without ultimate morbidity.[1-4, 8]

B. Criteria for diagnosis of *suspected* NEC include (1) one or more perinatal stress factors, (2) systemic manifestations (temperature instability, lethargy, apnea, or bradycardia), (3) gastrointestinal manifestations (poor feeding, increasing gastric aspirate, emesis, mild abdominal disten-tion, or occult blood in the stool), and (4) radiographic signs of ileus.[3]

C. Criteria for diagnosis of *definite* NEC include (1) any of the criteria in Comment B, (2) gastrointestinal manifestations (occult or gross bleeding, marked abdominal distention, (3) radiographic manifestations (significant ileus, bowel wall edema, ascites, unchanging or persistent rigid bowel loops, pneumatosis intestinalis, or portal vein gas).[3]

D. Criteria for diagnosis of *advanced* NEC include (1) any of the criteria in Comments B and C, (2) deterioration of vital signs, (3) septic shock, (4) marked gastrointestinal bleeding, and (5) pneumoperitoneum.[3]

E. Nonoperative therapy consists of (1) restoring the circulating blood volume, (2) placing the bowel at rest, and (3) giving system antibiotics for enteric flora. This results in a 64 to 100 per cent survival rate.[1-4, 8]

F. Resection and anastomosis carry a prohibitive mortality rate.[11] The enterostomy is performed immediately proximal to the resected margin. The type of enterostomy used (end enterostomy with mucous fistula, Mikulicz, Bishop-Koop, or Santulli) is largely a matter of preference. Rarely, a single ileal perforation may be closed primarily.

Characteristically, total parenteral feedings are needed for 7 to 30 days, and hospitalization for 4 to 8 weeks. The enterostomy is usually closed after 1 to 3 months.

G. Nonoperative therapy for advanced cases is uniformly fatal. Simple drainage of the perforated area without enterostomy or resection has occasionally been successful.[12]

H. Mortality occurs because of sepsis, intraventricular and intrapulmonary hemorrhage, prematurity, respiratory distress, and complications that result from parenteral nutrition.[1-4, 8]

I. Morbidity includes (1) bowel dysfunction due to brush border alterations that result in lactose deficiency and diarrhea and (2) intestinal stricture (7 per cent of cases). Treatment includes parenteral feeding and resection of the stricture. Seventy-four per cent of strictures are of the large bowel and are of insidious onset, with a median of 22 days and a range of 10 days to 4½ months. When the stricture is resected without prior diverting enterostomy the mortality rate is 29 per cent, but with prior diverting enterostomy it is only 8 per cent.[1-4, 8, 10, 13-16]

J. Recovery from the acute episode usually takes 7 to 14 days.

K. In addition to the morbidity already noted in Comment I, there may be progressive necrosis and perforation, wound dehiscence, evisceration, and disseminated intravascular coagulopathy.[1-4, 8]

L. This highly selected group represents 33 per cent of the total cases of NEC.[1-4, 8]

M. All these infants, who have either an enterostomy or a resected bowel, have significant morbidity and all are prone to complications as outlined in Comments H and I. In addition there may be ileostomy dysfunction and bowel insufficiency. In order to maintain life, 15 cm. of the small bowel is necessary if the ileocecal valve remains, and if it is absent 40 cm. is necessary.[17]

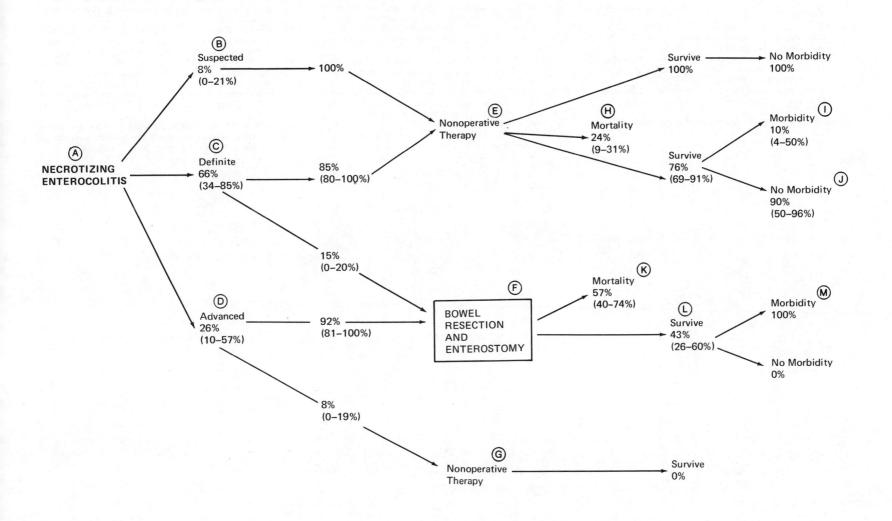

NEONATAL NECROTIZING ENTEROCOLITIS (NEC) *Continued*

References

1. Dudgeon, D. L., et al.: Surgical management of acute necrotizing enterocolitis in infancy. J. Pediatr. Surg., 8:607, 1973.
2. O'Neill, J. A., Jr., Stahlman, M. T., and Meng, H. C.: Necrotizing enterocolitis in the newborn: Operative indications. Ann. Surg., 182:274, 1975.
3. Bell, M. J., et al.: Neonatal necrotizing enterocolitis: Therapeutic decisions based upon clinical staging. Ann. Surg., 187:1, 1978.
4. Bell, M. J., et al.: Neonatal necrotizing enterocolitis: Prevention of perforation. J. Pediatr. Surg., 8:601, 1973.
5. Santulli, T. V., et al.: Acute necrotizing enterocolitis in infancy: A review of 64 cases. Pediatrics, 55:376, 1975.

6. Torma, M. J., DeLemos, R. A., and Rogers, J. R.: Necrotizing enterocolitis in infants. Analysis of 45 consecutive cases. Am. J. Surg., 126:758, 1973.
7. Hutter, J. J., Jr., Hathaway, W. E., and Wayne, E. R.: Hematologic abnormalities in severe neonatal necrotizing enterocolitis. J. Pediatr., 88:1026, 1976.
8. Kosloske, A. M.: Necrotizing enterocolitis in the neonate. Surg. Gynecol. Obstet., 148:259, 1979.
9. Touloukian, R. J.: Neonatal necrotizing enterocolitis: An update on etiology, diagnosis and treatment. Surg. Clin. North Am., 56:281, 1976.
10. Krasna, I. H., et al.: Colonic stenosis following enterocolitis of the newborn. J. Pediatr. Surg., 5:200, 1970.
11. Cummins, G. E.: Necrotizing enterocolitis. Med. J. Aust., 1:376, 1977.
12. Ein, S. H., Marshall, D. G., and Girvan, D.: Peritoneal drainage under local anesthesia for perforations from

necrotizing enterocolitis. J. Pediatr. Surg., 12:963, 1977.
13. Chiba, T., Watanabe, I., and Kasai, M.: Colonic atresia following necrotizing enterocolitis. J. Pediatr. Surg., 10:965, 1975.
14. Stein, H., Kavin, I., and Faerber, E. N.: Colonic strictures following nonoperative management of necrotizing enterocolitis. J. Pediatr. Surg., 10:943, 1975.
15. Bell, M. J., et al.: Intestinal stricture in necrotizing enterocolitis. J. Pediatr. Surg., 11:319, 1976.
16. Lloyd, D. A., and Cyrves, S.: Intestinal stenosis and enterocyst formation as late complications of neonatal necrotizing enterocolitis. J. Pediatr. Surg., 8:479, 1973.
17. Wilmore, D. W.: Factors correlating with a successful outcome following extensive intestinal resection in newborn infants. J. Pediatr. Surg., 80:88, 1972.

NEONATAL JAUNDICE

NEONATAL JAUNDICE BY JOHN LILLY, M.D.

Comments

A. This discussion excludes hemolytic, metabolic, and infectious causes of jaundice, which with recent diagnostic advances can usually be differentiated from cholestasis. The surgeon's concern is delineation of intrahepatic and extrahepatic causes of cholestasis. This usually requires operative cholangiography, which should not be postponed beyond 3 months of age.

B. Neonatal hepatitis and biliary atresia probably are different manifestations of the same disease. In hepatitis extrahepatic bile ducts are patent and therefore operation offers nothing; its prognosis is better than that for atresia.

C. Alpha$_1$-antitrypsin deficiency (AAT) is associated with intrahepatic cholestasis in 5 per cent of afflicted infants. Hepatocytes of such infants with $P_1{}^{zz}$ allele contain an amorphous material within the dilated lumen of the endoplasmic reticulum that is probably responsible. Special stains of needle biopsy specimens of such patients may make operative cholangiography unnecessary. Most such patients are asymptomatic; about 7 per cent die in infancy because of cholestatic disease and 10 to 15 per cent develop cirrhosis in childhood that requires portacaval shunts. Hepatic transplant in one patient returned AAT levels to normal.

D. Previously, patients with paucity of intrahepatic ducts were believed to have a form of biliary atresia. In fact, the extrahepatic biliary system, although diminutive (probably from disuse), is patent. Such children often live to adolescence and then die of complications of cirrhosis.

E. Preference between excision or internal drainage of the cyst remains controversial.[3]

	CYST EXCISION	CYST DRAINAGE	CHI SQUARE
Mortality	7%	10%	ns°
Morbidity	8%	50%	0.01
Reoperation	0%	30%	0.01

°ns = Not significant

F. Biliary hypoplasia is not a disease entity but a radiographic finding. If the diminutive ducts are due to disuse secondary to intrahepatic cholestasis (i.e., neonatal hepatitis, AAT deficiency, or paucity of the intrahepatic bile ducts), the prognosis is that of the primary disease. If the duc-

tal hypoplasia is a manifestation of a biliary structural abnormality (i.e., biliary atresia or choledochal cyst), ductal patency may improve, stabilize, or be lost. The ultimate prognosis in the latter cases depends on the severity of the basic disease.[1]

G. "Correctable" biliary atresia is a condition in which the proximal bile ducts are patent but the distal bile ducts are obliterated. Theoretically, 100 per cent cure should be obtained if the diagnosis is made early enough and if biliary obstruction is relieved. Unfortunately, whether because of delay in operation or coexistent intrahepatic biliary duct disease, only about 50 per cent of infants with this condition have a protracted survival. Death is usually due to progressive liver cirrhosis.[6]

H. Previously, the average survival for "noncorrectable" biliary atresia was 18 months and 92 per cent were dead after 3 years. Kasai's operation, in which a defunctionalized limb of jejunum is anastomosed to the transected bile ducts at the liver hilum, has revolutionized the treatment of this disease. Biliary obstruction is relieved in about two thirds of patients under 4 months of age who have the operation, and about half of these pa-

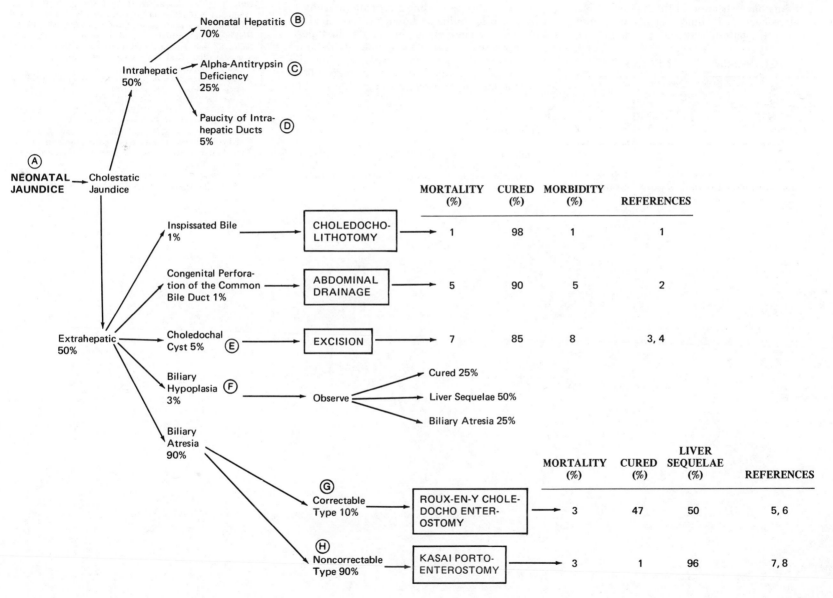

(A) **NEONATAL JAUNDICE** → Cholestatic Jaundice

Intrahepatic 50%
- → Neonatal Hepatitis (B) 70%
- → Alpha-Antitrypsin Deficiency (C) 25%
- → Paucity of Intra-hepatic Ducts (D) 5%

Extrahepatic 50%

	MORTALITY (%)	CURED (%)	MORBIDITY (%)	REFERENCES
Inspissated Bile 1% → CHOLEDOCHO-LITHOTOMY	1	98	1	1
Congenital Perforation of the Common Bile Duct 1% → ABDOMINAL DRAINAGE	5	90	5	2
Choledochal Cyst 5% (E) → EXCISION	7	85	8	3, 4

Biliary Hypoplasia (F) 3% → Observe
- → Cured 25%
- → Liver Sequelae 50%
- → Biliary Atresia 25%

Biliary Atresia 90%

	MORTALITY (%)	CURED (%)	LIVER SEQUELAE (%)	REFERENCES
(G) Correctable Type 10% → ROUX-EN-Y CHOLEDOCHO ENTEROSTOMY	3	47	50	5, 6
(H) Noncorrectable Type 90% → KASAI PORTO-ENTEROSTOMY	3	1	96	7, 8

tients have sustained bile drainage. Operative success is almost totally dependent upon the patient's age at operation.

AGE (Months)	SUCCESS (%)
< 2	90
2–3	40
3–4	10
> 4	0

The operative mortality has been zero in 43 patients who had Kasai's operation at my institution. Almost all patients achieving bile drainage, however, have had recurrent cholangitis during the first postoperative year. Moreover, with rare exceptions, survivors have varying degrees of permanent liver damage. Thus the long-term prognosis is guarded.[7]

References

1. Lilly, J. R., and Altman, R. P.: The surgery of the liver and bile ducts. *In* Ravitch, M. M., et al. (eds.): Pediatric Surgery, 3rd ed. Chicago, Year Book Medical Publishers, 1978.
2. Lilly, J. R., Weintraub, W. H., and Altman, R. P.: Spontaneous perforation of the extrahepatic bile ducts and bile peritonitis in infancy. Surgery, 75:664–673, 1974.
3. Flanigan, P. D.: Biliary cysts. Ann. Surg., *182*:635, 1975.
4. Saito, S., and Ishida, M.: Congenital choledochal cyst (cystic dilation of the common bile duct). Prog. Pediatr. Surg., 3:604, 1968.
5. Kasai, M.: Treatment of biliary atresia with special reference to hepatic portoenterostomy and its modifications. Prog. Pediatr. Surg., 6:5, 1974.
6. Izant, R. J., Jr., et al.: Biliary atresia survey. Surgery Section, Am. Acad. Pediatrics, 1965.
7. Kasai, M., Watanabe, I., and Ohi, R.: Followup studies of long-term survivors after hepatic portoenterostomy for "noncorrectable" biliary atresia. J. Pediatr. Surg., *10*:173, 1975.
8. Lilly, J. R., and Javitt, N. B.: Biliary lipid excretion after hepatic portoenterostomy. Ann. Surg., *184*:369, 1976.

HIRSCHSPRUNG'S DISEASE

HIRSCHSPRUNG'S DISEASE BY NINH N. TRAN, M.D.

Comments

A. Diagnosis may be facilitated by absence of meconium within the first 24 hours of life, which occurs in 90 per cent of cases of Hirschsprung's disease.[4,19] Barium enema is unreliable in the very young[4] and when very short or very long segments are involved.[19] Error rate in the first month is 23 per cent; in patients 1 to 12 months old it is 12.7 per cent; and after age one it is 6.5 per cent.[19]

B. Associated malformations include cardiac defects (3 per cent), esophageal atresia (± 1 per cent), urinary defects (megaloureter, reflux, and others) (5 per cent), genital defects (± 3 per cent), mongolism (2–5 per cent), and Laurence-Biedl-Moon disease. The overall incidence of malformations is 15 to 20 per cent.[4, 13, 19, 20] Sexual modified multifactorial inheritance is responsible for 3.5 per cent of cases; 2.6 per cent of index cases are male patients and 7.2 per cent are female patients.

C. Nonoperative management consists primarily of colonic irrigations for wash-out. Complications[15, 19] include perforation, which has an incidence of 5 per cent and a mortality rate of ± 33 per cent; obstruction, with a rate of 32 per cent in the newborn and 23 per cent in infants; and enterocolitis.[5, 8, 15, 19, 30] Incidence of enterocolitis in the first 3 months of life is 24 per cent and overall is 15 per cent. Mortality rate without colostomy is 30 to 55 per cent and with colostomy is 4 per cent.

D. Biopsy must be obtained at multiple levels. Hematoxylin and eosin stain accuracy is 98 per cent.[1, 4, 19] The purpose is to establish the diagnosis and determine the proximal level of the lesion,[1, 4, 6, 15, 19] which is the rectosigmoid area in 75 per cent of cases, the descending colon ± the transverse colon in 15 per cent, and the ascending colon ± the ileum in 10 per cent.

E. Ostomy performed proximal to the disease is not an absolute guarantee against enterocolitis.[20]

F. The two forms in children and adults are (1) classic constipation, gradual distention, and failure to thrive and (2) megarectum, involving intermittent resistent constipation of late onset.

G. Results of resection for classic Hirschsprung's megacolon are shown in the table below.

With persistent dilation and bowel training, nearly 90 per cent of patients have normal function 5 to 25 years following operation.[16, 20] Patients develop normal bowel habits in 89.7 per cent of cases; 3.2 per

TECHNIQUES	MORTALITY (%)		EARLY COMPLICATIONS (%)				LATE COMPLICATIONS (%)					
	Early	Late	Intestinal Obstruction	Incomplete Resection	Leak	Enterocolitis	Stricture	Constipation	Diarrhea	Soiling	Urinary	Genital
Swenson's rectosigmoidectomy pull-through[4, 12, 14, 16, 20]	3.8	2.5	3	4.6	7.3	16.4	7.2	12.3 or less	7.2 or less	3.2–12.8	0–2.7	0
Soave's endorectal pull-through[4, 16]	3.3	—	1.3	2.2	0.2	—	8.2[a]	6.2	6.0	5.0	0	0
Duhamel's retrorectal pull-through[2, 4, 6, 16]	4.3	3.5	5	0.8	0.5	8.0	0[b]	7.6	—	3.5	0	0
State's anterior resection[15, 18]	6.4	—	—	—	0.5	—	0	10	0.5	0	0	0
Martin's long laterolateral ileoproctostomy and coloproctostomy[11, 15]	See footnote c.					75.0	See footnote d.					

[a]There were 4 cases of rectal prolapse.
[b]Late complications were (1) persistence of spur, (2) pouch and fecaloma (10.0 per cent), and (3) fistula-in-ano (3.5 per cent).
[c]This procedure is performed only in cases of total colonic aganglionosis. Because of the small number of cases there are no adequate statistics.
[d]Late complications include (1) considerable diarrhea and (2) vitamin B_{12} deficiency.

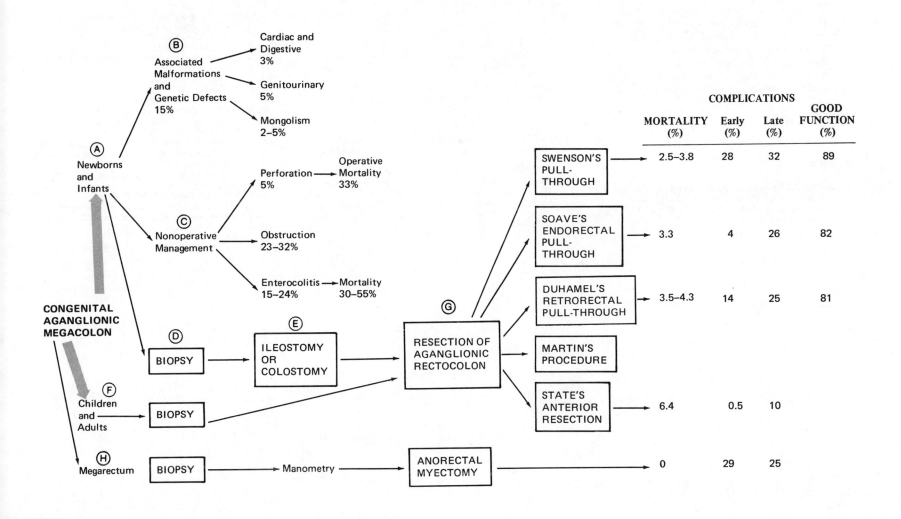

cent have permanent soiling, and 1.4 per cent need permanent colostomy.

H. The existence of this lesion is controversial.[20] It allegedly consists of a very short aganglionic segment of the rectum. Biopsy and manometry are essential for diagnostic proof. Operation consists of excising a small strip of rectal muscle ± the internal sphincter up to normal ganglion cells (frozen sections).[3, 9]

References

1. Bodian, M., Stephens, F. D., and Ward, B. C. H.: Hirschsprung's disease. *Lancet*, 1:19–22, 1950.
2. Kleinhaus, S., et al.: Hirschsprung's disease. J. Pediatr. Surg., 14:S88–197, 1979.
3. Duhamel, B.: Les Achalasies Recto-Anales. Ann. Chir. Infant., 6:345–347, 1965.
4. Ehrenpreis, T.: Hirschsprung's disease. Chicago, Year Book Medical Publishers, 1970.
5. Fraser, G. C., and Berry, C.: Mortality in neonatal Hirschsprung's disease with particular reference to enterocolitis. J. Pediatr. Surg., 2:205–211, 1967.
6. Grosfeld, J. L., Ballantyne, T. V. N., and Csicsko, J. F.: A critical evaluation of the Duhamel operation for Hirschsprung's disease. Arch. Surg., 113:454–460, 1978.
7. Lawson, J. O. N., and Nixon, H. H.: Anal canal pressure in the diagnosis of Hirschsprung's disease. J. Pediatr. Surg., 2:544–552, 1967.
8. Leenders, E., et al.: Aganglionic megacolon in infancy. Surg. Gynecol. Obstet., 131:424–430, 1970.
9. Lynn, H. B., and Van Heerden, J. A.: Rectal myectomy in Hirschsprung's disease. Arch. Surg., 110:991–994, 1975.
10. Madsen, C. M., and Nielsen, O. H.: Hirschsprung's disease: Long-term results in nonoperated cases. Prog. Pediatr. Surg., 10:103–110, 1967.
11. Martin, L. W.: Surgical management of Hirschsprung's disease involving the small intestine. Arch. Surg., 97:183–188, 1968.
12. Nielsen, O. H., and Madsen, C. M.: Thirteen to 25 years' follow-up after Swenson's operation for Hirschsprung's disease. Prog. Pediatr. Surg., 10:97–104, 1977.
13. Passarge, E.: The genetics of Hirschsprung's disease. Evidence for heterogenous etiology and a study of 63 families. N. Engl. J. Med., 276:138–163, 1967.
14. Puri, P., and Nixon, H. H.: Long-term results of Swenson's operation for Hirschsprung's disease. Prog. Pediatr. Surg., 10:87–96, 1977.
15. Sieber, W. K.: Hirschsprung's disease. Curr. Probl. Surg., 15(6):5–76, 1978.
16. Soave, F.: Megacolon: Long-term results of surgical treatment. Prog. Pediatr. Surg., 10:161–169, 1977.
17. Soave, F.: Extramucosal endorectal pull-through. Curr. Probl. Surg., 15(6):77–93, 1978.
18. State, D.: Surgical treatment for idiopathic congenital megacolon (Hirschsprung's disease). Surg. Gynecol. Obstet., 95:201–212, 1952.
19. Swenson, O., Sherman, J. O., and Fisher, J. H.: Diagnosis of congenital megacolon. An analysis of 501 patients. J. Pediatr. Surg., 8:587–591, 1973.
20. Swenson, O., et al.: The treatment and postoperative complications of congenital megacolon. A 25-year followup. Ann. Surg., 182:266–273, 1975.

INTUSSUSCEPTION

INTUSSUSCEPTION BY MORDANT E. PECK, M.D.

Comments

A. Intussusception is reported in major children's hospitals of the United States and Canada from 5 to 35 times a year. Nevertheless, it is one of the most common abdominal surgical emergencies of infancy and childhood. There is a geographic variation in incidence. England and the Scandinavian countries report an occurrence of approximately 2.5 per thousand live births.[2, 3] Seventy per cent of cases occur in children less than 1 year old, 9 per cent in those less than 3 months old, and 61 per cent in those 3 to 9 months old.[3, 11] Ratio of occurrence is 2:1 male:female.[2, 3, 8, 11] The underlying pathologic condition may be polyps (0.8 per cent of patients), neoplasm (0.2 per cent), Meckel's diverticulum (3.5 per cent), or bowel reduplication (0.2 per cent).[1]

Occurrence of intussusception has been associated with upper respiratory infections, gastroenteritis, mesenteric lymphadenitis, and lymphoid hyperplasia secondary to viral infections,[11] but these are probably of minor contributory importance.[12] Why 95 per cent of all intussusceptions begin at or near the ileocecal valve is not known.

B. The mortality rate in untreated cases is not definitely known. Occasionally the gangrenous intussusceptum will autolyze and be expelled.[2]

C. Early therapy, either by barium enema or by operation, lowers mortality.

D. Barium enema produces diagnostic errors in ileoileal intussusception that does not involve the large bowel. In such cases the barium enema will not reduce the intussusception.

References

1. Ladd, W. E., and Gross, R. E.: Abdominal Surgery of Infancy and Childhood. Philadelphia, W. B. Saunders, 1947.
2. Ravitch, M. M.: Intussusception in Infants and Children. Springfield, Ill., Charles C Thomas, 1959.
3. Ravitch, M. M.: Intussusception. In Benson, C. D., et al. (eds.): Pediatric Surgery, Vol. II. Chicago, Year Book Medical Publishers, 1962.
4. Packard, G. B., and Allen, R. P.: Results in the treatment of intussusception of infants and children. Surgery, 41:567, 1957.
5. Packard, G. B., and Allen, R. P.: Intussusception. Surgery, 45:496, 1959.
6. Benson, C. D., Lloyd, J. R., and Fischer, H.: Intussusception in infants and children. Arch. Surg., 86:745, 1963.
7. Peck, D. A., Lloyd, H. B., and DuShane, J. W.: Intussusception in children. Surg. Gynecol. Obstet., 116:398, 1963.
8. Ein, S. H., and Stephens, C. A.: Intussusception: 354 cases in 10 years. J. Pediatr. Surg., 6:16, 1971.
9. Larsen, E., and Miller, R. C.: Clinical aspects of intussusception. Am. J. Surg., 124:69, 1972.
10. Gierup, J., Jowlf, H., and Lividitis, A.: Management of intussusception in infants and children: A survey based on 288 consecutive cases. Pediatrics, 50:535, 1972.
11. Freund, H., Hurvitz, H., and Schiller, M.: Etiologic and therapeutic aspects of intussusception in childhood. Am. J. Surg., 134:272, 1977.
12. Schenken, J. R., Kruger, R. L., and Schultz, L.: Papillary lymphoid hyperplasia of the terminal ileum: An unusual cause of intussusception and gastrointestinal bleeding in childhood. J. Pediatr. Surg., 10:259, 1975.

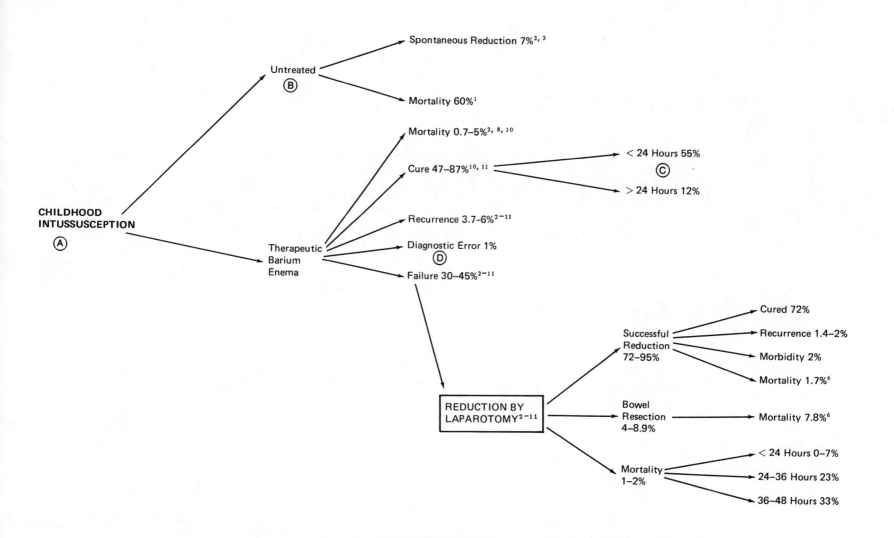

Section **I**

Breast

SOLITARY BREAST NODULE BY ROBERT M. PASH, M.D.

Comments

A. In children under age 12, care should be taken not to diagnose developing breast buds as tumors, because surgical excision may lead to cosmetic deformity. Primary breast cancer in young girls (age 10 to 20) is so rare as to be a surgical oddity. True breast carcinoma in the younger ages is of a distinct juvenile histologic type. Occasional reports of mortality vary from 100 per cent 5-year survival to death within 2 years.[6, 14] Frequency of benign breast lesions in children and young girls (to age 20) is shown in the following table.

LESION	FREQUENCY (%)
Fibroadenoma	76.4
Mastopathies	10.5
Intraductal papillomatosis	5.5
Gross cysts	3.4
Inflammatory lesions	2.9

B. Approximately one per 100 breast biopsies in this age group is malignant. This is less than 2 per cent of all breast cancers. Survival figures in young women with breast cancer are comparable to those of the older age groups if the regional lymph nodes are free of disease. Once the regional nodes are involved by metastases the 10-year survival rate is less than 20 per cent.[18]

C. It is difficult to determine the prevalence of benign breast disease in the population. Although most benign breast lesions are not associated with malignancy, several studies have shown a 4- to 5-fold increased risk of breast cancer in women with biopsy-proven cystic mastitis and epithelial hyperplasia. Fifteen per cent of women undergoing mastectomy for carcinoma will have chronic cystic mastitis in the specimen. It may be that some benign breast lesions and breast carcinoma are caused by similar factors.[5] Frequency and median age for some benign breast lesions in women are shown in the following table.

LESION	FREQUENCY (%)	MEDIAN AGE (Years)
Chronic cystic mastitis and its components	34	41
Fibroadenoma	27	27
Fibrous mastopathy	16	34
Acute and chronic inflammation	13	26
Miscellaneous	10	41

D. The percentage may vary with selected patient populations and with the use of xeromammography and other screening procedures.[3] The probability of the biopsy being positive for cancer depends upon patient selection, use of xeromammography, heredity, and hormonal and environmental influence.

History of breast cancer, early menarche, and late menopause increase the cancer risk; pregnancy prior to 30, early surgical menopause, and small body size decrease the probability. The overall risk of breast cancer is 5.5 to 6 per cent in women.[4, 11, 13] Median age at diagnosis is 48 years. The delay in diagnosis averages 9 months.

E. Lymph node metastases and survival in patients with Paget's disease are shown in the table below.[12, 15]

F. These highly curable lesions include noninfiltrating duct carcinoma, lobular carcinoma *in situ,* and infiltrating duct or lobular carcinomas 1 cm. or less in diameter that present in the outer half of the breast. Despite reports of 52 per cent residual cancer remaining in the breast tissue after wide local excision and of axillary node metastases in 16 per cent of such patients, there is a 98 per cent 5-year survival rate and a 95 per cent 10-year survival rate. Increased use of screening xeromammography increases the number of minimal carcinomas found.[9, 21]

G. Prognosis relates to both tumor size and

LOCATION	NODES	10-YEAR SURVIVAL (%)	10-YEAR CUMULATIVE SURVIVAL (%)
Nipple only (40%)	—	83–95	87–94
	+(0–17%)	50	
With breast mass (50%)	—	67	35–38
	+(45–65%)	35	

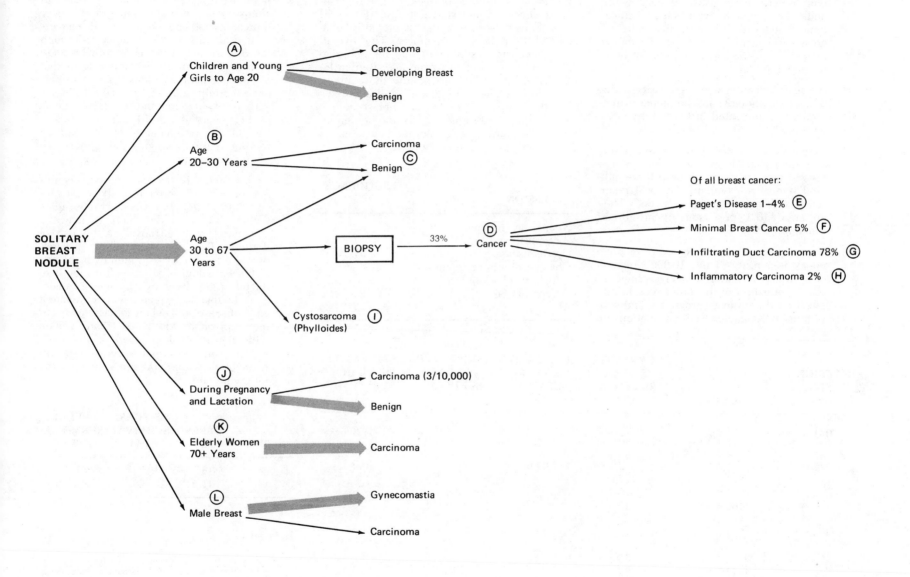

SOLITARY BREAST NODULE *Continued*

lymph node metastases. Axillary lymph node involvement with small primary tumors suggests a biologically more aggressive cancer. Survival relative to size of lesion and nodal metastases is shown in the table below.

H. Because 5-year survival is a rarity, radiation, chemotherapy, and hormonal manipulation are indicated instead of operative excision.[19]

I. These occur in the younger age group and often attain huge size without metastases. Eighty per cent of these fibroepithelial tumors are benign, but local recurrence occurs following excision.[7] They are rare (0.3 per cent of all breast tumors).

J. Breast cancer that develops during pregnancy is a rarity (3 per 10,000 pregnancies) and is considered solely coincidental. Termination of the pregnancy has no effect on the ultimate prognosis, and subsequent pregnancies have no relationship to the recurrence of disease. The high incidence of metastatic disease (60 to 74 per cent positive nodes) is probably related to delay in diagnosis. The overall prognosis is similar to that for nonpregnant women of the same age. Benign lesions in this group include those breast changes due to pregnancy and abscesses that usually occur in breast-feeding mothers.[1, 4] Frequency of some benign lesions during pregnancy and lactation is shown in the following table.

LESION	FREQUENCY (%)
Neoplasms (lipoma, fibroma, papilloma)	37
Cystic disease	31
Changes due to pregnancy (galactocele, lobular hyperplasia)	22
Abscess	7

K. A breast lump in a woman 70 years old almost always is malignant. Breast cancer represents 30 per cent of all cancer-related deaths in the elderly. Although the disease may grow more slowly, node metastases occur at the same rate as that of younger patients. Considering an operative mortality rate of 1 per cent in breast surgery of the aged and life expectancies of 13.9 years at age 70 and 8.2 years at age 80, the treatment of choice will be the one that will provide the highest rate of 10-year survival.[10]

L. Breast cancer in men is a rarity, accounting for only 0.7 per cent of all breast cancers.[16] In young men it is most often idiopathic, but in older men it may be associated with cirrhosis or the use of digitalis. The highest incidence of carcinoma of the breast is in men over the age of 60. Pathologically the malignancy is of ductal origin. Prognosis for men is analogous to that for women with equivalent early disease, but when metastases occur men appear to do worse than women with the equivalent stage of disease.[16] Nodal metastases and survival rates in male breast carcinoma are shown in the following table.

LESION SIZE (cm.)	NODES	AGE-CORRECTED 5-YEAR SURVIVAL (%)	CUMULATIVE 5-YEAR SURVIVAL (%)	AGE-CORRECTED 10-YEAR SURVIVAL (%)	CUMULATIVE 10-YEAR SURVIVAL (%)
0–1.9	− +(32.7%)	86 45	63.6	81 27	48.3
2–2.9	− +(51%)	83 65	64.6	70 47	40.0
3–3.9	− +(63.8%)	76 45	46.7	64 34	29.1
4–5.9	− +(68.8%)	78 38	43.3	75 20	24.4
6+	− +(71%)	55 26	28.5	49 13	17.0

NODES	CASES (%)	5-YEAR SURVIVAL (%)	10-YEAR SURVIVAL (%)
−	38	79	56.3
+	41.5	28	10

References

1. Byrd, B. F., et al.: Treatment of breast tumors associated with pregnancy and lactation. Ann. Surg., 155:940–947, 1962.

2. Correa, P.: The epidemiology of cancer of the breast. Am. J. Clin. Pathol., *64*:720–727, 1975.
3. Degenshein, G. A., et al.: Breast biopsies. Ratio of malignant to benign. N.Y. State J. Med., *76*:1538–1539, 1976.
4. Donegan, W. L.: Mammary carcinoma and pregnancy. *In* Spratt, J. S., and Donegan, W. L.: Cancer of the Breast. Philadelphia, W. B. Saunders Co., 1967, pp. 170–178.
5. Donnelly, P., et al.: Benign breast lesions and subsequent breast carcinoma in Rochester, Minnesota. Mayo Clin. Proc., *50*:650–666, 1970.
6. Farrow, J., and Ashikari, H.: Breast lesions in young girls. Surg. Clin. North Am., *49*:261–269, 1969.
7. Hajdu, D. I., Espinoza, M. N., and Robbins, G. F.: Recurrent cystosarcoma phyllodes. Cancer, *38*:1402–1406, 1976.
8. Handley, R. S.: Cancer of the breast. Am. Surg., *41*:667–670, 1975.
9. Hutter, R.: The interpretive art/science of pathology CA, *28*:141–145, 1978.
10. Kesseler, H. J., and Seton, J. Z.: Treatment of operable breast carcinoma in the aged. Am. J. Surg., *135*:664–666, 1978.
11. Leis, H. P.: Present knowledge of breast cancer. Minerva Chir., *131*:1297–1312, 1976.
12. Maier, W. P., et al.: Paget's disease in the female breast. Surg. Gynecol. Obstet., *128*:1253–1263, 1969.
13. Mambo, N., and Gallager, H. S.: Carcinoma of the breast: The prognostic significance of extranodal extension of axillary disease. Cancer, *39*:2280–2285, 1977.
14. McDivitt, R. W., and Stewart, F. W.: Breast carcinoma in children. JAMA, *195*:144–146, 1966.
15. Nance, F. C., et al.: Paget's disease of the breast. Ann. Surg., *171*:864–874, 1970.
16. Ribeiro, G. G.: Carcinoma of the male breast: A review of 200 cases. Br. J. Surg., *64*:381–383, 1977.
17. Say, C., and Donegan, W.: Invasive carcinoma of the breast: Prognostic significance of tumor size and involved axillary lymph nodes. Cancer, *34*:468–471, 1974.
18. Schwartz, G. F., and Zeok, J. V.: Carcinoma of the breast in young women. Am. J. Surg., *131*:570–574, 1976.
19. Stocks, L. H., and Patterson, F. M.: Inflammatory carcinoma of the breast. Surg. Gynecol. Obstet., *143*:885–889, 1976.
20. Urban, J. A., Papachristou, D., and Taylor, J.: Bilateral breast cancer: Biopsy of the other breast. Cancer, *40*:1968–1973, 1977.
21. Wanebo, H., Huvos, A. G., and Urban, J. A.: Treatment of minimal breast cancer. Cancer, *33*:349–357, 1974.

411

BREAST CANCER BY ROGER S. WOTKYNS, M.D.

Comments

A. Only 20 to 30 per cent of patients with an early diagnosis of breast cancer will have a normal life expectancy. Only one quarter of these patients have axillary lymph node involvement on examination of the surgical specimen. Continued critical assessment of current treatment practice is mandatory.

B. The relationship of site of breast cancer to axillary lymph node metastasis is as follows:[1] outer upper quadrant (51 per cent), outer lower quadrant (39 per cent), inner upper quadrant (36 per cent), inner lower quadrant (33 per cent), and within 1 cm. of nipple (47 per cent).

C. The significance of metastasis in different axillary lymph node groups is as follows:[1] Subclavicular metastasis (one or more nodes) has a 16 per cent 10-year survival rate; scapular, central, interpectoral, or axillary vein metastasis (4 or more nodes) has a 30 per cent 10-year survival rate. The greater the number of nodes involved, the more ominous the significance. Twenty-five per cent of cases in clinical stages I and II will have internal mammary lymph node metastasis. Internal mammary node involvement usually occurs only after axillary node involvement. The more numerous the axillary node involvement, the greater likelihood that there will be internal mammary node involvement. In reviewing pathologic specimens, 22 per cent of lymph nodes recut after having been reported free of tumor will be found to contain tumor on multiple section.

D. Size of primary tumor as related to axillary lymph node metastasis is shown in the following table.

SIZE (cm.)	AXILLARY LYMPH NODE METASTASIS (%)
Not palpable	19
<1	22
1 to 3	28
3 to 5	48
5 to 8	52
>8	52

E. Cell type as related to rate of treatment failure is shown in the following table.[2]

HISTOLOGIC TYPE	FREQUENCY (%)	GROSS TREATMENT FAILURE (%)
Infiltrating duct cell (IDC)	50	36
Combined (IDC+ tubular or IDC+ invasive lobular)	36	25
Lobular, invasive	5.4	29
Medullary	4.6	21
Mucinous	2	1
Tubular	1	6
Lobular, in-situ	1	1

Infiltrating duct cell tumors have an incidence of bilaterality (metachronous) that increases at a rate of about 1 per cent a year. Lobular, medullary, mucinous, and tubular tumors with noninvasive cell types tend to have a high (20 to 30 per cent) risk of bilaterality. Forty-eight per cent of well differentiated tumors metastasize to regional lymph nodes, and 70 per cent of anaplastic tumors metastasize to regional nodes.

Inflammatory carcinomas may be any of the aforementioned cell types; differentiated only by invasion of lymphatic channels, which produces the inflammatory sign. Survival is less than 2 years.

F. Breast cancer is more common in nulliparous women over the age of 35. The incidence of cancer decreases with parity.[1] The effect, if any, of breast feeding on the development of breast cancer is controversial, as is the possible role of oral contraceptives in breast cancer development. The effect of pregnancy and lactation on prognosis is shown in the following table.

STAGE	10-YEAR SURVIVAL (%)
I	60
II	27
III	12
IV	0

G. Prognosis related to patient's age for all stages of breast cancer is shown in the following table.[1]

AGE (Years)	10-YEAR SURVIVAL (%)
<30	40
30 to 64	63
>64	57

H. About 10 per cent of patients with carcinoma of the breast have a mother or a sister with carcinoma of the breast.[1]

I. Mammography[4, 6] adds an extra dimension to the clinical evaluation of breast masses. Two features of the x-ray picture — ductal prominence and dysplasia — are keys to diagnosis and more im-

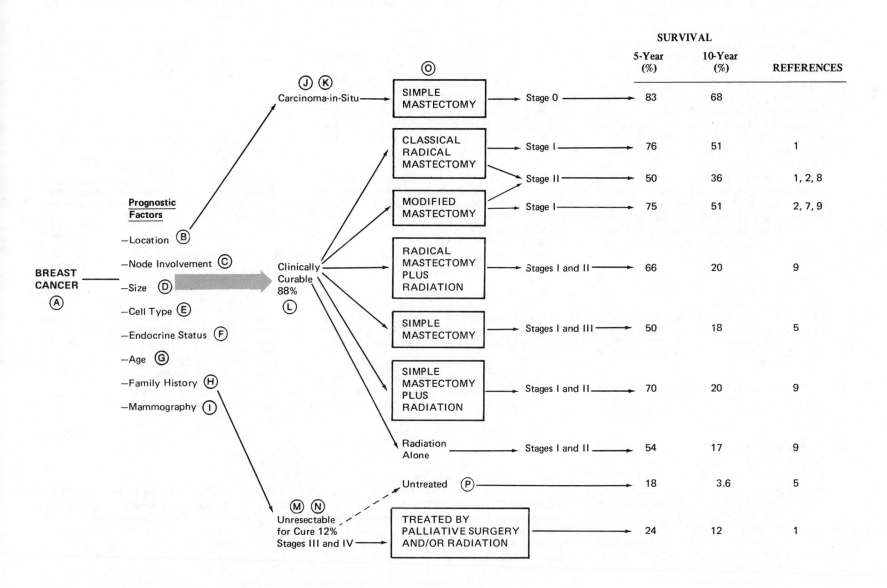

			SURVIVAL		
			5-Year (%)	10-Year (%)	REFERENCES
	Carcinoma-in-Situ (J) (K)	SIMPLE MASTECTOMY (O)	Stage 0	83	68	
		CLASSICAL RADICAL MASTECTOMY	Stage I	76	51	1
			Stage II	50	36	1, 2, 8
		MODIFIED MASTECTOMY	Stage I	75	51	2, 7, 9
Prognostic Factors		RADICAL MASTECTOMY PLUS RADIATION	Stages I and II	66	20	9
—Location (B)	Clinically Curable 88% (L)	SIMPLE MASTECTOMY	Stages I and III	50	18	5
—Node Involvement (C)		SIMPLE MASTECTOMY PLUS RADIATION	Stages I and II	70	20	9
—Size (D)		Radiation Alone	Stages I and II	54	17	9
—Cell Type (E)		Untreated (P)		18	3.6	5
—Endocrine Status (F)	Unresectable for Cure 12% Stages III and IV (M) (N)	TREATED BY PALLIATIVE SURGERY AND/OR RADIATION		24	12	1

BREAST CANCER (A)

—Age (G)

—Family History (H)

—Mammography (I)

413

portant, to the *prediction of women at risk*.

In detecting malignant lesions 11 per cent of mammograms give false positive results and 6 per cent give false negative results.

In patients younger than 50, the prominent duct pattern (P_2) is associated with a very high relative cancer risk, and DY (severe dysplasia) carries a smaller increased risk. P_1, P_2, and DY women account for 57 per cent of the population. In these women 93 per cent of breast cancer is found. Women in the N1 group (fatty breast tissue) are 43 per cent of the population. In this group only 7.5 per cent of breast cancers are found. After age 50 there is little variation in breast cancer prevalence among women with different parenchymal patterns.

J. There are multiple foci of cancer in 54 per cent of breasts studied. It is for this reason that any operation less than simple mastectomy for carcinoma *in situ* is not advocated.

K. Survival parallels the natural survival curve (see Comment P).

L. It is common to see recurrence of breast cancer 15 to 20 years after apparently successful treatment. This makes the definition of *cure* difficult.

M. The classification system of the American Joint Committee on Cancer Staging and End Results Reporting for breast cancer is as follows:

T_1 = Tumor 2 cm. or less in size, skin not involved, no local attachment, no Paget's disease.

T_2 = Tumor larger than 2 cm. or with skin attachment; nipple retraction. No pectoral muscle, or chest wall involvement.

T_3 = Tumor of any size with any of the following: Skin infiltration, ulceration, peau d'orange, or muscle or chest wall attachment.

N_0 = No clinically palpable axillary nodes.

N_1 = Clinically palpable nonfixed homolateral lymph nodes.

N_2 = Clinically palpable homolateral or infraclavicular nodes that are fixed to one another or to other structures.

M_0 = No distant metastasis.

M_1 = Clinical or radiologic evidence of metastasis in areas other than homolateral or infraclavicular lymph nodes.

Stage I = $T_{1-2}N_0M_0$
Stage II = $T_{1-2}N_1M_0$
Stage III = $T_3N_0M_0$ or $T_{1-2}N_2M_0$
Stage IV = Any clinical stage with M_1

N. Patients with lesions that are unresectable for cure should be offered less operations with or without radiation and chemotherapy to improve the quality of their lives during the course of their disease.

O. Mortality of radical mastectomy is 1.8 per cent, of modified mastectomy, 1.0 per cent, and of simple mastectomy, less than 1 per cent.[1] Morbidity is shown in the table below.

P. A comparison of patients with carcinoma of the breast in various stages of the disease is shown in Figure 1.[1, 3, 5, 7]

References

1. Haagensen, C. D.: Diseases of the Breast, 2nd ed. Philadelphia, W. B. Saunders Co., 1971.
2. Cooperman, A. M., and Esselstyn, C. B.: Breast cancer. Surg. Clin. North Am., 58:659, 1977.
3. MacKay, E. M., and Sellers, A. H.: Breast Cancer at the Ontario Cancer Clinics, 1938–1956: A Statistical Review. Medical Statistics Branch, Ontario Department of Health (1965).
4. Wolf, J. N.: Risk of breast cancer development by mammographic parenchymal pattern. Cancer, 37:2486, 1976.
5. Bloom, H. J. G., Richardson, W. W., and Harries, E. J.: Natural history of untreated breast cancer (1805–1933). Br. Med. J., 213:5299, 1962.
6. Peyster, R. G., Kalisher, L., and Cole, P.: Mammographic parenchymal patterns and the prevalence of breast cancer. Radiology, 125:387, 1977.
7. Shimkim, M. D., et al.: Simple and radical mastectomy for breast cancer: A re-analysis of Smith and Meyer's report from Rockford, Illinois. J. Natl. Cancer Inst., 27:1197–1215. 1961.
8. Handley, R. S., and Thackray, A. C.: The internal mammary lymph node chain in carcinoma of the breast: Study of 50 cases. Lancet, 2:276–278, 1949.
9. Swartz, S. I.: Principles of Surgery. New York, McGraw-Hill Book Co., 1969.

TREATMENT	RESTRICTION OF MOTION	EDEMA	POST-OPERATIVE SEROUS COLLECTIONS	SKIN LOSS	COSMETIC DEFECT	NERVE INJURY
Radical mastectomy	++	++	+++	++	++++	++
Modified mastecomy	+	++	++	+	+	+
Simple mastectomy	+	−	+	±	+	−
Radiation	++	+++	−	++	+	+

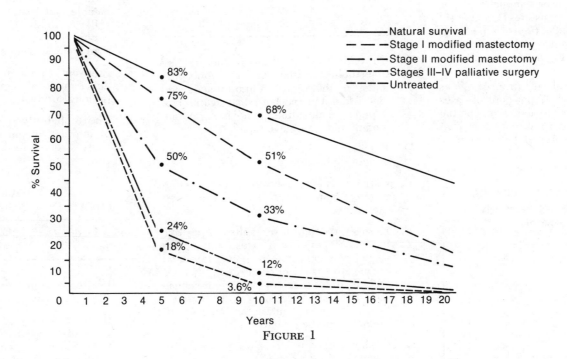

FIGURE 1

POSTMASTECTOMY RECURRENT BREAST CANCER BY JOHN C. HEISER, M.D.

Comments

A. Sites of first recurrence of breast cancer following mastectomy include skeletal (27 per cent of cases), local (26 per cent), regional (15 per cent), axillary (2 per cent), pulmonary (21 per cent), digestive (4 per cent), hemic or lymphatic (4 per cent), and miscellaneous sites (1 per cent).[5] Mean survival from the time of appearance of the first recurrence ("modern" treatment) is shown in Figure 1.[1]

B. Radiation for local recurrences gives complete control in 67 per cent of cases that lasts 32 months, and gives partial control in 24 per cent of cases that lasts 11 months.[7] The interval between mastectomy and local recurrence is shown in the following table.[6]

RECURRENCE INTERVAL
(Months)

STAGE	Parasternal	Chest Wall
A	50	41
B	36	26

C. Currently available drugs include the antimetabolites Adriamycin, cyclophosphamide, methotrexate, 5-fluorouracil, and vincristine and the hormonal agents clomiphene, nafoxidine, tamoxifen, aminoglutethimide, and levodopa.

D. FAC is 5-fluorouracil, Adriamycin, and cyclophosphamide.

E. CMFVP is cyclophosphamide, methotrexate, 5-fluorouracil, vincristine, and prednisone.

F. Estrogen receptor test results are positive in 70 to 85 per cent of cases, with a 55 to 60 per cent objective response rate, and are negative in 15 to 30 per cent of cases, with a 10 per cent objective response rate. Estrogen receptor values from either primary or metastatic tumors will predict response equally well.

G. Oophorectomy is of value primarily in premenopausal women.

H. Response to adrenalectomy was seen in 22 to 42 per cent of patients who did not respond to oophorectomy.[12]

I. All data on prolonged survival and response are confused by frequent simultaneous use of radiation and various types of chemotherapy.

THERAPY FOR ADJUVANT BREAST CANCER

J. Indications for adjuvant therapy are debatable but mainly include (1) positive axillary nodes, (2) inner quadrant and central lesions, and (3) lesions greater than 3 cm. in diameter.

K. Adjuvant radiation decreases the incidence of local recurrence but does not prolong survival.

L. The probability of positive involvement of internal mammary nodes in these lesions is shown in the following table.[6]

LOCATION	OVERALL INCIDENCE	POSITIVE AXILLARY NODES
Inner quadrant	29–31%	54%
Central	47%	49%

If disease is present in parasternal nodes, 10-year survival is 13 to 15 per cent.[6]

M. If the axillary nodes are involved, the value of radiation is debatable.[6] There is less controversy when large or many axillary nodes are involved.

N. The primary benefit of adjuvant chemotherapy is for women less than 50 years old or premenopausal.[13]

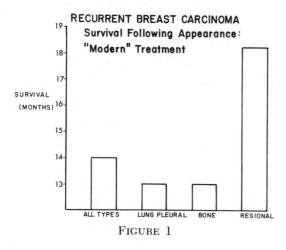

FIGURE 1

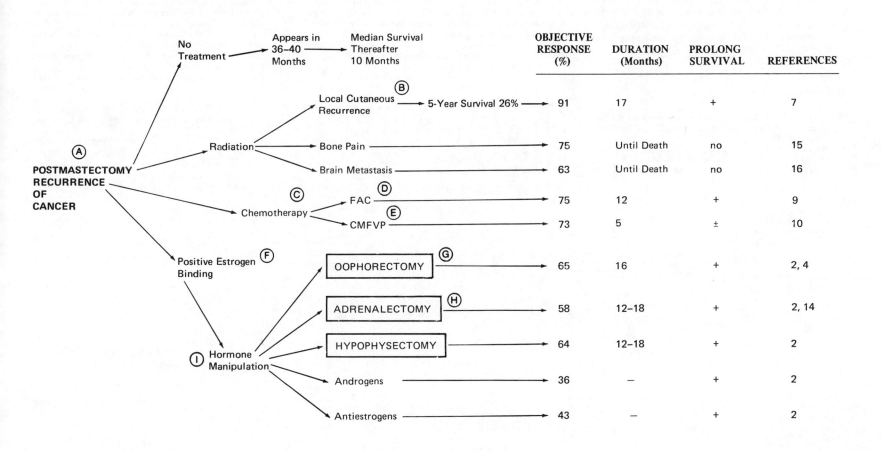

	OBJECTIVE RESPONSE (%)	DURATION (Months)	PROLONG SURVIVAL	REFERENCES
Local Cutaneous Recurrence (B) → 5-Year Survival 26%	91	17	+	7
Bone Pain	75	Until Death	no	15
Brain Metastasis	63	Until Death	no	16
FAC (D)	75	12	+	9
CMFVP (E)	73	5	±	10
OOPHORECTOMY (G)	65	16	+	2, 4
ADRENALECTOMY (H)	58	12–18	+	2, 14
HYPOPHYSECTOMY	64	12–18	+	2
Androgens	36	—	+	2
Antiestrogens	43	—	+	2

No Treatment → Appears in 36–40 Months → Median Survival Thereafter 10 Months

(A) POSTMASTECTOMY RECURRENCE OF CANCER

Radiation

(C) Chemotherapy

(F) Positive Estrogen Binding

(I) Hormone Manipulation

O. L-PAM is L-phenylalanine mustard. CMF is cyclophosphamide, methotrexate, and 5-fluorouracil.

P. Although hormone manipulation is of benefit in treating recurrence, there are no hard data to prove its value in adjuvant therapy.[8, 18] Surgical removal of the ovaries provides a quicker and more dependable castration than radiation.[19]

References

1. DeVitt, J. E.: Effect of palliative treatment on the survival of patients with breast cancer. Can. J. Surg., *20*:46–50, 1977.
2. McQuire, W. L.: Current status of estrogen receptors in human breast cancer. Cancer, *36*:638–644, 1975.
3. Chamberlain, A., et al.: Efficacy of adrenalectomy for metastatic cancer of the breast. Surg. Gynecol. Obstet., *138*:891–895, 1974.
4. Veronesi, U., Pizzocaro, G., and Rossi, A.: Oophorectomy for advanced carcinoma of the breast. Surg. Gynecol. Obstet., *141*:569–570, 1975.
5. Fisher, B., et al.: Postoperative radiotherapy in the treatment of breast cancer: Results of NSABP clinical trial. Ann. Surg., *172*:711–732, 1970.
6. Haagenson, C. D.: Diseases of the Breast, 2nd ed. Philadelphia, W. B. Saunders Co., 1971.
7. Chu, F. C., et al.: Locally recurrent carcinoma of the breast: Results of radiation therapy. Cancer, *37*:2677–2681, 1976.
8. Ravdin, R. G.: Results of a clinical trial concerning the worth of prophylactic oophorectomy for breast cancer. Surg. Gynecol. Obstet., *131*:1055–1064, 1970.
9. Blumenschein, G. R.: FAC chemotherapy for breast cancer. Proc. Am. Soc. Clin. Oncol., March 1974.
10. Carter, S. K.: Single and combination nonhormonal chemotherapy in breast cancer. Cancer, *30*:1543–1555, 1972.
11. Fletcher, G. H.: Textbook of Radiotherapy. Philadelphia, Lea & Febiger, 1973.
12. Yonemoto, R. H.: Randomized sequential hormonal therapy vs. adrenalectomy for metastatic breast carcinoma. Cancer, *39*:547–555, 1977.
13. Bonadonna, G., et al.: The CMF program for operable breast cancer with positive axillary nodes. Cancer, *39*:2904–2915, 1977.
14. Wilson, R. E.: Evaluation of adrenalectomy and hypophysectomy in the treatment of metastatic cancer of the breast. Cancer, *24*:1322–1330, 1969.
15. Guttman, R.: Radiotherapy in locally advanced cancer of the breast. Cancer, *20*:1046, 1967.
16. Chao, J. H.: Roentgen therapy of cerebral metastasis. Cancer, *7*:682–689, 1954.
17. Fisher, B.: L-Phenylalanine mustard in the management of primary breast cancer. Cancer, *39*:2883–2903, 1977.
18. Legha, S. J.: Hormonal therapy of breast cancer: New approaches and concepts. Ann. Intern. Med., *88*:69–77, 1978.
19. Fracchia, A. A.: Castration for primary inoperable or recurrent breast carcinoma. Surg. Gynecol. Obstet., *128*:1226–1234, 1969.

418

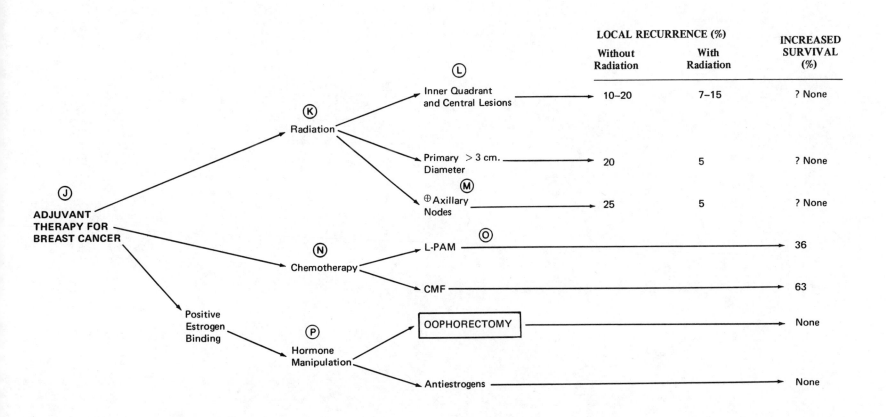

	LOCAL RECURRENCE (%)		INCREASED SURVIVAL (%)
	Without Radiation	With Radiation	
Inner Quadrant and Central Lesions	10–20	7–15	? None
Primary > 3 cm. Diameter	20	5	? None
⊕ Axillary Nodes	25	5	? None
L-PAM			36
CMF			63
OOPHORECTOMY			None
Antiestrogens			None

Section J

Soft Tissue

MAJOR BURNS BY CHARLES A. BUERK, M.D.

Comments

A. Major burns include (1) all third degree burns of more than 10 per cent of the body surface area (BSA), (2) all second degree burns of more than 25 per cent BSA in adults and of more than 20 per cent BSA in children, (3) all burns involving the hands, face, eyes, ears, feet, and perineum, (4) all burns associated with inhalation injury, (5) all electrical burns, and (6) all burns complicated by fracture or other major trauma or by illness.[1]

B. Critical burns are second and third degree burns totalling over 40 per cent of BSA.[2]

C. Severe burns are those that total between 20 and 40 per cent of BSA.[2]

D. Moderate burns are those that total less than 20 per cent of BSA.[2]
   Survival statistics in these categories depend on both age and percentage of body surface area burned (see Figure 1).

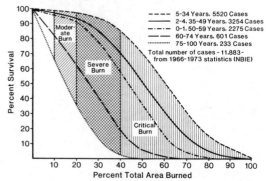

FIGURE 1. (Modified from: Feller et al.[6])

Survival Curves Fit By Probit Analysis For Age Groups

- - - - 5-34 Years, 5520 Cases
——— 2-4, 35-49 Years, 3254 Cases
——— 0-1, 50-59 Years, 2275 Cases
— · — 60-74 Years, 601 Cases
········· 75-100 Years, 233 Cases
Total number of cases - 11,883 - from 1966-1973 statistics (NBIE)

E. A few (±2 per cent) will die within the first few hours of smoke inhalation or associated injuries.

F. The early phase of treatment, 0 to 5 days, primarily involves resuscitation, maintenance of proper fluid and electrolyte balance, and prophylaxis against subsequent infection.

G. Hypovolemia occurs with delayed resuscitation; depressed cardiac output perhaps is caused by a toxic depressant factor produced by the burn.

H. Acute tubular necrosis (ATN) is rare (less than 3 per cent of cases), occurring with sepsis and electrical burns, when there is severe associated trauma, or following inadequate resuscitation.

I. Pulmonary insufficiency occurs in 40 per cent of severely burned patients[4] and has a mortality rate of between 15 and 70 per cent.[5]

J. Expected 5-day survival is 85 per cent for critical burns, 90 per cent for severe burns, and 95 per cent for moderate burns.

K. Early excision (within 2 to 7 days) reduces the duration of hospitalization but does not affect the chance of ultimate survival[6] (see Figure 2).

L. Allografts characteristically survive 5 to 14 days as temporary biologic dressings; xerografts from pigs last about 5 to 10 days.

M. Standard therapy consists of topical antibiotics until eschar separation plus intermediate débridement.

N. The increased energy expenditure created by thermal burns requires forced

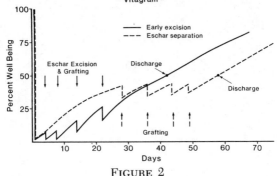

Well Being Following Major Burn
Early Escharectomy vs Awaiting Spontaneous Separation
- Vitagram -

——— Early excision
- - - - Eschar separation

FIGURE 2

feeding of an equivalent number of calories by mouth or intravenously to avoid malnutrition.

O. Diffuse gastritis occurs in 80 per cent of patients with burns of more than 30 per cent of body surface area.[7] In 1970, true ulceration occurred in 10 per cent of patients with 30 per cent body surface burns. Ulceration occurred in 60 per cent of patients with burns of more than 60 per cent BSA, and mortality was 70 per cent.[8] This incidence seems to be reduced by the use of antacids and H-2 blocking agents, better nutrition, and better respiratory care.

P. Thirty per cent of severely burned children develop hypertension and, despite the administration of antihypertensive drugs, a few develop acute encephalopathy.[9]

Q. Acute acalculous cholecystitis usually is associated with sepsis, biliary or gastrointestinal stasis, or dehydration.[10]

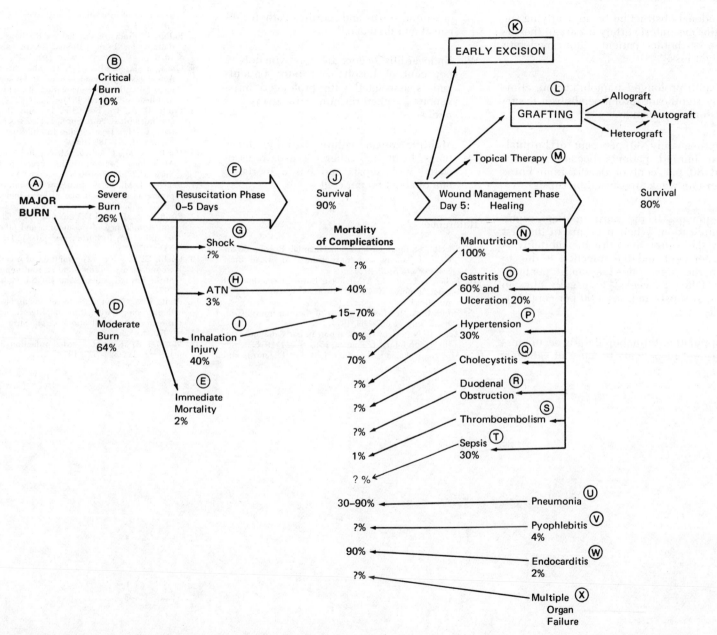

R. Duodenal obstruction by an overlying superior mesenteric artery occurs in the supine asthenic patient after moderate weight loss.[11]

S. Despite prolonged immobilization, clinically significant thromboembolism is surprisingly uncommon.[12]

T. Approximately 30 per cent of hospitalized burned patients become septic,[13] and 80 per cent of deaths from burns after one week are caused by sepsis.

U. Pneumonia is the most frequent septic complication. When it occurs in the first few days after the burn the mortality is 30 per cent and the infection is due to airborne organisms. Late-onset pneumonia (after 2 weeks) is usually due to wound sepsis and has a 90 per cent mortality rate.

V. Suppurative thrombophlebitis occurs in 4 per cent of patients because of catheters or wound sepsis and requires catheter removal and drainage.[14]

W. Endocarditis occurs in approximately 2 per cent of hospitalized burn patients and is associated with prolonged intravenous catheterization. Recovery is rare.[15]

X. Multiple organ failure (kidney, liver, lungs, heart, and others) is usually associated with sepsis and has a mortality rate of about 60 per cent.

References

1. Specific Optimal Criteria for Hospital Resources for Care of Patients with Burn Injury. American Burn Association, April 1976.
2. Feller, I. L., et al.: A Michigan burn information and triage system. Michigan Hospitals, December 1977, pp. 10–15.
3. Pruitt, B. A., Jr.: Complications of thermal injury. Clin. Plast. Surg., 1:667–669, 1974.
4. Agee, R. N., et al.: Use of xenon in early diagnoses of inhalation injury. J. Trauma, 16:218–224, 1976.
5. Moylan, J. A., and Alexander, L. G. J.: Diagnosis and treatment of inhalation injury. World J. Surg., 2:218–291, 1978.
6. Feller, I., Flora, J., and Bawol, R.: Baseline results of therapy for burn patients. JAMA, 236:1943–1947, 1976.
7. Czaja, A. J., McAlhany, J. C., and Pruitt, B. A., Jr.: Acute gastroduodenal disease following thermal injury: An endoscopic evaluation of incidence and natural history. N. Engl. J. Med., 291:925–929, 1964.
8. Pruitt, B. A., Jr., Foley, F. D., and Moncrief, J. A.: Curling's ulcer. Ann. Surg., 172:523–536, 1970.
9. Lowry, G. H.: Hypertension in children with burns. J. Trauma, 4:481–485, 1964.
10. Muster, A. M., Goodwin, M. N., and Pruitt, B. A., Jr.: Acalculous cholecystitis in burned patients. Am. J. Surg., 122:591–593, 1971.
11. Reckler, J. M., et al.: Superior mesenteric artery syndrome as a consequence of burn injury. J. Trauma, 12:979–985, 1972.
12. Pruitt, B. A., Jr., and DiVincenti, F. C.: The occurrence and significance of pneumonia and other pulmonary complications in burned patients. J. Trauma, 10:519–531, 1970.
13. Loebl, E. C., et al.: The method of quantitative burn-wound biopsy cultures and its routine use in the care of the burned patient. Am. J. Clin. Pathol., 61:20–24, 1974.
14. Pruitt, B. A., Jr., et al.: Intravenous therapy in burn patients: Suppurative thrombophlebitis and other life-threatening complications. Arch. Surg., 100:399–404, 1970.
15. Munster, A. M., et al.: Cardiac infections in burns. Am. J. Surg., 122:524–527, 1971.

MALIGNANT MELANOMA

MALIGNANT MELANOMA BY GREGORY VAN STIEGMANN, M.D.

Comments

A. Incisional biopsy, though not theoretically preferable, does not alter prognosis.[14]

B. Clinical staging is based on physical examination; pathologic staging is based on microscopic node analysis.[11]
Regional node involvement in clinical stage I is 20 to 30 per cent and in clinical stage II is 80 per cent.

C. Depth of tumor invasion is predictive of regional node involvement and therefore of the value of prophylactic node excision in stage I disease.[4] Tumors with less than 1 mm. invasion rarely have node involvement and have a 100 per cent 5-year survival rate.[1, 2] Tumors with more than 1 mm. invasion have progressively increasing involvement of nodes and correspondingly worse prognosis.[23] There is no conclusive evidence that prophylactic excision of nodes improves survival in stage I disease.[6, 22] The following table shows survival with extremity lesions.[10, 24]

LEVEL	% WITH POSITIVE REGIONAL NODES	5-YEAR NED° SURVIVAL (%)
I Tumor above basement membrane	0	100
II Invasion of loose tissue of papillary dermis	0–5	95–100
III Tumor at junction of papillary and reticular dermis	10–20	80–85
IV Invasion of reticular dermis	30–40	65
V Invasion of subcutaneous tissue	50–70	20–30

° No evidence of disease.

D. Malignant melanoma may be classified into three types with different clinical characteristics, biologic behavior, and prognosis.[4]

TYPE	RELATIVE INCIDENCE (%)	MORTALITY (%)
Superficial spreading	55	30
Nodular	30	55
Lentigo maligna Malignant melanoma	15	10

Further prognostic variables include (1) location (in descending order of prognosis): (a) lower extremity, (b) upper extremity, (c) head and neck, (d) trunk, and (e) oropharynx, genitalia, and anorectum;[14, 19] (2) unknown site of primary (2 to 4 per cent of all cases), which usually presents with established metastases and poor prognosis;[5] (3) sex: women fare better than men; (4) size: lesions less than 3 cm. in diameter have a better prognosis than those greater than 3 cm; and (5) infiltration of capillaries and lymphatics at the site of the primary, which indicates poor prognosis.[9]

E. Nonspecific systemic immunotherapy in stage II disease is experimental. It appears occasionally to delay recurrence and may prolong survival.[8]

F. In-continuity mode dissection does not improve prognosis, nor does asynchronous wide excision and node dissection.[7]

G. The 30 to 40 per cent complication rate following groin dissection include necrosis of skin edges, lymph leakage, and leg edema.[12] Twenty per cent of patients undergoing node dissection develop stasis or "in transit" metastases. These metastases occur between the site of the primary excision and the site of the regional node dissection.[18]

H. The isolated limb is perfused with high concentrations of L-phenylalanine mustard, using hyperthermia to increase tumor cell destruction.[15, 21] Five-year survival in one series of stage I lesions was 85 per cent.[17]

I. Eighty per cent of all recurrences occur within the first 2 years. Melanoma has been known to recur, however, as many as 17 years following the original diagnosis.[14] (See Figure 1.)

J. Various drugs used for stage III disease include vinblastine, vincristine, BCNU, and DTIC. DTIC alone has a 20 per cent objective response rate (50 per cent reduction in tumor size for at least 1 month).[3] The combination of BCNU, vincristine, and DTIC has a 28 per cent response rate; however, the increased mor-

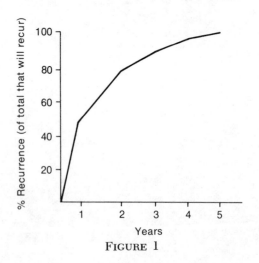

FIGURE 1

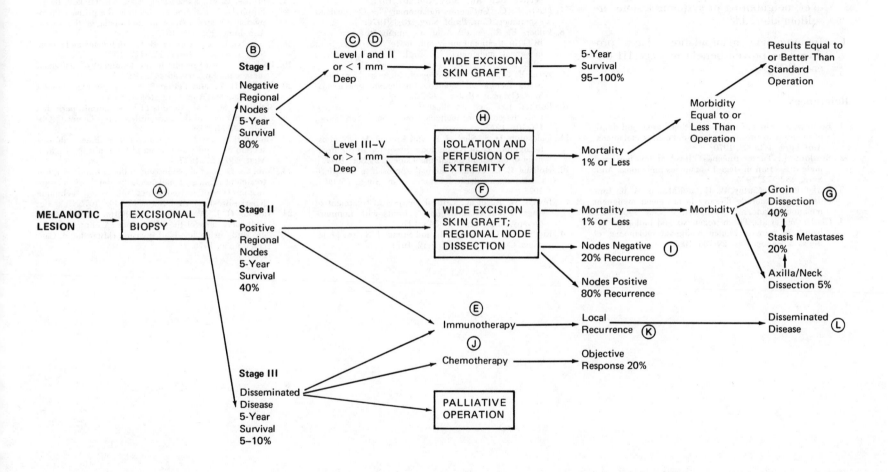

bidity of the added agents makes DTIC as a single drug the agent of choice.[16]

K. Recurrent lesions may regress when injected directly with BCG vaccine; however, neighboring or systemic lesions are seldom altered.[16]

L. Immunologic manipulations have produced no proven benefit in stage III disease.[13, 20]

References

1. Breslow, A.: Thickness, cross sectional area, and depth of invasion in the prognosis of cutaneous melanoma. Ann. Surg., 172:902, 1970.
2. Breslow, A.: Tumor thickness, level of invasion, and node dissection in stage I cutaneous melanoma. Ann. Surg., 182:572, 1975.
3. Burke, P. J., McCarthy, W. H., and Milton, M. B.: Imidazole carboxamide therapy in advanced malignant melanoma. Cancer, 27:744, 1971.
4. Clarke, W., et al.: The histogenesis and biological behavior of primary human malignant melanomas of the skin. Cancer Res., 29:705, 1969.
5. Das Gupta, T. K., Bowden, L., and Berg, J.: Malignant melanoma of unknown primary origin. Surg. Gynecol. Obstet., 117:341, 1963.
6. Das Gupta, T. K.: Results of treatment of 269 patients with primary cutaneous melanoma: A 5-year prospective study. Ann. Surg., 186:201, 1977.
7. Davis, N. C.: Cutaneous melanoma: The Queensland experience. Curr. Probl. Surg., 13:1, 1976.
8. Eilber, F. R., et al.: Adjuvant immunotherapy with BCG in treatment of lymph node metastases from malignant melanoma. N. Engl. J. Med., 294:237, 1976.
9. Elias, E. G., et al.: A clinicopathologic study of prognostic factors in cutaneous malignant melanoma. Surg. Gynecol. Obstet., 144:327, 1977.
10. Fortner, J. G., et al.: Biostatistical basis of elective node dissection for malignant melanoma. Ann. Surg., 186:101, 1977.
11. Goldsmith, H. S., Shah, J. P., and Kim, D. H.: Prognostic significance of lymph node dissection in the treatment of malignant melanoma. Cancer, 26:606, 1971.
12. Holmes, E. C., et al.: A rational approach to the surgical management of melanoma. Ann. Surg., 186:481, 1977.
13. Jewell, W. R., et al.: Critical analysis of treatment of stage II and III melanoma patients with immunotherapy. Ann. Surg., 183:543, 1976.
14. Knutson, C. O., Hori, J. M., and Spratt, J. S., Jr.: Melanoma. Curr. Probl. Surg., 8:12, 1971.
15. Krementz, E. T., and Ryan, R. F.: Chemotherapy of melanoma of the extremities by perfusion: 14 years' clinical experience. Ann. Surg., 175:900, 1972.
16. Luce, J. K.: Chemotherapy of malignant melanoma. Cancer, 30:1604, 1972.
17. McBride, C. M., Sugarbaker, E. V. and Hickey, R. C.: Prophylactic isolation-perfusion as the primary therapy for invasive malignant melanoma of the limbs. Ann. Surg., 182:316, 1975.
18. Moore, G. E., and Gerner, R. E.: Malignant melanoma. Surg. Gynecol. Obstet., 132:427, 1971.
19. Pack, G. T.: End results in the treatment of malignant melanoma. Surgery, 46:447, 1959.
20. Seigler, H. F., and Fetter, B. F.: Current management of melanoma. Ann. Surg., 186:1, 1977.
21. Stehlin, J. S., et al.: Results of hyperthermic perfusion for melanoma of the extremities. Surg. Gynecol. Obstet., 140:339, 1975.
22. Veronesi, U., et al.: Inefficacy of immediate node dissection in stage I melanoma of the limbs. N. Engl. J. Med., 297:627, 1977.
23. Wanebo, H. J., et al.: Selection of the optimum surgical treatment of stage I melanoma by depth of microinvasion: Use of the combined microstage technique (Clarke-Breslow). Ann. Surg., 182:302, 1975.
24. Wanebo, H. J., Woodruff, J., and Fortner, J. G.: Malignant melanoma of the extremities: A clinicopathologic study using levels of invasion (Microstage). Cancer, 35:666, 1975.

SOFT TISSUE SARCOMA

SOFT TISSUE SARCOMA BY S. REPLOGLE, M.D., AND R. GERNER, M.D.

Comments

A. These represent 1 to 2 per cent of all malignancies. Eighteen per cent[4] of patients have a second neoplasm that developed prior to the sarcoma and 50 per cent[5] develop a second neoplasm after the sarcoma. Cell type classification has been radically improved by electron microscopic studies. The commonest type of sarcoma in adults is now suggested to be malignant fibrous histiocytoma.[11]

B. The high rate of local recurrence excludes local excision alone.

C. Wide excision removes a 5 to 6 cm. 3-dimensional margin of normal tissue including the insertions of involved muscles and major vessels within the area, using grafts if necessary.[3] If the lesion is within 10 to 15 cm. of the regional nodes, regional lymphatic dissection is added.[5]

D. Thirty-three per cent of lesions are histologically sterilized by radiation (3000 to 4000 rads preoperatively or up to 6000 rads); 72 per cent of lesions regress at least 25 per cent. Liposarcoma is the most radiosensitive cell type.[7]

E. Amputation is the indicated treatment if wide excision (see Comment C) is not possible or feasible, as is the case in tumors near a joint.

F. Regional node dissection is performed when there are (1) clinically positive nodes, (2) nodal drainage within 10 to 15 cm. of primary, and (3) cell types (rhabdomyosarcoma and synovioma) that have a high rate of nodal spread.[4]

G. Factors affecting survival include (1) cell type: Fibrosarcoma has a 70 per cent 5-year survival rate versus a 45 per cent survival of 5 years or less for rhabdomyosarcoma and synovioma; (2) histologic grade (frequency of mitotic figures): The table shows prognosis related to grade.

GRADE	24 MONTHS DISEASE-FREE	5-YEAR SURVIVAL
I (Low)	86%	74%
II	51%	
III (High)	17%	20–46%

(3) Tumor size: Patients with tumors smaller than 5 cm. have a 63 to 67 per cent 5-year survival rate, compared with 35 to 46 per cent for tumors larger than 5 cm.; (4) location: In lesions of the thigh, the 5-year survival rate is 51 per cent; of the leg, 65 per cent; and of the foot, 75 per cent; (5) nodal involvement: With positive inguinal nodes, 5-year survival is 18 per cent;[6, 8-10] (6) other factors indicating poor prognosis include short tumor doubling time, involvement of skin or periosteum, and younger age of patient.

H. Fifty-six per cent of recurrences occur within one year and 85 per cent within two years. Of these, 59 per cent die of sarcoma.[1]

I. Eighty per cent of distant metastases are pulmonary or pleural; 71 per cent appear within one year and 82 per cent within two years.[4]

J. Repeated wide excision or amputation of the limb for local recurrence has the same probability of tumor recurrence as the original excision if the tumor is still localized. Because of the approximately 30 per cent likelihood of distant metastases after local recurrence, some physicians advise amputation instead of a second wide excision.[5]

K. Single-agent chemotherapy, including actinomycin D, vincristine, and cyclophosphamide, has a response rate of 15 to 20 per cent.
Response to DTIC is 18 per cent and to Adriamycin, 28 per cent
Combined therapy with DTIC and Adriamycin has a 10 to 50 per cent response rate.[2]

L. If the primary tumor is controlled, pulmonary resection of a metastasis or metastases may be indicated if these are the only metastases, if pulmonary function is adequate, and if the tumor doubling time is more than 40 days.[6]

M. Radiation therapy may provide various degrees of tumor regression and pain relief in patients with nonresectable tumors, particularly liposarcomas and rhabdomyosarcomas.[2]

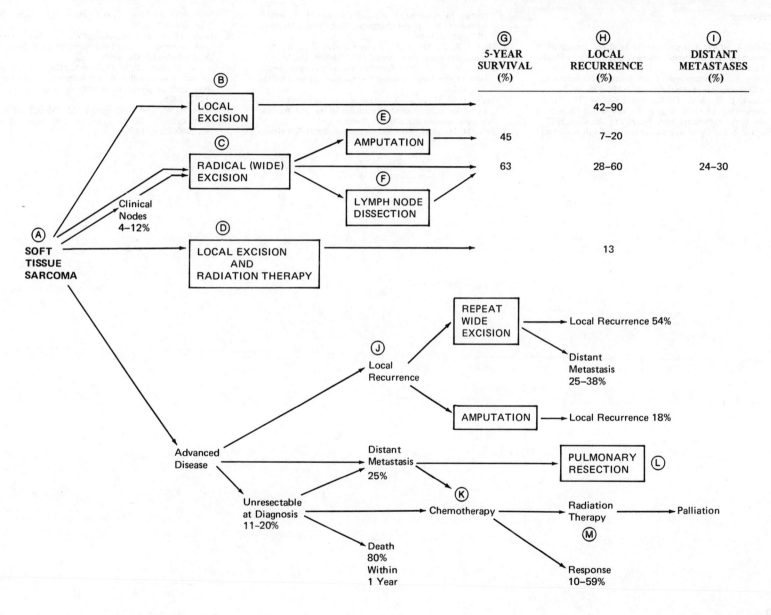

SOFT TISSUE SARCOMA *Continued*

References

1. Cantin, J., et al.: The problem of local recurrence after treatment of soft tissue sarcoma. Ann. Surg., *168*:47–53, 1968.
2. Chang, P.: Management of soft tissue sarcomas: Current status. Am. J. Med. Sci., *273*:244–258, 1977.
3. Fortner, J. G., Kim, D. K., and Shin, M. H.: Limb-preserving vascular surgery for malignant tumors of the lower extremity. Arch. Surg., *112*:391–394, 1977.
4. Fortner, J. G.: Operative management of soft tissue sarcomas. *In* Najarian, J. S., and Delaney, J. P. (eds.): Advances in Cancer Surgery. New York, Stratton, 1976, pp. 393–399.
5. Gerner, R. E., Moore, G. E., and Pickerell, J. W.: Soft tissue sarcomas. Ann. Surg., *181*:803–808, 1975.
6. Joseph, W. L.: Criteria for resection of sarcoma metastatic to the lung. Cancer Chemother. Rep., *58*:285–290, 1974.
7. McNeer, G. P., et al.: Effectiveness of radiation therapy in the management of sarcoma of the soft somatic tissues. Cancer, *22*:390–397, 1968.
8. Shin, M. H., et al.: Surgical treatment of 297 soft tissue sarcomas of the lower extremity. Ann. Surg., *182*:597–602, 1975.
9. Simon, M. A., and Enneking, W. F.: Management of soft tissue sarcomas of the extremities. J. Bone Joint Surg., *58A*:317–327, 1976.
10. Snit, H. D., Russell, W. O., and Martin, R. G.: Sarcoma of soft tissue: Clinical and histopathologic parameters and response to treatment. Cancer, *35*:1478–1483, 1975.
11. Weiss, S. W., and Enzinger, F. M.: Malignant fibrous histiocytoma: An analysis of 200 cases. Cancer, *41*:2250–2266, 1978.

HODGKIN'S DISEASE

HODGKIN'S DISEASE BY WINONA MACKEY, M.D.

Comments

A. Diagnosis is based on the identification of Sternberg-Reed cells according to the Rye classification, which correlates with stage and has prognostic significance.[1, 2]

B. Ann Arbor staging classification in Hodgkin's disease is as follows:

Stage I: Involvement of a single lymph node region (I) or of a single extralymphatic organ or site (I_E).

Stage II: Involvement of two or more lymph node regions or of an extralymphatic organ or site on the same side of the diaphragm (II_E).

Stage III: Involvement of lymph node regions on both sides of the diaphragm (III); may be accompanied by involvement of the spleen (III_S) or by localized involvement of an extralymphatic organ or site (III_E) or both (III_{SE}).

Stage IV: Diffuse or disseminated involvement of one or more extralymphatic organs or tissues, with or without associated lymph node involvement.

An *A* suffix indicates no systemic symptoms. A *B* suffix indicates fever above 38° C, night sweats or unexplained loss of 10 per cent or more of body weight in the 6 months preceding diagnosis, or a combination of these.[3]

C. The lymphangiogram is valuable and should be used prior to the staging laparotomy to detect para-aortic disease, for continued surveillance of the area, and for the delineation of the radiotherapeutic fields.[4, 5]

D. Vascular invasion in the spleen (20 per cent of cases) and, questionably, in the lymph nodes (6 to 14 per cent) is associated with early relapse, bone marrow involvement, and shortened survival. It may indicate disseminated extranodal disease. Its significance is under investigation.[6, 7]

E. Exploratory laparotomy is a valuable adjunct to modern drug therapy because it alters therapy in one third of patients. About 25 per cent of patients with clinically negative spleens actually have involvement. Evaluation of lymph nodes and liver may be incorrect 31 per cent and 12 per cent of the time, respectively. Lymph nodes outside the traditional radiation portals (mesenteric and porta hepatis) may be involved with tumor 7 per cent of the time.[2, 4, 8, 9]

F. Significant morbidity associated with exploratory laparotomy includes infection, wound dehiscence, and thrombophlebitis more than 9 per cent of the time and more severe complications, such as pulmonary embolism, ulcers with GI hemorrhage, and problems requiring re-exploration, in 2.2 per cent of cases. Approximately 0.5 per cent of complications contribute to death. The overall complication rate is 12.8 per cent.[2, 9]

G. Splenectomy is reported to increase hematopoietic tolerance to radiotherapy and perhaps to chemotherapy.[4]

H. General principles of radiotherapy for Hodgkin's disease are (1) 3500 to 4000 rads in 3½ to 4½ weeks is the required tumoricidal dose. (2) Local involved fields may be used for stage I_A or II_A high cervical or mediastinum-limited nodes or for inguinal or femoral nodes only (lymphocytic or nodular sclerosis type) when results of lymphangiogram and exploratory laparotomy are negative. (3) Extended fields or total nodal radiation is used for other situations except stage IV disease, for which chemotherapy or a combination is used.[10]

I. No difference in survival rates between the use of localized and extended fields of radiation has been shown in stage I or II disease. More local recurrences are seen when localized fields are used; and more complications (about twice as many) occur when extended fields are used.[11, 12]

J. Major complications of radiotherapy include (1) radiation pneumonitis (6 to 10 per cent), (2) pericarditis (6 to 7 per cent), (3) myelitis (0.15 per cent), (4) thyroid abnormalities (13 per cent), (5) sustained marrow depression (approximately 1 per cent), and (6) Lhermitte's syndrome (11 per cent). Acute morbidity includes nausea, vomiting, anorexia, diarrhea, dysphagia, and fatigue.[5, 10]

K. Multiple drug chemotherapy, especially MOPP, has improved complete remission rates from 10 to 30 per cent with single agents to 60 to 80 per cent, with duration of remission in excess of 3 years.[13, 14]

L. Relapses occur in 30 to 60 per cent of

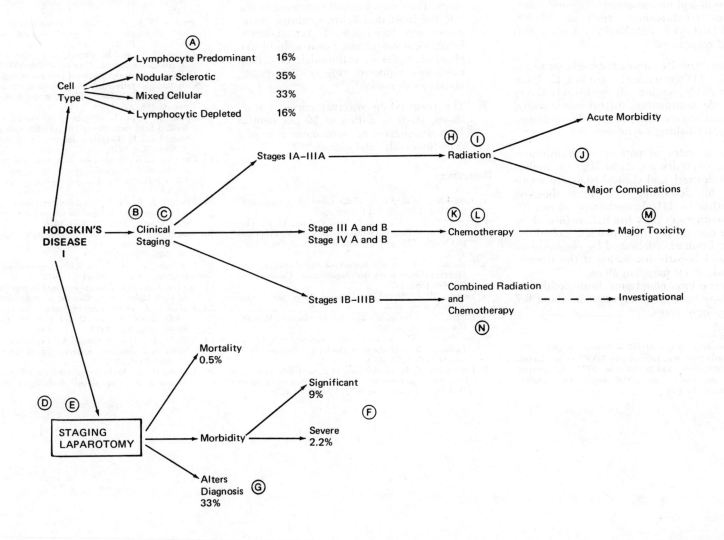

Ⓐ
Lymphocyte Predominant 16%
Nodular Sclerotic 35%
Mixed Cellular 33%
Lymphocytic Depleted 16%

Cell
Type

HODGKIN'S
DISEASE
I

Ⓑ Ⓒ
Clinical
Staging

Stages IA–IIIA

Stage III A and B
Stage IV A and B

Stages IB–IIIB

Ⓗ Ⓘ
Radiation

Ⓐcute Morbidity

Major Complications
Ⓙ

Ⓚ Ⓛ
Chemotherapy

Major Toxicity
Ⓜ

Combined Radiation
and
Chemotherapy

Investigational

Ⓝ

Ⓓ Ⓔ
STAGING
LAPAROTOMY

Mortality
0.5%

Morbidity

Significant
9%

Severe
2.2%

Ⓕ

Alters
Diagnosis
33%
Ⓖ

cases, and emphasis at the present is on determining the optimum duration of remission and on increasing response rates. Other combinations, such as MVPP, ABVD, CAVe and MOPP*, have given good responses.[10]

M. Major toxicity from chemotherapy includes (1) nausea and vomiting, (2) bone marrow depression, (3) cystitis, (4) alopecia, (5) neuropathy, (6) cardiomyopathy, (7) pulmonary fibrosis, (8) GI symptoms, and (9) Cushing's syndrome.[5, 10]

N. Relapse rates of patients with intermediate stage disease (I_B to III_B) are higher than desired, and clinical trials are ongoing to determine the best therapy, whether by (1) chemotherapy alone, (2) chemotherapy plus irradiation (low dose to areas of previous disease), (3) high dose irradiation followed by chemotherapy and hepatic irradiation if the liver is at risk, or (4) radiation alone.

Secondary neoplasms from combined therapy have been reported in about 9.7 per cent of cases.[15, 16]

*Chemotherapy agents: MOPP = Mustargen (HN_2), Oncovin, procarbazine, and prednisone; MVPP = Mustargen, Velban, procarbazine, and prednisone; ABVD = Adriamycin, bleomycin, Velban, and DTIC; and CAVe = CCNU, Adriamycin, and Velban.

O. Relapses generally occur early: 87 per cent within 3 years and 97 per cent by 5 years. They may be true recurrences (inside the irradiated field); marginal recurrences (on the edge of the irradiated field); local extensions (same side of diaphragm), nodal or extranodal; or distant extensions (opposite side of diaphragm), nodal or extranodal.[17-19]

P. The relapse-free survival curve, for all stages, starts to flatten at 50 per cent at 10 years, suggesting permanent cure of a once invariably fatal illness.[10, 20]

References

1. Lukes, R. J., et al.: Report of the nomenclature committee. Cancer Res. 26:1311, 1966.
2. Young, R. C., Anderson, T., and DeVita, V. T.: The treatment of Hodgkin's disease. *In* Current Problems in Cancer. Chicago, Year Book Medical Publishers, 1977.
3. Carbone, P. P., et al.: Report of the committee on Hodgkin's disease staging classification. Cancer Res., 31:1860–1861, 1971.
4. Lacher, M. J.: Hodgkin's Disease. New York, John Wiley & Sons, 1976.
5. Kaplan, H. S.: Hodgkin's Disease. Cambridge, Harvard University Press, 1972.
6. Kirschner, R. H., et al.: Vascular invasion and hematogenous dissemination of Hodgkin's disease. Cancer, 34:1159–1162, 1974.
7. Lamoureax, K. B., et al.: Lack of identifiable vascular invasion in patients with extranodal dissemination of Hodgkin's disease. Cancer, 31:824–825, 1973.
8. Piro, A. J., Hellman, S., and Moloney, W. C.: The influence of laparotomy on management decisions in Hodgkin's disease. Arch. Intern. Med., 130:844, 1972.
9. Meeker, W. R., et al.: Critical evaluation of laparotomy and splenectomy in Hodgkin's disease. Arch. Surg., 1:105, Aug, 1972.
10. Kaplan, H. S., and Rosenberg, S. A.: The management of Hodgkin's disease. Cancer, 36:796–803, 1975.
11. Collaborative study: Survival and complications of radiotherapy following involved and extended field therapy of Hodgkin's disease, stages I and II. Cancer, 38:288–305, 1976.
12. Miller, J. B., et al.: Results of involved field and extended field radiotherapy in patients with pathologic stage I and II Hodgkin's disease. Am. J. Roentgenol., 127:833–839, 1976.
13. Prosnitz, L. R., et al.: Low dose radiation therapy and combination chemotherapy in the treatment of advanced Hodgkin's disease. Radiology, 107:187–193, 1973.
14. Prosnitz, L. R., et al.: Long term remissions with combined modality therapy for advanced Hodgkin's disease. Cancer, 37:2826–2833, 1976.
15. Rosenberg, S. A., et al.: Combination chemotherapy and radiotherapy for Hodgkin's disease. Cancer, 30:1505–1510, 1972.
16. Goodman, R., et al.: Results of continued modality treatment. Cancer, 40:84–89, 1977.
17. Weller, S. A., et al.: Initial relapses in previously treated Hodgkin's disease. Cancer, 37:2840–2846, 1976.
18. Weller, S. A., et al.: Initial relapse in previously treated Hodgkin's disease, II. Int. J. Radiat. Oncol. Biol. Phys., 2:863–872, 1977.
19. Mill, W. B., et al.: Extended field radiation therapy in Hodgkin's disease: Analysis of failures. Cancer, 40:2896–2904, 1977.
20. Kaplan, H. S.: Multidisciplinary contributions to the conquest of a neoplasm. Radiology, 123:551–558, 1977.

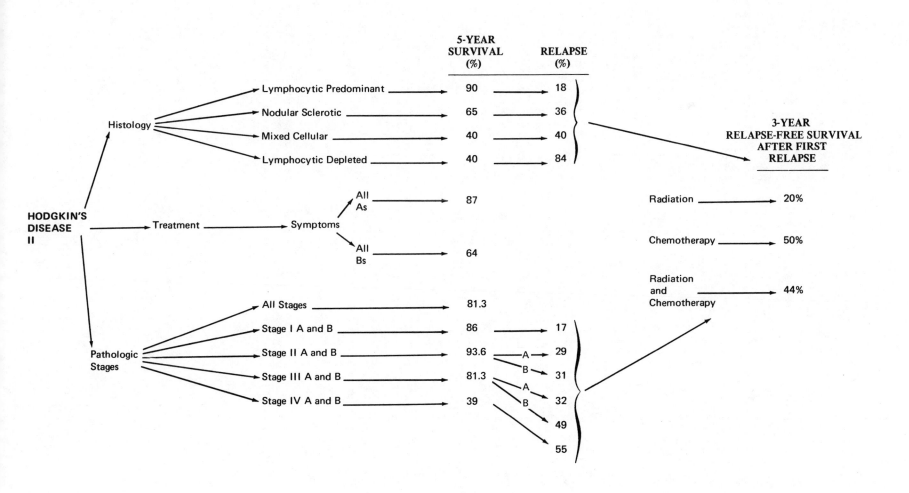

Section **K**

Urologic

WILMS' TUMOR BY RICHARD R. AUGSPURGER, M.D.

Comments

A. Wilms' tumor has an incidence 0.8 to 1 case per 100,000 live births. Female children are affected more often than male children, and 90 per cent of cases occur before age 10. Associated diseases include aniridia (1 to 2 per cent), hemihypertrophy (3 per cent), and GU anomalies (4 to 7 per cent).[3, 4, 6, 8, 10]

B. Prognosis depends on three variables: age, grade, and stage.[2, 3, 5, 6, 10-12]

C. Mesoblastic nephroma should be differentiated from Wilms' tumor. It occurs in children less than 6 months old and is benign.[4]

D. Since 92 per cent of deaths or recurrences occur within 2 years, survival is based on 2-year disease-free status.[1]

E. No standardized grading system has been adopted, although prognosis is dependent on this variable.[1-3, 10, 12]
   Grade I: Well differentiated. Parenchyma has well formed tubules and glomeruli constituting $\geq$ 50 per cent of the tumor; myxomatous stroma; few spindle cells.
   Grade II: Moderately well differentiated. Less than 50 per cent of the tumor has parenchymal elements; poorly formed tubules; abortive glomeruli; myxomatous stroma and increased spindle cells.
   Grade III: Poorly differentiated. Spindle cells predominate; little parenchymatous differentiation; rare abortive glomeruli and tubular elements.

F. The national Wilms' tumor study staging system is as follows:[4]
   Group I: Tumor limited to kidney; capsule intact.
   Group II: Tumor extends beyond kidney or into blood vessels, including the vena cava, but does not involve adjacent organs or regional lymph nodes; completely resectable.
   Group III: Residual nonhematogenous tumor confined to the abdomen but not involving the liver; includes those ruptured during operation; incompletely resectable.
   Group IV: Hematogenous metastasis (lung, liver, bone, or brain).
   Group V: Bilateral renal involvement.

G. Preoperative radiation therapy is advocated by Lemerle[9, 10, 12, 13] because of the decreased incidence of tumor spillage at surgery. However, a 5 per cent incidence[6, 7] of preoperative error in diagnosis is the reason it is not employed routinely in the United States.

H. Radical nephrectomy, with biopsy of lymph nodes and visual exploration of the opposite kidney, is the primary treatment and has a mortality rate of 1 per cent.[1, 15]

I. Combination chemotherapy with vincristine and actinomycin D is more effective than either agent alone. Adriamycin is added in treating groups III and IV. Preoperative chemotherapy has not been efficacious.[6]

J. Radiation therapy to the tumor bed in group II disease and to the entire abdomen in groups III and IV disease is employed.[5, 6, 9, 10, 13] Local radiation in "localized" group III disease is as effective as radiation to the entire abdomen.

K. A 3 per cent mortality rate is associated with combined radiation and chemotherapy.[6]

L. Group I patients who are more than two years old may benefit from postoperative radiation therapy.[6]

M. Bilateral Wilms' tumor requires individualization of treatment, employing complete resection of the tumor with combinations of nephrectomy — partial nephrectomy or bilateral partial nephrectomy — followed by chemotherapy and radiation therapy. If the tumor is unresectable, biopsy only, followed by a 2 to 3 month course of chemotherapy and radiotherapy, is the treatment used. At that point, a "second look" operation and attempts at resection have yielded good results.[14]

References

1. Beckwith, T. B., et al.: Histopathology and prognosis of Wilms' tumor: Results from the first National Wilms' Tumor Study. Cancer, 41:1937, 1978.
2. Kheir, S., et al.: Histologic grading of Wilms' tumor as a potential prognostic factor: Results of retrospective study of 26 patients. Cancer, 41:1199, 1978.
3. Breslow, N. E., et al.: Wilms' tumor: Prognostic factors for patients without metastases at diagnosis. Result of

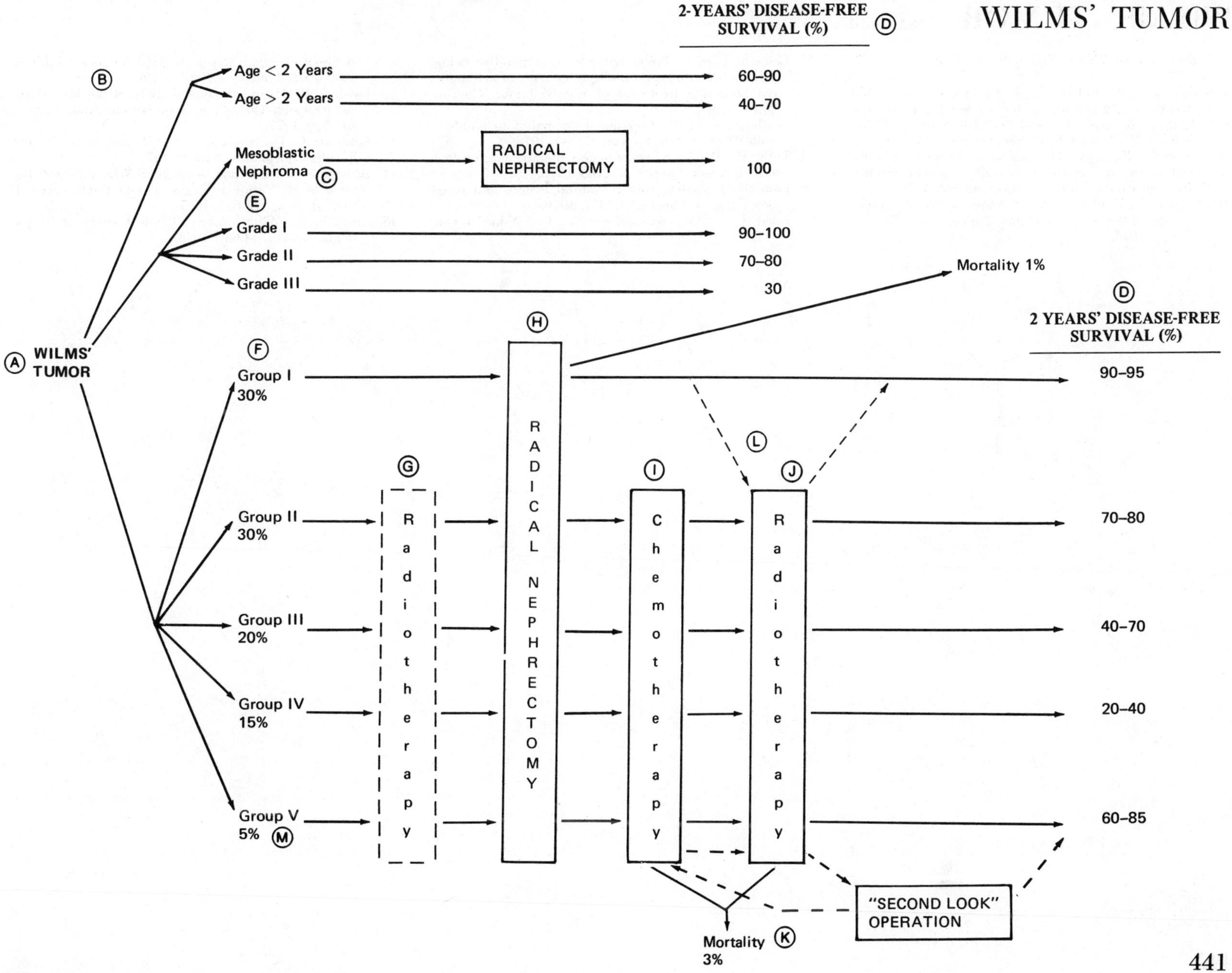

WILMS' TUMOR

2-YEARS' DISEASE-FREE SURVIVAL (%) Ⓓ

Age < 2 Years	60–90
Age > 2 Years	40–70

Ⓑ

Mesoblastic Nephroma Ⓒ → RADICAL NEPHRECTOMY → 100

Ⓔ

Grade I	90–100
Grade II	70–80
Grade III	30

Ⓐ WILMS' TUMOR

Mortality 1%

Ⓓ 2 YEARS' DISEASE-FREE SURVIVAL (%)

Ⓕ Group I 30% → 90–95

Ⓗ RADICAL NEPHRECTOMY

Ⓖ Radiotherapy

Ⓘ Chemotherapy

Ⓙ Radiotherapy

Ⓛ

Group II 30%	70–80
Group III 20%	40–70
Group IV 15%	20–40
Group V 5% Ⓜ	60–85

"SECOND LOOK" OPERATION

Mortality 3% Ⓚ

441

the National Wilms' Tumor Study. Cancer, *41*:1577, 1978.

4. Gilchrist, G. S., and Kelalis, P. P.: Tumors and related disorders: Kidney and ureter. *In* Kelalis, P. P., and King, L. R. (eds.): Clinical Pediatric Urology. Philadelphia, W. B. Saunders, 1976, pp. 896–915.

5. Cassady, J. R., et al.: The increasing importance of radiation therapy in the improved prognosis of children with Wilms' tumor. Cancer, *39*:825, 1977.

6. D'Angio, G. J., et al.: The treatment of Wilms' tumor: Results of the National Wilms' Tumor Study. Cancer, *38*:633, 1976.

7. Lemerle, J., et al.: Preoperative vs. postoperative radiotherapy and single vs. multiple courses of actinomycin D in the treatment of Wilms' tumor. Cancer, *38*:647, 1976.

8. Pendergrass, T. W.: Congenital anomalies in children with Wilms' tumor. Cancer, *37*:403, 1976.

9. Tefft, M.: Postoperative radiation therapy for residual Wilms' tumor. Cancer, *37*:2768, 1976.

10. Lemerle, J.: Wilms' tumor: Natural history and prognostic factors. Cancer, *37*:2557, 1976.

11. Bond, J. V.: Prognosis and treatment of Wilms' tumor at Great Ormond Street Hospital for Sick Children, 1960–1972. Cancer, *36*:1202, 1975.

12. Lawler, W.: Histopathological study of the first Medical Research Council nephroblastoma trial. Cancer, *40*:1519, 1977.

13. Lemerle, J.: The management of Wilms' tumor. Recent Results Cancer Res., *62*:206, 1977.

14. Bishop, H. C.: Survival in bilateral Wilms' tumor: Review of 30 National Wilms' Tumor Study cases. J. Pediatr. Surg., *12*:631, 1977.

15. Aron, B. S.: Wilms' tumor: Clinical study of 81 patients. Cancer, *33*:637, 1974.

NEUROBLASTIC TUMORS

NEUROBLASTIC TUMORS BY RICHARD R. AUGSPURGER, M.D.

Comments

A. *Neuroblastoma* is a term often used to encompass the spectrum of neurocrest tumors.[7]

B. The apparent increased survival with thoracic and other sites is probably due to earlier recognition. For a given stage, anatomic location does not alter prognosis.[1, 3, 5] Tumor has an abdominal site in 60 per cent of cases (40 per cent adrenal and 20 per cent in other abdominal sites), a thoracic site in 15 per cent, and other sites in 25 per cent.

C. Ganglioneuromas are benign; 25 per cent are found incidentally at autopsy.[7]

D. Ganglioneuroblastoma is less malignant than neuroblastoma; however, stage for stage the prognosis is similar.[7]

E. Neuroblastoma has a high rate of spontaneous regression. Surgical removal of the primary tumor seems to promote spontaneous regression.[7, 8, 12, 13, 15]

F. Thirty per cent of patients present with surgically excisable nonmetastatic lesions.

G. Surgical excision has a mortality rate of 6 per cent and an unreported incidence of morbidity.[14]

H. Radiotherapy is employed for residual tumor (macroscopic in stages III and IV and microscopic in stage III and possibly in stage II) and palliation (stage IV). No increase in survival has been noted in stage II disease.[1, 2, 6, 7, 9]

I. Chemotherapy has not improved survival rates but has prolonged remission times. It is recommended for treating residual tumor (stage III and possibly II) and metastatic disease (stage IV) and for decreasing the size of unresectable tumors (stages III and IV). Primary agents, used alone or in combination, include Cytoxan, vincristine, DTIC, Adriamycin, and nitrogen mustard.[4, 7, 10, 11]

J. Staging of neuroblastoma is as follows:[3]
Stage I: Tumor contained in organ of origin.
Stage II. Tumor in continuity but beyond organ of origin and not across the midline; regional nodes may be involved.
Stage III: Tumor extends in continuity across the midline; bilateral regional nodes affected.
Stage IV: Disseminated disease.
Stage IVs: Disseminated disease without cortical bone involvement.

K. Prognosis depends on the stage of tumor and the age of the patient.[1-5, 10-13]

TWO YEARS' DISEASE-FREE SURVIVAL (%)

STAGE	<1 Year Old	1–2 Years Old	>2 Years Old	Overall
I	80–100	75–90	50–70	80
II	70–90	40–70	30–50	60
III	30–50	20–50	10–20	30
IV	10–20	0–5	0–5	5
IVs	90	30–50	30–40	75
Overall	70	25	10	25

L. Stage IVs is a special category, usually occurring in patients younger than 1 year old. It has a high incidence of spontaneous regression and a survival rate between those of stages I and II. Surgical excision is recommended. Radiotherapy and adjunctive chemotherapy are employed, depending on the clinical response of the patient and age.

M. No data are available to evaluate the results of "second look" surgical exploration and resection.

References

1. Gilchrist, G. S., and Tank, E. S.: Tumors of the adrenal medulla and sympathetic chain. *In* Kelalis, P. P. and King, L. R. (eds.): Clinical Pediatric Urology, Philadelphia, W. B. Saunders, 1976, pp. 975–987.
2. Leape, L. L.: Diagnosis and management of Wilms' tumors and neuroblastomas. *In* Skinner, D. G. and deKernion, J. B.: Genitourinary Cancer. Philadelphia, W. B. Saunders, 1978, pp. 179–199.
3. Evans, A. E., et al.: A proposed staging for children with neuroblastoma. Cancer, 27:374, 1971.
4. Evans, A. E., et al.: Cyclophosphamide treatment of patients with localized and regional neuroblastoma. Cancer, 38:655, 1976.
5. Evans, A. E., et al.: Factors influencing survival of children with nonmetastatic neuroblastoma. Cancer, 38:661, 1976.
6. Evans, A. E.: Diagnosis and treatment of neuroblastoma. Pediatr. Clin. North Am., 23:161, 1976.
7. Hassenbusch, S., et al.: Prognostic factors in neuroblastic tumors. J. Pediatr. Surg., 11:287, 1976.
8. Bernstein, I. D.: Immunology and immunotherapy of childhood neoplasia. Pediatr. Clin. North Am., 23:102, 1976.
9. Koop, C. E. et al.: The management of abdominal neuroblastoma. Cancer, 35:905, 1975.
10. Leikin, S.: The impact of chemotherapy on advanced neuroblastoma. Survival of patients in 1956, 1962, 1966–68 in children's cancer study. A. J. Pediatr., 84:131, 1974.
11. Grosfeld, J. L.: Metastatic neuroblastoma factors influencing survival. J. Pediatr. Surg., 13:59, 1978.
12. Jaffe, N.: Neuroblastoma: Review of the literature and examination of factors contributing to its enigmatic character. Cancer Treat. Rev., 3:61, 1976.
13. Kinner, L. M. K., et al.: Neuroblastoma: Its natural history and prognosis. A study of 487 cases. Br. Med. J., 3:301, 1974.
14. Koop, C. E., et al.: Neuroblastoma: An assessment of therapy in reference to staging. J. Pediatr. Surg., 6:595, 1971.
15. Marcus, R.: Present strategy of treatment of neuroblastoma. Recent Results Cancer Res., 62:210, 1977.

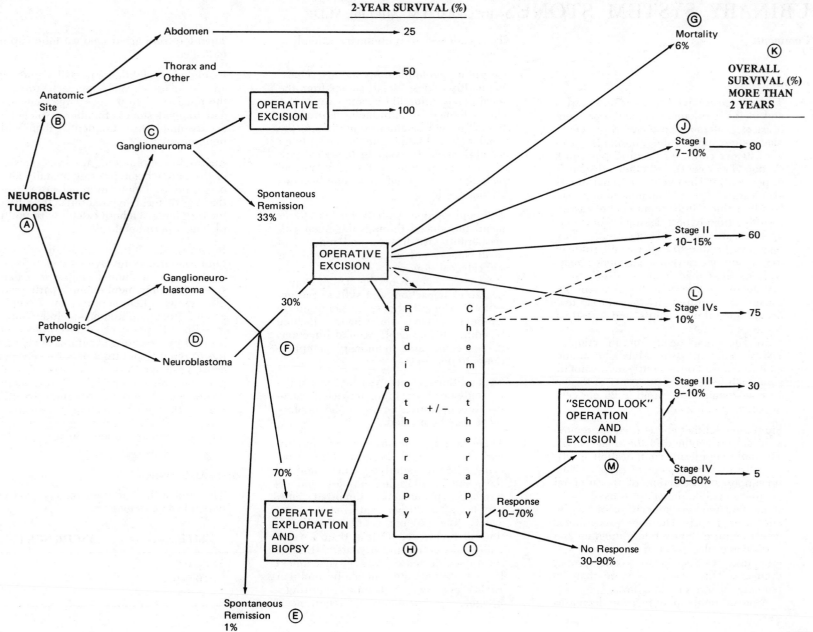

2-YEAR SURVIVAL (%)

Abdomen → 25

Thorax and Other → 50

OPERATIVE EXCISION → 100

NEUROBLASTIC TUMORS

Ⓐ

Anatomic Site Ⓑ

Ⓒ Ganglioneuroma

Spontaneous Remission 33%

Pathologic Type

Ganglioneuro-blastoma

Ⓓ

Neuroblastoma

30%

Ⓕ

70%

OPERATIVE EXCISION

Spontaneous Remission 1% Ⓔ

OPERATIVE EXPLORATION AND BIOPSY

Radiotherapy Ⓗ

+ / −

Chemotherapy Ⓘ

Response 10–70%

No Response 30–90%

"SECOND LOOK" OPERATION AND EXCISION Ⓜ

Ⓖ Mortality 6%

Ⓚ OVERALL SURVIVAL (%) MORE THAN 2 YEARS

Ⓙ Stage I 7–10% → 80

Stage II 10–15% → 60

Ⓛ Stage IVs 10% → 75

Stage III 9–10% → 30

Stage IV 50–60% → 5

445

URINARY SYSTEM STONES BY GERALD M. MILLER, M.D.

Comments

RENAL STONES

A. The composition of renal stones varies and includes calcium oxalate (73 per cent of cases), calcium phosphate (8 per cent), magnesium ammonium phosphate (struvite) (9 per cent), uric acid (7 per cent), cystine (1 per cent), and other substances (2 per cent).[19] The etiology of renal stones also varies.[2, 4, 5, 8, 12] Calcium stones may be idiopathic (70 to 80 per cent of cases), resulting from hypercalciuria (30 per cent) or hyperuricosuria (25 per cent). They may also be due to hyperparathyroidism (5 per cent of cases) or to anatomic abnormalities (less than 5 per cent of cases).

Calcium oxalate stones[12] may result because of acquired hyperoxaluria that occurs after ileitis, colitis, and intestinal bypass surgery.[9]

Struvite stones result from infection in 100 per cent of cases. Metabolic abnormalities cause 60 per cent[20] and anatomic abnormalities cause 5 per cent[12] of these. Uric acid stones are found in 25 per cent of patients with gout.

B. Simple pyelolithotomy is used for removal of calculi confined to the renal pelvis. The only significant complication is urinary fistula (25 per cent of cases).[13] This presupposes obstruction of the ureteral or ureteropelvic junction caused by a stone fragment or stenosis secondary to edema or fibrosis. Drainage exceeding 2 weeks requires an excretory urogram and cystoscopic placement of a ureteral catheter into the pelvis to assure proper drainage. This results in more than 95 per cent closure in 2 to 3 days.

A dorsal lumbotomy incision decreases the incidence of pulmonary complications.

C. Coagulum pyelolithotomy aids in removing multiple loose, small stones from the renal pelvis, infundibula, and calyces.[14] A clot is formed by introducing fibrinogen, thrombin, and calcium chloride into the renal pelvis. Plasma can be substituted for fibrinogen. Incision in the renal pelvis is made to remove the resultant gel with the encased calculi. Complications are negligible.

D. The nephroscope (with Water-Pik attachment) introduced through the renal pelvis permits visualization and removal of small, loose, and impacted infundibular and calyceal stones.

Success depends on the size of stones, degree of impaction, and skill of the operator.[21] Complications, in addition to failure to remove the calculus, include bleeding (10 per cent), wound infections (2 per cent), and pulmonary complications (10 per cent).

E. Nephrolithotomy involves incision of the renal tissue down to an impacted calculus. Intraoperative x-rays or the nephroscope may be needed.

F. There is a high recurrence rate for urinary tract calculi because they have many different underlying causes and are the result of multiple, complex, and interrelated phenomena. Reported rates vary from 9 to 80 per cent,[1] but the average is 40 to 50 per cent.[7, 10-12] Average time of recurrence is less than 7 years with peaks at 1.5 and 8 years.[2, 7] Risk of recurrence decreases year by year unless there is an untreated metabolic problem. Eighty per cent of patients requiring a lithotomy[2, 12] develop a recurrence.[10]

Therefore prolonged medical followup is indicated.

G. Extended pyelolithotomy (Gil-Vernet) is an extraparenchymal approach through the renal sinus to remove large branched and trapped stones. Significant bleeding occurs much less frequently than with nephrotomy.[16]

H. Anatrophic nephrotomy involves incision of the parenchyma intersegmentally after occlusion of the main renal artery and the use of local hypothermia. It is used for very large staghorn calculi with multiple small peripheral calculi.[15]

I. Removal of multiple impacted or staghorn calculi may involve various types of nephrotomy, including simple or extensive anatrophic nephrotomy, partial nephrectomy, or heminephrectomy. Complications from nephrotomy include initial bleeding (15 per cent), delayed bleeding (caused by loosening of sutures or sloughing of renal tissue from necrosis) (10 per cent), prolonged urine drainage (15 to 25 per cent), retained calculi (approximately 25 per cent), recurrence of stones (15 to 25 per cent), wound infection (5 per cent), progressive renal failure (2 per cent), and pulmonary complications (30 per cent).[13, 15]

URETERAL STONES

J. The probability of spontaneous passage depends on diameter.

SIZE (cm.)	INCIDENCE (%)
<0.5	80
0.5–0.8	15
>0.8	5

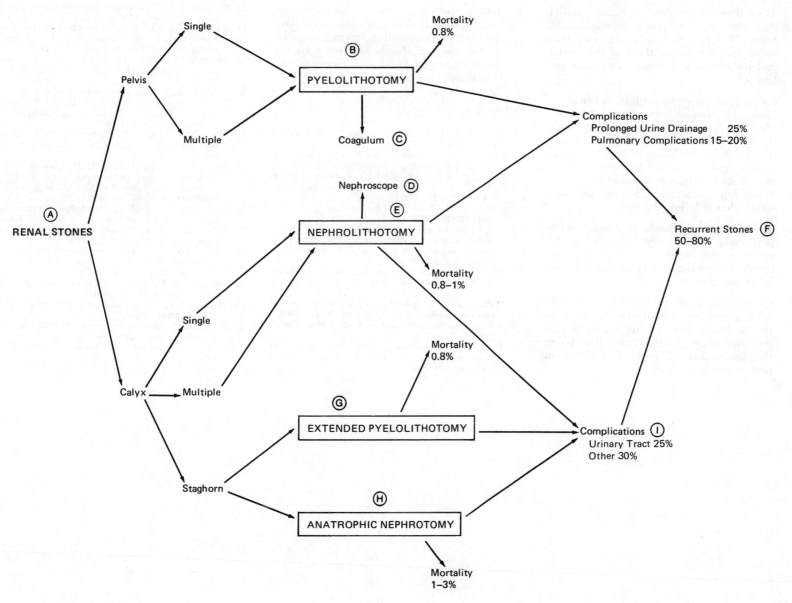

More than 95 per cent of stones smaller than 0.5 cm. will pass spontaneously. Stones 0.5 to 0.8 cm. in diameter may move into the lower third of the ureter and be amenable to endoscopic manipulation.

K. Indications for open surgical removal include (1) stones larger than 0.8 cm., (2) *impacted* stones of any size above the true bony pelvis, (3) unsuccessful attempts at manipulation of lower ureteral calculi, and (4) disease processes rendering basket extraction impossible, e.g., fused hips, urethral stricture, and ureteral stricture below the stone.

L. The surgical approach is usually extraperitoneal. The choice of incision depends on the location of the stone in the ureter. Hospitalization is for about 7 days following surgery.

M. Cystoscopic stone manipulation is limited to stones less than 0.8 cm. in diameter in the lower third of the ureter within the true bony pelvis. Above that point, the probability of ureteral avulsion or perforation is too high.

N. The probability of successful endoscopic stone removal depends upon stone size, amount of surrounding edema, and skill of the operator. The newer stone baskets have improved yield and reduced complications.

References

1. Malek, R. S.: Renal lithiasis: A practical approach. J. Urol., *118*:893, 1977.
2. Coe, F. L., Keck, J., and Norton, E.: The natural history of calcium urolithiasis. JAMA, *238*:1519, 1977.
3. Furlow, W. L., and Bucchiere, J. J.: Surgical fate of ureteral calculi: Review of Mayo Clinic experience. J. Urol., *116*:559, 1976.
4. Epstein, F. H.: Time to cut for the stone. N. Engl. J. Med., *298*:105, 1978.
5. Coe, F. L.: Treated and untreated recurrent calcium nephrolithiasis in patients with idiopathic hypercalciuria, hyperuricosuria or no metabolic disorder. Ann. Intern. Med., *87*:404, 1977.
6. Sleight, M. W., and Wickham, J.: Long-term followup of 100 cases of renal calculi. Br. J. Urol., *49*:601, 1977.
7. Williams, R. E.: Long-term survey of 538 patients with upper urinary tract stone. Br. J. Urol., *35*:416, 1963.
8. Williams, H.: Nephrolithiasis. N. Engl. J. Med., *290*:33, 1974.
9. Piuto, B., and Bernshtam, J.: Diethylaminoethanol cellulose in treatment of absorptive hyperoxaluria. J. Urol., *119*:630, 1978.
10. Williams, R. E.: The results of conservative surgery for stone. Br. J. Urol., *44*:292, 1972.
11. Almby, B., Meirik, O., and Schönebeck, J.: Incidence, morbidity and complications of renal and ureteral calculi. Scand. J. Urol. Nephrol., *9*:249, 1975.
12. Marshall, V., White, R. H., and Blandy, J. P.: Natural history of renal and ureteral calculi. Br. J. Urol., *47*:117, 1975.
13. Smith, D. R., Schulte, J. W., and Smart, W. K.: Surgery of the kidney. *In* Campbell M. F., and Harrison, J. H. (eds.): Urology, 3rd ed. Vol. 3. Philadelphia, W. B. Saunders, 1970, p. 2143.
14. Marshall, S., Lyon, R. P., and Scott, M. P., Jr.: Further simplifications for coagulum pyelolithotomy. J. Urol., *119*:588, 1978.
15. Boyce, W. H., and Harrison, L. H.: Complications of renal stone surgery. *In* Smith, R. B., and Skinner, D. G. (eds.): Complications of Urologic Surgery. Philadelphia, W. B. Saunders, 1976, p. 87.
16. Gil-Vernet, J.: Extended pyelolithotomy for removal of staghorn calculus. *In* Scott, R., et al. (eds.): Current Controversies in Urologic Management. Philadelphia, W. B. Saunders, 1972, p. 321.
17. Boyarsky, S.: Ureteral surgery: Management of ureteral calculosis. Glenn, J. F.: Urologic Surgery, p. 209. New York, Harper & Row, 1975.
18. Anderson, E. E.: Management of ureteral calculi. Urol. Clin. North Am., *1*:357, 1974.
19. Herring, L. C.: Observations of 10,000 urinary calculi. J. Urol., *88*:445, 1962.
20. Smith, L. H.: Medical evaluation of urolithiasis: Urol. Clin. North Am., *1*:241, 1974.
21. Gittes, R. F.: Operative nephroscopy. J. Urol., *116*:148, 1976.

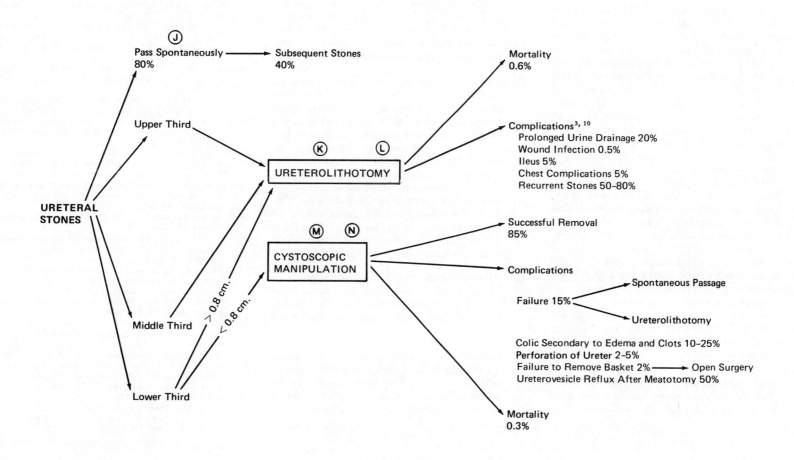

Ⓙ

Pass Spontaneously ⟶ Subsequent Stones
80%   40%

Mortality
0.6%

Upper Third

Complications[3, 10]
   Prolonged Urine Drainage 20%
   Wound Infection 0.5%
   Ileus 5%
   Chest Complications 5%
   Recurrent Stones 50–80%

Ⓚ   Ⓛ

URETEROLITHOTOMY

URETERAL
STONES

Successful Removal
85%

Ⓜ   Ⓝ

CYSTOSCOPIC
MANIPULATION

Complications

Spontaneous Passage

Failure 15%

Ureterolithotomy

Middle Third

> 0.8 cm.

< 0.8 cm.

Colic Secondary to Edema and Clots 10–25%
Perforation of Ureter 2–5%
Failure to Remove Basket 2% ⟶ Open Surgery
Ureterovesicle Reflux After Meatotomy 50%

Lower Third

Mortality
0.3%

449

RENAL CELL CARCINOMA BY RONALD R. PFISTER, M.D.

Comments

A. Renal cell carcinoma has an incidence of 3.5 cases per 100,000 per year[15] and rarely occurs before age 20.[16] The manifestations of renal cell tumor can be varied and include[12] genitourinary signs (hematuria, mass) (65 per cent), varicocele (0.6 to 11 per cent), GI symptoms (61 per cent), hematologic manifestations (most frequently anemia [30 per cent] and erythrocytosis [1 to 5 per cent]), endocrinologic signs (hypercalcemia [5 to 15 per cent) and ectopic ACTH production), and fever (10 to 20 per cent). Fever is the sole presenting symptom in 2 to 4 per cent of cases.

Bilateral renal cell carcinoma is rare.[14] The prognosis is poor: 72 per cent of patients die within 6 months.[2] Survival after radical nephrectomy (with node dissection compared with survival after simple nephrectomy (without node dissection) is greater by a percentage identical to the incidence for each corresponding grade.[13] Increasing lymph node involvement corresponds to increasing tumor grade: In grade I it is 12 per cent, in grade II, 28 per cent, and in grade III, 34 per cent. Grading of the tumor along with staging can help predict survival.[13]

B. Single metastases, especially if they occur after the nephrectomy, have a fairly good 5-year survival rate (35 per cent).[5] The later the appearance of the metastasis, the better the chance for survival.

C. Periodic reports of spontaneous regression have appeared. Of the 40 reported by Bloom,[10] all but 2 had pulmonary metastasis and 80 per cent were male. Johnson reported an increased survival rate when metastasis was limited to bone.[11]

D. Radical nephrectomy includes removal of Gerota's fascia, early ligation of the renal artery followed by ligation of the renal vein, and ipsilateral dissection of regional lymph nodes. Preoperative radiation has no influence on survival, although it reduced the incidence of residual tumor or recurrence in the renal fossa.[9] Bone pain may be relieved by irradiation, but otherwise radiotherapy is of no real value. Various chemotherapeutic agents, such as progesterone, vinblastine, and hormonal agents, and radiation have been used without predictable responses.[2]

E. Fibrosarcomas, the most common sarcomas, usually come from the renal capsule. They are reported to invade rapidly, with 40 per cent involving the renal vein.[2, 3]

F. Patients with leiomyosarcoma, only about 40 of which have been reported, rarely survive 5 years.[4] The tumor occurs twice as often in women as in men and most commonly presents as a metastasis.

References

1. Gupta, O. P., and Dube, M. K.: Rare primary renal sarcoma. Br. J. Urol., 43:546, 1971.
2. Skinner, D. G., and DeKernion, J. B.: Genitourinary Cancer. Philadelphia, W. B. Saunders Co., 1978, pp. 107–133.
3. Demming, C. L., and Harvard, B. M.: Tumors of the kidney. In Campbell, M. F., and Harrison, J. H. (eds.): Urology, 3rd ed. Philadelphia, W. B. Saunders Co. 1970, pp. 885–976.
4. Loomis, R. C.: Primary leiomyosarcoma of the kidney: Report of a case and review of the literature. J. Urol., 107:559, 1972.
5. Tolia, B. M., and Whitmore, W. W.: Solitary metastases for renal cell carcinoma. J. Urol., 114:836, 1975.
6. Katz, S. A., and Davis, J. E.: Renal adenocarcinoma: Prognostics and treatment reflected by survival. Urology, 10:10, 1977.
7. Riches, E.: The natural history of renal tumors. In Riches, E. (ed.): Tumors of the Kidney and Ureter. Baltimore, Williams & Wilkins Co., 1964, pp. 124–134.
8. Skinner, D. G., Vermillion, C. D., and Colom, R. B.: The surgical management of renal cell carcinoma. J. Urol., 107:705, 1972.
9. Van der Werf-Messing, B.: Carcinoma of the kidney. Cancer, 32:1056, 1973.
10. Bloom, H. J. G.: Hormone-induced and spontaneous regression of metastatic renal cancer. Cancer, 32:1066, 1973.
11. Johnson, D. E., Kaesler, K. E., and Samuels, M. C.: Is nephrectomy justified in patients with metastatic renal carcinoma? J. Urol., 114:27, 1975.
12. Gibbons, R. P., et al.: Manifestations of renal cell carcinoma. Urology, 8:201, 1976.
13. Skinner, D. G., et al.: Diagnosis and management of renal cell carcinoma. Cancer, 28:1165, 1971.
14. Vermillion, C. D., Skinner, D. G., and Pfister, R. C.: Bilateral renal cell carcinoma. J. Urol., 108:219, 1972.
15. MacDonald, E. J.: The present incidence and survival picture in cancer and the promise of improved prognosis. Bull. Am. Coll. Surg., 33:75, 1948.
16. Ward, J. S., and Middleton, R. G.: Renal cell carcinoma in children. Urology, 2:50, 1973.

RENAL CELL CARCINOMA

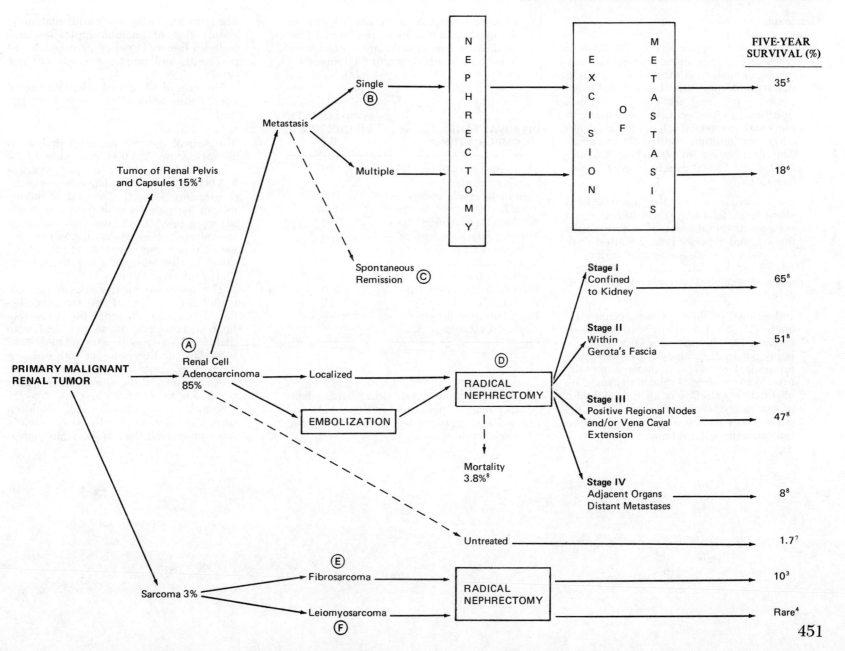

FIVE-YEAR SURVIVAL (%)

Tumor of Renal Pelvis and Capsules 15%[2]

Metastasis

Single ⒷN E P H R E C T O M Y — EXCISION OF METASTASIS — 35[5]

Multiple — 18[6]

Spontaneous Remission Ⓒ

PRIMARY MALIGNANT RENAL TUMOR

Ⓐ Renal Cell Adenocarcinoma 85%

Localized — RADICAL NEPHRECTOMY Ⓓ

EMBOLIZATION

Mortality 3.8%[8]

Stage I Confined to Kidney — 65[8]

Stage II Within Gerota's Fascia — 51[8]

Stage III Positive Regional Nodes and/or Vena Caval Extension — 47[8]

Stage IV Adjacent Organs Distant Metastases — 8[8]

Untreated — 1.7[7]

Sarcoma 3%

Fibrosarcoma Ⓔ — RADICAL NEPHRECTOMY — 10[3]

Leiomyosarcoma Ⓕ — Rare[4]

451

RENAL TRANSPLANTATION BY RICHARD WEIL, III, M.D.

Comments

A. Causes of the approximately 10,000 new cases of end-stage renal disease that develop annually in the USA include nephritis (45 per cent of cases), unknown causes (8 per cent), diabetes (7 per cent), infections (6 per cent), hypertension (5 per cent), congenital causes (5 per cent), and other (multiple) causes (24 per cent). The cost of treatment (80 per cent federally funded) for 55,000 patients was $800 million in 1978.[1, 2]

B. For vascular access the arteriovenous shunt is preferable to the external shunt because of the absence of extracorporeal devices and superior patency; arteriovenous grafts (bovine heterograft artery or fabric) are less successful but necessary when autogenous vessels are not suitable.[3]

C. Indications for bilateral nephrectomy include (1) severe renin-dependent hypertension, (2) chronic renal infection, (3) large polycystic kidneys with no space for transplant, and (4) massive proteinuria. Marked ureteral dilatation caused by obstruction or reflux is an indication for ureterectomy. Hypersplenism with WBC count lower than 4000 per cu. mm. is an indication for splenectomy.

D. Chronic hemodialysis means 5 hours on the machine 2 to 3 times per week.[4] Disadvantages and complications of chronic hemodialysis are shown in the table.

DISADVANTAGE/ COMPLICATION	APPROXIMATE INCIDENCE (%)
Time-consuming travel to dialysis center	100
Pain from needle punctures	100
Anemia	95
Weakness following dialysis	>50
Muscle cramps, or nausea during dialysis	30
Symptomatic renal osteodystrophy	25
Intractable hypertension	<10
Pericarditis	10
Hospitalization for new/ revised vascular access	<once/year

E. Approximately 3000 kidney transplants per year are performed in the U.S.A., and to date, approximately 40,000 have been done world-wide.

F. The late morbidity of transplantation is mainly that of immunosuppression and includes tumors (4 per cent), cataracts (20 per cent), and aseptic necrosis (20 per cent).

The rate of vocational rehabilitation of nondiabetic males after 1 year is 88 per cent.[2]

G. The annual cost for in-center dialysis is approximately $25,000 per patient; for home dialysis the cost per year is $15,000. Kidney transplantation costs approximately $20,000. The cost of follow-up care for patients with successful transplants is low.[5] The major cause of death in dialysis patients is cardiovascular disease (30 per cent of cases), and the major cause of death after kidney transplantation is infection (50 per cent).

The prognosis for diabetics is approximately 85 per cent of that for nondiabetics. For young diabetics the 2-year patient survival rate is 45 per cent with dialysis, 75 per cent with related-donor transplant, and 65 per cent with cadaver-donor transplant.[6] HLA matching has not greatly improved the rate of cadaver graft survival in the U.S.[7]

Kidney transplantation for children more than 2 years old has been slightly more successful than kidney transplanta-

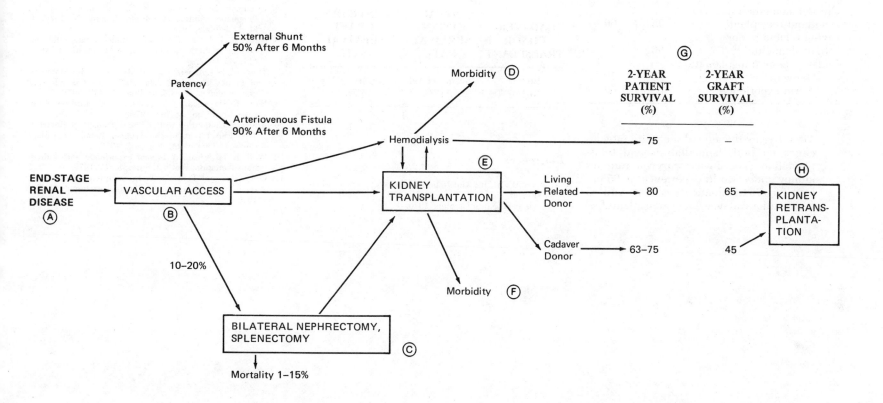

External Shunt
50% After 6 Months

Patency

Arteriovenous Fistula
90% After 6 Months

Morbidity (D)

(G)

	2-YEAR PATIENT SURVIVAL (%)	2-YEAR GRAFT SURVIVAL (%)
Hemodialysis	75	—

END-STAGE RENAL DISEASE
(A)

VASCULAR ACCESS
(B)

KIDNEY TRANSPLANTATION
(E)

Living Related Donor — 80 — 65

Cadaver Donor — 63–75

(H)

KIDNEY RETRANS-PLANTA-TION

45

10–20%

BILATERAL NEPHRECTOMY, SPLENECTOMY
(C)

Morbidity (F)

Mortality 1–15%

tion in adults.[8] Survival data are shown in the following table.

TREATMENT	PATIENT SURVIVAL (%)	
	2 Years	4 Years
Chronic hemodialysis without transplant[1]	75	60
Living related donor transplantation[9, 10]	80	75
Cadaver donor transplantation		
Denver[10]	75	70
World experience[9]	63	53

After 4 years the annual mortality rate declines for both hemodialysis and transplantation. The 2-year survival rate for kidney grafts (world experience) is 65 per cent for related-donor transplants and 45 per cent for cadaver-donor transplants.[9]

H. The main cause of kidney transplant failure is rejection (60 per cent). After graft loss the patient may elect to have hemodialysis or retransplantation. Prognosis for retransplantation is shown in the following table.[11]

CADAVER-DONOR TRANSPLANT	2-YEAR PATIENT SURVIVAL RATE	2-YEAR GRAFT SURVIVAL RATE
2nd	Same as 1st	Same as 1st
3rd or 4th	51%	17%

References

1. Bryan, F. A., Jr.: The National Dialysis Registry. Final Report. Research Triangle Institute. Research Triangle Park, North Carolina, 1976.
2. Simmons, R. G., Klein, S. D., and Simmons, R. L.: Gift of Life: The Social and Psychological Impact of Organ Transplantation. New York, John Wiley & Sons, 1977.
3. Butt, K. M., Friedman, E. A., and Kountz, S. L.: Angioaccess. Curr. Probl. Surg., 13(9):1–67, 1976.
4. Massry, S. G., and Sellers, A. L.: Clinical Aspects of Uremia and Dialysis. Springfield, Ill., Charles C Thomas, 1976.
5. Friedman, E. A., Delano, B. G., and Butt, K. M. H.: Pragmatic realities in uremic therapy. N. Engl. J. Med., 298:368, 1978.
6. Najarian, J. S., et al.: Kidney transplantation for the uremic diabetic patient. Surg. Gynecol. Obstet., 114:682, 1977.
7. Terasaki, P. I., Opelz, G., and Mickey, M. R.: Summary of kidney transplant data, 1977 — Factors affecting graft outcome. Transplant. Proc., 10:417, 1978.
8. Weil, R. III, et al.: Transplantation in children. Surg. Clin. North Am., 56:467, 1976.
9. Advisory Committee to the Renal Transplant Registry: The 13th report of the Human Renal Transplant Registry. Transplant. Proc., 9:9, 1977.
10. Weil, R. III, et al.: A 14-year experience with kidney transplantation. World J. Surg., 1:145, 1977.
11. Opelz, G., and Terasaki, P. I.: Recipient selection for renal retransplantation. Transplantation, 21:483, 1976.

ADRENAL TUMORS

ADRENAL TUMORS BY CHARLES W. VAN WAY, III, M.D.

Comments

A. Bilateral adrenalectomy reliably and quickly cures Cushing's disease, but about 10 per cent of patients will develop Nelson's syndrome, which is the development of a pituitary tumor following adrenalectomy. Management of this tumor may be difficult (see Comment C).[4-6]

B. Orthovoltage or cobalt irradiation is most commonly used, but these probably are less effective than alpha-particle beam irradiation, which is available only with a research particle accelerator. Interstitial irradiation is most effective but requires operative implantation. All forms induce panhypopituitarism. Response requires 6 to 12 months.[4-6]

C. About 10 per cent of patients have an enlarged sella, hence, a pituitary tumor. These patients must have pituitary resection. Recent work indicates that a high proportion of patients with so-called bilateral adrenal hyperplasia may have a tiny pituitary adenoma that is amenable to microsurgical removal. This can be done without inducing panhypopituitarism. This therapy is very new but may be the therapy of choice in the future.[7-9]

D. The most common ACTH-producing tumor is lung cancer, although other tumors are associated with this condition. The prognosis of this disease is that of the underlying malignant tumor that is producing the ACTH. The incidence varies widely in the literature, apparently depending on the aggressiveness with which diagnosis is sought.

E. Malignant pheochromocytoma cannot be diagnosed histologically; criteria are local invasion, metastases, and recurrence following adequate excision. If unresectable, it invariably kills. The treatment is to control hypertension by using alpha-adrenergic blockade as palliation. Chemotherapy and radiotherapy are useless.

F. Bilateral hyperplasia is probably better treated medically than surgically. The hypertension is usually mild and easily controlled, and the surgical cure rate is not good, even with total adrenalectomy.[12, 13]

G. These are rare tumors. Half or more of those reported are carcinomas.[1-3]

456

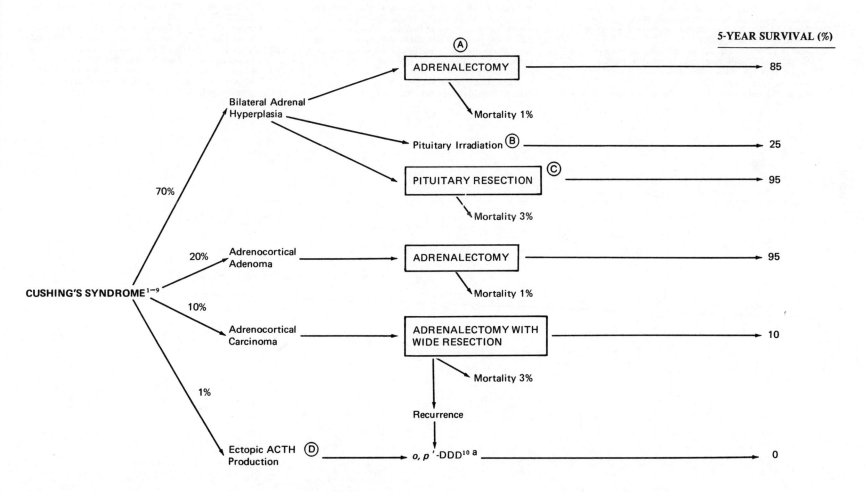

5-YEAR SURVIVAL (%)

Ⓐ ADRENALECTOMY — 85
Mortality 1%

Bilateral Adrenal Hyperplasia

Pituitary Irradiation Ⓑ — 25

Ⓒ PITUITARY RESECTION — 95
Mortality 3%

70%

CUSHING'S SYNDROME[1-9]

20% Adrenocortical Adenoma — ADRENALECTOMY — 95
Mortality 1%

10% Adrenocortical Carcinoma — ADRENALECTOMY WITH WIDE RESECTION — 10
Mortality 3%

Recurrence

1% Ectopic ACTH Production Ⓓ — o, p'-DDD[10] [a] — 0

[a] 2,2-Bis (2-chlorophenyl-4-chlorophenyl)-1, 1-dichloroethane), Mitotane; Lysodren

457

ADRENAL TUMORS *Continued*

References

1. Harrison, T., et al.: Surgical Disorders of the Adrenal Gland. New York, Grune & Stratton, 1975.
2. O'Neal, L. W.: Surgery of the Adrenal Glands. St. Louis, C. V. Mosby, 1968.
3. Glenn, F., Peterson, R. E., and Mannix, H. Surgery of the Adrenal Gland. New York, Macmillan, 1968.
4. Temple, T. E., Jr., et al.: Treatment of Cushing's disease. N. Engl. J. Med., 281:801, 1969.
5. Orth, D. N., and Liddle, G. W.: Results of treatment in 108 patients with Cushing's syndrome. N. Engl. J. Med., 285:243, 1971.
6. Jennings, A. S., Liddle, G. W., and Orth, D. N.: Results of treating childhood Cushing's disease with pituitary irradiation. N. Engl. J. Med., 297:957, 1977.
7. Bigos, S. T., et al.: Cure of Cushing's disease by transsphenoidal removal of a microadenoma from a pituitary gland despite a radiographically normal sella turcica. J. Clin. Endocrinol. Metabol., 45:1251, 1977.
8. Tyrrell, J. B., et al.: Cushing's disease: Selective transsphenoidal resection of pituitary microadenomas. N. Engl. J. Med., 298:753, 1978.
9. Daughaday, W. H.: Cushing's disease and basophilic microadenomas. (Editorial). N. Engl. J. Med., 298:793, 1978.
10. Van Way, C. W., III, et al.: Pheochromocytoma. Curr. Prob. Surg., June 1974, pp. 1–59.
11. Manger, W. M., and Gifford, R. W., Jr.: Pheochromocytoma. New York, Springer-Verlag, 1977, pp. 304–344.
12. Melby, J. C.: Solving the adrenal lesion of primary aldosteronism. N. Engl. J. Med., 294:441, 1976.
13. Delarue, N. C., et al.: Hypertension due to "primary" hyperaldosteronism — Surgical considerations. Surgery, 80:289, 1976.

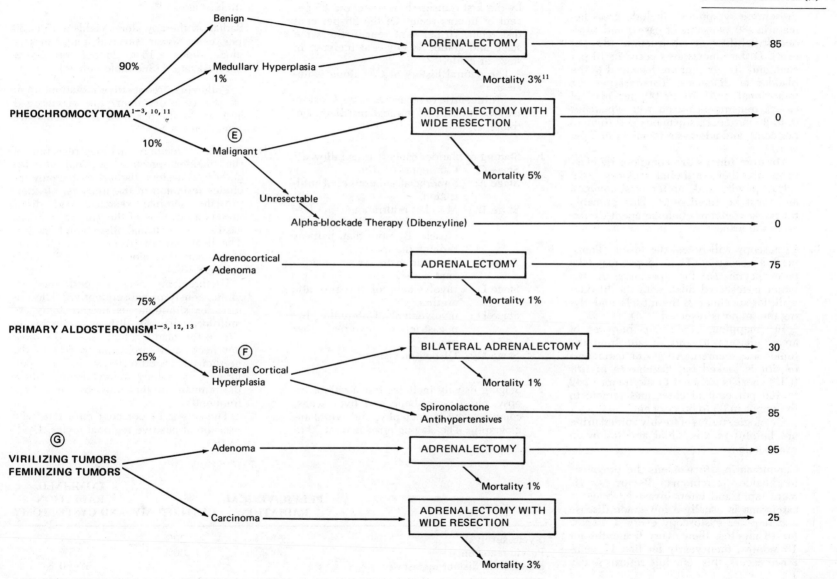

PHEOCHROMOCYTOMA[1-3, 10, 11]

90% → Benign → ADRENALECTOMY → 85

Medullary Hyperplasia 1% → Mortality 3%[11]

10% → (E) Malignant → ADRENALECTOMY WITH WIDE RESECTION → 0

Mortality 5%

Unresectable → Alpha-blockade Therapy (Dibenzyline) → 0

PRIMARY ALDOSTERONISM[1-3, 12, 13]

75% → Adrenocortical Adenoma → ADRENALECTOMY → 75

Mortality 1%

25% → (F) Bilateral Cortical Hyperplasia → BILATERAL ADRENALECTOMY → 30

Mortality 1%

Spironolactone Antihypertensives → 85

(G) VIRILIZING TUMORS FEMINIZING TUMORS

Adenoma → ADRENALECTOMY → 95

Mortality 1%

Carcinoma → ADRENALECTOMY WITH WIDE RESECTION → 25

Mortality 3%

459

CANCER OF THE BLADDER BY ROBERT DONOHUE, M.D., AND NORMAN PETERSON, M.D.

Comments

A. Presenting symptoms[14] include gross hematuria (80 per cent of cases) and bladder irritability or obstruction (33 per cent). Distant metastases occur in 10 per cent, and 70 per cent are localized to the bladder at diagnosis. Tumor types are transitional cell (76 to 90 per cent of cases), transitional mixed with squamous (6 to 20 per cent), squamous cell (6 to 13 per cent), and adenocarcinoma (1 to 2 per cent).[15, 16]

Multiple tumors are common. Involvement of other urothelial surfaces — the calyx, pelvis, and ureter — is common and must be ruled out.[23] This probably reflects a common etiologic agent excreted in the urine.[17]

B. Cystoscopy will reveal the lesion. Transurethral resection (TUR) biopsy may take two specimens: for specimen A the tumor is resected flush with the bladder wall; for specimen B the muscle underlying the tumor is resected.

In "mapping," cold cup biopsies of areas adjacent to and distant from the tumor are secured. Atypia or carcinoma *in situ* is looked for. Carcinoma *in situ* (CIS) coexists adjacent to the tumor in 42 to 100 per cent of cases and remote to the tumor in 33 to 55 per cent.

Cytologic studies of freshly voided urine are helpful in the initial and follow-up examinations.

C. Carcinoma *in situ* worsens the prognosis in bladder carcinoma. Recurrence is more rapid and often invasive.[1] Stage A carcinoma is usually a low-grade disease and requires cystoscopy every 3 months for 18 months, then every 6 months for 18 months, then yearly for life. If recurrence occurs, this schedule returns to day 1.

D. Fifteen per cent of patients are cured by the first transurethral resection; 85 per cent of tumors recur. Of the 85 per cent that recur, 70 per cent remain the same stage and grade; 30 per cent increase in stage or grade.[2]

The natural history of CIS alone is unclear.

Multicentric or recurrent stage A lesions may be treated by topical instillation of thiotepa.[18]

E. Staging of bladder cancers is as follows:[17]
Stage O: Carcinoma *in situ*.
Stage A: Superficial subepithelial infiltration.
Stage B: Muscle infiltration: B_1 less than halfway through the muscle, B_2 more than halfway through the muscle.
Stage C: Penetration to serosa or adjacent tissue.
Stage D_1:   Involvement of the prostatic urethra.
Stage D_2:   involvement of obturator, hypogastric, or external iliac nodes.
Stage D_3:   Distant metastases.

F. Staging usually includes transurethral biopsy, chest x-ray, bone and liver scans, computerized tomography, and lymphangiography. The staging error is from 30 to 55 per cent, and generally the tumor is understaged.[4, 19]

G. Radiation therapy alone yields a 15 to 30 per cent 5-year survival rate. Surgery alone yields a 15 to 25 per cent 5-year survival rate.[20] (See table below.)

Following preoperative radiation, up to 66 per cent of tumors are downstaged and up to 33 per cent of patients are tumor-free.[20, 21, 24, 25]

H. Simple cystectomy includes resection of the bladder, prostate, seminal vesicles and distal ureters. Radical cystectomy includes resection of the urachus, bladder, prostate, seminal vesicles, and distal ureters as well as of the obturator, hypogastric, and external iliac lymph nodes. The ileal conduit (Bricker procedure) is the urinary diversion of choice. (See table on page 462.)

Urethrectomy may be performed simultaneously or subsequently.[22] The criteria for simultaneous urethrectomy are multifocal disease, diffuse carcinoma *in situ* of the bladder, tumor near the bladder neck, and carcinoma *in situ* of the urethra. If urethrectomy is not performed, endoscopy and cytologic study of the remnant urethra must be carried out frequently.

There is a 14 per cent cure rate with excision of positive regional nodes (D_2).[6]

	PELVIC/VESICAL RADIATION	CYSTECTOMY	COMBINED RADIATION AND CYSTECTOMY
5-year survival	20%	20%	40%
Pelvic recurrence	30%	30%	15%
Death from distant metastases			50–60%

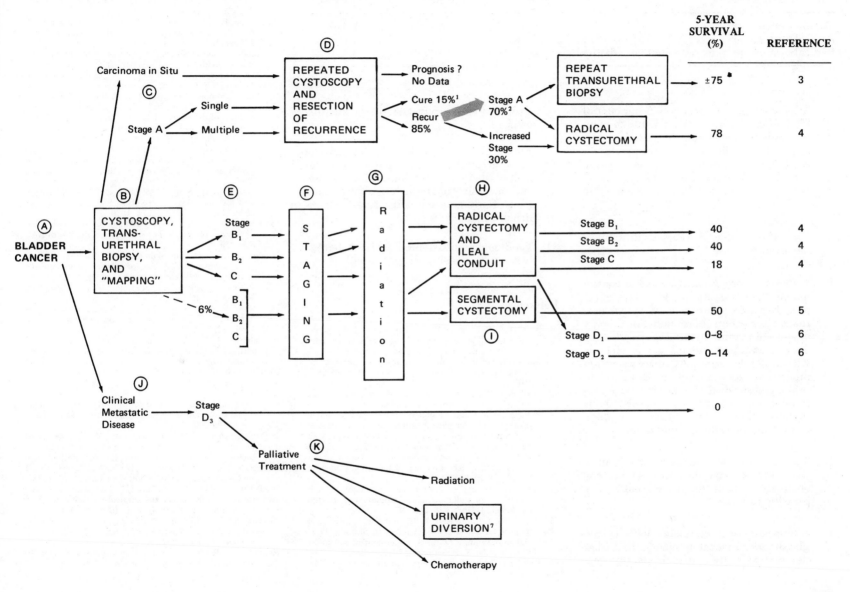

	5-YEAR SURVIVAL (%)	REFERENCE

Ⓓ

Carcinoma in Situ ⟶ REPEATED CYSTOSCOPY AND RESECTION OF RECURRENCE ⟶ Prognosis ? No Data

Ⓒ

Stage A ⟶ Single ⟶
⟶ Multiple ⟶

Cure 15%[1]
Recur 85%

Stage A 70%[2] ⟶ REPEAT TRANSURETHRAL BIOPSY ⟶ ±75 · — 3

Increased Stage 30% ⟶ RADICAL CYSTECTOMY ⟶ 78 — 4

Ⓐ
BLADDER CANCER

Ⓑ
CYSTOSCOPY, TRANS-URETHRAL BIOPSY, AND "MAPPING"

Ⓔ
Stage B₁
B₂
C

6% → B₁ B₂ C

Ⓕ
S T A G I N G

Ⓖ
R a d i a t i o n

Ⓗ
RADICAL CYSTECTOMY AND ILEAL CONDUIT

Stage B₁ — 40 — 4
Stage B₂ — 40 — 4
Stage C — 18 — 4

Ⓘ
SEGMENTAL CYSTECTOMY — 50 — 5

Stage D₁ — 0–8 — 6
Stage D₂ — 0–14 — 6

Ⓙ
Clinical Metastatic Disease ⟶ Stage D₃ ⟶ 0

Palliative Treatment

Ⓚ
⟶ Radiation
⟶ URINARY DIVERSION[7]
⟶ Chemotherapy

461

CANCER OF THE BLADDER *Continued*

TREATMENT	MORTALITY	MORBIDITY	REFERENCE
Simple cystectomy	5%	0–59%	3, 4, 6
Radical cystectomy	8%		
Radical cystectomy plus preoperative radiation	1.0–16%	28–59%	3, 4, 6

I. After staging, approximately 6 per cent of bladder carcinomas are amenable to curative radical, segmental, or partial cystectomy.[5] The criteria are a single tumor area, first occurrence, a 2-cm. margin available, no evidence of carcinoma *in situ* elsewhere, and location 2 cm from the bladder neck.

J. No patients live 5 years with clinical metastatic disease.[4, 6]

K. Radiation therapy may be used to control hemorrhage from the bladder. It is effective, but late recurrence of the hemorrhage often occurs. Local radiation therapy to areas of painful metastases can alleviate the pain.[20] Chemotherapy is not effective with systemic disease.[7] Urinary diversion procedures for obstruction do not yield prolonged survival. Urinary diversion performed for palliation with subsequent radiation therapy for irritative symptoms of the bladder helps to give relief.

L. Squamous cell carcinoma is usually invasive, with a high incidence of ureteral obstruction. It is often associated with parasitic infection.[8]

M. Adenocarcinoma correlates with cystitis glandularis, urachal remnants, and bladder exstrophy. It is usually deeply invasive, and the survival statistics are dismal.[9]

N. Eighty per cent of bladder diverticula show atypical changes. Three to 7 per cent of bladder diverticula contain tumor, and one third of these tumors are squamous. Early invasion is the rule in diverticular tumors.[10, 11]

O. Papilloma is considered to be a benign tumor with a malignant potential.[12, 13]

References

1. Althausen, A. F., Prout, G. R., and Daley, J. J.: Noninvasive papillary carcinoma of the bladder associated with carcinoma *in situ*. J. Urol., *116*:575, 1976.
2. Barnes, R. W., et al.: Bladder carcinoma: Survival following transurethral resection. Cancer Res., 37:2895, 1977.
3. Whitmore, W. F., Jr.: The treatment of bladder tumors. Surg. Clin. North Am., *49*:349, 1969.
4. Skinner, D. G., and Kaufmann, J. J.: Management of invasive and highgrade bladder cancer. *In* Skinner, D. G. and deKernion, J. B. (eds.): Genitourinary Cancer. Philadelphia, W. B. Saunders, 1978, pp. 262–282.
5. Utz, D. C., et al.: A clinicopathologic evaluation of partial cystectomy for carcinoma of the urinary bladder. Cancer, 32:1075, 1973.
6. Whitmore, W. F., et al.: Radical cystectomy with or without prior radiation in the treatment of bladder carcinoma. J. Urol., *118*:184, 1977.
7. deKernion, J. B., Stewart, B. H., and Yagoda, A.: Treatment of advanced bladder cancer. *In* Skinner, D. G. and deKernion, J. B. (eds.): Genitourinary Cancer. Philadelphia, W. B. Saunders, 1978, p. 284.
8. Richie, J. P., et al.: Squamous carcinoma of the bladder: Treatment by radical cystectomy. J. Urol., *115*:670, 1976.
9. Jacobo, E., et al.: Primary adenocarcinoma of the bladder: A retrospective study of 20 patients. J. Urol., *117*:54, 1977.
10. Kelalis, P., and McLean, P.: Treatment of diverticulum of the bladder. J. Urol., 98:349, 1967.
11. Knappenberger, S. T., Uson, A. C., and Melicow, M. M.: Primary neoplasm occurring in vesical diverticula — A report of 18 cases. J. Urol., 83:153, 1960.
12. Lerman, R. I., Hutter, R. V., and Whitmore, W. F.: Papilloma of the urinary bladder. Cancer, 25:333, 1970.
13. Lerman, R. I., et al.: The association of benign papilloma with cancers of sites other than the bladder and ureter. J. Urol., *104*:418, 1970.
14. Massey, B. D., et al.: Carcinoma of the bladder — A 20-year experience in private practice. J. Urol., 93:212, 1965.
15. Friedell, G. H., Soto, E. A., and Nagy, G. K.: Cytologic and histopathologic study of bladder cancer patients. Urol. Clin. North Am., *3*:71, 1976.
16. Friedell, G. H., et al.: Histopathology and classification of urinary bladder carcinoma. Urol. Clin. North Am., *3*:53, 1976.
17. deKernion, J. B., and Skinner, D. G.: The epidemiology, diagnosis and staging of bladder carcinoma. *In* Skinner, D. G., and deKernion, J. B. (eds.): Genitourinary Cancer. Philadelphia, W. B. Saunders, 1978, p. 213–231.
18. Veenema, R. J., et al.: Thiotepa bladder installations: Therapy and prophylaxis for superficial tumors. J. Urol., *101*:711, 1969.
19. Schmidt, J. D., and Weinstein, S. H.: Pitfalls in the clinical staging of bladder cancer. Urol. Clin. North Am., *3*:107, 1976.
20. Caldwell, W. L.: Radiotherapy: Definitive, integrated, and palliative therapy. Urol. Clin. North Am., *3*:129, 1976.
21. deWeerd, J. H., and Colby, M.: Bladder carcinoma treated by irradiation and surgery. Interval report. J. Urol., *109*:409, 1973.
22. Schellhammer, P. F., and Whitmore, W. F.: Transitional cell carcinoma of the urethra in men having cystectomy for bladder carcinoma. J. Urol., *115*:56, 1976.
23. Batata, M., and Grabstald, H.: Upper urinary tract urothelial tumors. Urol. Clin. North Am., *3*:79, 1976.
24. Prout, G., Slack, N., and Bross, I.: Preoperative irradiation as an adjuvant in the surgical management of invasive bladder cancer. J. Urol., *105*:223, 1971.
25. Van der Werf-Messing, B.: Carcinoma of the bladder treated by preoperative irradiation followed by cystectomy. Cancer, 32:1084, 1973.
26. Prout, G. R., Jr.: The surgical management of bladder carcinoma. Urol. Clin. North Am., *3*:149, 1976.

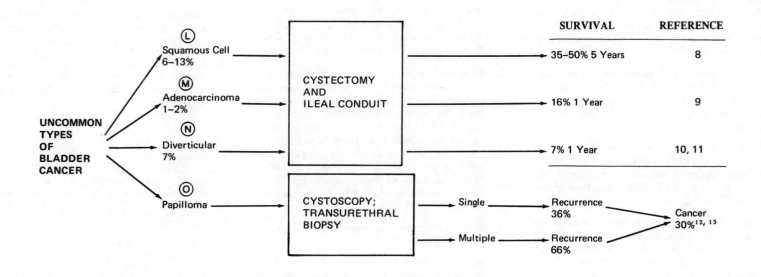

SURVIVAL	REFERENCE
35–50% 5 Years	8
16% 1 Year	9
7% 1 Year	10, 11

UNCOMMON
TYPES
OF
BLADDER
CANCER

Ⓛ Squamous Cell 6–13%

Ⓜ Adenocarcinoma 1–2%

Ⓝ Diverticular 7%

Ⓞ Papilloma

CYSTECTOMY
AND
ILEAL CONDUIT

CYSTOSCOPY;
TRANSURETHRAL
BIOPSY

Single → Recurrence 36%

Multiple → Recurrence 66%

Cancer 30%[12, 13]

GERMINAL TESTIS TUMORS BY J. WETTLAUFER, M.D., AND NORMAN E. PETERSON, M.D.

Comments

A. "Markers" are alpha$_1$-fetoprotein (AFP) and beta–human chorionic gonadotropin (β-HCG). Radioimmunoassay is specific for these glycoproteins. AFP is never elevated in seminoma, and βHCG rarely is elevated in pure seminoma. Either or both markers are elevated in 90 per cent of cases of stage II and III nonseminoma. There have been no known false positive elevations. Subsequent metastases develop in 67 per cent of patients with preoperative marker elevations and in only 4 per cent of those with negative preoperative markers.[1, 2]

B. Most of these tumors are seminoma, and 20 per cent occur in the contralateral normally descended testis. The incidence of malignancy is unaltered by orchidopexy.[3-6]

C. Most bilateral testis tumors are seminomas and are successive. The probability of developing a second contralateral primary testis tumor is 500 times that of the general population.[7, 8]

D. There are 3 pathologic types of seminoma. Classic pure seminoma is the most common. Ten per cent of seminomas are anaplastic and account for most of the metastasizing seminomas. They are the least radiosensitive and have a poor prognosis (70 per cent survival). Spermatocytic seminomas (9 per cent) occur in older people and do not commonly metastasize. The pure and spermatocytic types are highly radiosensitive.[7, 9]

E. Staging is based on clinical-pathologic extent of disease. Stage I is a tumor confined to the testis; stage II has metastases to the subdiaphragmatic retroperitoneal lymphatics; and stage III is a tumor that has spread beyond the retroperitoneal lymph nodes above or below the diaphragm, i.e., visceral or disseminated disease.[10, 11]

F. Radiation is the primary treatment for stage I and II disease. Dose is 2000 to 4000 rads, depending on the extent of tumor spread to ipsilateral ilioinguinal and bilateral para-aortic lymphatics. Radiation to the mediastinum and supraclavicular ports in stage I disease is optional. For localized stage III disease, 2500 to 3000 rads is the usual dose.[12-14]

G. Effective single agents are chlorambucil, cyclophosphamide, and cis-platinum or combination therapy with Bleo-Comf. or actinomycin D, vincristine, and Cytoxan.[10, 15] The initial response rates to these agents are good, but there is a high recurrence rate. High-dose cyclophosphamide is promising as an adjunct to radiation for advanced bulky seminoma.[16] To obtain optimum benefit, chemotherapy should precede radiation.

H. Survival figures represent 2 to 3 years' disease-free status.[17]

I. Approximately 40 per cent of nonseminomas are mixed, with more than one cell type. About 75 per cent of teratocarcinomas are a combination of teratoma and embryonal carcinoma. Pure choriocarcinoma has a very poor prognosis, with only an isolated case surviving.[7]

J. The survival in stage I disease with retroperitoneal lymph node dissection (RLND) alone approximates 90 per cent and may be increased to 98 per cent with limited adjuvant chemotherapy using actinomycin D.[20]

K. The survival rate for microscopic or minimal stage II disease is increased by adjuvant chemotherapy.[19, 20] The 3-year survival rate for bulk stage II disease is lower (73 per cent), and such patients should probably receive preoperative cytoreductive chemotherapy as well as postoperative chemotherapy.[20-22]

L. The complete response rate (50 to 75 per cent) is much higher using combination chemotherapy with Velban or vincristine and bleomycin and cis-platinum.[10, 21-23]

M. Judicious thoracotomy with excision of stable, resectable solitary pulmonary lesions will increase the survival rate.[20, 21, 24]

References

1. Lange, P. H., and Fraley, E. E.: Serum alpha fetoprotein and human chorionic gonadotropin in the treatment of patients with testicular tumors. Urol. Clin. North Am., 4:393, 1977.
2. Scardino, P., et al: The value of serum markers in the staging and prognosis of germ cell tumors of the testis. J. Urol., 118:994, 1977.
3. Johnson, D. E.: Testicular Tumors, Flushing, N.Y., Medical Examination Publishing Co., 1971.
4. Notter, G., and Ranudd, N. E.: Treatment of malignant testicular tumors. A report on 355 patients. Acta Radiol. [Ther.] (Stockh), 2:273, 1964.
5. Dow, J. A., and Mostofi, F. K.: Testicular tumors following orchiopexy. South. Med. J., 60:193, 1967.
6. Batata, M. A., Whitmore, W. F., Jr., and Hilaris, B. S.: Cancer of the undescended or maldescended testis. Am. J. Roentgenol., 126:302, 1976.
7. Mostofi, F. K., and Price, E. B., Jr.: Tumors of the male genital system. In Atlas of Tumor Pathology. Washington, D.C., Armed Forces Institute of Pathology, 2nd Series, Fasc. 8, 1973.
8. Hamilton, J. B., and Gilbert, J. B.: Studies in malignant

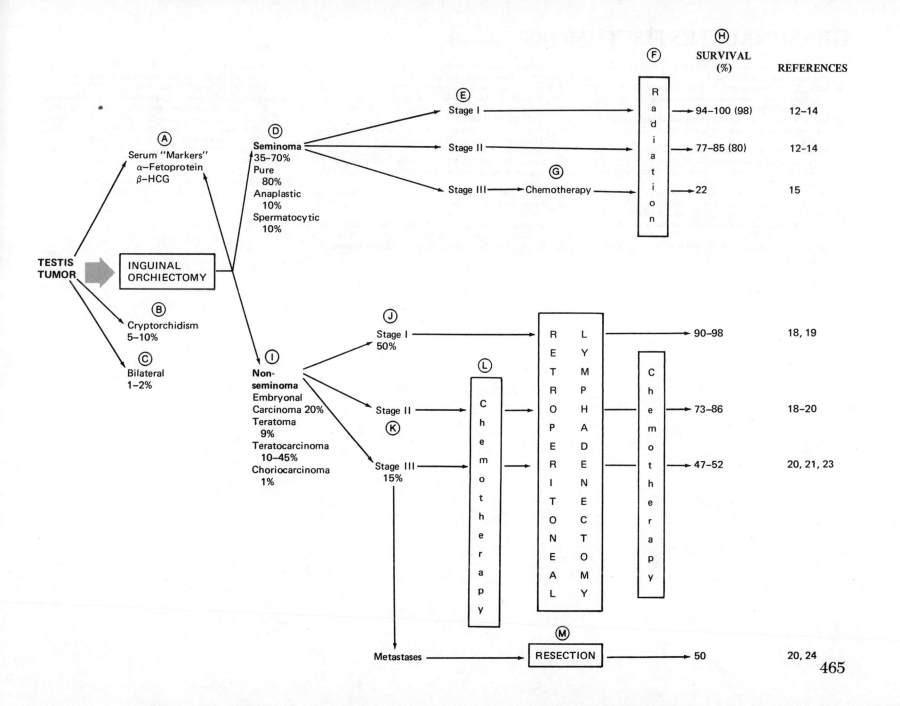

GERMINAL TESTIS TUMORS *Continued*

tumors of the testis. IV. Bilateral testicular cancer. Cancer Res., 2:125, 1942.

9. Maier, J. G., Mittemeyer, B. T., and Sulak, M. H.: The treatment and prognosis in seminoma of the testis. J. Urol., 99:72, 1968.

10. Samuels, M. D., et al.: Combination chemotherapy in germinal cell tumors. Cancer Treat. Rev., 3:185, 1976.

11. Skinner, D. G.: Non-seminomatous testis tumors: A plan of management based in 96 patients to improve survival in all stages by combined therapeutic modalities. J. Urol., 115:65, 1976.

12. Maier, J. G., and Sulak, M. H.: Radiation therapy in malignant testis tumors. Cancer, 32:1212, 1973.

13. Doornbos, J. F., Hussey, D. H., and Johnson, D. E.: Radiotherapy for pure seminoma of the testis. Radiology, 116:401, 1975.

14. Earle, J. D., Bagshaw, M. A., and Kaplan, H. S.: Super-voltage radiation therapy of the testicular tumors. Am. J. Roentgenol., 117:633, 1973.

15. Smith, R. B.: Management of testicular seminoma. *In* Skinner, D. G., and de Kernion, J. B. (eds.): Genitourinary Cancer. Philadelphia, W. B. Saunders Co., 1978, pp. 460–469.

16. Weitzman, S. A., Carey, R. W.: High dose cyclophosphamide as an adjunct to radiotherapy for advanced seminoma. J. Urol., 117:613, 1977.

17. Nefzger, M., and Mostofi, F.: Survival after surgery for germinal malignancies of the testis. Cancer, 30:1225, 1972.

18. Staubitz, W. J., et al.: Survival treatment of nonseminomatous germinal testis tumors. Cancer, 32:1206, 1973.

19. Donohue, J. P.: Retroperitoneal lymphadenectomy. Urol. Clin. North Am., 4:509, 1977.

20. Skinner, D. E.: Management of nonseminomatous tumors of the testis. *In* Skinner, D. E., and de Kernion, J. B. (eds.): Genitourinary Cancer. Philadelphia, W. B. Saunders Co., 1978, pp. 470–493.

22. Merrin, C., Beckley, S., and Takita, N.: Multimodal treatment of advanced testicular tumor with radical reductive surgery and multisequential chemotherapy with cisplatinum, bleomycin, vinblastine, vincristine and actinomycin D. J. Urol., 120:73, 1978.

23. Cuitkovic, E., et al.: Germ cell tumor chemotherapy update. American Society of Clinical Oncologists (ASCO) Abstracts, 18:324, 1972.

24. Wettlaufer, J. N.: Stage III germinal testis tumors: Aggressive approach. J. Urol., 116:593, 1976.

PROSTATISM

PROSTATISM BY EUGENE HELLER, M.D.

Comments

A. In addition to prostatic hyperplasia, bladder neck contracture, "median bar" prostatic enlargement, and carcinoma of the prostate can produce symptoms similar to those of prostatism. Enlargement of the middle and two lateral lobes produces obstruction.[6] "Middle lobe" enlargement produces contracture of the bladder neck or "median bar" formation.[15] From the evidence it can be concluded that some testicular hormone or hormones other than testosterone is the cause of hyperplasia of the prostate in dogs. It is widely accepted that the development of benign prostatic hypertrophy (BPH) requires the presence of the testes.

B. Seventy-five per cent of males over age 70 years will have BPH on physical examination.[21] Seldom is it seen in patients younger than 40,[15] and it usually requires 15 to 20 years to become clinically symptomatic.[1]

C. Despite remission or stabilization of symptoms, there is no regression of hyperplasia.[15]

D. See also the table following this algorithm.

E. The incidence of recurrence of prostatism following prostatectomy is 2 per cent (0.3 per cent after perineal prostatectomy and 7 per cent after transurethral resection).

Time of recurrence is 3 to 10 years, postoperatively.

The mortality and morbidity of reoperation for recurrence will depend on the same factors that influenced the original survey.

F. The incidence of cancer following prostatectomy in patients over 50 years is 7 to 58 per cent; in patients 70 to 80 it is 41 per cent; and in patients over 80 it is 57 percent.[23]

References

1. Brendler, H.: Benign prostatic hyperplasia: Natural history. *In* Benign Prostatic Hyperplasia — A Workshop sponsored by the Kidney Disease and Urology Program of the National Institute of Arthritis, Metabolism, and Digestive Diseases. Washington, D.C., U.S. Government Printing Office, 1975.
2. Caine, M.: The late results and sequelae of prostatectomy. Br. J. Urol., 26:205–226, 1954.
3. Harrison, J. H., et al. (eds.): Campbell's Urology, 4th ed., vol. 3. Philadelphia, W. B. Saunders Co., 1979.
4. Emmett, J. L., and Whitten, D. M.: Clinical Urography, 3rd ed. Philadelphia, W. B. Saunders Co., 1970, p. 569.

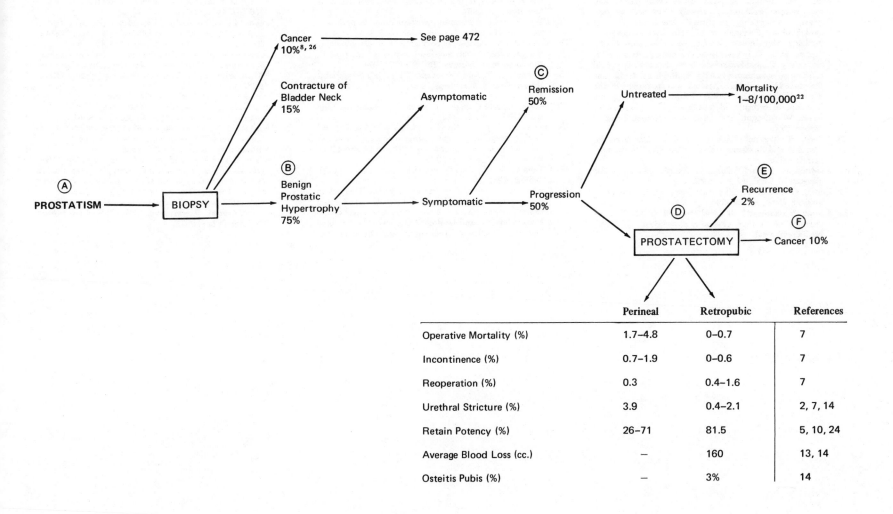

Cancer
10%[8, 26] ──────────→ See page 472

Contracture of
Bladder Neck
15%

Ⓒ Remission
50%

Ⓐ
PROSTATISM ──────→ BIOPSY

Asymptomatic

Untreated ──────→ Mortality
1–8/100,000[22]

Ⓑ
Benign
Prostatic
Hypertrophy
75%

Symptomatic ──────→ Progression
50%

Ⓔ
Recurrence
2%

Ⓓ
PROSTATECTOMY ──→ Cancer 10%

Ⓕ

	Perineal	Retropubic	References
Operative Mortality (%)	1.7–4.8	0–0.7	7
Incontinence (%)	0.7–1.9	0–0.6	7
Reoperation (%)	0.3	0.4–1.6	7
Urethral Stricture (%)	3.9	0.4–2.1	2, 7, 14
Retain Potency (%)	26–71	81.5	5, 10, 24
Average Blood Loss (cc.)	—	160	13, 14
Osteitis Pubis (%)	—	3%	14

5. Finkle, A. L., and Prian, D. V.: Sexual potency in elderly men before and after prostatectomy. JAMA, *196*:139, 1966.

6. Franks, L.: Benign prostatic hyperplasia: Gross and microscopic anatomy. *In* Benign Prostatic Hyperplasia — A workshop sponsored by the Kidney Disease and Urology Program of the National Institute of Arthritis, Metabolism, and Digestive Diseases. Washington, D.C., U.S. Government Printing Office, 1975.

7. Grayhack, J. T., and Sadlowski, R. W.: Results of surgical treatment of benign prostatic hyperplasia. *In* Benign Prostatic Hyperplasia — A workshop sponsored by the Kidney Disease and Urology Program of the National Institute of Arthritis, Metabolism, and Digestive Diseases. Washington, D.C., U.S. Government Printing Office, 1975.

8. Jewett, H.: Present status of radical prostatectomy for stages A and B prostatic cancer. Urol. Clin. North Am., 2:105, 1975.

9. Kaufman, J. J., and Schutz, J.: Needle biopsy of the prostate. J. Urol., 87:164, 1962.

10. Lilien, O. M., et al.: The case for perineal prostatectomy. J. Urol., 99:79, 1968.

11. Lytton, B., Emery, J. M., and Harvard, B. M.: The incidence of benign prostatic obstruction. J. Urol., 99:639–45, 1968.

12. Melchior, J., et al.: TURP: Computerized analysis of 2223 consecutive cases. J. Urol., *112*:643, 1974.

13. Millin, T.: Retropubic prostatectomy. *In* Campbell, M., and Harrison, J. H. (eds.): Urology. Philadelphia, W. B. Saunders Co., 1954.

14. Millin, T., et al.: Retropubic prostatectomy: Experiences based on 757 cases. Lancet, *1*:381–385, 1949.

15. Moore, R. A.: Benign hypertrophy and carcinoma of the prostate. Occurrence and experimental production in animals. Surgery, *16*:152–167, 1944.

16. Nauninga, J. B., and O'Connor, V. J., Jr.: Suprapubic prostatectomy: A review, 1966-70. J. Urol., *102*:723. 1969.

17. Nesbitt, R., and Conger, K.: Studies of blood loss during TURP. J. Urol., *46*:713, 1941.

18. O'Connor, V. J., Jr., Bulkley, G. J., and Sokol, J. K.: Low suprapubic prostatectomy: Comparison of results with standard operations in 2 groups of 142 patients. J. Urol., *90*:301, 1963.

19. O'Connor, V. J., Jr.: Campbell's Urology, Vol. III, 1965, p. 1963.

20. Paulson, D.: Benign prostatic hyperplasia: Evaluation and assessment of bladder neck obstruction. *In* Benign Prostatic Hyperplasia — A workshop sponsored by the Kidney Disease and Urology Program of the National Institute of Arthritis, Metabolism, and Digestive Diseases. Washington, D.C., U.S. Government Printing Office, 1975.

21. Perrin, P., Barnes, R. H., and Bergman, R. T.: Forty years of transurethral prostatic resections. J. Urol., *116*:757, 1976.

22. Rotkin, I.: Epidemiology of benign prostatic hypertrophy: Review and speculations. *In* Benign Prostatic Hyperplasia — A workshop sponsored by the Kidney Disease and Urology Program of the National Institute of Arthritis, Metabolism, and Digestive Diseases. Washington, D.C., U.S. Government Printing Office, 1975.

23. Scott, R., et al.: J. Urol., *101*:602–7, 1969.

24. Stearns, D. B.: Retropubic prostatectomy, 1947-1960: A critical evaluation. J. Urol., *85*:322–328, 1961.

25. Valk, W. L.: TUR Prostate for BPH. Presented at a conference on BPH, New York, October 31, 1974.

26. Whitmore, W.: A.J.M., *21*:967, 1956.

27. Wilson, J., Walsh, P., and Suteri, P.: Studies on the pathogenesis of benign prostatic hypertrophy in the dog. *In* Benign Prostatic Hyperplasia — A workshop sponsored by the Kidney Disease and Urology Program of the National Institute of Arthritis, Metabolism, and Digestive Disease. Washington, D.C., U.S. Government Printing Office, 1975.

PROSTATECTOMY FOR PROSTATISM

	Transurethral	Suprapubic	References
Operative Mortality *(%)*	0.3–1.3	1–2	7, 21
Incontinence *(%)*	0.4–1.4	0–1.2	7
Reoperation *(%)*	6.4–7.0	0–0.7	7
Urethral Stricture *(%)*	2.7–5.1	5.1	2, 7
Retained Potency *(%)*	98	61–87	2, 5, 10
Hemorrhage *(%)*	2.8	3.5–4.2	12, 16, 18
Epididymitis *(%)*	0.5–2.1	3.5	12, 16, 18
Fibrinolysis *(%)*	0.5		12, 16, 18
Myocardial Infarction *(%)*	0.8	0.7	12, 16, 18
Extravasation *(%)*	0.6		12, 16, 18
Pyelonephritis *(%)*	0	0	12, 16, 18
Average Weight Tissue Removed *(gm.)*	18.5	68	19
Average Blood Loss *(ml.)*	169 (< 100: 49%) (> 250: 22%)		17
Osteitis Pubis *(%)*		3	14

CANCER OF THE PROSTATE BY ROBERT DONOHUE, M.D.

Comments

A. This is the second most common neoplasm in men (60,000 per year in the U.S.). The incidence of prostatic cancer discovered at autopsy (random selection) is shown in the following table.[1]

AGE (Years)	INCIDENCE (%)
30–39	1
40–49	4
50–59	7
60–69	12
70–79	18
80	26

B. The incidence of discovery at transurethral prostatectomy (TURP) is 6 to 20 per cent.[2]

Two per cent of patients with stage A adenocarcinoma die of the disease, and only 10 per cent develop clinical evidence of disease.[3]

Repeat transurethral biopsy 3 months after initial resection of stage A lesions shows 28 per cent residual cancer.[4]

C. The accuracy of transperineal needle biopsy is 73 per cent; of transrectal needle biopsy, 81 per cent; and of transurethral biopsy, 70 per cent.[5-7]

D. Full staging costs about $2000, takes 5 days, and includes (1) microscopic grading, (2) serum acid phosphatase determination, (3) bone survey, (4) bone marrow acid phosphatase determination (optional), (5) bone scan, (6) excretory urogram (IVP), (7) cystoscopic examination, (8) lymphangiogram (optional), and (9) lymph node dissection.

E. Staging and distribution of the various stages are as follows:[8]

A_1 = 1, 2, or 3 foci of well differentiated tumor (overall incidence, 13 per cent).

A_2 = More than 50 per cent of the specimen contains tumor, or the tumor is high grade (11 per cent).

B_1 = Nodule occupying less than 1 lobe; the other lobe is normal (11 per cent).

B_2 = Prostatic nodule occupying one entire lobe or abnormality detected in both lobes; biopsy proven (16 per cent).

C = Local extension to pelvic walls or seminal vesicles (4.3 per cent).

D = Metastatic; extends beyond the prostate and the seminal vesicles (28 per cent).

D_1 = Metastatic to pelvic lymph nodes.

D_2 = Metastatic beyond pelvic lymph nodes.

Pelvic lymphadenectomy of the obturator, hypogastric, and external iliac nodes in cases of early, potentially curable cancer demonstrated 25 per cent of stage B cancers and 60 per cent of stage C cancers that had involved nodes, making them in actuality stage D_1.[9]

F. For radical prostatectomy of stage A_2 tumors, the mortality rate is 3 per cent. Complications include rectal injury (9 per cent), pelvic recurrence (9 per cent), stress incontinence (42 per cent), total incontinence (15 per cent), anastomosis stricture (9 per cent), and impotence (± 100 per cent).[10]

Of nodules detected on rectal exam and biopsied, 50 per cent are malignant and 50 per cent are benign.[11]

Radical perineal prostatectomy for a 1 to 1.5 cm. nodule in one lobe without evidence of other disease demonstrated 16 per cent seminal vesicle involvement (stage C). There were no 15-year survivors. In 11 per cent disease was confined to one lobe (stage B_1 pathologically). In 73 per cent there was disease in the other lobe (stage B_2 pathologically).

Stages B_1 and B_2 have a 33 per cent 15-year survival rate.

G. For radical prostatectomy of stage B_2 tumors the mortality rate is 1 per cent. Complications include perineal fistula (13 per cent), temporary incontinence (21 per cent), permanent incontinence (10 per cent), bladder neck contracture (6 per cent), wound infection (3 per cent), osteitis pubis (1.5 per cent), urethral stricture (9 per cent), and impotence (100 per cent).[12, 13]

H. In discussing the complications of external beam radiation therapy, stages B_1 and B_2 are combined into one category and stage C is considered as a separate category.[14, 15]

The complications are cystitis (2 to 41 per cent), proctitis (2 to 41 per cent), stricture (0 to 4 per cent), lymphedema of the leg (6 per cent), lymphedema of the penis (6 per cent), and positive post-therapy biopsy (15 to 55 per cent).

Impotency occurs in approximately 40 per cent of patients treated with external beam radiation therapy.

I. Early hormonal therapy for the asymptomatic patient is not beneficial in stage C disease.[16] Five-year survival rates of patients with stage C lesions are as follows: with estrogen therapy, 50 per cent; with orchiectomy, 56 per cent; with both estrogen and orchiectomy, 44 per cent; and with placebo, 58 per cent.[16]

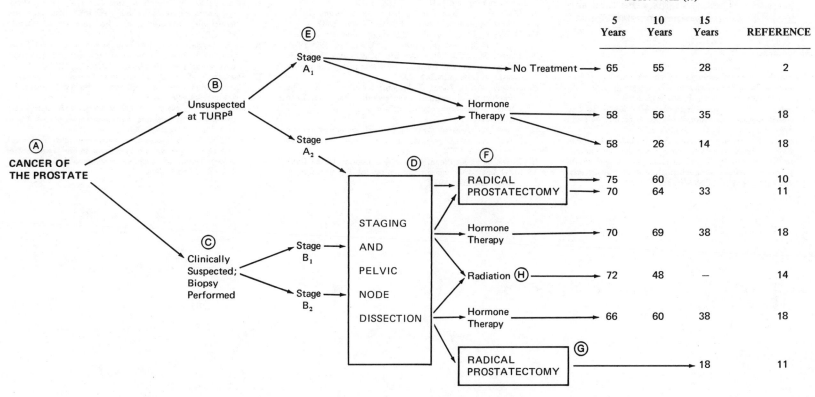

SURVIVAL (%)

	5 Years	10 Years	15 Years	REFERENCE
No Treatment	65	55	28	2
Hormone Therapy	58	56	35	18
	58	26	14	18
RADICAL PROSTATECTOMY	75	60		10
	70	64	33	11
Hormone Therapy	70	69	38	18
Radiation (H)	72	48	–	14
Hormone Therapy	66	60	38	18
RADICAL PROSTATECTOMY			18	11

(A) CANCER OF THE PROSTATE

(B) Unsuspected at TURP[a]

(E) Stage A₁

Stage A₂

(C) Clinically Suspected; Biopsy Performed

Stage B₁

Stage B₂

(D) STAGING AND PELVIC NODE DISSECTION

(F) RADICAL PROSTATECTOMY

(G)

[a] TURP = Transurethral prostatectomy

J. In Stage D disease the response does not correlate with serum testosterone concentrations.

K. Some patients with stage C disease treated by estrogen and orchiectomy showed a marked response of the tumor to rectal palpation. These patients were then subjected to radical perineal prostatectomy.[19]

References

1. Scott, R., et al.: Carcinoma of the prostate in elderly men — Incidence, Growth, Characteristics, and Clinical Significance. J. Urol., *101*:602, 1969.
2. Heaney, J. A., et al.: Prognosis of clinically undiagnosed prostatic carcinoma and the influence of endocrine therapy. J. Urol., *118*:283, 1977.
3. Byar, D. P., and the Veterans' Administration Cooperative Urologic Research Group: Survival of patients with incidentally found microscopic cancer of the prostate: Results of a clinical trial of conservative treatment. J. Urol., *108*:908, 1972.
4. Wettlaufer, J. N., and McMillen, S. M.: The role of repeat transurethral biopsy in stage A carcinoma of the prostate. J. Urol., *116*:759, 1976.
5. Bissada, N. K., Roundtree, G. A., and Sulieman, J. S.: Factors affecting accuracy and morbidity in transrectal biopsy of the prostate. Surg. Gynecol. Obstet., *145*:869, 1977.
6. Fortunoff, S.: Needle biopsy of the prostate: A review of 346 biopsies. J. Urol., *87*:159, 1962.
7. Kaufman, J. J., and Schultz, J. I.: Needle biopsy of the prostate: A reevaluation. J. Urol., *87*:164, 1962.
8. Donohue, R. E., et al.: Staging of prostatic carcinoma — A different distribution. J. Urol., *122*:327, 1979.
9. Barzell, W., et al.: Prostatic adenocarcinoma: Relationship of grade and local extent to the pattern of metastases. J. Urol., *118*:278, 1977.
10. Nichols, R. T., Barry, J. M. and Hodges, C. V.: The morbidity of radical prostatectomy for multifocal stage I prostatic adenocarcinoma. J. Urol., *117*:83, 1977.
11. Jewett, H.: Present status of radical prostatectomy for stage A and B prostatic cancer. Urol. Clin. North Am., 2:105, 1975.
12. Boxer, R. J., Kaufman, J. J., and Goodwin, W. E. Radical prostatectomy for carcinoma of the prostate. J. Urol., *117*:208, 1977.
13. Jewett, H. J., Eggleston, J. C., and Yawn, D. H.: Radical prostatectomy, the management of carcinoma of the prostate: Probable cause of some therapeutic failure. J. Urol., *107*:1034, 1972.
14. Bagshaw, M.: Radiation therapy for cancer of the prostate. *In* Skinner, D. G., and deKernion, J. B. (eds.): Genitourinary Cancer. Philadelphia, W. B. Saunders, 1978, pp. 355–378.
15. Rhany, R. K., Wilson, S. K., and Caldwell, W. L.: Biopsy-proven tumor following definitive irradiation for resectable carcinoma of the prostate. J. Urol., *107*:627, 1972.
16. V. A. Cooperative Urological Research Group: Treatment and survival of patients with cancer of the prostate. Surg. Gynecol. Obstet., *124*:1011, 1967.
17. Shearer, R. J., et al.: Plasma testosterone: An accurate monitor of hormone treatment in prostatic cancer. Br. J. Urol., *45*:668, 1973.
18. Barnes, R. W., Hirst, A., and Rosenquist, R.: Early carcinoma of the prostate: Comparison of stages A and B. J. Urol., *115*:404, 1976.
19. Scott, W. W.: Evaluation of endocrine control therapy and radical penile prostatectomy in the treatment of selected cases of advanced carcinoma of the prostate. J. Urol., 77:521, 1957.

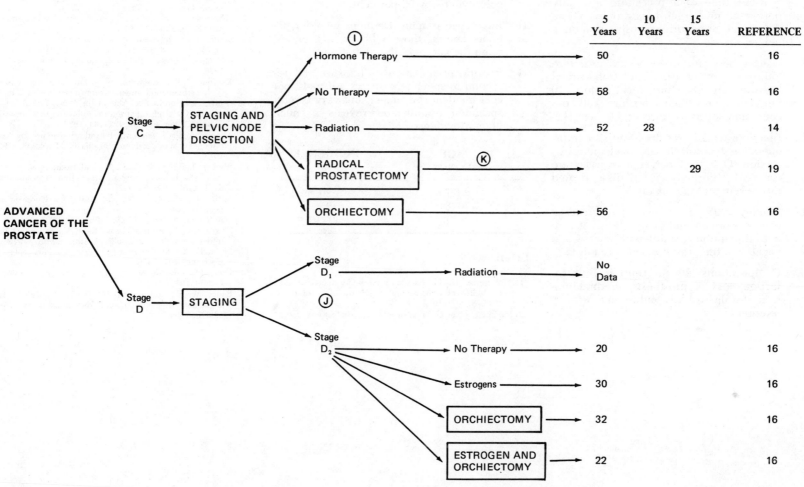

SURVIVAL (%)

	5 Years	10 Years	15 Years	REFERENCE
Hormone Therapy ⓘ	50			16
No Therapy	58			16
Radiation	52	28		14
RADICAL PROSTATECTOMY ⓚ			29	19
ORCHIECTOMY	56			16
Stage D₁ → Radiation	No Data			
Stage D₂ → No Therapy	20			16
Estrogens	30			16
ORCHIECTOMY	32			16
ESTROGEN AND ORCHIECTOMY	22			16

TRANSURETHRAL PROSTATECTOMY BY ALFRED JOHN DeFALCO, M.D.

Comments

A. Among the specific factors that influence prognosis is preoperative renal function. For instance, azotemia increases mortality 3 to 9 times. The procedure is usually performed for benign hypertrophy. These data refer to recurrent obstruction in a benign gland.

B. Causes of death include cardiac failure (50 per cent of cases), gastrointestinal bleeding (10 per cent), renal factors (10 per cent), respiratory failure (90 per cent), and sepsis (3 per cent).[1]

C. Bleeding usually results from poor intraoperative hemostasis and inadequate resection. One to 2 per cent of cases are caused by fibrinolysis and disseminated intravascular coagulopathy.[3]

D. Usually ± 95 per cent of cases bleeding can be stopped endoscopically. If it cannot, suprapubic control with suture and packing of the prostatic bed is required.[3]

E. Complications (20 per cent) include infection, loss of prosthesis, urethral erosion, fistula, osteitis pubis, and urinary retention.[7]

F. Office visits for dilatation are needed every 2 to 4 months for life.

G. Previous or intraoperative ligation of the vas deferens reduces the incidence of epididymitis by 50 per cent.

H. Impotence is more frequent in older patients and in those who do not understand the nature of the operation.[13]

I. Routine examination of transurethral resection to specimens shows a 9 to 12 per cent incidence of cancer, but very careful specimen examination reveals a much higher incidence.[2, 14, 15]

AGE (Years)	INCIDENCE (%)
≤65	20
70–80	25
>80	30–40

References

1. Holtgrewe, H. L.: Factors influencing mortality and morbidity of transurethral resection of prostate. J. Urol., 87:450, 1962.
2. Melchior, J., et al.: Transurethral prostatectomy: Computerized analysis of 2223 consecutive cases. J. Urol., 112:634, 1974.
3. Kirkman, N. S.: Post-prostatectomy hematuria. Br. J. Surg., 54:1026, 1967.
4. Hewitt, C. D., Overholts, E. L., and Finder, R. J.: Gram-negative septicemia in urology. Trans. Am. Assoc, Genitourin. Surg., 56:131, 1964.
5. Schumer, W.: Steroids in the treatment of septic shock. Ann. Surg., 184:333, 1976.
6. Smith, R.: Complications of transurethral surgery. In Smith, R., and Skinner, D. (eds.): Complications of Urologic Surgery. Philadelphia, W. B. Saunders Co., 1976, p. 296.
7. Kaufman, J. J., and Raz, S.: Passive urethral compression with a silicone gel prosthesis for the treatment of male urinary incontinence. Mayo Clin. Proc., 51:373, 1976.
8. Lentz, H. C.: Urethral strictures following transurethral prostatectomy. J. Urol., 117:194, 1977.
9. Abrams, J. I.: Treatment of urethral stricture by free thickness skin graft urethroplasty. Urology, 1:93, 1973.
10. Renker, J. R., Hancock, C. V., and Henderson, W. D.: Prophylactic vasectomy in prevention of epididymitis. J. Urol., 104:303, 1970.
11. Antila, L., Markkula, N., and Iisalo, E.: Geriatric aspects of patients with benign prostatic hypertrophy. Acta Chir. Scand., 357:95, 1966.
12. Nicolaides, A., Field, E., and Kaka, V.: Prostatectomy in deep vein thrombosis. Br. J. Surg., 59:487, 1972.
13. McMadiosky, M. C.: Post-prostatectomy impotence. J. Urol., 115:401, 1976.
14. Dias, R., Lowengood, R., and Gaetz, H.: Urology, 11:599, 1978.
15. Bauer, W. C., McGaveran, N. H., and Carlin, M. L.: Unsuspected carcinoma of the prostate. Cancer, 13:370, 1960.

TRANSURETHRAL PROSTATECTOMY

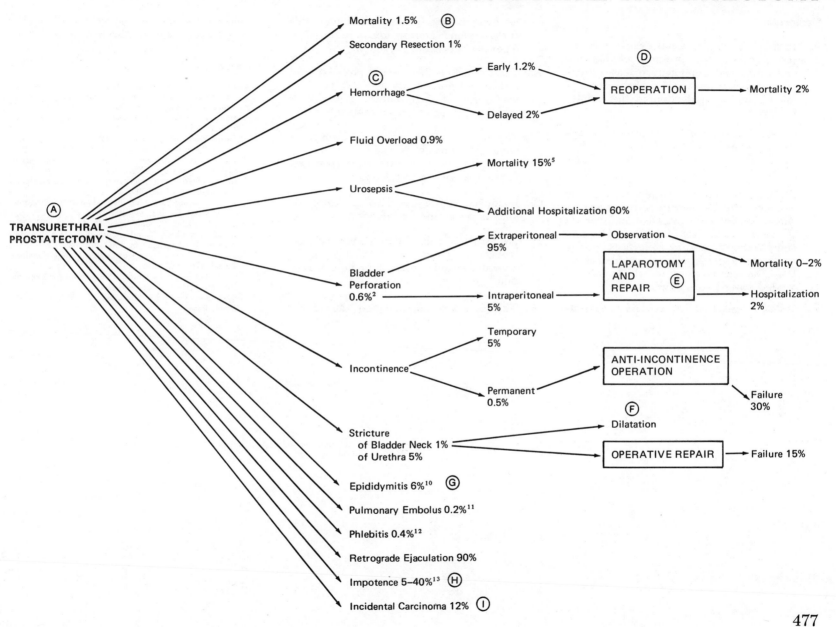

NEPHRECTOMY BY Alfred John De Falco, M.D.

Comments

A. In addition to the usual factors such as age, nutrition, and presence of diabetes or cardiac and pulmonary disease, prognosis depends on function of the remaining kidney and infection in the kidney removed.

B. Common indications include trauma, hydronephrosis, pyelonephritis, calculus, renal artery stenosis, and donor kidney graft.

C. Radical or extended nephrectomy is characteristically performed for cancer. It can be performed transabdominally or via a thoracoabdominal incision. Thoracic complications such as atelectasis, pneumothorax, and hydrothorax are almost totally limited to cases in which the extended procedure is employed.

D. Initial vascular pedicle control and isolated ligation largely have eliminated this complication.[9] Transfusion is required in 5 per cent of cases.

E. There is a 40 to 50 per cent probability of serious left renal injury and a 10 per cent probability of right kidney injury with specific rupture following trauma.

F. This occurs mainly when the thoracoabdominal approach is used, but it may occur inadvertently with high subcostal incision or with rib refraction.[5]

G. Incidence is increased when nephrectomy is performed for infection.[5]

H. AV fistula is a rare complication of mass pedicle ligation and infection that may be recognized only years following operation.[9]

I. This is a rare complication caused not only by a retained sponge or an iatrogenic foreign body but also by a stone.

References

1. Robson, C. J., Churchill, B. M., and Anderson, W.: Result of radical nephrectomy for renal stone carcinoma. Trans. Assoc. Genitourin. Surg., *60*:122, 1968.
2. Bergan, J. J.: Donor nephrectomy. Transplant. Proc., 5:1131, 1972.
3. Uehling, D. T., Malek, J. H., and Wear, J. D.: Complications of donor nephrectomy. J. Urol., *111*:7, 45; 1974.
4. Viner, N., et al.: Bilateral nephrectomy—Analysis of 100 cases. J. Urol., *113*:291, 1975.
5. Penn, I.: The use of living donors in kidney transplantation. Arch. Surg., *101*:226, 1970.
6. Barry, J., and Hodges, C.: Subcostal approach to kidney and adrenal. J. Urol., *114*:666, 1975.
7. Smith, D., Schulte, J., and Smart, W.: Surgery of the kidney: *In* Campbell, M. (ed.): Urology, 2nd ed. Philadelphia, W. B. Saunders Co., 1963, p. 2362.
8. Spanos, P.: Complications of related kidney donation. Surgery, 76:741, 1974.
9. Cole, J.: The subcostal modification of thoracoabdominal incision. J. Urol., *112*:168, 1974.
10. Goldstream, A.: Post-nephrectomy AV fistula. J. Urol., 98:44, 1968.

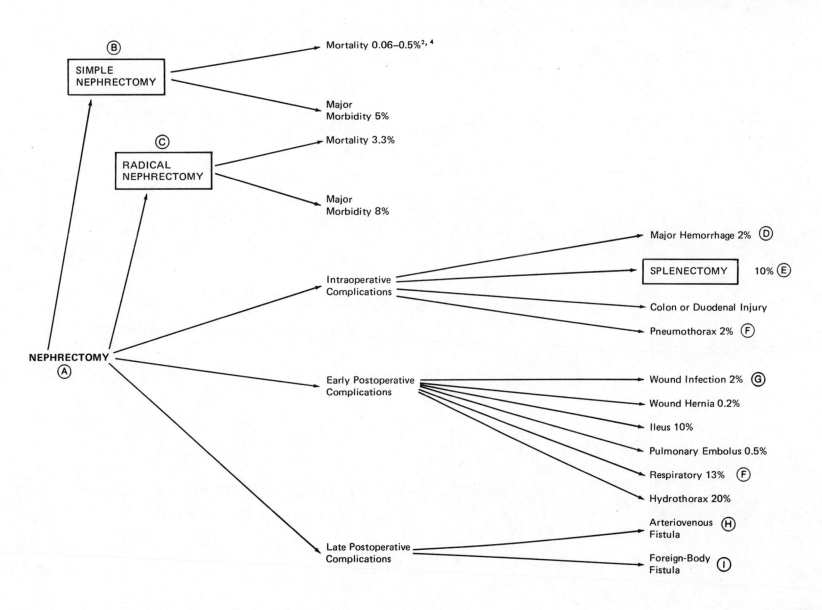

SIMPLE NEPHRECTOMY Ⓑ

Mortality 0.06–0.5%[2, 4]

Major Morbidity 5%

RADICAL NEPHRECTOMY Ⓒ

Mortality 3.3%

Major Morbidity 8%

NEPHRECTOMY Ⓐ

Intraoperative Complications

Major Hemorrhage 2% Ⓓ

SPLENECTOMY 10% Ⓔ

Colon or Duodenal Injury

Pneumothorax 2% Ⓕ

Early Postoperative Complications

Wound Infection 2% Ⓖ

Wound Hernia 0.2%

Ileus 10%

Pulmonary Embolus 0.5%

Respiratory 13% Ⓕ

Hydrothorax 20%

Late Postoperative Complications

Arteriovenous Ⓗ Fistula

Foreign-Body Ⓘ Fistula

479

Section L

Orthopedic

FRACTURE OF THE CERVICAL SPINE BY JEROME D. WIEDEL, M.D.

Comments

A. Slightly more than 50 per cent of all spinal fractures involve the cervical region. Causes include[8] vehicular accidents (46.5 per cent), sports and recreation (26.4 per cent), falls (17.3 per cent), and penetrating wounds (6.3 per cent), with 3.5 per cent from other causes.

   Males predominate (82 per cent), with peak incidence between ages 20 to 29 and 40 to 45.[9]

B. Nonindustrial accidents account for 89 per cent of penetrating injuries that fracture the cervical spine. Almost all of these patients have some neurologic deficit.[1, 3, 7, 9]

C. Laminectomy simply decompresses the spinal cord. Most surgeons do not advocate its use in open injuries because it almost never improves the pre-existing deficit, and it increases the incidence of infection and spinal fluid fistula.[4, 6] Operative mortality from laminectomy is less than 1 per cent, and wound complications occur in ± 10 per cent of cases.

D. Closed treatment consists of traction, plaster cast, and halo cast or vest for immobilization, until the fragments are stable. Average hospitalization is 16 days.[5]

E. An incomplete spinal cord injury is indicated by the presence, however altered, of voluntary muscle function or sensation below the level of cord injury. Total loss of sensation and absence of voluntary muscle function suggest a complete spinal cord injury.[2]

F. The primary advantage of open reduction and internal fixation plus fusion is stabilization of the spine, which permits earlier mobilization even though hospitalization time may not be decreased.

G. Once a quadriplegic reaches an acute trauma unit, the mortality rate is ± 5 per cent. A decubitus ulcer will occur in 10 per cent of cases during the first hospitalization and in 20 per cent overall. It costs $8000 to treat one bed sore.

   Urologic complications are the main cause of late mortality. One hundred per cent of quadriplegics with indwelling catheters will have bladder infections but, with good care and the absence of a high pressure system, infection of the kidneys is no more likely than in the normal population.[9] Some complications of quadriplegia in the initial hospitalization period are thrombophlebitis (± 70 per cent of cases), bleeding stress ulcer (± 80 per cent are minor; ± 5 per cent become major), pulmonary complications (± 40 per cent), and urinary tract infection (± 60 per cent).

   The cost for the original hospitalization is about $22,000 (102 days). Lifetime care cost averages about $400,000. Life expectancy is normal except for respirator cases, who have a mortality rate of ± 65 per cent in the first year.

   Sexual function in the male is 0 per cent, although a reflex erection is present.

   Female patients retain 100 per cent of sexual function.

References

1. Bosch, A., Stauffer, E. S., and Nickel, V. L.: Incomplete traumatic quadriplegia. A 10-year review. JAMA, *216*:473–478, 1971.
2. Bohlman, H.: The pathology and current treatment concepts of cervical spine injuries. A critical review of 300 cases. J. Bone Joint Surg., *54A*:1353–1354, 1972.
3. Meyer, P. R., Jr., et al.: Fracture-dislocation of the cervical spine: Transportation, assessment, and immediate management. A.A.O.S. Instructional Course Lectures, *25*:171–183, 1976.
4. Stauffer, E. S., Kelly, E. G., and Wood, R. W.: Civilian gunshot wounds of the spine: Is laminectomy indicated? J. Bone Joint Surg., *58A*:727, 1976.
5. Forsyth, H. F., Alexander, E., Jr., and Underdal, R.: The advantages of early spine fusion in the treatment of fracture-dislocation of the cervical spine. J. Bone Joint Surg., *41A*:17–36, 1959.
6. Yashon, D., Jane, J. A., and White, R. J.: Prognosis and management of spinal cord and cauda equina bullet injuries in 65 civilians. J. Neurosurg., *32*:163–170, 1970.
7. Morgan, T. H., Wharton, G. W., and Austin, G. N.: The results of laminectomy in patients with incomplete spinal cord injuries. Paraplegia, *9*:14–23, 1971.
8. Young, J. S.: Selected statistical summaries of SCI data for 1973–1977. Proceedings of the National Spinal Cord Injury Model Systems' Conference. Phoenix, Arizona, April 20–21, 1978.
9. Personal communications: Robert R. Jackson, M.D., Project Director, Rocky Mountain Regional Spinal Cord Injury Care Center, Inc., and Medical Director, Craig Hospital, Englewood, Colorado.
10. Thomas, J. P.: Rehabilitation services administration model system concept. Proceedings of the National Spinal Cord Injury Model Systems' Conference. Phoenix, Arizona, April 20–21, 1978.

FRACTURE OF THE CERVICAL SPINE

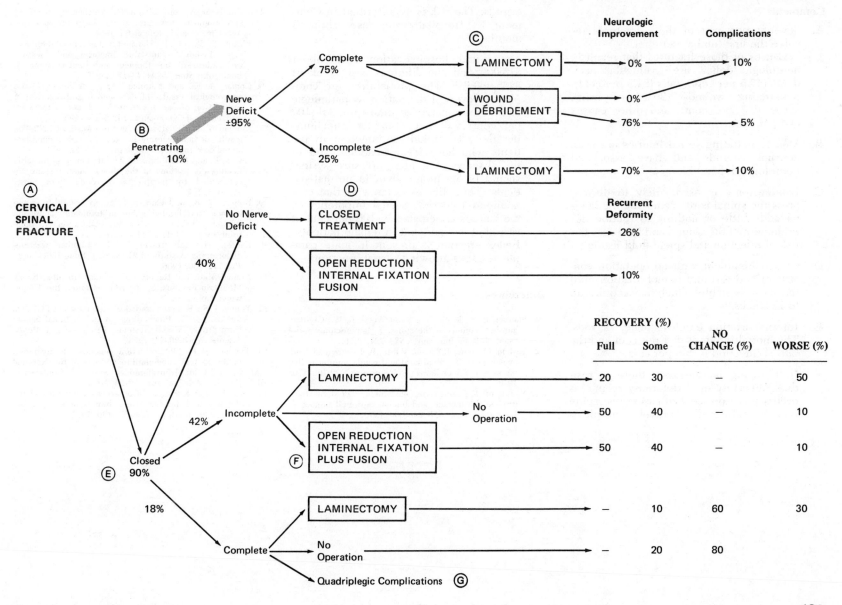

FRACTURE OF THE LUMBAR SPINE by Jerome D. Wiedel, M.D.

Comments

A. Seventy per cent of these fractures involve the first lumbar vertebra.

Causes of those fractures that result in neurologic deficit are[12] vehicular accidents (47.5 per cent), falls (24.9 per cent), penetrating wounds (20.9 per cent), sports (2.3 per cent), and other causes (4.4 per cent).

B. Most penetrating spinal injuries are from gunshot wounds and have associated neurologic deficit.[1,2]

C. Laminectomy is used solely to decompress the spinal cord. Removing the lamina adds little or nothing to routine débridement of the wound and increases the risk of infection and spinal fluid fistula.[1]

D. Closed treatment with no operation consists of bed rest and immobilization until the spine is stable, which may require up to 12 weeks.

E. Internal fixation employs plates or rods. The mortality rate is ± 1 per cent and the rate of infection is ± 5 per cent.

F. If following laminectomy there is residual deformity or if deformity recurs (as occurs in 70 per cent of cases), the spine must be stabilized operatively with plates or rods. The risk is as described in Comment E. Hospitalization lasts about 3 months.[3, 6-10]

G. The initial hospitalization costs about $15,000 and the lifetime cost is about $225,000.[11, 13] The probability for complete recovery if the patient is paraplegic on first examination is almost nil. All (100 per cent) will have bladder infections, but the rate of kidney infection in patients who have ideal treatment and in the absence of a high pressure system should be no higher than in normal patients. Their life expectancy is that of a noninjured control. Sexual impotency in the male is anticipated in 100 per cent of cases but is 0 per cent in female patients. Reflex erection is present in male paraplegics, thus allowing sexual function.

References

1. Stauffer, E. S., Kelly, E. G., and Wood, R. W.: Civilian gunshot wounds of the spine: Is laminectomy indicated? J. Bone Joint Surg., 58A:727, 1976.
2. Yashon, D., Jane, J. A., and White, R. J.: Prognosis and management of spinal cord and cauda equina bullet injuries in 65 civilians. J. Neurosurg., 32:163–170, 1970.
3. Young, M. H.: Long-term consequences of stable fractures of the thoracic and lumbar vertebral bodies. J. Bone Joint Surg., 55B:295–300, 1973.
4. Westerborn, A., and Olsson, O.: Mechanics, treatment and prognosis of fractures of the dorso-lumbar spine. Acta Chir. Scand., 102:59–83, 1951.
5. Flesch, J. R., et al.: Harrington instrumentation and spine fusion for unstable fractures and fracture-dislocations of the thoracic and lumbar spine. J. Bone Joint Surg., 59A:143–153, 1977.
6. Comar, A. E., and Kaufman, A. A.: A survey of the neurological results of 858 spinal cord injuries; A comparison of patients treated with and without laminectomy. J. Neurosurg., 13:95–106, 1956.
7. Morgan, T. H., Wharton, G. W., and Austin, G. N.: The results of laminectomy in patients with incomplete spinal cord injuries. Paraplegia, 9:14–23, 1971.
8. Lewis, J., and McKibbin, B.: The treatment of unstable fracture-dislocations of the thoracolumbar spine accompanied by paraplegia. J. Bone Joint Surg., 56B:603, 1974.
9. Roberts, J. B., and Curtiss, P. H., Jr.: Stability of the thoracic and lumbar spine in traumatic paraplegia following fracture or fracture-dislocation. J. Bone Joint Surg., 52A:1115–1130, 1970.
10. Kaufer, H., and Hayes, J. T.: Lumbar fracture-dislocations. A study of 21 cases. J. Bone Joint Surg., 48A:712–730, 1966.
11. Annual Statistical Report, 1977. Craig Hospital, Rocky Mountain Regional Spinal Injury Center, Inc. Englewood, Colorado.
12. Young, J. S.: Selected statistical summaries of SCI data for 1973–1977. Proceedings of the National Spinal Cord Injury Model Systems' Conference. Phoenix, Arizona, April 20–21, 1978.
13. Thomas, J. P.: Rehabilitation services administration model system concept. Proceedings of the National Spinal Cord Injury Model Systems' Conference. Phoenix, Arizona, April 20–21, 1978.
14. Day, B., and Kokan, P.: Compression fractures of the thoracic and lumbar spine from compensable injuries. Clin. Orthop., 124:173–176, 1977.

FRACTURE OF THE LUMBAR SPINE

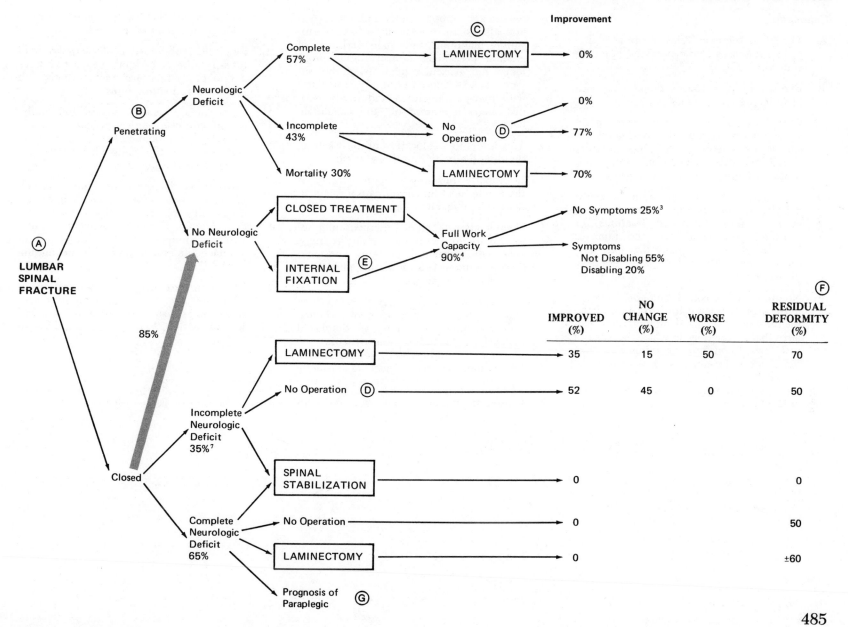

Improvement

Ⓒ

LUMBAR SPINAL FRACTURE Ⓐ

Penetrating Ⓑ

Neurologic Deficit
- Complete 57% → LAMINECTOMY → 0%
- Incomplete 43% → No Operation Ⓓ → 0% / 77% ; → LAMINECTOMY → 70%
- Mortality 30%

No Neurologic Deficit
- CLOSED TREATMENT
- INTERNAL FIXATION Ⓔ
→ Full Work Capacity 90%[4]
→ No Symptoms 25%[3]
→ Symptoms: Not Disabling 55%, Disabling 20%

85%

Closed
- Incomplete Neurologic Deficit 35%[7]
- Complete Neurologic Deficit 65%
- Prognosis of Paraplegic Ⓖ

Ⓕ

	IMPROVED (%)	NO CHANGE (%)	WORSE (%)	RESIDUAL DEFORMITY (%)
LAMINECTOMY	35	15	50	70
No Operation Ⓓ	52	45	0	50
SPINAL STABILIZATION	0			0
No Operation	0			50
LAMINECTOMY	0			±60

485

FRACTURES ABOUT THE SHOULDER BY M. H. SUSMAN, M.D.

Comments

A. The "four-segment" classification of displaced fractures of the proximal humerus is used.[6, 7]

B. Figures in parentheses denote approximate incidence of injury.[8]

C. Closed treatment may vary from simple sling immobilization with graduated unsupervised activity to manipulation under anesthesia, immobilization, and prolonged supervised physical therapy.[6-8]

D. This may consist of open reduction internal fixation of fracture fragments, as is done in most three-part fractures, or prosthetic replacement of the humeral head, as is done in many four-part fractures and most four-part fracture-dislocations.

E. Nonunion of proximal humeral fractures most often is related to distraction of the fracture site by closed methods, particularly that of traction or a hanging type of cast. Displaced greater tuberosity fractures can go to nonunion if displacement is greater than 1 cm., which also produces subacromial impingement and cuff deficiency.

F. Significant complications include infection after open treatment, adhesive capsulitis, malunion with pain and loss of motion, occasional neurovascular problems, and avascular necrosis of the humeral head — most frequently associated with four-part fractures and rarely with displaced fractures of the anatomic neck.[2, 6-8]

G. This refers to the location of the fracture, dividing the bone into three sections.

H. Improperly performed open surgery is the single most important causal factor in nonunion of clavicular fractures.[3]

I. Complications include neurovascular injury, malunion with angulation or excessive callus formation or both, and pain with or without loss of motion, particularly in distal fractures.[4, 5, 8, 10]

J. Open reduction is rarely indicated in clavicle fracture management. Indications include reduction of displaced distal-third fractures, neurovascular involvement (middle-third), soft tissue interposition, and the occasional cosmetic concern.

K. Closed treatment of clavicular fractures can be accomplished by a great number of different retention devices.[8]

L. Regardless of location, all scapular fractures require considerable causative trauma, among which are pneumothorax, rib fractures, and spinal injury.

M. Os acromiale, usually present bilaterally, can be confused with acromion fractures. An axillary roentgenogram is necessary to visualize well the coracoid fractures and some glenoid injuries.

N. Indications for open treatment include displaced split-socket glenoid fractures, displaced coracoid fractures with or without acromioclavicular separation, neurovascular injury, markedly angulated or displaced fractures, and the rare nonunion.[1, 9, 11]

O. The high percentage of complications is explained by the very common occurrence of persistent postfracture pain and loss of motion, here regarded as complications.

Note: Some percentage figures are the author's estimates in cases where no exact figures could be found.

		CLOSED TREATMENT (%)	OPEN TREATMENT (%)	SATISFACTORY TO EXCELLENT RESULTS (%)	NONUNION (%)	COMPLICATIONS (%)	REFERENCES
Nondisplaced (80%) Ⓑ		100	0	95–100	0	0–1	6, 8
Two-part Fracture (10%)	Anatomic Neck	99–100	0–1	99	< 1	1–5 Ⓕ	
	Surgical Neck	95–100	0–5	90	1–5 Ⓔ	5–10	
	Greater Tuberosity	95–100	0–5	90	1–2	1–5	6–8
	Lesser Tuberosity	100	0	95	< 1	< 1	
Three-part Fracture (3%)	Greater Tuberosity and Neck	30 Ⓒ	70 Ⓓ	48	15 Ⓔ	31	6–8
	Lesser Tuberosity and Neck	38	62	31	15	31	6–8
Four-part Fracture (4%)		37	63	37	13	20	6–8
Fracture Dislocations; Articular Surface Fractures (3%)	Two-part	99	1	99	< 1	1–5	
	Three-part	32	68	60	15	31	
	Four-part	11	89	65	13	20	2, 6–8

PROXIMAL HUMERUS Ⓐ

FRACTURES ABOUT THE SHOULDER *Continued*

References

1. Findlay, R. T.: Fractures of the scapula and ribs. Am. J. Surg., *38*:489–494, 1937.
2. Knight, R. A., and Mayne, J. A.: Comminuted fractures and fracture-dislocations involving the articular surface of the humeral head. J. Bone Joint Surg., *39A*:1343–1355, 1957.
3. Neer, C. S., II: Nonunion of the clavicle. JAMA, *172*:1006–1011, 1960.
4. Neer, C. S., II: Fracture of the distal clavicle with detachment of the coracoclavicular ligaments in adults. J. Trauma, *3*:99–110, 1963.
5. Neer, C. S., II: Fractures of the distal third of the clavicle. Clin. Orthop., *58*:43–50, 1968.
6. Neer, C. S., II: Displaced proximal humeral fractures. I. Classification and evaluation. J. Bone Joint Surg., *52A*:1077–1089, 1970.
7. Neer, C. S., II: Displaced proximal humeral fractures. II. Treatment of three-part and four-part displacement. J. Bone Joint Surg., *52A*:1090–1103, 1970.
8. Rockwood, C. A., Jr., and Green, D. P.: Fractures. Philadelphia, J. B. Lippincott, 1975.
9. Rowe, C. R.: Fractures of the scapula. Surg. Clin. North Am., *43*:1565–1571, 1963.
10. Rowe, C. R.: An atlas of anatomy and treatment of midclavicular fractures. Clin. Orthop., *58*:29–42, 1968.
11. Wilber, M. C., and Evans, E. B.: Fractures of the scapula. J. Bone Joint Surg., *59A*:358–362, 1977.
12. Zdravkovic, D., and Damholt, V. V.: Comminuted and severely displaced fractures of the scapula. Acta Orthop. Scand., *45*:60–65, 1974.

		Ⓒ CLOSED TREATMENT (%)	OPEN TREATMENT (%)	GOOD TO EXCELLENT RESULTS (%)	NONUNION (%)	COMPLICATIONS (%)	REFERENCES
Ⓖ	Middle Third (80%) Ⓚ	98–99	1–2	96–99	0.8[a] 3.7[b]	1–3 Ⓘ	4, 5, 8, 10
CLAVICLE	Distal Third (15%) Ⓙ	85–90	10–15	90	0–5	5–10	3–5, 10
	Proximal Third (5%)	99	1	98–99	0–1	1	8
Ⓛ SCAPULA	Upper (Acromion, Coracoid, Glenoid) Ⓜ	90	10 Ⓝ	15–20	0–1	80–85 Ⓞ	1, 8, 9, 11, 12
	Lower (Body, Neck, Spine)	98	2	95–100	0	0–5	8, 9, 11

[a]Closed treatment
[b]Open treatment

489

FOREARM FRACTURES OF ADULTS BY TRACY HICKS, M.D.

Comments

A. Because the forearm is a semirigid rectangle, when one bone breaks there usually is an accompanying fracture or dislocation.

B. Open (compound) fractures occur in 13 to 33 per cent of forearm fractures. After débridement, treatment results are as follows:

TREATMENT	GOOD TO EXCELLENT RESULTS	OSTEO-MYE-LITIS	NONUNION
Plaster Immobilization	28%	14%	2–7%
Internal Fixation	92%	10%	1%

If osteomyelitis develops, the internal fixation material can be removed and infection will clear in 95 per cent of cases. Meanwhile, the bones will have consolidated in position.[1]

C. Monteggia fracture is a fracture of the ulna (usually the proximal third) associated with dislocation of the proximal radial-ulnar joint.[9, 10, 13]

D. Galeazzie fracture is a fracture of the distal half of the radius associated with dislocation of the distal radial-ulnar joint.[9, 13]

E. Open reduction and fixation is the rule rather than the exception if there is any displacement because the procedure (1) has a higher incidence of good to excellent results, (2) has lower incidences of delayed union or nonunion, rotational displacement, muscle atrophy, and osteoporosis, and (3) allows earlier motion.[1, 4–6, 8–10, 12, 13] The estimated incidence of open reduction in adult forearm fractures is 60 per cent for fracture of a single bone, 85 per cent for fracture of a single bone plus dislocation, and 95 per cent for fracture of both bones. In children the incidence is approximately reversed.

Complications of open reduction include (1) wound infection (2 per cent of cases), (2) Volkmann's contracture (0.3 to 1 per cent), (3) failure of fixation (0.4 to 3 per cent), (4) re-fracture through screw holes (2.5 to 6 per cent), (5) causalgia (1 to 2 per cent), (6) iatrogenic injury to nerves or blood vessels (2 per cent), and (7) myositis ossificans (less than 1 per cent).[1, 4, 5, 8–11, 13]

F. Good to excellent results are defined as 80 per cent of normal supination and pronation, and 80 per cent restoration of strength.

Results with closed reduction and cast are shown in the table below.[2, 7, 9–11, 13, 14] Other complications of closed treatment are (1) compartment syndrome (1 per

TYPE OF FRACTURE	INITIAL REDUCTION (%)	MAINTAINED REDUCTION (%)	GOOD TO EXCELLENT RESULTS (%)	COMPLICATIONS (%)			
				NU[a]	MU[b]	CU[c]	Nerve Injury
Radial	27	80	14–35	20	4		9
Ulnar	70	65	22–40	22	9–30		5
Monteggia	15	65	6–8	22–35	10–35		3–7
Galeazzie	21	45	8–28	26–37	30–65		1–3
Both Bones:							
Proximal	55	60	29–50	14–41		4–10	
Middle	45	60	35–55	2–6		3–16	
Distal	85	75	41–61	6–17		6	

[a]NU = nonunion
[b]MU = malunion
[c]CU = cross-union

490

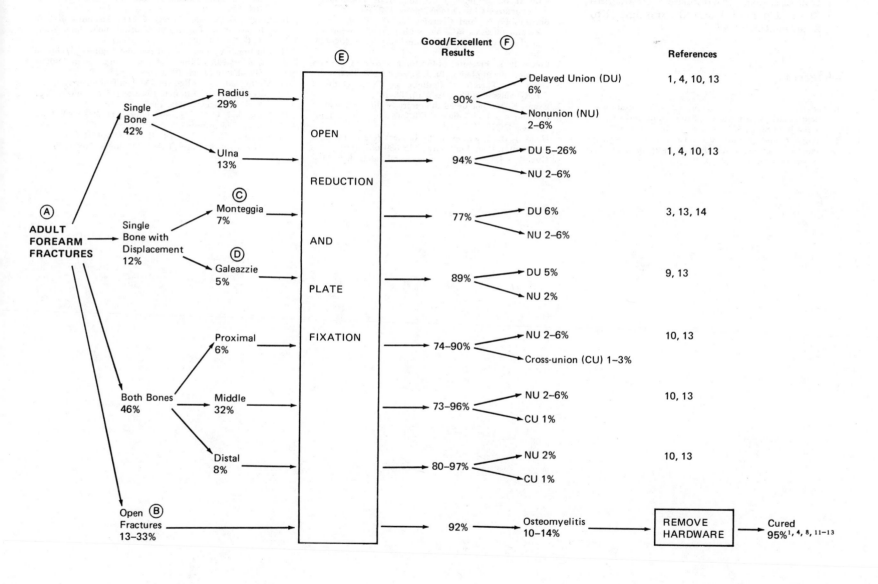

Good/Excellent Results (F)

References

ADULT FOREARM FRACTURES (A)

Single Bone 42%
- Radius 29% → OPEN → 90% → Delayed Union (DU) 6% / Nonunion (NU) 2–6% — 1, 4, 10, 13
- Ulna 13% → REDUCTION → 94% → DU 5–26% / NU 2–6% — 1, 4, 10, 13

Single Bone with Displacement 12%
- Monteggia (C) 7% → AND → 77% → DU 6% / NU 2–6% — 3, 13, 14
- Galeazzie (D) 5% → PLATE → 89% → DU 5% / NU 2% — 9, 13

Both Bones 46%
- Proximal 6% → FIXATION → 74–90% → NU 2–6% / Cross-union (CU) 1–3% — 10, 13
- Middle 32% → 73–96% → NU 2–6% / CU 1% — 10, 13
- Distal 8% → 80–97% → NU 2% / CU 1% — 10, 13

Open (B) Fractures 13–33% → 92% → Osteomyelitis 10–14% → REMOVE HARDWARE → Cured 95%[1, 4, 8, 11–13]

(E)

FOREARM FRACTURES OF ADULTS *Continued*

cent of cases), (2) Volkmann's contracture (0.3 to 1 per cent), and (3) causalgia (1 to 2 per cent).[2, 7, 9-11, 13, 14]

References

1. Anderson, L. D., et al.: Compression–plate fixation in acute diaphyseal fractures of the radius and ulna. J. Bone Joint Surg., 57A:287–297, 1975.
2. Bolton, H., and Quinlan, A. G.: The conservative treatment of fractures of the shaft of the radius and ulna in adults. Lancet, 2:700, 1952.
3. Boyd, H. B., and Boals, J. C.: Rigid fixation of Monteggia fractures. Clin. Orthop., 66:94–100, 1969.
4. Burwell, H. N., and Charnley, A. D.: Treatment of forearm fractures in adults with particular reference to plate fixation. J. Bone Joint Surg., 46B:404–425, 1964.
5. Cowie, R. S.: Fractures of the forearm treated by open reduction and plating. Br. J. Surg., 44:263, 1956.
6. Danis, R.: Theorie et Pratique de l'Osteosynthese. Paris, Masson et Cie., 1949, pp. 95–105.
7. Evans, E. M.: Rotational deformity in the treatment of fractures of both bones of the forearm. J. Bone Joint Surg., 27:373–379, 1945.
8. Hicks, J. H.: Fractures of the forearm treated by rigid fixation. J. Bone Joint Surg., 43B:680–687, 1961.
9. Hughston, J. C.: Fracture of the distal radial shaft: Mistakes in management. J. Bone Joint Surg., 39A:249–264, 1957.
10. Knight, R. A., and Purvis, G. D.: Fractures of both bones of the forearm in adults. J. Bone Joint Surg., 31A:755–764, 1949.
11. Lidstrom, A.: Fractures of the distal radius: A clinical and statistical study of end results. Acta Orthop. Scand., Suppl. 41, 1959.
12. Müller, M. E., Allgower, M., and Willenegger, H.: Technique of Internal Fixation of Fractures. New York, Springer-Verlag, 1965.
13. Rockwood, C. A., Jr., and Green, D. P. (eds.): Fractures. Philadelphia, J. B. Lippincott, 1975.
14. Speed, J. S., and Boyd, H. B.: Closed treatment of Monteggia fractures. JAMA, 115:1699–1704, 1940.

FRACTURES ABOUT THE WRIST

FRACTURES ABOUT THE WRIST BY DONALD FERLIC, M.D.

Comments

A. These include Colles' and Smith's fractures.

B. In Colles' fractures[4] the ulnar styloid is fractured in 47 per cent of cases. The ulnar head is fractured in 1.5 per cent of cases.

C. Unstable fractures may require skeletal fixation or percutaneous pinning.

D. Indications for open reduction include an impacted articular surface and nerve entrapment.

E. Complications of a distal radius fracture include (1) decreased palmar flexion (95 per cent of cases), (2) decreased range of motion (ROM) in the digits (48 per cent), (3) decreased grip strength (33 per cent), (4) delayed union (0.7 per cent), (5) nonunion (0.2 per cent), (6) persistent pain (2 per cent), (7) decreased ROM of shoulder (1 per cent), (8) traumatic neuritis (0.2 per cent), and (9) causalgia (0.1 per cent).

F. Resection of fracture fragment may be needed.[11]

G. Nonunion may produce instability of the radial-ulnar joint.

H. Unrecognized scaphoid fractures have a poorer prognosis and require open reduction in a greater percentage of cases.

I. This includes prosthetic replacement, fusion of the proximal row, wrist fusion, or another attempt at bone grafting.

J. Most of these fractures are associated with carpal injuries.[15]

K. Few fractures of the carpal bones are displaced.[11] Incidences of fracture of the individual carpal bones are as follows: scaphoid (70.8 per cent); triquetrum (14.3 per cent), of which 18 per cent are compression fractures and 82 per cent are avulsion type; capitate (2.4 per cent); lunate (5.6 per cent); hamate (2.1 per cent); pisiform (2.1 per cent); trapezium (2.1 per cent), and lesser multiangular bones (0.5 per cent).

L. Avulsion fractures heal with 4 to 6 weeks of immobilization therapy.[12]

M. Localized intercarpal arthritis is the major complication.[11, 12]

N. If the hook of the hamate is fractured, it should be excised.[6, 8]

References

1. Bacorn, R. W., and Kurtzke, J. F.: Colles' fracture: A study of 2000 cases from the New York State Workmen's Compensation Board. J. Bone Joint Surg., 50A:570–575, 1968.
2. Baumann, J. V., and Campbell, R. D., Jr.: Significance of architectural types of fractures of the carpal scaphoid and relation to timing of treatment. J. Trauma, 2:431–438, 1962.
3. Bizzaro, A. H.: Traumatology of the carpus. Surg. Gynecol. Obstet., 34:574–588, 1922.
4. Bohler, L.: The Treatment of Fractures, Vol. 1. New York, Grune & Stratton, 1956.
5. Bonnin, J. G., and Greening, W. P.: Fractures of the triquetrum. Br. J. Surg., 31:278, 1943.
6. Bowen, T. L.: Injuries of the hamate bone. Hand, 5:235–238, 1973.
7. Brown, P. E.,, and Dameron, T. B.: Surgical treatment for nonunion of the scaphoid. South. Med. J., 68:415–421, 1975.
8. Cameron, H. U., et al.: Fracture of the hook of the hamate. J. Bone Joint Surg., 57A:276–277, 1975.
9. Cassebaum, W. H.: Colles' fracture: A study of end results. JAMA, 143:963–965, 1950.
10. Cole, J. M., and Obletz, B. E.: Comminuted fractures of the distal end of the radius treated by skeletal transfixion in plaster cast: An end-result study of 33 cases. J. Bone Joint Surg., 48A:931–945, 1966.
11. Conwell, H. E., and Reynolds, F. C.: Management of Fractures, Dislocations and Sprains. St. Louis, C. V. Mosby Co., 1961.
12. Dobyns, J. H., and Linscheid, R. L.: Fractures and dislocations of the wrist. In Rockwood, C. A., Jr., and Green, D. P. (eds.): Fractures. Philadelphia, J. B. Lippincott Co., 1975, pp. 345–440.
13. Frywan, G.: Fracture of the distal radius including sequelae: Shoulder-hand-finger syndrome, disturbance in the distal radioulnar joint, and impairment of nerve function — A clinical and experimental study. Acta Orthop. Scand., 108(Suppl.):1–155, 1967.
14. Gartland, J. F., Jr., and Werley, C. W.: Evaluation of healed Colles' fractures. J. Bone Joint Surg., 33A:895–907, 1951.
15. Mazet, R., Jr., and Hohl, M.: Fractures of the carpal navicular: Analysis of 91 cases and review of the literature. J. Bone Joint Surg., 45A:82–112, 1963.
16. Muray, G.: End results of bone grafting for nonunion of the carpal navicular. J. Bone Joint Surg., 28:749–755, 1946.
17. Stewart, M. J.: Fractures of the carpal navicular. J. Bone Joint Surg., 36A:998–1006, 1954.
18. Russe, O.: Fracture of the carpal navicular. J. Bone Joint Surg., 42A:759–768, 1960.

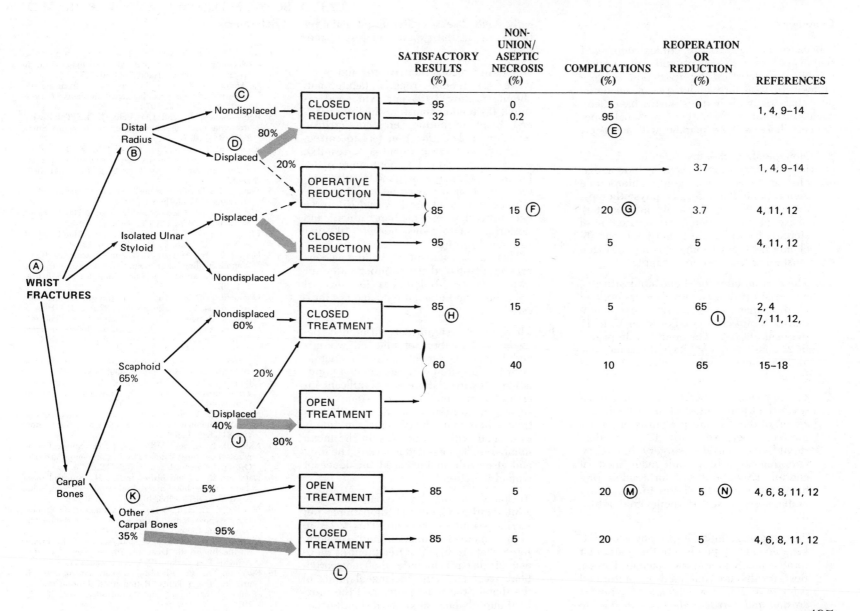

	SATISFACTORY RESULTS (%)	NON-UNION/ ASEPTIC NECROSIS (%)	COMPLICATIONS (%)	REOPERATION OR REDUCTION (%)	REFERENCES
Ⓒ Nondisplaced → CLOSED REDUCTION	95	0	5	0	1, 4, 9–14
	32	0.2	95 Ⓔ		
Ⓓ Displaced (20%) → OPERATIVE REDUCTION				3.7	1, 4, 9–14
	85	15 Ⓕ	20 Ⓖ	3.7	4, 11, 12
Displaced → CLOSED REDUCTION	95	5	5	5	4, 11, 12
Nondisplaced 60% → CLOSED TREATMENT	85 Ⓗ	15	5	65 Ⓘ	2, 4 7, 11, 12,
Displaced 40% → OPEN TREATMENT	60	40	10	65	15–18
Other Carpal Bones 35% (5%) → OPEN TREATMENT	85	5	20 Ⓜ	5 Ⓝ	4, 6, 8, 11, 12
(95%) → CLOSED TREATMENT	85	5	20	5	4, 6, 8, 11, 12

WRIST FRACTURES Ⓐ

Distal Radius Ⓑ

Isolated Ulnar Styloid

Carpal Bones

Scaphoid 65%

Other Carpal Bones 35% Ⓚ

Ⓙ 80%

Ⓛ

495

RHEUMATOID ARTHRITIS OF THE HAND AND WRIST

BY F. A. SCOTT, M.D., AND J. A. BOSWICK, JR., M.D.

Comments

Because of the variable clinical course of rheumatoid disease, quantitation of surgical results and statistical interpretation is very difficult. In areas for which there are no statistical analyses published, estimates have been made according to the authors' personal experience. These will be marked with an asterisk (°).

A. Nonoperative therapy includes (1) antiinflammatory agents (aspirin, indomethacin, corticosteroids, gold, chloroquine and D-penicillamine), (2) physiotherapy, (3) splints during the acute inflammatory phase, (4) intra-articular administration of steroids for the acute target joint, and (5) chemical synovectomy (using nitrogen mustard or thiotepa, for example).

B. There is no cure for rheumatoid arthritis, no certain way to achieve remission, and no drug that can regularly relieve symptoms.[17] Remission is achieved in 13 to 17 per cent of cases. The condition improves in 22 to 38 per cent, stays the same in 2 to 27 per cent, and worsens in 19 to 63 per cent.

C. The decision for operation depends upon severity of pain and disability plus localization of disease and prognosis of the indicated operative procedure. Seldom should one consider surgery before attempting to achieve adequate medical control. Exceptions are for tendon rupture or nerve compression in previously undiagnosed cases of rheumatoid arthritis.

D. The prognosis following synovectomy is variable and depends on the particular joint(s) involved and the stage of disease. Best results are obtained if performed *prior to finding any evidence of articular erosion and cartilage destruction* (i.e., in early-stage disease). Significant pain relief occurs at the expense of loss of motion.

E. Soft tissue reconstructive procedures include (1) tendon repairs (acute and chronic rupture)[13] (95 per cent good results); (2) tendon transfers (including lateral band re-routing, crossed intrinsic transfers, and tendon transfers to correct wrist rotation)[7] (75 per cent good results); (3) reconstruction for boutonnière deformity[15] (45 per cent good results); (4) reconstruction for swan-neck deformity[14] (45 per cent good results); and (5) nerve decompression for median, ulnar, and posterior interosseous nerves[6] (99 per cent good results).

There are no statistically valid data confirming results; these numbers are our own estimates. References for surgical procedures and general outcome are indicated.

F. There is no significant difference between the numbers of infected wounds and hematoma formation in rheumatoid arthritis compared with the general population. However, there is a significant increase in the incidence of wound edge separation in rheumatoid disease. Steroid treatment of more than 3 years' duration is associated with an increase in the mean number of days needed for wound healing and also with an increased incidence of wound infection.[8]

G. Fusion offers considerable pain relief and joint stability for almost all patients but sacrifices range of motion. This leads to improvement in function and strength. Joints that are fused in treatment of rheumatoid disease include the metacarpophalangeal and interphalangeal joints of the thumb, the wrist joints, and the proximal interphalangeal joints of the digits.

References

1. Ansell, B., and Harrison, S.: A 5-year followup of synovectomy of the proximal interphalangeal joint in rheumatoid arthritis. Hand, 7:34–36, 1975.
2. Beckenbaugh, R., et al: Review and analysis of silicone-rubber metacarpophalangeal implants. J. Bone Joint Surg., 58A:483, 1976.
3. Beckenbaugh, R., and Linscheid, R. L.: Total wrist arthroplasty: A preliminary report. J. Hand Surg., 2:337–344, 1977.
4. Ellison, M. R., Kelly, K. J., and Flatt, A. E.: The results of surgical synovectomy of the digital joints in rheumatoid disease. J. Bone Joint Surg., 53A:1041–1060, 1971.
5. Flatt, A. E.: The Care of the Rheumatoid Hand, 3rd ed. St. Louis, C.V. Mosby Co., 1974, p. 71.
6. Flatt, A. E.: The Care of the Rheumatoid Hand, 3rd ed. St. Louis, C. V. Mosby Co., 1974, pp. 79–82
7. Flatt, A. E.: The Care of the Rheumatoid Hand, 3rd ed. St. Louis, C.V. Mosby Co., 1974, pp. 120–133.
8. Garner, R. W., Mowat, A. G.., and Hazleman, B. L.: Wound healing after operations on patients with rheumatoid arthritis. J. Bone Joint Surg., 55B:134–144, 1973.
9. Granowitz, S., and Vainio, K.: Interphalangeal joint arthrodesis. Acta Orthop. Scand., 37:301–310, 1966.
10. Haber, J., Boswick, J. A., and Phelps, D. B.: The role of soft tissue reconstruction in flexible implant arthroplasty of the metacarpophalangeal joint. Clin. Orthop. 140:178–183, 1978.
11. Lipscomb, P. R.: Synovectomy of the wrist for rheumatoid arthritis. JAMA, 194:655–659, 1965.
12. Millender, L. H., and Nalebuff, E. A.: Preventive surgery–tenosynovectomy and synovectomy. Orthop. Clin. North Am., 6:766–768, 1975.
13. Nalebuff, E. A.: Surgical treatment of tendon rupture in the rheumatoid hand. Surg. Clin. North Am., 49A:811–822, 1969.
14. Nalebuff, E. A., and Millender, L. H.: Surgical treatment of swan-neck deformity in rheumatoid arthritis. Orthop. Clin. North Am., 6:733–752, 1975.
15. Nalebuff, E. A., and Millender, L. H.: Surgical treatment of the boutonnière deformity. Orthop. Clin. North Am., 6:753–763, 1975.
16. Nicolle, F. V., Holt, P. J. L., and Calnan, J. S.: Prophylactic synovectomy of the joints of the rheumatoid hand. Ann. Rheum. Dis., 30:476–480, 1971.
17. Rodnan, G. P., McEwen, C., and Wallace, S. L.: Primer on the Rheumatic Diseases, 7th ed. New York, The Arthritis Foundation, 1973, p. 34 (Table 7).
18. Swanson, A. B.: Flexible implant arthroplasty for arthritic finger joints: Rationale, technique and results of treatment. J. Bone Joint Surg., 54A:435–455, 1972.

RHEUMATOID ARTHRITIS OF THE HAND AND WRIST

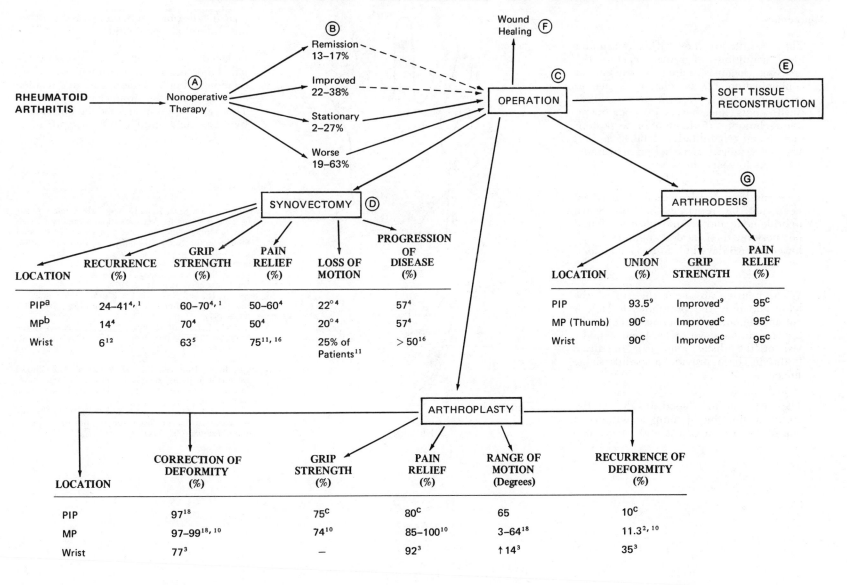

RHEUMATOID ARTHRITIS → (A) Nonoperative Therapy

- Remission 13–17% (B)
- Improved 22–38%
- Stationary 2–27%
- Worse 19–63%

→ OPERATION (C) → Wound Healing (F)

→ SOFT TISSUE RECONSTRUCTION (E)

SYNOVECTOMY (D)

LOCATION	RECURRENCE (%)	GRIP STRENGTH (%)	PAIN RELIEF (%)	LOSS OF MOTION	PROGRESSION OF DISEASE (%)
PIP[a]	24–41[4, 1]	60–70[4, 1]	50–60[4]	22°[4]	57[4]
MP[b]	14[4]	70[4]	50[4]	20°[4]	57[4]
Wrist	6[12]	63[5]	75[11, 16]	25% of Patients[11]	> 50[16]

ARTHRODESIS (G)

LOCATION	UNION (%)	GRIP STRENGTH	PAIN RELIEF (%)
PIP	93.5[9]	Improved[9]	95[c]
MP (Thumb)	90[c]	Improved[c]	95[c]
Wrist	90[c]	Improved[c]	95[c]

ARTHROPLASTY

LOCATION	CORRECTION OF DEFORMITY (%)	GRIP STRENGTH (%)	PAIN RELIEF (%)	RANGE OF MOTION (Degrees)	RECURRENCE OF DEFORMITY (%)
PIP	97[18]	75[c]	80[c]	65	10[c]
MP	97–99[18, 10]	74[10]	85–100[10]	3–64[18]	11.3[2, 10]
Wrist	77[3]	—	92[3]	↑14[3]	35[3]

[a]PIP = Proximal interphalangeal joint
[b]MP = Metacarpophalangeal joint
c = Authors' personal experience

497

FLEXOR TENDON INJURIES IN THE HAND BY C. A. LUEKENS, JR., M.D.

Comments

A. These results are those of experts under ideal conditions of repair. Factors decreasing prognosis include (1) crushing or contamination, (2) associated damage to joints and nerves, (3) inadequate facilities (instruments, anesthesia), (4) poor operative techniques, (5) inattention to postoperative and rehabilitative details,[6] and (6) age — the prognosis is better in patients less than 40 years old.[3]

B. Tendons lacerated less than 75 per cent need not be repaired, but the usual débridement and wound closure should be performed. Guarded motion is allowed after 6 days but no resistance for 3 weeks.[5]

C. When injuries are near the tip of the hand and only the profundus tendon is cut and tendon repair seems difficult, the tendon can be sewn to the bone (tenodesis) or the distal joint can be fused (arthrodesis) to provide a useful, stable finger.

D. The criterion for "good result" is the ability to flex the tip pulp to within 1.5 cm. of the palmar crease and have a less

than 30° flexion contracture of the proximal interphalangeal joint.[1]

E. Delayed primary repair or secondary repair following initial thorough wound irrigation and débridement can give results as good as those from primary repair. This is a good option for delaying definitive treatment until conditions are optimum for repair.

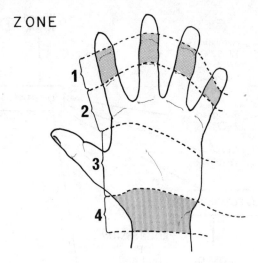

ZONE

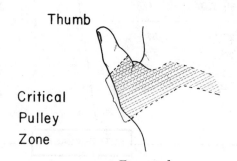

Thumb

Critical
Pulley
Zone

FIGURE 1

References

1. Kleinert, H. E., Kutz, J., and Cohen, M.: Primary repair of zone 2 flexor tendon lacerations. American Academy of Orthopaedic Surgeons' Symposium on Tendon Surgery in the Hand. St. Louis, C.V. Mosby Co., 1975, pp. 91–104.
2. Green, W., and Niebauer, J.: Results of primary and secondary flexor tendon repairs in no man's land. J. Bone Joint Surg., 56A:1216–1222, 1974.
3. Boyes, J. H., and Stark, H. H.: Flexor tendon grafts in the fingers and thumb. J. Bone Joint Surg., 53A:1332–1342, 1971.
4. Urbaniak, J. R., and Goldner, J. L.: Laceration of the flexor pollicis longus tendon: Delayed repair by advancement, free graft, or direct suture. J. Bone Joint Surg., 55A:1123–1148, 1973.
5. Wray, R. C., Holtman, B., and Weeks, P. M.: Clinical treatment of partial tendon lacerations without suturing and with early motion. Plast. Reconstr. Surg., 59:231–234, 1977.
6. Peacock, E. E., Madden, J. W., and Trier, W. C.: Postoperative recovery of flexor tendon function. Am. J. Surg., 122:686–692, 1971.

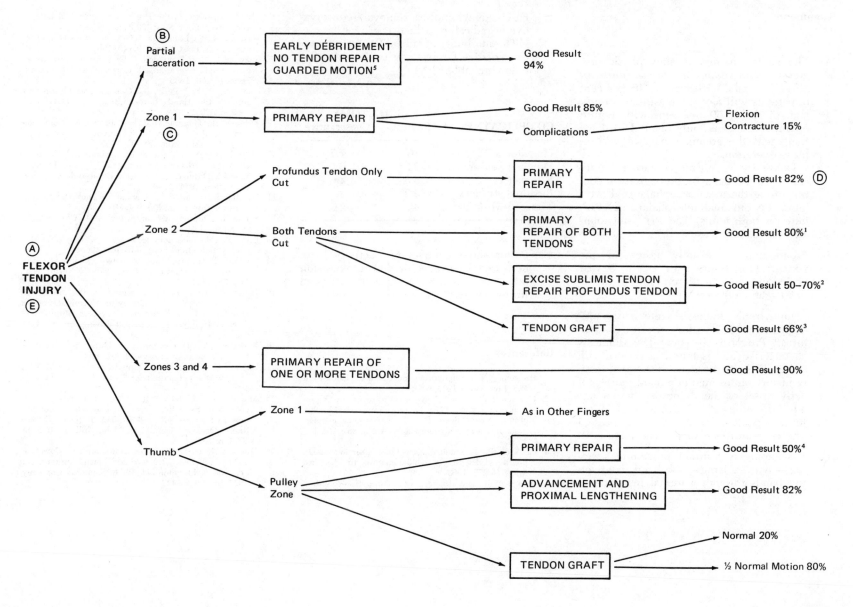

Ⓐ **FLEXOR TENDON INJURY** Ⓔ

Ⓑ Partial Laceration → EARLY DÉBRIDEMENT NO TENDON REPAIR GUARDED MOTION[5] → Good Result 94%

Zone 1 Ⓒ → PRIMARY REPAIR → Good Result 85% / Complications → Flexion Contracture 15%

Zone 2 → Profundus Tendon Only Cut → PRIMARY REPAIR → Good Result 82% Ⓓ

Both Tendons Cut → PRIMARY REPAIR OF BOTH TENDONS → Good Result 80%[1]

→ EXCISE SUBLIMIS TENDON REPAIR PROFUNDUS TENDON → Good Result 50–70%[2]

→ TENDON GRAFT → Good Result 66%[3]

Zones 3 and 4 → PRIMARY REPAIR OF ONE OR MORE TENDONS → Good Result 90%

Thumb → Zone 1 → As in Other Fingers

Pulley Zone → PRIMARY REPAIR → Good Result 50%[4]

→ ADVANCEMENT AND PROXIMAL LENGTHENING → Good Result 82%

→ TENDON GRAFT → Normal 20% / ½ Normal Motion 80%

DUPUYTREN'S CONTRACTURE BY IAN WINSPUR, M.D.

Comments

A. The natural history is slow phasic progression and remission over a course of 10 to 12 years.[10] Ultimately, 46 per cent of patients will have increasing deformity and, of those, 50 per cent will require operation.[4, 7] Thus, only about 1 in 4 patients with this common disease[16] will require operation.

Deformity requiring operation ("critical")[7, 14, 19] occurs with 30 degrees of contracture at the metacarpophalangeal (MP) joint, the proximal interphalangeal (PIP) joint, or both joints. The PIP joint tolerates contracture least well.[18]

B. Progression is usually faster in the young.[3] Progression over a 3 to 5 year period may be considered rapid in the 50 to 60 year age group.[8]

C. "Dupuytren's diathesis" refers to a predisposition to develop severe contractures.[1] Prognosis is poor. The diathesis characteristically is found in people with (1) Anglo-Saxon heritage,[8] (2) strong family history (autosomal dominant trait)[13], (3) early onset of the deformity (under age 40), (4) epilepsy,[12] (5) alcoholism,[9] (6) ectopic deposits,[3, 12, 17] and (7) early postoperative recurrence of the contracture.[2, 15]

D. Fasciotomy is a minor procedure severing — not excising — localized contracting bands through a formal incision.[10, 14]

E. Fasciectomy implies removal (conservative or radical) of palmar fascia.[3, 4, 10]

The morbidity of radical fasciectomy vs. conservative fasciectomy is shown in the following table.[6, 7, 9–11, 18]

COMPLICATION	FASCIECTOMY	
	Radical	Conservative
Hematoma (%)	16	7.7
Delayed healing (%)	22	6.2
Edema (%)	5.5	4.6
Residual stiffness (%)	3.2	2
Time off work (days)	42	21

F. Postoperative contracture ("activity") can be a true recurrence or due to extension into a new area. Sixty per cent will need further surgery.[5, 6, 10]

References

1. Hueston, J.T.: Dupuytren's contracture. Edinburgh, E.S. Livingston, 1963, p.51.
2. Hueston, J.T.: Digital Wolfe grafts in recurrent Dupuytren's contracture. Plast. Reconst. Surg., 29:342, 1962.
3. McIndoe, A., and Beare, R. L. B.: The surgical management of Dupuytren's contracture. Am. J. Surg., 95:197, 1958.
4. Clarkson, P.: The radical fasciectomy operation for Dupuytren's disease: A condemnation. Br. J. Plast. Surg., 16:273, 1963.
5. Dickie, W.R., and Hughes, N.C.: Dupuytren's contracture: A review of the late results of radical fasciectomy. Br. J. Plast. Surg., 20:311, 1967.
6. Hakstian, R.W.: Long-term results of extensive fasciectomy. Br. J. Plast. Surg., 19:140, 1966.
7. Shaw, H.M., and Eastwood, D.S.: Dupuytren's contracture: A selective approach to treatment. Br. J. Plast. Surg., 18:164, 1965.
8. Clarkson, P., and Pelly, A.: General and Plastic Surgery of the Hand. Philadelphia, F.A. Davis Co., 1962, p. 329.
9. Tubiana, R., Thomine, J.M., and Brown, S.: Complications in the surgery of Dupuytren's contracture. Plast. Reconstr. Surg., 39:603, 1967.
10. Millesi, H.: The clinical and morphological course of Dupuytren's disease. In Hueston, J.T., and Tubiana, R. (eds): Dupuytren's Disease. Edinburgh, Churchill Livingston, 1974, p. 49.
11. Hamlin, E.: Limited fasciectomy of Dupuytren's contracture. Ann. Surg., 135:194, 1952.
12. Skoog, T.: Dupuytren's contracture. Acta Chir. Scand., 96 (Suppl. 139), 1948.
13. Ling, R.S.M.: The genetic factor in Dupuytren's disease. J. Bone Joint Surg., 45B:709, 1963.
14. Tubiana, R.: Limited and extensive operations in Dupuytren's contracture. Surg. Clin. North Am., 44:1072, 1964.
15. Hueston, J.T.: Prognosis as a guide to the timing and extent of surgery in Dupuytren's contracture. In Hueston, J.T., and Tubiana, R. (eds.): Dupuytren's disease. Edinburgh, Churchill Livingston, 1974, p. 61.
16. Early, P.: Population studies in Dupuytren's contracture. J. Bone Joint Surg., 44B:602, 1962.
17. Gosset, J.: Maladie de Dupuytren et anatomie des aponeurosis palmodigitales. Ann. Chir., 21:9, 551, 1967.
18. Michon, J.: Operative difficulties and postoperative complications in the surgery of Dupuytren's contracture. In Hueston, J.T. and Tubiana, R. (eds.): Dupuytren's Disease. Edinburgh, Churchill Livingston, 1974, p. 101.
19. Hueston, J. T.: Dupuytren's contracture. In Converse, J. M. (ed.): Reconstructive and Plastic Surgery, 2nd ed., vol. 6. Philadelphia, W. B. Saunders Company, 1977, pp. 3403–3427.

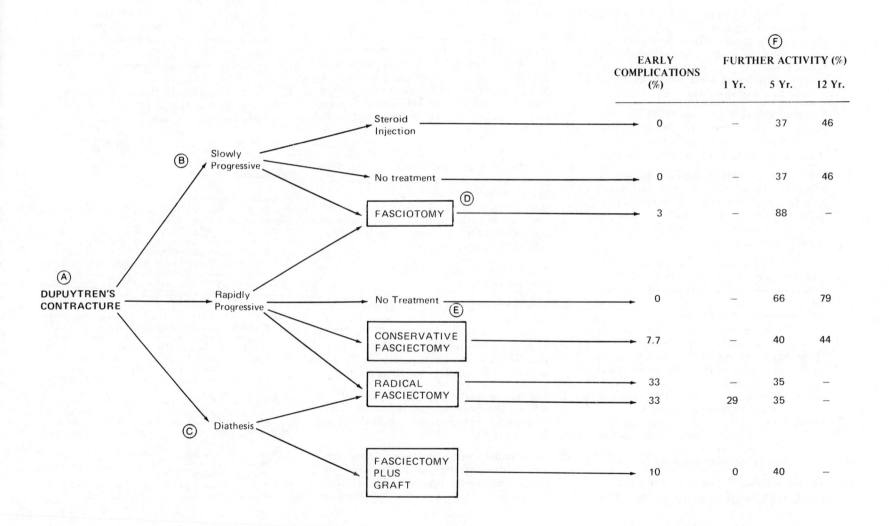

	EARLY COMPLICATIONS (%)	FURTHER ACTIVITY (%)		
		1 Yr.	5 Yr.	12 Yr.
Steroid Injection	0	—	37	46
No treatment	0	—	37	46
FASCIOTOMY	3	—	88	—
No Treatment	0	—	66	79
CONSERVATIVE FASCIECTOMY	7.7	—	40	44
RADICAL FASCIECTOMY	33	—	35	—
	33	29	35	—
FASCIECTOMY PLUS GRAFT	10	0	40	—

Ⓐ DUPUYTREN'S CONTRACTURE
Ⓑ Slowly Progressive
Ⓒ Diathesis
Ⓓ
Ⓔ
Ⓕ
Rapidly Progressive

REPAIR OF PERIPHERAL NERVES (Upper Extremity)

BY JOHN A. BOSWICK, JR., M.D., AND FRANK A. SCOTT, M.D.

Comments

A. Prognosis following repair is better when (1) patient is a child, (2) injury is minor, (3) repair is made within 6 months, (4) nerve ends are easily approximated (i.e., when there is no tension across the neurorrhaphy), and (5) a purely motor or sensory nerve is involved.

B. Suturing within 4 to 6 months of injury is equal to primary repair. Intrafascicular nerve grafts are also equivalent and are better than primary suture under tension.

C. Protective sensibility implies the ability to differentiate hot and cold and sharp and dull. Assessment of nerve recovery is difficult, and therefore results quoted out of context cannot be compared with those of other series.

D. The Nerve Committee of the British Medical Research Council's system for assessment of motor function is as follows:[10]

  Bad: M_0 = No contraction.
  M_1 = Perceptible contraction of proximal muscles.
  Poor: M_2 = Perceptible contraction of both proximal and distal muscles.
  Fair: M_3 = Muscles powerful enough to act against resistance.
  Good: M_4 = M_3 level plus return of synergistic and independent movements.
  M_5 = Complete recovery.

E. Thumb rotation is lost in one third of patients with median nerve injury.[2] One third of patients have mixed innervation (i.e., median and ulnar) of their thenar musculature.[5]

F. The muscle-tendon units available for transfer to restore thumb rotation are: (1) the flexor superficialis tendon (preferably from the ring finger) or (2) the extensor indicis proprius tendon to the dorsoulnar aspect of the thumb MP joint. Tendon transfer achieves good thumb rotation in 80 per cent of cases in our own experience.

G. Results of combined ulnar and median nerve injury and repair are generally poorer than those of isolated nerve repair. Because of cross-innervation in 26.3 per cent of patients, the rate of return of normal function is lower if both median and ulnar nerves are cut.[6]

H. Innervation of the forearm musculature is not involved.

I. The ring finger sublimis tendon is the one most commonly used for transfer to restore pinching ability, and the long finger sublimis tendon is used to improve grip.[3, 4] In our own experience, 75 per cent of these transfers are successful.

J. Capsulodesis shortens the volar plate of the metacarpophalangeal joints to compensate for hyperextension that develops in ulnar palsy.

K. Most radial nerve injuries are above the elbow. Because the radial nerve has predominantly motor function (thumb, wrist and finger dorsiflexion), the results of repair are generally good. If good motor function does not return, tendon transfers offer a substantial improvement in hand function. Radial sensory supply is variable and relatively unimportant for useful hand function. It is therefore not generally used in assessing results.

L. Wrist, finger, and thumb extension are restored in about 95 per cent of cases in both our own and others' experience.[8]

References

1. Boswick, J.A., Jr., Schneewind, J., and Stromberg, W., Jr.: Evaluation of peripheral nerve repairs below the elbow. Arch. Surg., 90:50–51, 1965.
2. Boswick, J.A., Jr., and Stromberg, W.B., Jr.: Isolated injury to the median nerve above the elbow. J. Bone Joint Surg., 49A:653–658, 1967.
3. Brown, P.W.: Reconstruction for pinch in ulnar intrinsic palsy. Orthop. Clin. North Am., 5:323–342, 1974.
4. Burkhalter, W.E.: Restoration of power grip in ulnar nerve paralysis. Orthop. Clin. North Am., 5:289–303, 1974.
5. Forrest, W.J.: Motor innervation of human thenar and hypothenar muscles in 25 hands. A study combining electromyography and percutaneous nerve stimulation. Can. J. Surg., 10:196–199, 1967.
6. Millesi, H., Meissl, G., and Berger, A.: Further experience with interfascicular grafting of median, ulnar, and radial nerves. J. Bone Joint Surg., 58A:209–218, 1976.
7. Nicholson, O.R., and Seddon, H.J.: Nerve repair in civil practice: Results of treatment of median and ulnar nerve lesions. Br. Med. J., 1065–1071, 1957.
8. Riordan, D.C.: Radial nerve paralysis. Orthop. Clin. North Am., 5:283–287, 1974.
9. Seddon, H.: Surgical Disorders of the Peripheral Nerves, 2nd ed. Edinburgh, Churchill Livingstone, 1975, pp. 303–314.
10. Peripheral Nerve Injuries. Special Report Series, Medical Research Council (London), No. 282, 1954.

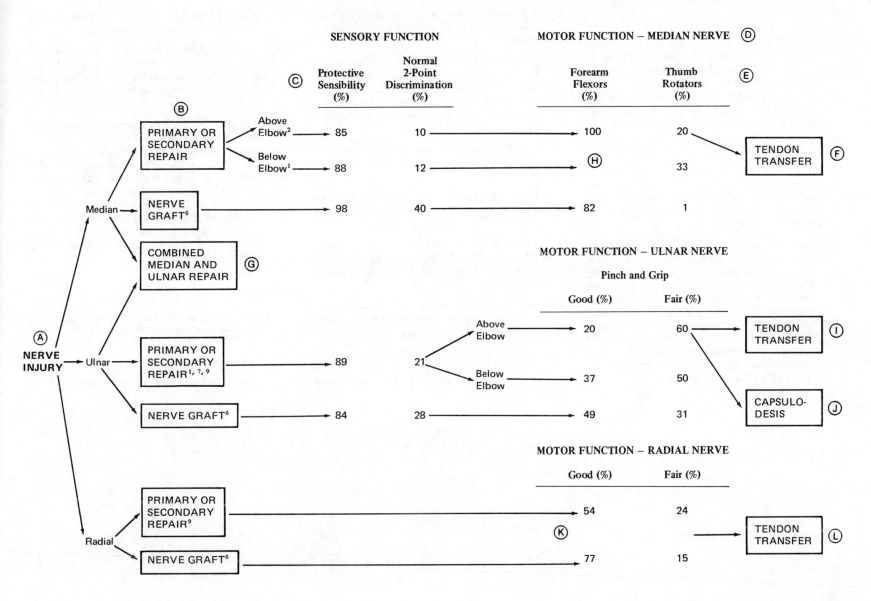

SENSORY FUNCTION

MOTOR FUNCTION – MEDIAN NERVE Ⓓ

Ⓒ Protective Sensibility (%)

Normal 2-Point Discrimination (%)

Forearm Flexors (%)

Thumb Rotators (%) Ⓔ

Ⓑ PRIMARY OR SECONDARY REPAIR

Above Elbow² → 85   10 → 100   20 → TENDON TRANSFER Ⓕ

Below Elbow¹ → 88   12 → Ⓗ   33

NERVE GRAFT⁶ → 98   40 → 82   1

COMBINED MEDIAN AND ULNAR REPAIR Ⓖ

MOTOR FUNCTION – ULNAR NERVE

Pinch and Grip

Good (%)   Fair (%)

Above Elbow → 20   60 → TENDON TRANSFER Ⓘ

Ⓐ NERVE INJURY

Median

Ulnar

PRIMARY OR SECONDARY REPAIR¹ ⁷ ⁹ → 89   21

Below Elbow → 37   50

NERVE GRAFT⁶ → 84   28 → 49   31   CAPSULO-DESIS Ⓙ

MOTOR FUNCTION – RADIAL NERVE

Good (%)   Fair (%)

Radial

PRIMARY OR SECONDARY REPAIR⁹ → 54   24

Ⓚ → TENDON TRANSFER Ⓛ

NERVE GRAFT⁶ → 77   15

503

PELVIC FRACTURES BY WILLIAM G. WINTER, M.D.

Comments

A. Mortality rate varies with age[11] and severity of associated injuries.[11, 18] Death is due to exsanguination or late complications of multiple organ failure.[4, 18] Mean blood requirement in an unstable injury is 3800 ml.; in a stable injury, 1600 ml., and in cases of pelvic crush, 4000 ml.

B. Stable fractures involve no disruption of the load-bearing regions of the sacrum or ilium. Stability is relative. Straddle (bilateral anterior ischiopubic) fractures are here considered stable but frequently are associated with visceral — particularly urologic — injury.[1, 13]

C. Posterior acetabular fracture-dislocations often produce significant sciatic nerve injury. Malgaigne hemipelvic fracture-dislocations, especially those involving multiple sacral foramina, may involve any portion of the lumbosacral plexus; the prognosis in this case is worse. While full vocational rehabilitation occurs 60 per cent of the time after pelvic fractures with neuropathy, complete neurologic return rarely, if ever, transpires.[5, 6, 12]

D. Supportive traction (5 to 20 lb.) diminishes pain and facilitates early joint motion.

E. Although most anterocentral acetabular fractures are benign,[16] they may produce late arthritis owing to articular surface injury. Sufficient protection by limited weight-bearing may improve the prognosis.

F. Crush injuries usually also involve intra-abdominal injury that requires laparotomy.[10, 13, 19]

G. Pelvic fractures with deep perineal or anal lacerations require diverting colostomy[10, 13, 19] and distal washout.

H. Traction of up to 50 lb. may be required for 3 months. Lateral vectors added by greater trochanter pins[18] are occasionally useful.

I. All acetabular fractures, regardless of treatment, are best protected by a period of limited weight-bearing.

J. Early reduction may minimize the possibility of subsequent avascular necrosis and arthritis.[16] Some physicians recommend emergent open reduction for all posterior fracture-dislocations.[3]

K. External skeletal fixation for unstable pelvic fractures is being evaluated. It decreases bleeding and allows earlier mobilization, but stabilization is not always rigid.

L. Arthritis of the hip after acetabular fracture results either from direct articular surface damage or from an incongruent reduction of the femoral head under the acetabular dome. Sacroiliac arthritis after hemipelvic fracture-dislocations results in low back and buttock pain. The degree of symptoms does not clearly correlate with the accuracy of reduction. Persistent superior iliac dislocation *will* result in leg length discrepancy.

References

1. Conolly, W. B., and Hedberg, E. L.: Observations on fractures of the pelvis. J. Trauma, 9:104–111, 1969.
2. Dunn, W., and Morris, H. D.: Fractures and dislocations of the pelvis. J. Bone Joint Surg., 50A:1639–1648, 1968.
3. Epstein, H. C.: Posterior fracture-dislocations of the hip. J. Bone Joint Surg., 43A:1079–1098, 1961.

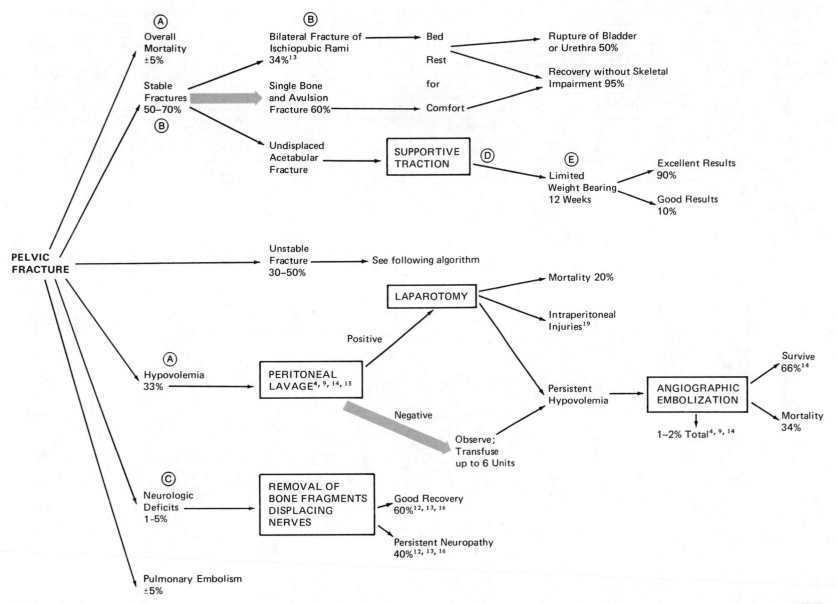

Ⓐ Overall Mortality ±5%

Ⓑ Bilateral Fracture of Ischiopubic Rami 34%[13]

Bed Rest for Comfort

Rupture of Bladder or Urethra 50%

Recovery without Skeletal Impairment 95%

Ⓐ
Ⓑ Stable Fractures 50–70%

Single Bone and Avulsion Fracture 60%

Undisplaced Acetabular Fracture

SUPPORTIVE TRACTION

Ⓓ Limited Weight Bearing 12 Weeks

Ⓔ Excellent Results 90%

Good Results 10%

PELVIC FRACTURE

Unstable Fracture 30–50% → See following algorithm

Ⓐ Hypovolemia 33%

PERITONEAL LAVAGE[4, 9, 14, 15]

Positive

LAPAROTOMY

Mortality 20%

Intraperitoneal Injuries[19]

Negative

Observe; Transfuse up to 6 Units

Persistent Hypovolemia

ANGIOGRAPHIC EMBOLIZATION

1–2% Total[4, 9, 14]

Survive 66%[14]

Mortality 34%

Ⓒ Neurologic Deficits 1–5%

REMOVAL OF BONE FRAGMENTS DISPLACING NERVES

Good Recovery 60%[12, 13, 16]

Persistent Neuropathy 40%[12, 13, 16]

Pulmonary Embolism ±5%

PELVIC FRACTURES *Continued*

4. Hawkins, L., Pomerantz, M., and Eiseman, B.: Laparotomy at the time of pelvic fracture. J. Trauma, *10*:619–623, 1970.
5. Holdsworth, F. W.: Dislocation and fracture-dislocations of the pelvis. J. Bone Joint Surg., *30B*:461–466, 1948.
6. Kane, W. J.: Fractures of the pelvis. *In* Rockwood, C. A., Jr., and Green, D. P. (eds.): Fractures, Vol. 2. Philadelphia, J. B. Lippincott Company, 1975.
7. Looser, K. G., and Crombie, H. D., Jr.: Pelvic fractures: An anatomic guide to severity of injury. Am. J. Surg., *132*:638–642, 1976.
8. Malgaigne, J. F.: Treatise on Fractures. Philadelphia, J. B. Lippincott, 1859.
9. Maull, K. I., and Sachatello, C. R.: Current management of pelvic fractures: A combined surgical-angiographic approach to hemorrhage. South. Med. J., 69:1285–1289, 1976.

10. Maull, K. I., Sachatello, C. R., and Ernst, C. B.: The deep perineal laceration, an injury frequently associated with open pelvic fractures: A need for aggressive surgical management. J. Trauma, *17*:685–696, 1977.
11. Patterson, F. P., and Morton, K. S.: The cause of death in fractures of the pelvis, with a note on treatment by ligation of the hypogastric (internal iliac) artery. J. Trauma, *13*:849–856, 1973.
12. Patterson, F. P., and Morton, K. S.: Neurologic complications of fractures of the pelvis. Surg. Gynecol. Obstet., *112*:702–706, 1961.
13. Peltier, L. F.: Complications associated with fractures of the pelvis. J. Bone Joint Surg., *47A*:1060–1069, 1965.
14. Ring, E. J., et al.: Angiography in pelvic trauma. Surg. Gynecol. Obstet., *139*:375–380, 1974.

15. Root, H. D., et al.: Diagnostic peritoneal lavage. Surgery, 57:633–637, 1965.
16. Rowe, C. R., and Lowell, J. D.: Prognosis of fractures of the acetabulum. J. Bone Joint Surg., *43A*:30–59, 1961.
17. Thompson, J. V., and Epstein, H. C.: Traumatic dislocation of the hip. J. Bone Joint Surg., *33A*:746–778, 1951.
18. Tipton, W. W., D'Ambrosia, R. D., and Ryle, G. P.: Nonoperative management of central fracture-dislocations of the hip. J. Bone Joint Surg., *57A*:888–893, 1975.
19. Trunkey, D. D., et al.: Management of pelvic fractures in blunt trauma injury. J. Trauma, *14*:912–923, 1974.
20. Watson-Jones, R.: Dislocations and fracture-dislocations of the pelvis. Br. J. Surg., 25:773–781, 1938.

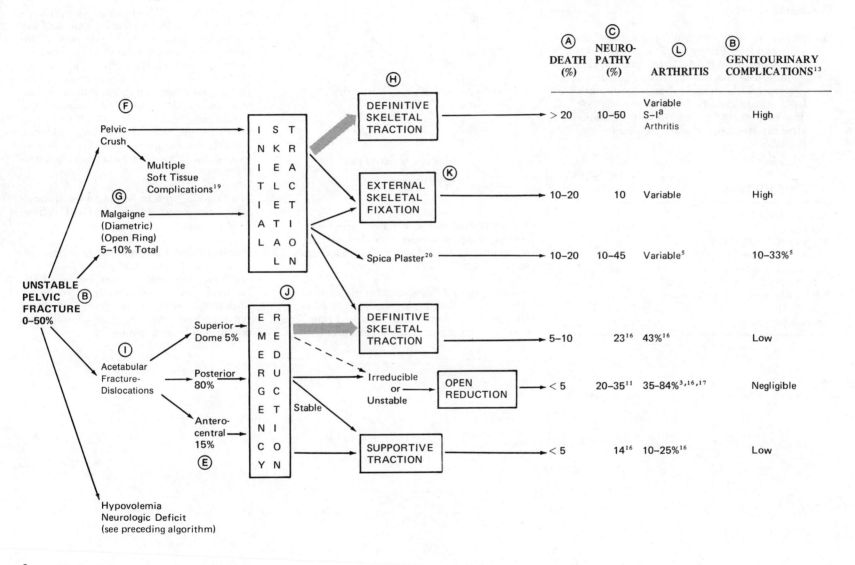

		A) DEATH (%)	C) NEURO-PATHY (%)	L) ARTHRITIS	B) GENITOURINARY COMPLICATIONS[13]
H) DEFINITIVE SKELETAL TRACTION		> 20	10–50	Variable S–I[a] Arthritis	High
EXTERNAL SKELETAL FIXATION K)		10–20	10	Variable	High
Spica Plaster[20]		10–20	10–45	Variable[5]	10–33%[5]
J) DEFINITIVE SKELETAL TRACTION		5–10	23[16]	43%[16]	Low
OPEN REDUCTION		< 5	20–35[11]	35–84%[3,16,17]	Negligible
SUPPORTIVE TRACTION		< 5	14[16]	10–25%[16]	Low

INITIAL TRACTION

EMERGENCY REDUCTION

F) Pelvic Crush

Multiple Soft Tissue Complications[19]

G) Malgaigne (Diametric) (Open Ring) 5–10% Total

UNSTABLE PELVIC FRACTURE 0–50% B)

I) Acetabular Fracture-Dislocations

Superior Dome 5%

Posterior 80%

Antero-central 15% E)

Stable

Irreducible or Unstable

Hypovolemia Neurologic Deficit (see preceding algorithm)

[a]S–I = Sacroiliac

507

HIP FRACTURES BY WILLIAM WINTER, M.D., AND R. ROKICKI, M.D.

Comments

A. Morbidity and mortality rates correlate with age (see Figure 1). The primary determinant of mortality is the pre-fracture condition of the patient. Institutionalized patients with organic brain syndromes have a particularly bleak prognosis.[20, 26] The incidences of medical complications after hip fracture are shown in the following table:

COMPLICATION	INCIDENCE (%)
Urinary tract infection	2–25
Pneumonia	3–7
Myocardial infarction	3–4
Gastrointestinal hemorrhage	3
Clinically apparent venous thrombosis	25
Clinically apparent pulmonary embolism	3
Decubitus ulcer	1–8

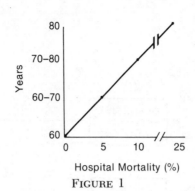

FIGURE 1

The morbidity rate is usually higher with nonoperative treatment.[7] Prophylactic administration of antibiotics decreased infection from 4.8 to 0.8 per cent in one series.[21]

The reported incidence of deep vein thrombosis following hip fracture is 40 to 60 per cent, depending on the criteria used for diagnosis (clinical examination, venography, ^{125}I fibrinogen, Doppler ultrasound, or other methods). One half are clinically silent. Six to 18 per cent of unprotected patients develop pulmonary emboli, of which 80 per cent are unsuspected, and 4 to 10 per cent are fatal. Although anticoagulant drugs reduce the incidence of deep vein thrombosis and pulmonary embolus, they result in a 10 to 20 per cent risk of bleeding into the wound, the complications of which may exceed the hoped-for benefits of anticoagulation.

B. "Pathologic" refers to fractures through bone weakened by neoplasia or diffuse osteoporosis.

C. Extracapsular fractures lie between the distal reflection of the hip capsule and the lesser trochanter. They include basilar neck and intertrochanteric fractures. Subcapital and transcervical fractures lying proximal to the synovial reflection are termed "intracapsular."

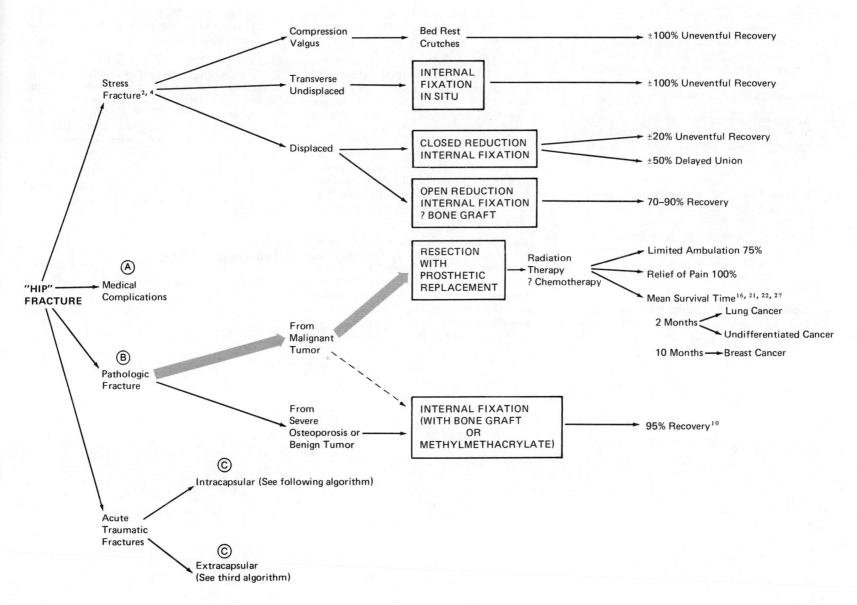

"HIP" FRACTURE

Stress Fracture[2, 4]
- Compression Valgus → Bed Rest Crutches → ±100% Uneventful Recovery
- Transverse Undisplaced → INTERNAL FIXATION IN SITU → ±100% Uneventful Recovery
- Displaced
  - CLOSED REDUCTION INTERNAL FIXATION → ±20% Uneventful Recovery / ±50% Delayed Union
  - OPEN REDUCTION INTERNAL FIXATION ? BONE GRAFT → 70–90% Recovery

Ⓐ Medical Complications

Ⓑ Pathologic Fracture
- From Malignant Tumor → RESECTION WITH PROSTHETIC REPLACEMENT → Radiation Therapy ? Chemotherapy
  - Limited Ambulation 75%
  - Relief of Pain 100%
  - Mean Survival Time[16, 21, 22, 27]
    - 2 Months → Lung Cancer / Undifferentiated Cancer
    - 10 Months → Breast Cancer
- From Severe Osteoporosis or Benign Tumor → INTERNAL FIXATION (WITH BONE GRAFT OR METHYLMETHACRYLATE) → 95% Recovery[10]

Acute Traumatic Fractures
- Ⓒ Intracapsular (See following algorithm)
- Ⓒ Extracapsular (See third algorithm)

D. Little soft tissue injury accompanies the low-velocity falls that produce most hip fractures. In contrast, upper femoral fractures following high-velocity injury have extensive soft tissue damage, resulting in a high incidence of nonunion, avascular necrosis, and failure of fixation.[15, 18, 23]

E. Nonoperative treatment of displaced fractures of the femoral neck is usually incompatible with rehabilitation. It may be indicated for terminally ill, aged, or nonambulatory patients.

F. Reported results of prosthetic replacement of the femoral head still vary widely.[14, 15, 17, 20, 24, 36] When used in high-risk, marginally ambulatory patients, the results are poor.[7, 15] It is usually reserved for those cases in which accurate reduction, fixation, or rehabilitation is very difficult.[15]

G. Nonunion usually results from inaccurate reduction, poor bony contact, or insecure fixation. Its incidence has decreased with the use of fixation devices that permit controlled "impaction" of the fracture fragments.[15]

H. Avascular necrosis (AVN) results from compromised blood supply to the femoral head through the capsular arteries. The incidence of AVN in displaced intracapsular fractures varies inversely with the quality of reduction and fixation.[3, 8, 15, 17] Significant prognostic data include (1) its incidence in intertrochanteric fractures: 0 to 1 per cent;[14] (2) the characteristic time from injury to radiologic diagnosis: more than 12 months;[15] and (3) the characteristic time until the first symptoms appear: 12 to 24 months.[15]

I. A *stable* fracture is minimally comminuted. Postoperative weight-bearing and muscular forces compress the fracture surfaces together when the fracture is properly reduced and fixed. By contrast, *unstable* fractures are significantly comminuted, especially posteriorly or medially. Comminution prevents load-bearing across the fracture region; the same forces often disrupt fixation and lead to varus collapse.[6]

J. Various types of operative procedures (impaction, osteotomies, methacrylate fixation, and others) may be used to align and fix unstable intertrochanteric fractures.[5, 6, 10, 11, 15, 19, 25] Prognosis appears to depend more on the skill and experience of the surgical team than on any single technique.

K. Extracapsular fractures usually unite after traction treatment, but the morbidity of prolonged bed rest in the aged is very high.[6]

References

1. Bentley, G.: Impacted fractures of the neck of the femur. J. Bone Joint Surg., *50B*:551, 1968.
2. Blickenstaff, L. D., and Morris, J. M.: Fatigue fractures of the femoral neck. J. Bone Joint Surg., *48A*:1031, 1966.
3. Boyd, H. B., and George, I. L.: Complications of frac-

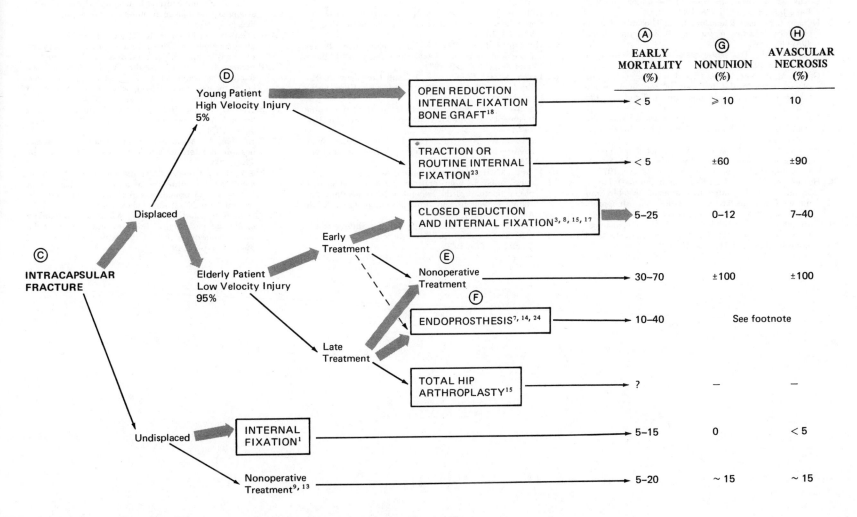

	(A) EARLY MORTALITY (%)	(G) NONUNION (%)	(H) AVASCULAR NECROSIS (%)
(C) INTRACAPSULAR FRACTURE			
(D) Young Patient High Velocity Injury 5%			
OPEN REDUCTION INTERNAL FIXATION BONE GRAFT[18]	< 5	≥ 10	10
TRACTION OR ROUTINE INTERNAL FIXATION[23]	< 5	±60	±90
Displaced			
Elderly Patient Low Velocity Injury 95%			
Early Treatment — CLOSED REDUCTION AND INTERNAL FIXATION[3, 8, 15, 17]	5–25	0–12	7–40
(E) Nonoperative Treatment	30–70	±100	±100
(F) ENDOPROSTHESIS[7, 14, 24]	10–40	See footnote	
Late Treatment — TOTAL HIP ARTHROPLASTY[15]	?	—	—
Undisplaced — INTERNAL FIXATION[1]	5–15	0	< 5
Nonoperative Treatment[9, 13]	5–20	~ 15	~ 15

±75% satisfactory; ±25% unsatisfactory (because of infection, migration, dislocation, and pain)

tures of the neck of the femur. J. Bone Joint Surg., 29:13, 1947.

4. Devas, M. B.: Stress fractures of the femoral neck. J. Bone Joint Surg., *47B*:728, 1965.

5. Dimon, J. H., and Hughston, J. C.: Unstable intertrochanteric fractures of the hip. J. Bone Joint Surg., *49A*:440, 1967.

6. Evans, E. M.: Trochanteric fractures. J. Bone Joint Surg., *33B*:192, 1951.

7. Garcia, A., Jr., Neer, C. S., II, and Ambrose, G. B.: Displaced intracapsular fractures of the neck of the femur. I. Mortality and morbidity. J. Trauma, *1*:128, 1961.

8. Garden, R. S.: Reduction and fixation of subcapital fractures of the femur. Orthop. Clin. North Am., 5:683, 1974.

9. Hansen, B. A. and Solgaard, S.: Impacted fractures of the femoral neck treated by early mobilization of weight-bearing. Acta Orthop. Scand., 49:180, 1978.

10. Harrington, K. D.: The use of methylmethacrylate as an adjunct in the internal fixation of unstable comminuted intertrochanteric fractures in osteoporotic patients. J. Bone Joint Surg., *57A*:744, 1975.

11. Harrington, K. D., and Johnston, J. O.: The management of comminuted intertrochanteric fractures. J. Bone Joint Surg., *55A*:1367, 1973.

12. Harrington, K. D., et al.: The use of methylmethacry-late as an adjunct in the internal fixation of malignant neoplastic fractures. J. Bone Joint Surg., *54A*:1665, 1972.

13. Hilleboe, J., et al.: The nonoperative treatment of impacted fractures of the femoral neck. South. Med. J., 63:1103, 1970.

14. Hinchey, J. J., and Day, P. L.: Primary prosthetic replacement in fresh femoral neck fractures. J. Bone Joint Surg., *46A*:223, 1964.

15. Lynch, M. H., Freeman, B. L., and Crenshaw, A. H.: Fractures of the femoral neck. J. Contin. Educ. Orthop., March 1978, p. 19.

16. Marcove, R. C., and Yang, D. J.: Survival time after treatment of pathologic fracture. Cancer, *20*:2154, 1967.

17. Metz, C. W., Jr., et al.: The displaced intracapsular fracture of the neck of the femur. J. Bone Joint Surg., *52A*:113, 1970.

18. Meyers, M. H., Harvey, J. P., and Moore, T. M.: The muscle pedicle bone graft in the treatment of displaced fractures of the femoral neck: Indications, operative technique and results. Orthop. Clin. North Am., 5:779, 1974.

19. Mulholland, R. C., and Gunn, D. R.: Sliding screw plate fixation of intertrochanteric femoral fractures. J. Trauma, *12*:581, 1972.

20. Niemann, K. M., and Mankin, H. J.: Fractures about the hip in an institutionalized patient population. J. Bone Joint Surg., *50A*:1327, 1968.

21. Parrish, F. F., and Murray, J. A.: Surgical treatment for secondary neoplastic fractures. J. Bone Joint Surg., *52A*:665, 1970.

22. Poigenfurst, J., Marcove, R. C., and Miller, T. R.: Surgical treatment of fracture through metastases in the proximal femur. J. Bone Joint Surg., *50B*:743, 1968.

23. Protzman, R. R., and Burkhalter, W. E.: Femoral neck fractures in young adults: A disaster. Paper presented at the 5th Annual Symposium of the Society of Military Surgeons, El Paso, Texas, 1973.

24. Salvati, E. A., et al.: Endoprosthesis in the treatment of femoral neck fractures. Orthop. Clin. North Am., 5:757, 1974.

25. Sarmiento, A.: Avoidance of complications of internal fixation of intertrochanteric fractures. Clin. Orthop., 53:47, 1967.

26. Sherk, H. H., Crouse, T. R., and Probst, C.: The treatment of hip fractures in institutionalized patients. A comparison of operative and nonoperative methods. Orthop. Clin. North Am., 5:543, 1974.

27. Zickel, R. E., and Mouradian, W. H.: Intramedullary fixation of pathological fractures and lesions of the subtrochanteric region of the femur. J. Bone Joint Surg., *58A*:1061, 1976.

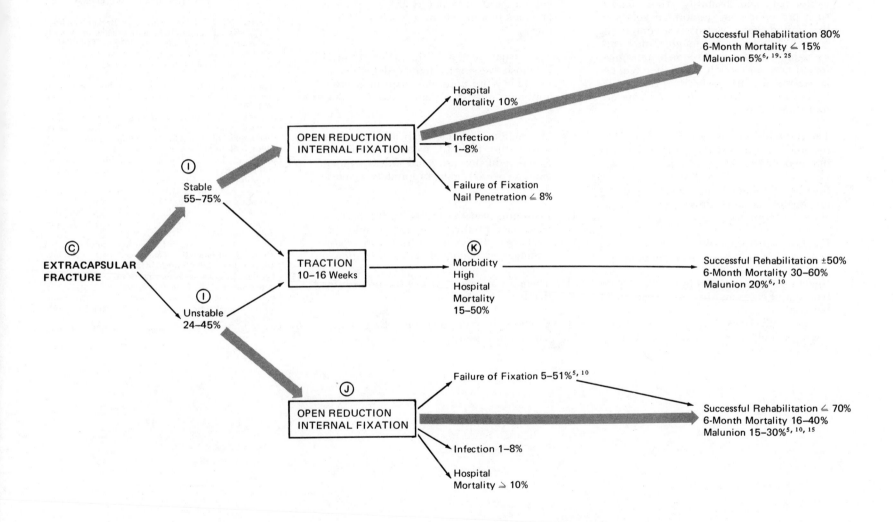

EXTRACAPSULAR FRACTURE Ⓒ

Ⓘ Stable 55–75%

Ⓘ Unstable 24–45%

OPEN REDUCTION INTERNAL FIXATION

Hospital Mortality 10%

Infection 1–8%

Failure of Fixation Nail Penetration ⩽ 8%

Successful Rehabilitation 80%
6-Month Mortality ⩽ 15%
Malunion 5%[6, 19, 25]

TRACTION 10–16 Weeks

Ⓚ Morbidity High Hospital Mortality 15–50%

Successful Rehabilitation ±50%
6-Month Mortality 30–60%
Malunion 20%[6, 10]

Ⓙ OPEN REDUCTION INTERNAL FIXATION

Failure of Fixation 5–51%[5, 10]

Infection 1–8%

Hospital Mortality ⩾ 10%

Successful Rehabilitation ⩽ 70%
6-Month Mortality 16–40%
Malunion 15–30%[5, 10, 15]

PROSTHETIC HIP REPLACEMENT BY MACK L. CLAYTON, M.D., AND W. HOWARD HUDSON, M.D.

Comments

A. Total hip arthroplasty is indicated primarily for pain and disability. About 65,000 such procedures are performed yearly in the United States. Sepsis is a contraindication.[1] Extraordinary lengths often are used in the operating room to minimize infection even though their effectiveness is statistically unproven.[18] Perioperative intravenous antibiotics commonly are administered also.

B. The mortality rate is primarily that of associated cardiovascular disease plus thromboembolism.[7]

C. Results of bilateral replacement are approximately as good. Prosthetic wear is as yet not a problem.

D. Fractures are primarily due to infection or loosening or to fracture at component.

E. Infection develops within 1 year in 66 per cent of cases and in 1 to 3 years in 24 per cent.

   Late infections are hematogenous. Such patients should take prophylactic antibiotics when at high risk (e.g., when having dental work).

   The probability of infection with a virgin hip is 0 to 6 per cent.[1, 7, 12] With a previous hip operation, it is 2.3 to 7.9 per cent.[1, 7, 12]

F. The usual restraints in using clinical diagnosis versus laboratory detection of thrombosis are pertinent. Aspirin is probably more effective than heparin or dextran.

G. Dislocation characteristically occurs within the first 10 weeks. Results of closed reduction are good unless components were inappropriately positioned.[1, 8, 16]

H. Loosening usually occurs on the femoral side. Contributing factors include patient's weight (over 175 lb.), varus positioning, and inadequate cement fixation.

I. There is increased risk with procedures that lengthen the limb.[13]

J. Fractures may occur at operation or as a late complication.[18, 20]

References

1. Wilson, P. D., Jr., et al.: Total Prosthetic Replacement of the Hip, 1977. J. Contin. Educ. Orthop., 5:23, 1978.
2. Coventry, M. B., Nolan, D. R., and Beckenbaugh, R. D.: "Delayed" prophylactic anticoagulation. A study of results and complications in 2012 total hip arthroplasties. J. Bone Joint Surg., 55A:1487, 1973.
3. Davis, W. H., et al.: Comparison of warfarin, low molecular weight dextran, aspirin, and subcutaneous heparin in prevention of venous thromboembolism following total hip replacement. J. Bone Joint Surg., 56A:1552, 1974.
4. Jennings, J. J., Harris, W. H., and Sarmiento, A.: A clinical evaluation of aspirin prophylaxis of thromboembolic disease after total hip arthroplasty. J. Bone Joint Surg., 58A:926, 1976.
5. Poss, R., et al.: Complications of total hip replacement arthroplasty in patients with rheumatoid arthritis. J. Bone Joint Surg., 58A:1130, 1976.
6. American Academy of Orthopaedic Surgeons: Instructional Course Lectures, 23:136–265, 1974.
7. Fitzgerald, R. H., et al.: Bacterial colonization of wounds and sepsis in total hip arthroplasty. J. Bone Joint Surg., 55A:1251, 1973.
8. Coventry, M. B., et al.: 2012 total hip arthroplasties: A study of postoperative course and early complications. J. Bone Joint Surg., 56A:273, 1974.
9. Charnley, J.: Fracture of femoral prosthesis in total hip replacement. Clin. Orthop., 111:105, 1975.
10. Charnley, J., and Cupic, Z.: The 9 and 10 year results of the low friction arthroplasty of the hip. Clin. Orthop., 95:9, 1973.
11. Fitzgerald, R. A.: Deep wound sepsis following total

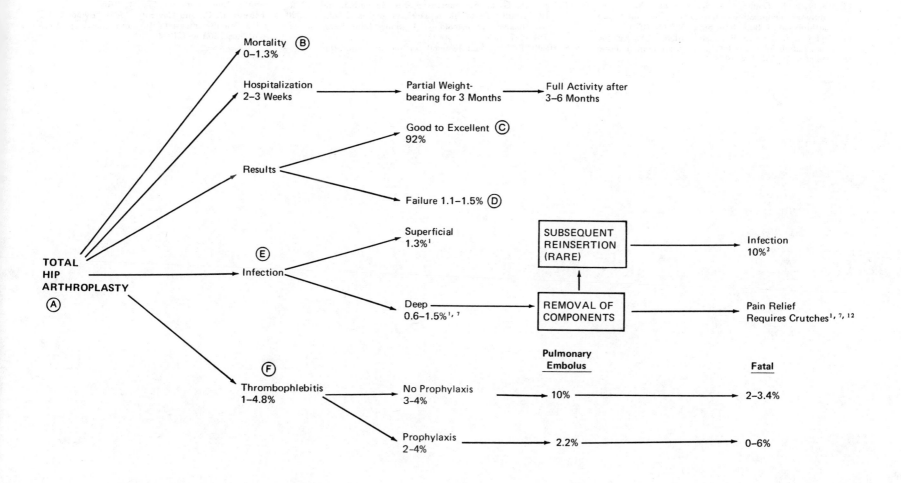

Mortality (B)
0–1.3%

Hospitalization
2–3 Weeks

Partial Weight-
bearing for 3 Months

Full Activity after
3–6 Months

Good to Excellent (C)
92%

Results

Failure 1.1–1.5% (D)

Superficial
1.3%[1]

(E)
Infection

SUBSEQUENT
REINSERTION
(RARE)

Infection
10%[2]

Deep
0.6–1.5%[1, 7]

REMOVAL OF
COMPONENTS

Pain Relief
Requires Crutches[1, 7, 12]

**TOTAL
HIP
ARTHROPLASTY**
(A)

**Pulmonary
Embolus**

Fatal

(F)
Thrombophlebitis
1–4.8%

No Prophylaxis
3–4%

10%

2–3.4%

Prophylaxis
2–4%

2.2%

0–6%

hip arthroplasty. J. Bone Joint Surg., 59A:847–855, 1977.

12. Hunter, G., and Dandy, D.: The natural history of the patient with an infected total hip replacement. J. Bone Joint Surg., 59B:293, 1977.

13. Weber, E. R., Daube, J. S., and Coventry, M. B.: Peripheral neuropathies associated with total hip arthroplasty. J. Bone Joint Surg., 58A:66, 1976.

14. Taylor, A. R., Kamdar, B. A., and Arden, G. P.: Ectopic ossification following total hip replacement. J. Bone Joint Surg., 58B:124, 1976.

15. Riegler, H. F., and Harris, C. M.: Heterotopic bone formation after total hip arthroplasty. Clin. Orthop., 117:209, 1976.

16. Ritter, M. A.: Dislocation and subluxation of the total hip replacement. Clin. Orthop., 121:92, 1976.

17. Parker, H. G., et al.: Comparison of the immediate and later results of total hip replacement with and without trochanteric osteotomy. J. Bone Joint Surg., 56A:1537, 1974.

18. Heath, R. L., et al.: Femoral fracture in conjunction with total hip replacement. J. Bone Joint Surg., 57A:494, 1975.

19. Brady, L. P., Enneking, W. F., and Franeo, J. A.: The effect of operating room environment on the infection rate after Charnley low friction total hip replacement. J. Bone Joint Surg., 57A:80, 1975.

20. McElfresh, E. C., and Coventry, M. B.: Femoral and pelvic fracture after total hip arthroplasty. J. Bone Joint Surg., 56A:483, 1974.

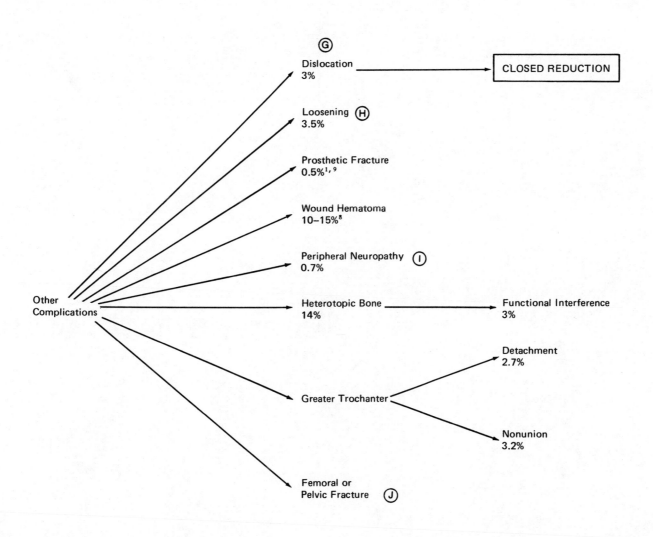

Section M

General

TOTAL PARENTERAL NUTRITION BY J. S. SIMON, M.D.

Comments

A. Although as many as 31 per cent of patients given total parenteral nutrition (TPN) die in the hospital, this figure obviously reflects the severity of the cause for using TPN and not the mortality of TPN itself.[1]

B. Once the techniques of venipuncture, catheter insertion, and sterility are perfected there is insignificant difference between the use of the supraclavicular and the infraclavicular approaches to the subclavian vein and the use of the internal jugular vein.[2, 3]

C. Pneumothorax accounts for the majority of pleural space complications, with hemothorax and hydrothorax representing a smaller precentage.[5]

D. Characteristically, catheter embolism occurs when the catherer tip is sheared off while it is being withdrawn through the needle. The tip may lodge anywhere in the central veins, the lungs, or, paradoxically, in the arterial tree. The catheter is usually retrieved with a transverse guide-wire snare technique done using fluroscopy.

E. Postmortem studies reveal that up to 25 per cent of patients have thrombosis of the innominate or subclavian vein. Up to 10 per cent of autopsied patients show pulmonary emboli and a higher number have septic thrombosis.[10]

F. Septic thrombosis is seen most commonly in burn patients.[6]

G. This refers to sepsis in TPN patients that has no other focus and that responds to catheter removal. Mortality is about 0.5 per cent. Proper, meticulous sterile technique and maintenance minimize infection. Frequency of changing the catheter and the use of different veins affect the incidence of sepsis.[1, 11]

H. A relatively high percentage (20 to 50 per cent) of infections are caused by Candida. Blood cultures of Candida or Staphylococcus suggest the catheter as the source of infection.[5]

I. K^+ is the major intracellular cation lost in negative nitrogen balance. Approximately 3 mEq of K^+ are lost for each gram of nitrogen.[8]

J. This may occur within 10 days of beginning TPN. Clinically the condition presents as peripheral paresthesias, lethargy, obtundation, and dysesthesia.[9]

K. Magnesium is important in the transfer of high-energy phosphate radicals to and from ADP. It is commonly depleted in starvation and decreases further with restitution of nitrogen stores.

L. This is less frequent when acetate is substituted for chloride.

M. Hyperammonemia occurs predominantly in patients with liver disease receiving casein hydrolysate.

N. Only one third of these patients are diabetic.[7] Symptoms include lethargy, seizure, and coma, with hyperglycemia (1000 mg. per 100 ml.) and serum osmolarity of 350 mOsm per liter.[5]

References

1. Ryan, J. A., et al.: Catheter complications in total parenteral nutrition: A prospective study of 200 consecutive patients. N. Engl. J. Med., 290:757, 1974.
2. Parsa, M. H., et al.: Experiences with central venous nutrition: Problems and their prevention. In Proceedings of the 57th Annual Clinical Congress of American College of Surgeons, Atlantic City, October 1971.
3. James, D. M., and Myers, R. T.: Central venous pressure monitoring: Misinterpretation, abuses, indications and a new technique. Ann. Surg., 176:693, 1972.
4. Bernard, R. W., and Stahl, W. M.: Subclavian vein catherization — A prospective study: Noninfectious complications. Ann. Surg., 173:184, 1971.
5. Fischer, J. E.: Total Parenteral Nutrition. Boston, Little, Brown, 1976.
6. Pruitt, B. A., et al.: Intravenous therapy in burn patients — Suppurative thrombophlebitis and other life-threatening complications. Arch. Surg., 100:399, 1970.
7. McCurdy, D. K.: Hypersomolar hyperglycemic nonketotic diabetic coma. Med. Clin. North Am., 54:683, 1970.
8. Dudruit, S. J., et al.: Parenteral hyperalimentation: Metabolic problems and solutions. Ann. Surg., 176:259, 1972.
9. Ruberg, R. L., et al.: Hypophosphatemia with hypophosphaturia in hyperalimentation. Surg. Forum, 22:87, 1971.
10. Popp, M. D., Law, E. J., and MacMillan, B. G.: Parenteral nutrition in the burned child: A study of 29 patients. Ann. Surg., 179:219, 1974.
11. Goldman, D. A., and Maki, D. G.: Infection control in parenteral nutrition. JAMA, 223:1360, 1973.

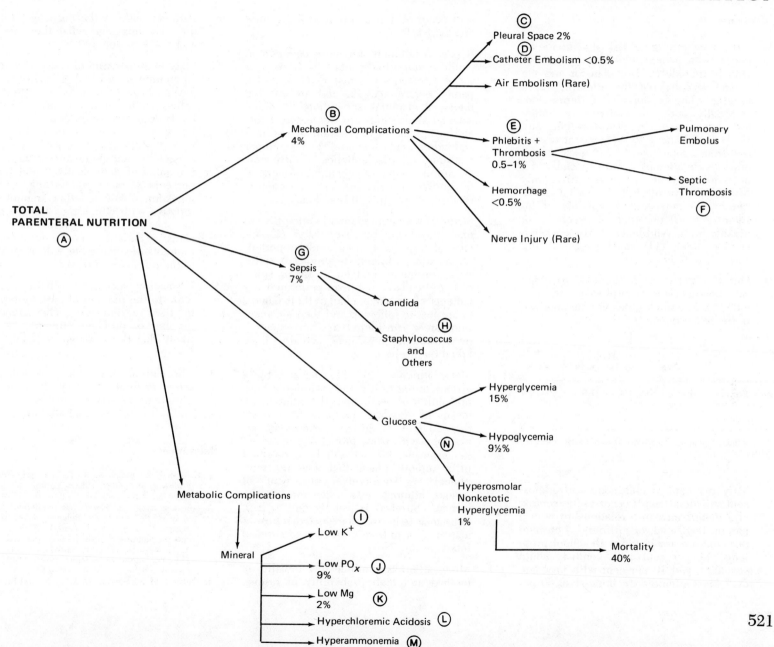

THE SUICIDAL PATIENT BY STEVEN L. DUBOVSKY, M.D.

Comments

A. Factors increasing the risk of a suicide attempt by a patient who has thoughts of suicide include[1-11] (1) a plan for and the means to carry out the attempt;[2] (2) a feeling of hopelessness;[3,4] (3) depression, especially with "vegetative (psychomotor) signs" (e.g., appetite, weight, and sleep disturbances);[3,5,6] (4) recent separation from a loved one;[3,4,7] (5) past history of a suicide attempt[3,8] and especially of 2 or more previous attempts;[1] (6) family history of suicide;[4,10] (7) social isolation;[4,9] (8) persistent complaints of insomnia;[7,11] (9) presence of psychosis or organic brain syndrome;[4,9] (10) a written suicide note;[9] (11) male[9] over age 40;[7] and (12) poor health.[4,8,11]

B. One to 5 per cent of childhood psychiatric disorders are complicated by suicide.[25] U.S. suicide rates are summarized in the following table.[4,12,13,16]

| | AGE | | | |
	<10	10–15	15–19°	Adult
Suicide rate per 100,000 population	Extremely rare	1%	4–7.3%	10–12%

° Suicide is one of the 3 leading causes of death in this age group.

Sixty per cent of childhood and adolescent suicide attempts occur in the context of a disturbance in a relationship with a parent, boyfriend, or girlfriend. Fourteen per cent are associated with school problems, 14 per cent with conflicts about sexuality, and 10 per cent with pregnancy.[19] Most attempts are impulsive: 50 per cent occur within 3 minutes of an emotional crisis.[17]

C. Repeated attempts are more common in children and adolescents who have poor social interactions, a history of loss of a parent before age 12, and an ongoing threat of parental separation.[12-15] Many suicidal adolescents are depressed. Signs and symptoms of depression in children and adolescents include[13,17] (1) temper tantrums, (2) disobedience, (3) truancy, (4) running away, (5) accident-proneness, (6) antisocial behavior, (7) promiscuity, (8) drug abuse, and (9) boredom.

D. Statistics concerning suicide attempts are often unreliable because[9,15,16,20] (1) suicide attempts are often under-reported; (2) suicide is difficult to predict because it is infrequent, and long-term prospective studies have not been performed; (3) patients often move, change their names, or are lost to followup and then are inappropriately considered as "no suicide," even though they may actually have killed themselves.

E. Major attempts are characterized by a serious intent to die and combine a high probability of death from the attempt (by means of shooting, jumping from more than 20 feet, hanging, or drowning, for example) with a low probability of rescue (for example, the act will be committed in a remote place that has no telephone).[9,23] Twenty-five per cent of serious attempts use ingestion as the means.[11] Survival is usually due to happenstance (e.g., the unexpected return of a spouse) or to timely medical or surgical intervention.[7,22]

F. Minor attempts combine low lethality of method and high probability of rescue. Patients without the conscious intent to die may misjudge what they are doing and die accidentally.[7,22]

G. Sixty to 80 per cent of successful suicides communicate suicidal thoughts to others within 1 to 12 months of killing themselves.[4,11] If others do not respond positively, the risk of suicide is increased.[1] Up to 82 per cent of successful suicides visit a physician with vague complaints (e.g., aches and pains or insomnia) within 6 months of their deaths,[11] and up to 55 per cent of those committing suicide by ingestion obtain a lethal amount of the sedative with which they kill themselves in one prescription from their physicians.[8] Patients may not volunteer thoughts of suicide but will usually admit to them if asked directly.[3,23]

H. Ultimately successful suicide is related more to the number of past attempts than to their seriousness. The greater the number of previous attempts, the more likely that the next one will be successful.

I. The patient is less likely to make subsequent attempts if his family, friends, and physicians respond positively to him[21] and if he obtains psychotherapy.[24]

References

1. Eisenthal, S., Faberow, N. L., and Schneidman, E.: Followup of neuropsychiatric patients in suicide observation status. Pub. Health Rep., 81:977–990, 1966.
2. Griest, J. H., et al.: Suicide risk prediction: A new approach. Life-Threatening Behavior, 4:212–222, 1974.
3. Faberow, N. L., and MacKinnon, D.: Prediction of suicide in neuropsychiatric hospital patients. In Beck, A. T., Resnick, H. L. P., and Lettieri, D. J. (eds.): The Prediction of Suicide. Bowie, Md., Charles Press Publishers, 1974, pp. 186–229.
4. Weiss, J. M. A.: Suicide. In Arieti, S., and Brody, E. B.:

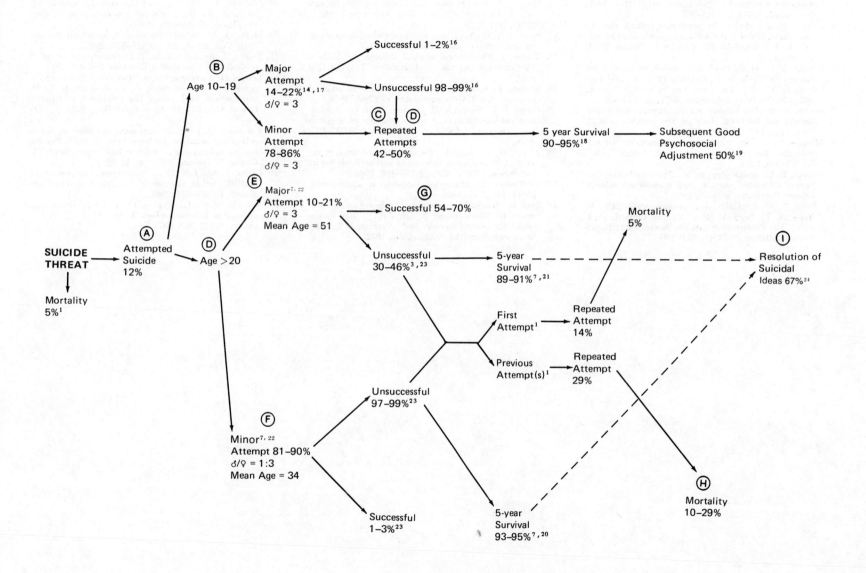

Ⓐ Attempted Suicide 12%

SUICIDE THREAT

Mortality 5%[1]

Ⓑ Age 10–19

Major Attempt 14–22%[14,17] ♂/♀ = 3

Successful 1–2%[16]

Unsuccessful 98–99%[16]

Minor Attempt 78–86% ♂/♀ = 3

Ⓒ Ⓓ Repeated Attempts 42–50%

5 year Survival 90–95%[18]

Subsequent Good Psychosocial Adjustment 50%[19]

Ⓓ Age >20

Ⓔ Major[7,22] Attempt 10–21% ♂/♀ = 3 Mean Age = 51

Ⓖ Successful 54–70%

Unsuccessful 30–46%[3,23]

5-year Survival 89–91%[7,21]

First Attempt[1]

Previous Attempt(s)[1]

Repeated Attempt 14%

Repeated Attempt 29%

Mortality 5%

Ⓘ Resolution of Suicidal Ideas 67%[24]

Ⓕ Minor[7,22] Attempt 81–90% ♂/♀ = 1:3 Mean Age = 34

Unsuccessful 97–99%[23]

Successful 1–3%[23]

5-year Survival 93–95%[7,20]

Ⓗ Mortality 10–29%

THE SUICIDAL PATIENT *Continued*

American Handbook of Psychiatry, vol. 3. New York, Basic Books, 1974, pp. 743–765.

5. Litman, R. E.: Models for predicting suicide risk. *In* Neuringer, C. (ed.): Psychological Assessment of Suicide Risk. Springfield, Ill., Charles C Thomas, 1974, pp. 18–24.

6. Litman, R. E., et al.: Prediction models of suicidal behaviors. *In* Beck, A. T., Resnick, H. L. P., and Lettieri, D. J. (eds.): The Prediction of Suicide. Bowie, Md., Charles Press Publishers, 1974, pp. 141–159.

7. Rosen, D. H.: The serious suicide attempt: Epidemiological and followup study of 886 patients. Am. J. Psychiatry, *127*:764–770, 1970.

8. Murphy, G. E.: The physician's responsibility for suicide. II. Errors of omission. Ann. Intern. Med., *82*:305–309, 1975.

9. Dorpat, T. L., and Ripley, H. S.: The relationship between attempted suicide and committed suicide. Compr. Psychiatry, 8:74–79, 1967.

10. Zung, W. W. K.: Index of potential suicide (IPS). *In* Beck, A. T., Resnick, H. L. P., and Lettieri, D. J. (eds.): The Prediction of Suicide. Bowie, Md., Charles Press Publishers, 1974, pp. 221–249.

11. Murphy, G. E.: The physician's responsibility for suicide. I. An error of commission. Ann. Intern. Med., *82*:301–304, 1975.

12. Bakwin, R. M.: Suicide in children and adolescents. J. Am. Med. Wom. Assoc., *28*:643–659, 1973.

13. Toolan, J.: Suicide and suicidal attempts in children and adolescents. Am. J. Psychiatry, *118*:719–723, 1962.

14. Stanley, E. J., and Barter, J. T.: Adolescent suicidal behavior. Am. J. Orthopsychiatry, *40*:87–96, 1970.

15. Barter, J. T., Swaback, D. O., and Todd, D.: Adolescent suicide attempts. A followup study of hospitalized patients. Arch. Gen. Psychiatry, *19*:523–527, 1968.

16. Faigel, H. C.: Suicide among young persons. A review of its incidence and causes and methods for its prevention. Clin. Pediatr., 5:187–190, 1966.

17. Jacobinzer, J.: Attempted suicides in adolescence. JAMA, *191*:7–11, 1965.

18. Otto, U.: Suicidal behaviour in childhood and adolescence. *In* Waldenstrom, J., Larsson, T., and Ljungstedt, N. (eds.): Suicide and Attempted Suicide. Stockholm, Nordiska Bokhandelns, 1972.

19. Mattson, A., Seese, L., and Hawkins, J.: Suicidal behavior as a child psychiatric emergency. Arch. Gen. Psychiatry, *20*:100–109, 1969.

20. Motto, J. A.: Suicide attempts: A longitudinal view. Arch. Gen. Psychiatry, *13*:516–520, 1965.

21. Brown, T. R., and Sheran, T. J.: Suicide prediction: A review. Life Threatening Behavior, 2:67–93, 1972.

22. Lester, D.: Demographic vs. clinical prediction of suicidal behaviors. *In* Beck, A. T., Resnick, H. L. P., and Lettieri, D. J. (eds.): The Prediction of Suicide. Bowie, Md., Charles Press Publishers, 1974, pp. 71–84.

23. Freeman, D. J., et al.: Assessing intention to die in self-injury behavior. *In* Neuringer, C. (ed.): Psychological Assessment of Suicide Risk. Springfield, Ill., Charles C Thomas, 1974, pp. 18–42.

24. Greer, S., and Lee, H. A.: Subsequent progress of potentially lethal attempted suicides. Acta Psychiatr. Scand., *43*:361–371, 1967.

25. Ackerly, W. C.: Latency-age children who threaten or attempt to kill themselves. J. Am. Acad. Child Psychiatry, 6:242–261, 1967.

SPINAL ANESTHESIA

SPINAL ANESTHESIA BY E. GOLDMAN, M.D.

Comments

A. Cardiovascular complications may be caused by systemic drug absorption or sympathetic denervation. Contributing factors include decreased previous blood volume, atherosclerotic cardiovascular disease, sick sinus syndrome, autonomic imbalance, drug therapy (with digitalis or propranolol), position, incorrect or excessive sedation, drug overdose, too high a level, other disease states, age, pregnancy, and respiratory obstruction. These complications are most common in the first 10 minutes following injection. A block given above T5 will paralyze the cardiac sympathetic fibers, producing bradycardia.[1-3]

B. Hypocarbia is a contributing cause. Diazepam is partially protective because it doubles the convulsant dose of lidocaine.[4]

C. Preventive measures include premedication with diazepam, use of minimal dosage or maximum dilution, use of epinephrine, aspiration before injection of total dose, and use of a test dose.

D. The incidence of these is directly proportional to the sensory level, which determines the resulting level of sympathectomy and hypotension.

E. Headache is the most common complication of spinal anesthesia. Contributing factors include (1) volume of cerebrospinal fluid lost; (2) age (incidence is 10 per cent in the first decade, 15 per cent for ages 20 to 40, and 8 per cent over age 40[5]); (3) sex (7 per cent incidence in men, 14 per cent in women[5]); (4) time of onset (1 day in 29 per cent, 2 days in 21 percent of cases[5]); (5) time of disappearance (53 per cent within 4 days[5]); (6) needle gauge used[6] (see table); (7) number of needle punctures made; (8) hydration; and (9) abdominal pressure. Injection of autologous blood quickly cures 95 to 97 per cent of patients and is safe.

NEEDLE GAUGE (#)	INCIDENCE (%)
19	22
22	6
24–26	1
32	0.4

F. This is a rare complication with accompanying severe headache that appears 3 to 12 days after even simple lumbar punctures. Paresis is never complete, and prognosis is good.[7, 8]

G. These are usually associated with postural headache.[9]

H. The syndrome is usually associated with adhesive arachnoiditis and ischemia of the spinal cord.[7]

I. Deficit is usually restricted to lumbar and sacral dermatomes.[9]

J. Thirteen per cent of cases occur during puncture and 0.1 per cent postoperatively, lasting up to several months.[8]

K. Amnesia resolves spontaneously within 24 hours.[7]

L. Most such cases occur when spinal anesthesia is inappropriately given to those with active neurologic disease.

M. The mortality rate is variously reported as 0 to 0.78 per cent.[11, 12] The cause of the rare death is hypotension due to drug overdose or to reaching too high a level of anesthesia.

References

1. Moore, D. C., and Bridenbaum, L. D.: Spinal block: A review of 11,574 cases. JAMA, 195:907, 1966.
2. Wetstone, D. L., and Wong, K. C.: Sinus bradycardia and asystole in spinal anesthesia. Anesthesiology, 41:87, 1974.
3. Perez-Tamayo, L., Velez, B. L., and Aldrete, J. A.: Sensory level of subarachnoid block: Influence of dose, height, and sitting height. Regional Anesthesia, 2:2, 1977.
4. de Jong, R. H.: Toxicity of local anesthetics. Regional Anesthesia, 2:8, 1977.
5. Vandam, L. D., and Dripps, R. D.: Long-term followup of patients who received 10,098 spinal anesthetics. Syndrome of decreased intracranial pressure. JAMA, 161:586, 1956.
6. Kennedy, W. J., Jr.: Effects of baricity, position, and equipment on successful spinal anesthesia. Regional Anesthesia, 3:1, 1978.
7. Lee, J. A., and Bryce-Smith, R.: In Practical Regional Anesthesia. New York, American Elsevier, 1976, p. 197.
8. Vandam, L. D., and Dripps, R. D.: Long-term followup of patients who received 10,098 spinal anesthetics. IV. Neurological disease incident to traumatic lumbar puncture during spinal anesthesia. JAMA, 172:1483, 1960.
9. Dripps, R. D., Eckenhoff, J. E., and Vandam, L. D.: Introduction to Anesthesia, 5th ed. Philadelphia, W. B. Saunders, 1977, p. 275.
10. Moore, D. C.: Effects of various anesthetics drugs, vasoconstrictors, and continuous techniques on the duration of spinal anesthesia. Regional Anesthesia, 3:3, 1978.
11. Marx, G. F., Mateo, C. V., and Orkin, L. R.: Computer analysis of postanesthetic deaths. Anesthesiology, 39:54, 1973.
12. Noble, A. B., and Murray, J. G.: A review of the complications of spinal anesthesia with experiences in Canadian teaching hospitals from 1959 to 1969. Can. Anaesth. Soc. J., 18:5, 1971.

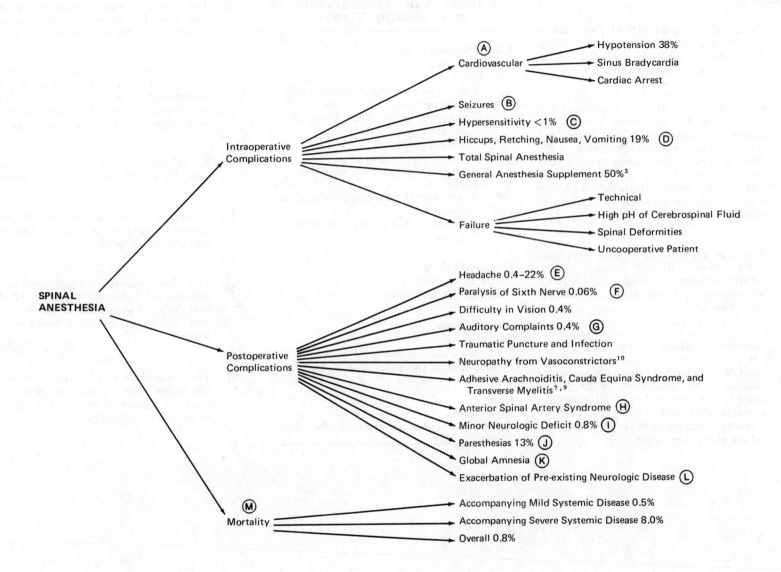

SPINAL ANESTHESIA

Intraoperative Complications

Cardiovascular (A)
→ Hypotension 38%
→ Sinus Bradycardia
→ Cardiac Arrest

Seizures (B)
Hypersensitivity <1% (C)
Hiccups, Retching, Nausea, Vomiting 19% (D)
Total Spinal Anesthesia
General Anesthesia Supplement 50%[3]

Failure
→ Technical
→ High pH of Cerebrospinal Fluid
→ Spinal Deformities
→ Uncooperative Patient

Postoperative Complications

Headache 0.4–22% (E)
Paralysis of Sixth Nerve 0.06% (F)
Difficulty in Vision 0.4%
Auditory Complaints 0.4% (G)
Traumatic Puncture and Infection
Neuropathy from Vasoconstrictors[10]
Adhesive Arachnoiditis, Cauda Equina Syndrome, and Transverse Myelitis[7,9]
Anterior Spinal Artery Syndrome (H)
Minor Neurologic Deficit 0.8% (I)
Paresthesias 13% (J)
Global Amnesia (K)
Exacerbation of Pre-existing Neurologic Disease (L)

Mortality (M)
Accompanying Mild Systemic Disease 0.5%
Accompanying Severe Systemic Disease 8.0%
Overall 0.8%

LOCAL ANESTHESIA BY LILIA J. USUBIAGA, M.D.

Comments

A. Factors affecting the rate of complication include pharmacologic properties of the drug, site of injection, and skill of the physician performing the block.

B. Systemic toxicity is dose-dependent and may be due to inadvertent intravascular injection, administration of a block in a very vascular site, fast absorption of the drug, overdose of the drug (true or relative), or direct access of the local anesthetic to the cerebral circulation. A systemic reaction may appear in any type of block[1, 2]

C. True allergic reaction to local anesthetic is uncommon, variously manifest by dermatitis, urticaria, itching, conjunctivitis, bronchospasm, hypotension, or anaphylactic shock.[3-5]

D. Immediate toxicity (seconds to minutes following injection) consists of simultaneous CNS, respiratory, and cardiovascular collapse with immediate death.[6-9] Delayed toxicity occurs 5 to 30 minutes after injection with cortical signs first, then respiratory collapse, followed by cardiovascular toxicity (see table).

SYSTEMIC TOXIC MANIFESTATIONS OF LOCAL ANESTHETIC DRUGS[11]

Central Nervous System
Stimulation of
  Medulla
    Cardiovascular center: Hypertension, tachycardia
    Respiratory center: Tachypnea, rhythm variation
    Vomiting center
Depression of
  Cortex: Unconsciousness; convulsions
  Medulla
    Vasomotor: Hypotension, tachycardia, syncope
    Respiratory: Variations, respiration, apnea

Peripheral Effects
Heart: Bradycardia
Vasomotor: Vasodilation

Allergic Effects
Skin: Urticaria
Respiratory and vasomotor centers:
  Anaphylactic shock (very rare)

Other
Psychogenic
Reaction to vasoconstrictors and other drugs

E. The toxicity of vasoconstrictors resembles and may be confused with the early stages of reaction to local anesthetics.[6]

F. Swelling, abscess, gangrene, or ulceration at the site of topical or infiltration local administration is uncommon. Bleeding is usually minor, but a large hematoma with neurologic complications may occur.

G. No reliable data about the incidence of mortality exist in the medical literature.

H. Absorption from mucous membranes is almost as rapid as intravenous absorption, and toxicity is similar.

I. Bier block consists of intravenous administration of local anesthetic distal to a tourniquet. Complications occur in the first 5 minutes following tourniquet release.[6]

J. The most common of all the sympathetic blockades, the stellate ganglion block (anterior approach) has a low percentage of serious complications.[11]

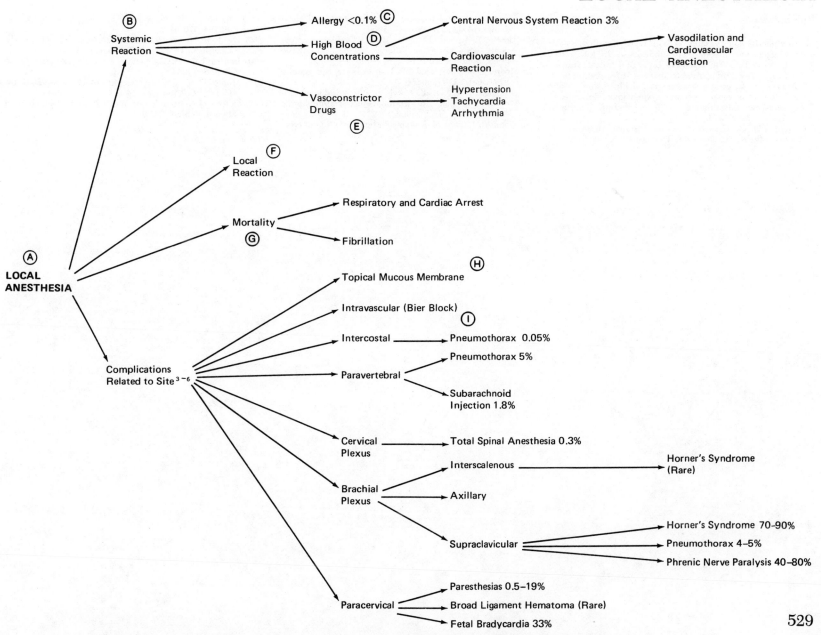

Ⓑ Systemic Reaction → Allergy <0.1% Ⓒ
→ High Blood Concentrations Ⓓ → Central Nervous System Reaction 3%
→ Cardiovascular Reaction → Vasodilation and Cardiovascular Reaction
→ Vasoconstrictor Drugs → Hypertension Tachycardia Arrhythmia
Ⓔ

Ⓐ LOCAL ANESTHESIA

Ⓕ Local Reaction

Mortality Ⓖ → Respiratory and Cardiac Arrest
→ Fibrillation

Complications Related to Site [3–6]
Ⓗ → Topical Mucous Membrane
→ Intravascular (Bier Block) Ⓘ
→ Intercostal → Pneumothorax 0.05%
→ Paravertebral → Pneumothorax 5%
→ Subarachnoid Injection 1.8%
→ Cervical Plexus → Total Spinal Anesthesia 0.3%
→ Brachial Plexus → Interscalenous → Horner's Syndrome (Rare)
→ Axillary
→ Supraclavicular → Horner's Syndrome 70-90%
→ Pneumothorax 4–5%
→ Phrenic Nerve Paralysis 40–80%
→ Paracervical → Paresthesias 0.5–19%
→ Broad Ligament Hematoma (Rare)
→ Fetal Bradycardia 33%

529

LOCAL ANESTHESIA *Continued*

References

1. Covino, B., and Vasallo, H. G.: Local anesthetics — Mechanisms of action and clinical use. *In* Kitz and Laver (eds.): The Scientific Basis of Clinical Anesthesia, New York, Grune & Stratton, 1976, chapter 6.
2. Aldrete, J. A., et al.: Reverse arterial blood flow as a pathway for central nervous system toxic responses following injection of local anesthetics. Anesth. Analg., 57(4), 1978.
3. Moore, D. C.: Complications of Regional Anesthesia. Springfield, Ill., Charles C Thomas, 1955, chapter 2.
4. Aldrete, J. A., and Johnson, D.: Allergy to local anesthetics. JAMA, 207:356–357, 1969.
5. Aldrete, J. A., and O'Higgins, J. W.: Evaluation of patients with history of allergy to local anesthetic drugs. South. Med. J., 64:118, 1971.
6. Moore, D. C.: Regional Block Anesthesia, Springfield, Ill., Charles C Thomas, 1977.
7. Usubiaga, J. E., et al.: Local anesthetic-induced convulsions in man: An electroencephalographic study. Anesth. Analg., 45(5), 1966.
8. Wikinski, J., et al.: Local anesthetic depression of electrically induced seizures in man. Anesth. Analg., 49:504–510, 1970.
9. De Jong, R. H.: Local Anesthetics. Springfield, Ill., Charles C Thomas, 1977, chapter 14.
10. Bonica, J. J.: Management of Pain. Philadelphia, Lea & Febiger, 1953.
11. Moore, D. C.: Stellate Ganglion Block. Springfield, Ill., Charles C Thomas, 1954.
12. Collins, J.: Principles of Anesthesiology. Philadelphia, Lea & Febiger, 1976.

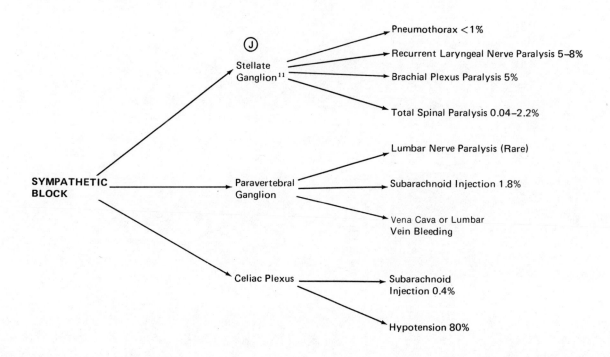

SYMPATHETIC
BLOCK

Ⓙ

Stellate
Ganglion[11]

Pneumothorax <1%

Recurrent Laryngeal Nerve Paralysis 5–8%

Brachial Plexus Paralysis 5%

Total Spinal Paralysis 0.04–2.2%

Paravertebral
Ganglion

Lumbar Nerve Paralysis (Rare)

Subarachnoid Injection 1.8%

Vena Cava or Lumbar
Vein Bleeding

Celiac Plexus

Subarachnoid
Injection 0.4%

Hypotension 80%

Section N

Life Expectancy Table

LIFE EXPECTANCY – 1975 (Years)

Age	Both Sexes	Male	Female	Age	Both Sexes	Male	Female	Age	Both Sexes	Male	Female
0	72.5	68.7	76.5	28	47.0	43.6	50.4	56	22.3	19.5	25.0
1	72.7	68.9	76.6	29	46.0	42.6	49.5	57	21.6	18.8	24.2
2	71.8	68.0	75.6	30	45.1	41.7	48.5	58	20.8	18.1	23.4
3	70.8	67.0	74.7	31	44.2	40.8	47.5	59	20.1	17.4	22.6
4	69.9	66.1	73.7	32	43.2	39.9	46.6	60	19.4	16.8	21.8
5	68.9	65.1	72.8	33	42.3	39.0	45.6	61	18.7	16.1	21.0
6	47.9	64.2	71.8	34	41.4	38.1	44.7	62	18.0	15.5	20.2
7	67.0	63.2	70.8	35	40.4	37.1	43.7	63	17.3	14.9	19.5
8	66.0	62.2	69.8	36	39.5	36.2	42.8	64	16.6	14.3	18.7
9	65.0	61.2	58.9	37	38.6	35.3	41.8	65	16.0	13.7	18.0
10	64.0	60.3	67.9	38	37.4	34.4	40.9	66	15.3	13.1	17.3
11	63.0	59.3	56.9	39	36.7	33.5	40.0	67	14.7	12.5	16.5
12	62.0	58.3	55.9	40	35.8	32.6	39.0	68	14.0	12.0	15.8
13	61.1	57.3	64.9	41	34.9	31.7	38.1	69	13.4	11.4	15.1
14	60.1	56.3	53.9	42	34.0	30.8	37.2	70	12.8	10.9	14.4
15	59.1	55.4	63.0	43	33.1	30.0	36.3	71	12.3	10.4	13.7
16	58.2	54.4	62.0	44	32.2	29.1	35.4	72	11.7	9.9	13.1
17	57.2	53.5	61.0	45	31.4	28.3	34.5	73	11.2	9.5	12.5
18	56.3	52.6	60.1	46	30.5	27.4	33.6	74	10.6	9.0	11.9
19	55.3	51.7	59.1	47	29.6	26.6	32.7	75	10.2	8.6	11.3
20	54.4	50.8	58.1	48	28.8	25.7	31.8	76	9.7	8.2	10.7
21	53.5	49.9	57.2	49	27.9	24.9	30.9	77	9.2	7.8	10.2
22	52.6	49.0	56.2	50	27.1	24.1	30.1	78	8.8	7.5	9.7
23	51.6	48.1	55.2	51	26.3	23.3	29.2	79	8.4	7.1	9.2
24	50.7	47.2	54.3	52	25.5	22.5	28.3	80	8.0	6.8	8.7
25	49.8	46.3	53.3	53	24.7	21.8	27.5	81	7.6	6.5	8.3
26	48.8	45.4	52.3	54	23.9	21.0	26.6	82	7.2	6.2	7.9
27	47.9	44.5	51.4	55	23.1	20.3	25.8	83	6.9	6.0	7.4
								84	6.5	5.7	7.1
								85	6.2	5.4	6.7